T0295050

Spinal Cord Injury

Spinal Cord Injury

Board Review

Edited by

Blessen C. Eapen, MD

Chief
Physical Medicine and Rehabilitation
VA Greater Los Angeles Health Care System
Los Angeles, California
United States

Associate Clinical Professor
Department of Medicine
Division of Physical Medicine and Rehabilitation
David Geffen School of Medicine at UCLA
Los Angeles, California
United States

David X. Cifu, MD

Associate Dean for Innovation and Systems Integration
Eminent Scholar, Herman J. Flax Professor and Chairman
Department of Physical Medicine and Rehabilitation
Virginia Commonwealth University School of Medicine
Richmond, Virginia
United States

Senior TBI Specialist
U.S. Department of Veterans Affairs
Washington, Washington DC
United States

Principal Investigator
Long-term Impact of Military-relevant Brain Injury Consortium (LIMBIC-CENC)

Senior Consultant
Sheltering Arms Institute
Richmond, Virginia
United States

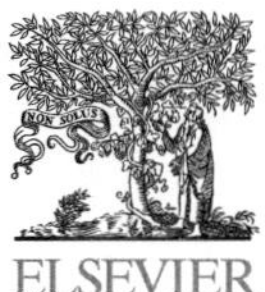

ELSEVIER

Elsevier
1600 John F. Kennedy Blvd.
Suite 1800
Philadelphia, PA 19103-2899

SPINAL CORD INJURY: BOARD REVIEW 978-0-323-83389-9

Content Strategist: Humayra R. Khan
Senior Content Development Specialist: Priyadarshini Pandey
Publishing Services Manager: Shereen Jameel
Senior Project Manager: Manikandan Chandrasekaran
Design Direction: Patrick Ferguson

Printed in India

Last digit is the print number: 9 8 7 6 5 4 3 2 1

To my devoted parents, Chacko Eapen and Aleyamma Eapen and all my family for your unwavering support, love, prayers, and always believing in me! To my loving wife, Tracy, and my sons, Elijah and Ayden, for inspiring me to be a better person, husband, father and for teaching me to take one day at a time and to cherish every moment we have together. To my VA Greater Los Angeles-PM&R family for pushing me to be a better academician, researcher, and physician.Finally, and most importantly, I would like to thank God, without whom none of this would be possible.

—Blessen C. Eapen, MD

I would like to dedicate this book to the people in my life who give me joy and make me a better person—the Cifu, Pushkin, and Freeman families, my beloved wife, Hilary, and our children, Gabriella, Isabelle, Spencer, and Kayla — and to the members of my Department, my research teams and my colleagues in Richmond and nationally who give me support and make me a better academician. Let's take the time to find meaning in everything we do, to appreciate all that we are fortunate to have, and to strive to make the world we share a better place for every person, animal, and living thing. We are all better together.

—David X. Cifu, MD

Section Editors

Elisabeth K. Acker, DO
Attending Physician
Spinal Cord Injury and Disorders Service
Central Virginia VA Health Care System;
Assistant Professor
Department of Physical Medicine and Rehabilitation
Virginia Commonwealth University
Richmond, Virginia
United States

Jordan Adler, MD
Assistant Professor
Department of Physical Medicine and Rehabilitation
University of Rochester Medical Center
Rochester, New York
United States

Camilo Castillo, MD, MBA
Director
Spinal Cord Injury Medicine Program
Associate Professor
Division of Physical Medicine and Rehabilitation
Department of Neurological Surgery
University of Louisville Health Frazier Rehabilitation
University of Louisville School of Medicine
University of Louisville Physicians Restorative Neuroscience
Louisville, Kentucky
United States

David Coons, MD
Chief
VA SCI/D Center
Rocky Mountain Regional VA;
Assistant Professor
Physical Medicine and Rehabilitation
University of Colorado
Aurora, Colorado
United States

Henry S. York, MD, ABPMR-SCI
Chief
Spinal Cord Injury/Disorder Service
VA San Diego Health Care System;
Health Sciences Clinical Assistant Professor
Department of Neurosciences
University of California - San Diego School of Medicine
San Diego, California
United States

Contributors

Andrea T. Aguirre, MD
Clinical Assistant Professor
Department of Physical Medicine
and Rehabilitation
University of Florida Health
Gainesville, Florida
Unites States
7. Neurological Assessment and Classification
10. Functional Assessments

Heather Asthagiri, MD
Associate Professor
Department of Physical Medicine and
Rehabilitation
University of Virginia
Charlottesville, Virginia
United States
8. Neuroimaging

Katelyn Barley, MS, CCC-SLP
Speech-Language Pathologist
Physical Medicine and Rehab
Central Virginia VA Health Care System
Richmond, Virginia
United States
18. Dysphagia and Common GI Issues After SCI
47. Communication and Spinal Cord Injury

Lisa A. Beck, APRN, CNS, MS
Assistant Professor Nursing
Physical Medicine and Rehabilitation
Mayo Clinic
Rochester, Minnesota
United States
42. Healthcare Maintenance for Patients With Spinal Cord Injuries/Disorders: Primary, Preventive, and Promotive Care

Kathryn Beckner, MS, OTR/L
Occupational Therapist
Spinal Cord Injury Clinical Specialist
Central Virginia VA Health Care System
Richmond, Virginia
United States
46. Activities of Daily Living

Mohammed B.A. Bhuiyan, MD, MPH
Attending Physician
Spinal Cord Injury/Disorder (SCI/D)
Central Virginia VA Health Care System;
Assistant Professor
Physical Medicine and Rehabilitation
School of Medicine
Virginia Commonwealth University
Richmond, Virginia
United States
42. Healthcare Maintenance for Patients With Spinal Cord Injuries/Disorders: Primary, Preventive, and Promotive Care

Derek Bui, DO
Resident Physician
Physical Medicine and Rehabilitation Residency
Department of Medicine, Division of PM&R
UCLA/VA Greater Los Angeles Healthcare System
Los Angeles, California
United States
9. Electrodiagnostics in Spinal Cord Injury

Keith Burau, MD
Adjunct/Assistant Professor
Department of Rehabilitation Medicine
UT Health San Antonio
Long School of Medicine
San Antonio, Texas
United States
18. Dysphagia and Common GI Issues After SCI

Philippines Cabahug, MD, FAAPMR
Director, Spinal Cord Injury Medicine Fellowship
Physical Medicine and Rehabilitation
Johns Hopkins SOM; Kennedy Krieger Institute
Assistant Professor
Physical Medicine and Rehabilitation
Johns Hopkins SOM
Baltimore, Maryland
United States
42. Healthcare Maintenance for Patients With Spinal Cord Injuries/Disorders: Primary, Preventive, and Promotive Care

Caitlin P. Campbell, PsyD
Rehabilitation Psychologist
SCI/D Center
Central Virginia VA Health Care System
Richmond, Virginia
United States
38. Psychological Aspects of Spinal Cord Injury

William Carter, MD, MPH
Assistant Professor
Physical Medicine and Rehabilitation
Virginia Commonwealth University
Richmond, Virginia
United States
12. Cardiovascular Issues in Spinal Cord Injury: Neurogenic Shock, Spinal Shock, and Orthostatic Hypotension
36. Infections With Spinal Cord Injury

Deborah Caruso, MD
Staff Physician
Physical Medicine and Rehabilitation
Assistant Professor
Central Virginia VA Health Care System
Richmond, Virginia
United States
23. Musculoskeletal Disorders

Camilo Castillo, MD, MBA
Director
Spinal Cord Injury Medicine Program
Associate Professor
Division of Physical Medicine and Rehabilitation
Department of Neurological Surgery
University of Louisville Health Frazier Rehabilitation
University of Louisville School of Medicine
University of Louisville Physicians Restorative Neuroscience
Louisville, Kentucky
United States
41. Myelopathy Without Specified Etiology

Teodoro Castillo, MD
Assistant Professor
Physical Medicine and Rehabilitation
Medical College of Virginia/Virginia Commonwealth University
Richmond, Virginia
United States
14. Pulmonary Issues After Spinal Cord Injury
15. Sleep Disorders in Individuals With Spinal Cord Injury

Rajbir Chaggar, MD
Resident Physician
Physical Medicine and Rehabilitation
Virginia Commonwealth University Medical Center
Richmond, Virginia
United States
19. Neurogenic Bladder

Audrey Chun, MD
Assistant Professor, Attending Physician
Department of Physical Medicine and Rehabilitation
Indiana University School of Medicine
Indianapolis, Indiana
United States
24. Heterotopic Ossification

Ellia Ciammaichella, DO, JD
Assistant Clinical Professor
University of Nevada School of Medicine;
Spinal Cord Injury / Disorder Program Director
Renown Rehabilitation
Reno, Nevada
United States
49. Rehabilitation Team

David Coons, MD
Chief
VA SCI/D Center
Rocky Mountain Regional VA;
Assistant Professor
Physical Medicine and Rehabilitation
University of Colorado
Aurora, Colorado
United States
4. Prevention of Spinal Cord Injury

Joanne M. Delgado-Lebron, MD
Physician
Physical Medicine and Rehabilitation
Memorial Healthcare System
Hollywood, Florida
United States
40. Nontraumatic Myelopathies

Karen DeMarco, MS, OTR/L
Occupational Therapist
Spinal Cord Injury Clinical Specialist
Central Virginia VA Health Care System
Richmond, Virginia
United States
46. Activities of Daily Living

David R. Dolbow, DPT, PhD, RKT
Associate Professor
Department of Physical Therapy
College of Osteopathic Medicine
William Carey University
Hattiesburg, Mississippi
United States
34. Nutritional and Body Composition Assessments After Spinal Cord Injury

Christina Draganich, DO
Resident Physician
Physical Medicine and Rehabilitation Department
University of Colorado
Denver, Colorado
United States
3. Epidemiology, Risk Factors, and Genetics

Linda R. Droste, MSN, RN, CWOCN, CBIS
Wound, Ostomy, Continence Nurse
Spinal Cord Injury and Disorder Units
Central Virginia VA Health Care System
Richmond, Virginia
United States
33. Pressure Ulcers/Injuries: Prevention, Treatment, and Management

Einat Engel-Haber, MD
Postdoctoral Fellow
Tim and Caroline Reynolds Center for Spinal Stimulation
Center for Spinal Cord Injury Research
Kessler Foundation
West Orange, New Jersey, United States;
Research Assistant Professor
Department of Physical Medicine and Rehabilitation
Rutgers New Jersey Medical School
Newark, New Jersey
United States
11. Outcomes After Traumatic Spinal Cord Injury

Blake Fechtel, MD, MSc
Resident Physician
Neurosurgery/ Division of Physical Medicine and Rehabilitation
University of Louisville
Louisville, Kentucky
United States
41. Myelopathy Without Specified Etiology

Justin Foley, MD
PM&R Resident
University of Utah School of Medicine
Salt Lake City, Utah
United States
10. Functional Assessments

Kevin Forster, DO
Physiatrist
Physical Medicine and Rehabilitation
VCU Health
Richmond, Virginia
United States
26. Spine Complications

Nicholas Gavern, MD
Resident Physician
Physical Medicine and Rehabilitation
University of Utah School of Medicine
Salt Lake City, Utah
United States
10. Functional Assessments

David H. Glazer, MD
Medical Director of Neurorehabilitation
Physical Medicine and Rehabilitation
Cincinnati VA Medical Center
Cincinnati, Ohio
United States
31. Traumatic Brain Injury and Spinal Cord Injury

Lance L. Goetz, MD
Associate Professor
Physical Medicine and Rehabilitation
Virginia Commonwealth University;
Staff Physician
Spinal Cord Injury and Disorders
Central Virginia VA Health Care System
Richmond, Virginia
United States
17. Neurogenic Bowel
19. Neurogenic Bladder
26. Spine Complications
28. Posttraumatic Syringomyelia

Jacob Goldsmith, MS, PhD
Postdoctoral Research Scientist
Spinal Cord Injury and Disorders Service
Central Virginia VA Health Care System
Richmond, Virginia
United States
35. Endocrine/Metabolic

Ashraf S. Gorgey, MPT, PhD, FACSM, FACRM
Director of SCI Research
Spinal Cord Injury and Disorders Service
Central Virginia VA Health Care System
Professor
Physical Medicine and Rehabilitation
Virginia Commonwealth University
Richmond, Virginia
United States
34. Nutritional and Body Composition Assessments After Spinal Cord Injury
35. Endocrine/Metabolic

Stacy Gross, MS, CCC-SLP
Speech-Language Pathologist
Physical Medicine and Rehab
Central Virginia VA Health Care System
Richmond, Virginia
United States
18. Dysphagia and Common GI Issues After SCI
47. Communication and Spinal Cord Injury

Andres Gutierrez, MD
Resident Physician
Physical Medicine and Rehabilitation
Memorial Healthcare System
Hollywood, Florida
United States
40. Nontraumatic Myelopathies

Mara C. Harris, DO
Resident Physician
Neurosurgery/Division of Physical Medicine and Rehabilitation
University of Louisville
Louisville, Kentucky
United States
41. Myelopathy Without Specified Etiology

Ricky Hawkins, PT, DPT, EP-C
Physical Therapist
Spinal Cord Injury and Disorders
Central Virginia VA Health Care System
Richmond, Virginia
United States
44. Exercise and Modalities

Stephanie Hendrick, MD
Attending Physician
Physical Medicine and Rehabilitation
Regional Medical Group;
Associate Program Director
Marianjoy Rehabilitation Hospital part of Northwestern Medicine
Wheaton, Illinois
United States
6. Prehospital Evaluation and Management

Isaac Hernandez Jimenez, MD
Assistant Professor
Department of Physical Medicine and Rehabilitation
McGovern Medical School
The University of Texas Health Science Center;
The Institute of Rehabilitation & Research (TIRR) Memorial Hermann, Houston, Texas
United States
39. Traumatic Myelopathy

Milissa L. Janisko, RD
Clinical Dietitian
Spinal Cord Injury and Disorder Unit
Central Virginia VA Health Care System
Richmond, Virginia
United States
34. Nutritional and Body Composition Assessments After Spinal Cord Injury

Jacob Jeffers, MD
Fellow
Department of Physical Medicine and Rehabilitation
McGovern Medical School – UTHealth
Houston, Texas
United States
4. Prevention of Spinal Cord Injury

Lavina Jethani, MD
Attending Physician
MultiCare Good Samaritan Hospital
Puyallup, Washington
United States
39. Traumatic Myelopathy

Kyle Jisa, MD
Resident Physician
Physical Medicine and Rehabilitation
Virginia Commonwealth University
Richmond, Virginia
United States
36. Infections With Spinal Cord Injury

Mahmut T. Kaner, MD
Attending Physician
Faith Regional Health Services
Norfolk, Nebraska
United States
39. Traumatic Myelopathy

Krysten Kasting, MD
Resident Physician
Physical Medicine and Rehabilitation
University of Colorado
Aurora Colorado
United States
2. Neuroanatomy

Allison Kessler, MD, MSc
Section Chief
Spinal Cord Injury Medicine
Shirley Ryan AbilityLab;
Assistant Professor
Physical Medicine and Rehabilitation
Northwestern University
Chicago, Illinois
United States
6. Prehospital Evaluation and Management

Steven Kirshblum, MD
Chief Medical Officer and Director of Spinal Cord Injury Services
Kessler Institute for Rehabilitation
Chief Medical Officer
Kessler Foundation
West Orange, New Jersey, United States;
Professor and Chair
Department of Physical Medicine and Rehabilitation
Newark, New Jersey, United States
11. Outcomes After Traumatic Spinal Cord Injury

Adam P. Klausner, MD
Professor, Director of Neurology and Voiding Dysfunction & Warren Koontz Professor of Urologic Research
Division of Urology
Virginia Commonwealth University;
Staff Urologist
Division of Urology
Central Virginia VA Health Care System
Richmond, Virginia
United States
20. Urological Conditions in Persons With Spinal Cord Injury

Heather Kloepping, MS, OTR/L
Occupational Therapist
Spinal Cord Injury Clinical Specialist
Central Virginia VA Health Care System
Richmond, Virginia
United States
46. Activities of Daily Living

Daniel Krasna, MD
Assistant Professor
Physical Medicine and Rehabilitation
Johns Hopkins University
Baltimore, Maryland
United States
31. Traumatic Brain Injury and Spinal Cord Injury

Sarah C. Krzastek, MD
Associate Chief of Urology
Division of Urology;
Central Virginia VA Health Care System;
Clinical Assistant Professor
Division of Urology
Virginia Commonwealth University
Richmond, Virginia
United States
20. Urological Conditions in Persons With Spinal Cord Injury

Shira Lanyi, BS
Medical Student
Virginia Commonwealth University School of Medicine
Richmond, Virginia
United States
20. Urological Conditions in Persons With Spinal Cord Injury

Venessa A. Lee, MD
Attending Physician
Spinal Cord Injury and Disorders
Physical Medicine and Rehabilitation
Saint Luke's Rehabilitation Institute
Overland Park, Kansas
United States
7. Neurological Assessment and Classification
10. Functional Assessments

Denise D. Lester, MD, FASAM
Pain Anesthesiologist, Addictionologist
Department of Physical Medicine and Rehabilitation
Central Virginia Veterans Health Care System
Richmond, Virginia
United States
37. Evaluation and Management of Pain After Spinal Cord Injury

Audrey Leung, MD
Assistant Professor
Physical Medicine and Rehabilitation
University of Washington
Seattle, Washington
United States
16. Thromboembolism/Deep Vein Thrombosis

Julie Mannlein, PT, MPT, ATP
OT/PT Supervisor
Wheelchair Seating Clinic
University of Michigan
Ann Arbor, Michigan
United States
45. Functional Mobility Following Spinal Cord Injury

George Marzloff, MD
Staff Physician
Spinal Cord Injuries and Disorders
Rocky Mountain Regional Veterans Affairs Medical Center;
Assistant Professor
Department of Physical Medicine and Rehabilitation
University of Colorado School of Medicine Anschutz Medical Campus
Aurora, Colorado
United States
1. Neurophysiology of the Spinal Cord

Sean McAvoy, MD
Assistant Professor
Spinal Cord Injury Medicine Fellowship Program Director
Physical Medicine and Rehabilitation
Virginia Commonwealth University;
Attending Physician
Spinal Cord Injury and Disorders
Central Virginia VA Health Care System
Richmond, Virginia
United States
29. Spasticity

Jean W. McCauley, BSPT, DPT, CCI, CWS
Physical Therapist
Wound Care Specialist
Physical Medicine and Rehabilitation SCI/D
Central Virginia VA Health Care System
Richmond, Virginia
United States
33. Pressure Ulcers/Injuries: Prevention, Treatment, and Management

William McKinley, MD
Professor
Physical Medicine and Rehabilitation
Director of SCI Medicine
Sheltering Arms Institute & Virginia Commonwealth University
Richmond, Virginia
United States
13. Autonomic Dysreflexia
32. Neuromodulatory and Disease-Modifying Agents

Brittni Micham, MD
Staff Physician
Spinal Cord Injury Service
VA Palo Alto Health Care System
Palo Alto, California
United States
30. Thermoregulation and Sweating

Derrick Miller, MD
Resident Physician
Department of Family Medicine
University of Maryland Capital Region
Largo, Maryland
United States
29. Spasticity

James Milligan, MD
Assistant Clinical Professor
Family Medicine, McMaster University
Hamilton, Ontario;
Director
Mobility Clinic
The Centre for Family Medicine
Kitchener, Ontario
Canada
42. Healthcare Maintenance for Patients With Spinal Cord Injuries/Disorders: Primary, Preventive, and Promotive Care

Brian Mutcher, PsyD
Clinical Psychologist
Spinal Cord Injury and Disorders
Central Virginia VA Health Care System
Richmond, Virginia
United States
38. Psychological Aspects of Spinal Cord Injury

Eduardo Nadal-Ortiz, MD
Physiatrist
Spinal Cord Injury Medicine Specialist
Guaynabo, Puerto Rico
Veterans Affairs Caribbean Healthcare System
San Juan, Puerto Rico
40. Nontraumatic Myelopathies

Anne Nastasi, MD
Associate Professor of Medicine
David Geffen School of Medicine, UCLA;
Staff Physician
Physical Medicine and Rehabilitation (PM&R) Department
UCLA/VA Greater Los Angeles Healthcare System
Los Angeles, California
United States
9. Electrodiagnostics in Spinal Cord Injury

Alden Newcomb, MD, MS
Resident Physician
Orthopaedic Surgery
Virginia Commonwealth University
Richmond, Virginia
United States
25. Spine Fractures, Dislocations, and Instability

Jed E. Olson, MD, FACP
Assistant Professor
Physical Medicine and Rehabilitation
University of Colorado;
Assistant Clinical Professor
General Internal Medicine
University of Colorado; Attending Physician
SCI/D Section
Rocky Mountain Regional VAMC
Aurora, Colorado
United States
5. Clinical and Basic Research

Michael Ray Ortiz, MD
Assistant Professor
Physical Medicine and Rehabilitation
Carolinas Rehabilitation
Charlotte, North Carolina
United States
43. Spinal Cord Injury and Aging

Hetal Patel, MD
Resident Physician
Physical Medicine and Rehabilitation
University of Washington
Seattle, Washington
United States
16. Thromboembolism/Deep Vein Thrombosis

Steven Peretiatko, MD, BS
Resident Physician
Physical Medicine and Rehabilitation,
Virginia Commonwealth University
Richmond, Virginia
United States
32. Neuromodulatory and Disease-Modifying Agents

Ricky Placide, MD, PT
Professor
Orthopedic Surgery
Virginia Commonwealth University
Medical College of Virginia
Richmond, Virginia
United States
25. Spine Fractures, Dislocations, and Instability

Justin Provo, MD
Resident Physician
Physical Medicine and Rehabilitation
University of Utah School of Medicine
Salt Lake City, Utah
United States
10. Functional Assessments

Stephanie Cowherd Ryder, MD
Attending Physician
Spinal Cord Injury/Disorders Center
Rocky Mountain Regional VA Medical Center;
Assistant Professor
Physical Medicine and Rehabilitation
University of Colorado School of Medicine
Aurora, Colorado
United States
2. Neuroanatomy

Scott Schubert, MD
Spinal Cord Injury Provider Section Chief
Rocky Mountain Regional VA Medical Center;
Assistant Professor
Physical Medicine and Rehabilitation
University of Colorado School of Medicine
Aurora, Colorado
United States
3. Epidemiology, Risk Factors, and Genetics

David R. Schulze, DO, MS
Resident Physician
Physical Medicine and Rehabilitation Residency
Department of Medicine, Division of PM&R
UCLA/VA Greater Los Angeles Healthcare System
Los Angeles, California
United States
9. Electrodiagnostics in Spinal Cord Injury

Lindsay A. Smith, MD
Resident Physician
Physical Medicine and Rehabilitation Residency
Department of Medicine, Division of PM&R
UCLA/VA Greater Los Angeles Healthcare System
Los Angeles, California
United States
9. Electrodiagnostics in Spinal Cord Injury

Ryan A. Smith, MD
Resident Physician
Physical Medicine and Rehabilitation Residency
Department of Medicine, Division of PM&R
UCLA/VA Greater Los Angeles Healthcare System
Los Angeles, California
United States
9. Electrodiagnostics in Spinal Cord Injury

Brittany Snider, DO
Clinical Chief of Outpatient Spinal Cord Injury Services
Kessler Institute for Rehabilitation
West Orange, New Jersey
United States;
Clinical Assistant Professor
Department of Physical Medicine and Rehabilitation
Rutgers New Jersey Medical School
Newark, New Jersey
United States
11. Outcomes After Traumatic Spinal Cord Injury

Vera Staley, MD
Physician
Physical Medicine and Rehabilitation
Denver Health Medical Center
Instructor
Department of Physical Medicine and Rehabilitation
University of Colorado School of Medicine
Aurora, Colorado
United States
1. Neurophysiology of the Spinal Cord

Tommy Sutor, MS, PhD
Postdoctoral Research Scientist
Spinal Cord Injury and Disorders Service
Central Virginia VA Health Care System
Richmond, Virginia
United States
35. Endocrine/Metabolic

Katharine Tam, MD
Staff Physician
Spinal Cord Injury/Disorder
St. Louis VA Healthcare System;
Assistant Professor
Department of Neurology
Division of Rehabilitation
Washington University
St. Louis, Missouri
United States
48. Participation/Living With Spinal Cord Injury

Robert J. Trainer, DO, MBA, FASAM
Pain Anesthesiologist, Addictionologist
Department of Physical Medicine and Rehabilitation
Central Virginia Veterans Health Care System
Richmond, Virginia
United States
37. Evaluation and Management of Pain After Spinal Cord Injury

Justin Tu, MD
Assistant Professor
Department of Orthopedics
Emory Healthcare
Atlanta, Georgia
United States
8. Neuroimaging

Jeffrey Tubbs, MD
Inpatient Section Chief
Spinal Cord Injury and Disorders
Central Virginia VA Health Care System;
Assistant Professor
Department of Physical Medicine and Rehabilitation
Virginia Commonwealth University
Richmond, Virginia
United States
27. Spinal Orthoses

Cody Unser, MPH
Founder
The Cody Unser First Step Foundation
Albuquerque, New Mexico
United States
42. Healthcare Maintenance for Patients With Spinal Cord Injuries/Disorders: Primary, Preventive, and Promotive Care

William R. Visser, MD
Physician
Division of Urology
Virginia Commonwealth University
Richmond, Virginia
United States
20. Urological Conditions in Persons With Spinal Cord Injury

Jennifer Wahl, DNP, MS, RN, CRRN
SCI/D Program Development Coordinator
Spinal Cord Injuries and Disorders
Rocky Mountain Regional Veterans Administration Medical Center
Aurora, Colorado
United States
5. Clinical and Basic Research

Jennifer Weekes, MD, MHSA
Staff Physician
Department of Physical Medicine and Rehabilitation
Mary Free Bed at Covenant
Saginaw, Michigan
United States
21. Sexuality and Reproduction After Spinal Cord Injury
22. Women's Health After Spinal Cord Injury

Cory Wernimont, MD
Assistant Professor
Physical Medicine and Rehabilitation
University of Michigan
Ann Arbor, Michigan,
United States
45. Functional Mobility Following Spinal Cord Injury

Oksana Witt, MD, MS
Physical Medicine and Rehabilitation (PM&R) Residency Program
Virginia Commonwealth University Health System
Richmond, Virginia
United States
15. Sleep Disorders in Individuals With Spinal Cord Injury

Elizabeth York, DO
PM&R Resident
University of Utah School of Medicine
Salt Lake City, Utah
United States
10. Functional Assessments

Preface

Spinal cord injury (SCI) was a death sentence until the 1950s, when Sir Ludwig Guttmann established the spinal unit at Stoke Mandeville Hospital in 1944 and introduced the innovation of comprehensive care and rehabilitation; revolutionizing the field and offering long life, and ultimately, a return to functioning for individuals with SCI. The system of care for individuals with SCI in the United States was sparked by federal government research and clinical initiatives to form dedicated systems of care from the federal government (the Department of Veterans Affairs, the National Institute of Disability and Rehabilitation Research) in the 1970s.

Spinal Cord Injury: Board Review offers a comprehensive and yet concise resource tool for anyone who is studying the field as part of their training or in preparation for certifying examinations, and for more experienced practitioners who desire to keep up to date with the most evidence-influenced clinical approaches to assessment and management. More than 120 of the nation's leading experts across the wide range of SCI medicine elements have been brought together in this book to create more than 50 chapters that offer authoritative yet practical approaches to diagnosis, acute management, and long-term care. The topics range from mainstream neurosurgical and trauma acute care of SCI to cutting-edge imaging, neuroimaging, and electrophysiologic assessment, and a diverse assortment of rehabilitation topics. The focus of the book is on identifying the clinically relevant core elements of each area so that a clinician or trainee can easily grasp these key components; however, there are also evidence-based recommendations and state-of-the-art research that will allow the reader to take their approach to the individual with acquired SCI to the next level.

Spinal Cord Injury: Board Review offers a unique approach that complements existing textbooks in the field by providing well-defined foundational clinical principles that allow the reader to both understand the essential information and integrate this information directly into practice. It is a resource that can be used by entry-level trainees and experienced, advanced practitioners to enhance their understanding and their effectiveness.

Acknowledgments

This book, *Spinal Cord Injury: Board Review*, represents the combined work of more than 120 authors with a range of healthcare backgrounds from across the United States and with varying interests and experiences in the practice of this specialty. This high number and diversity of experts were necessary to allow this text to reflect the full breadth of all that must be learned and applied to appropriately assess and manage individuals with traumatic spinal cord injury. Although we have attempted to capture as much of the scientific theory and knowledge related to both spinal cord injury and to spinal cord injury medicine as possible, the true art of healthcare is to take this vast corpus of knowledge and translate and integrate that into everyday practice. Although this evidence-based approach to care takes years of training, mentorship, and experience, the handbook offers a concise, useful, and informative resource that will give everyone from trainees to seasoned clinicians access to the key elements needed to move to expert status. We are indebted to the associate editors and all of the authors who worked so diligently to bring together the essential information relevant to the field in this single source. Although it is a handy and convenient reference that may be used for independent study, reviewing for certification exams, or to support practice, we urge all practitioners to rely on multiple sources of information and the oversight and advice of established practitioners. We would also like to acknowledge our academic and clinical institutions: the US Department of Veterans Affairs Physical Medicine and Rehabilitation Program Office and VA Medical Centers in Greater Los Angeles, Richmond; the University of California in Los Angeles; the Virginia Commonwealth University; and Sheltering Arms Institute.

Contents

CHAPTER 1

Neurophysiology of the Spinal Cord

Vera Staley and George Marzloff

OUTLINE

Introduction

This chapter serves to review the functional aspects of spinal cord anatomy. It is organized into three major sections: an overview of the sensory and motor systems, the spinal tracts, and the neurophysiology of the autonomic nervous system.

Sensory and Motor Systems

Sensory Information

The sensory nerve cell bodies are housed in the dorsal root ganglion, located just outside the intervertebral foramen. The dorsal root, carrying afferent sensory information, and ventral root, carrying efferent motor information, come together, forming the spinal nerve. The spinal nerve quickly branches into dorsal and ventral rami, which become peripheral nerves (Fig. 1.1).

Sensations including touch and proprioception, temperature, and pain are perceived peripherally by specialized receptors including mechanoreceptors, thermoreceptors, and nociceptors, respectively.[1]

Mechanoreceptors contain mechanosensitive ion channels that transmit physical distortion such as bending or stretching.[2] Rapidly adapting mechanoreceptors, including Pacinian corpuscles, Meissner corpuscles, and hair follicles, transmit signals quickly but then stop firing despite continued stimulus.[2] Other receptors including Ruffini corpuscles, Merkel receptors, and tactile discs fire slowly and provide a more sustained response, particularly to pressure and fine spatial details of texture.[2] Pacinian corpuscles transmit high-frequency vibration and tapping sensations and lie deep in subcutaneous tissue.[1] Meissner corpuscles lie more superficially in the dermis of nonhairy skin and transmit point discrimination, tapping, and low-frequency flutter.[1,3] Hair follicles contain receptors that detect movement of the hair and can transmit information about the velocity and direction of movement across the skin.[1] Ruffini corpuscles detect stretch and joint rotation and are located in the dermis and in joint capsules.[1] Merkel receptors and tactile discs detect vertical indentations in the skin.[1] Transmissions from mechanoreceptors travel from the peripheral nerve to the dorsal root ganglia through thickly myelinated Aβ fibers and enter the dorsal horn (Fig. 1.2).[2]

Thermoreceptors include warm and cold receptors that detect changes in skin temperature.[1] When cooler than 36°C, warm receptors are turned off and when warmer than 36°C, cold receptors are turned off. Extremes of temperature are transmitted through nociceptors.[1]

Nociceptors include multiple types of receptors that transmit mechanical stimuli, chemical stimuli, and extremes of temperature.[1] These signals are carried to the spinal cord via Aδ fibers, carrying fast and sharp pain, and C fibers, carrying slow, dull, and long-lasting pain.[2] These signals travel to the dorsal root ganglia and into the dorsal horn of the spinal cord.[2] They travel a short distance up and down the spinal cord in the zone of Lissauer and synapse in the lateral portion of the dorsal horn called the substantia gelatinosa.[2]

Motor Information

Signaling from the cortex to the periphery for muscle activation involves a series of motor neurons. Upper

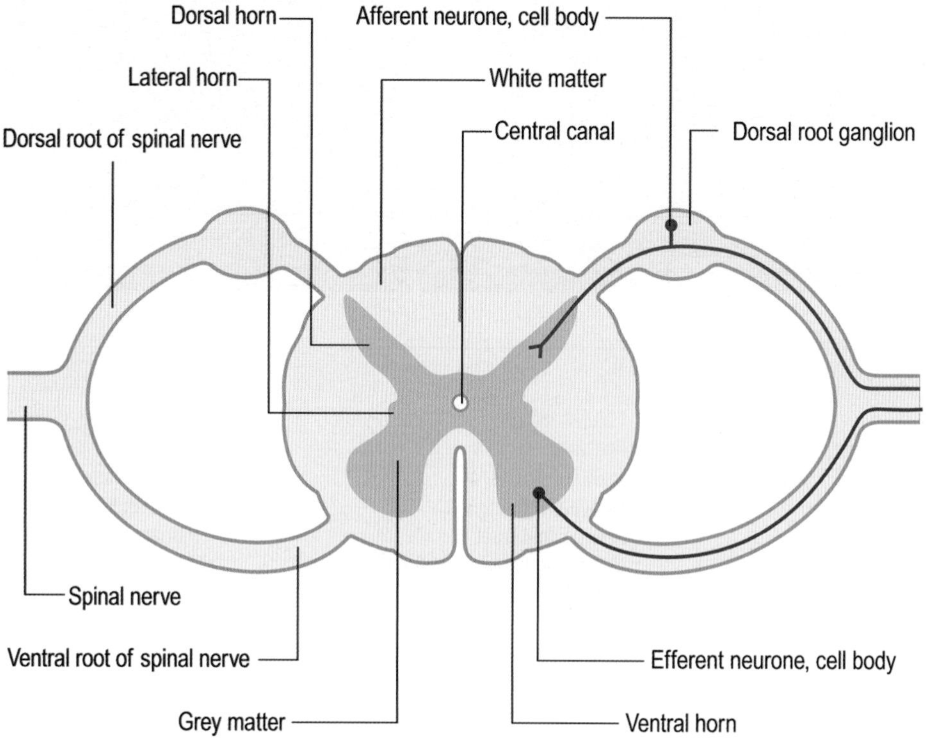

Dorsal horn
Afferent neurone, cell body
Lateral horn
White matter
Dorsal root of spinal nerve
Central canal
Dorsal root ganglion
Spinal nerve
Ventral root of spinal nerve
Efferent neurone, cell body
Grey matter
Ventral horn

Fig. 1.1 Organization of the Dorsal and Ventral Nerve Roots. (From Standring S, ed. *Gray's Anatomy*. 42nd ed. Elsevier; 2021 [Fig. 24.2].)

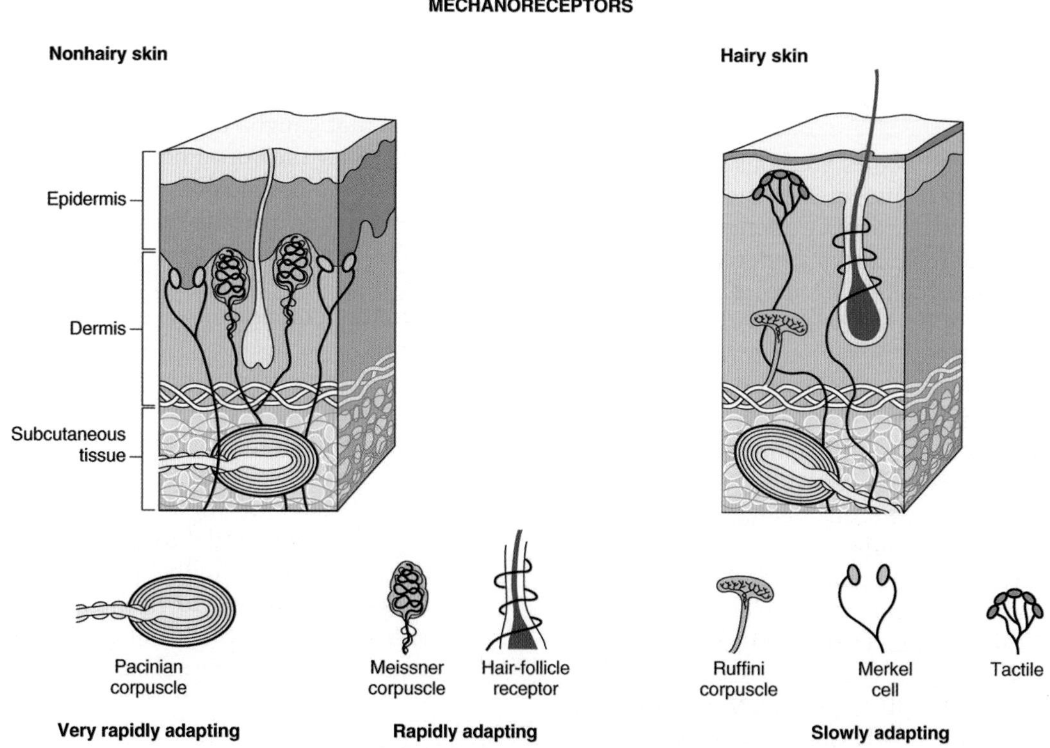

Fig. 1.2 Mechanoreceptors. (From Costanzo L, *Physiology*. 6th ed. Elsevier; 2018 [chapter 3, Fig. 3.9].)

motor neurons (UMN) in the cerebral cortex have axons that travel through the spinal cord to the ventral horns of the gray matter. The alpha motor neurons located in the ventral horns directly innervate skeletal muscle and are known as lower motor neurons (LMN). Alpha motor neurons exit the spinal cord in a dorsal root, through both the dorsal and ventral rami, into peripheral nerves and, ultimately, skeletal muscle fibers. Activation, contraction, and relaxation of skeletal muscles is under the control of a coordinated system of motor neurons and reflexes that are integrated in the spinal cord.[4]

Spinal Tracts

Gray and White Matter

The spinal cord is organized into gray matter centrally and white matter peripherally. The gray matter contains neurons and their glial cells, while the white matter contains the myelinated ascending and descending tracts.

The posterior (dorsal) horn contains neurons involved in sensory function. The anterior (ventral) horn contains both motor neurons and interneurons involved in skeletal muscle function. The neurons of the ventral horn are organized somatotopically with flexor motor neurons located dorsally and extensor motor neurons located ventrally (Fig. 1.3). Additionally, the motor neurons carrying information to the trunk are more medial and those carrying information to the limbs are more peripheral. In each thoracic and the superior two lumbar spinal cord segments, there is a lateral horn that carries preganglionic sympathetic neurons.

The white matter is divided into three main areas (anterior, lateral, and posterior), also termed *funiculi.* Within each funiculus, there are different bundles of fibers that traverse the spinal cord together that are known as tracts.

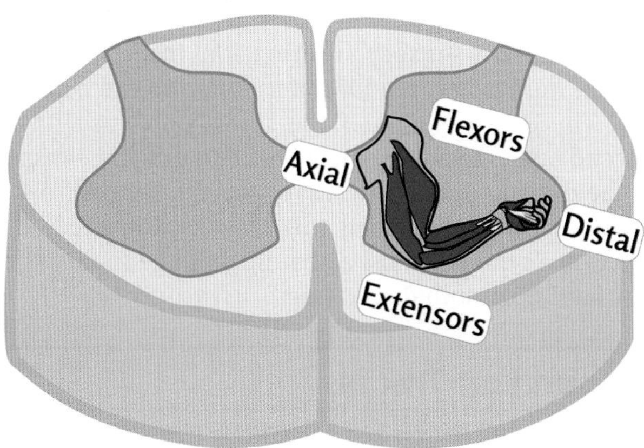

Fig. 1.3 Somatotopic Organization of the Ventral Horns.

Ascending Tracts

This section will review the key ascending tracts of the spinal cord, including the posterior funiculus (including the gracile and cuneate tracts), the lateral and anterior spinothalamic tracts, and the posterior spinocerebellar tract (Fig. 1.4).

Also known as the dorsal column medial lemniscus pathway, the posterior funiculus containing the **gracile and cuneate tracts** carries sensory information for position sense and discriminative touch (Fig. 1.5). Some of these sensory stimuli, including vibration, two-point discrimination, and light touch, are not specific to the posterior funiculus and are also carried by parallel tracts such as the spinocervical thalamic tract and the anterior spinothalamic tract.[4] Other sensations, such as the direction of movement of a joint, are carried only by the gracile and cuneate tracts.[4] The loss of joint position sense due to injury to the posterior funiculus can result in significantly impaired motor function.[4]

The gracile tract contains fibers from levels below the sixth thoracic segment and travels medially within the spinal cord. The cuneate tract contains fibers from levels above the sixth thoracic segment and travels more laterally within the posterior aspect of the spinal cord. The fibers are organized somatotopically within the spinal cord with sacral fibers medial and cervical fibers lateral. These fibers ascend ipsilaterally to the caudal medulla and synapse on the gracile and cuneate nuclei, decussate, and ascend as the medial lemniscus to the ventral posterolateral nucleus of the thalamus. The thalamic neurons project to the cerebral cortex.

Lateral and Anterior Spinothalamic Tracts

Pain and temperature sensory information is carried primarily by the **lateral spinothalamic tract**. Nerve fibers enter the spinal cord, synapse on the dorsal horn, cross the midline via the anterior white commissure, ascend one to two levels, and enter the contralateral lateral spinothalamic tract (Fig. 1.5). This tract lies in the lateral aspect of the spinal cord and is organized somatotopically, with sacral fibers laterally and cervical fibers medially. These fibers ascend and terminate on the ventral posterolateral nucleus of the thalamus.

Injury to the lateral spinothalamic tract will result in loss of pain and temperature to the contralateral side starting one to two levels below the lesion. If there is a lesion of the anterior white commissure, which can occur in syringomyelia, then pain and temperature can be affected bilaterally at the level of the lesion.

The **anterior spinothalamic tract** carries light touch and pain information, which enter the spinal canal via the dorsal root, pass through the dorsal horn, and

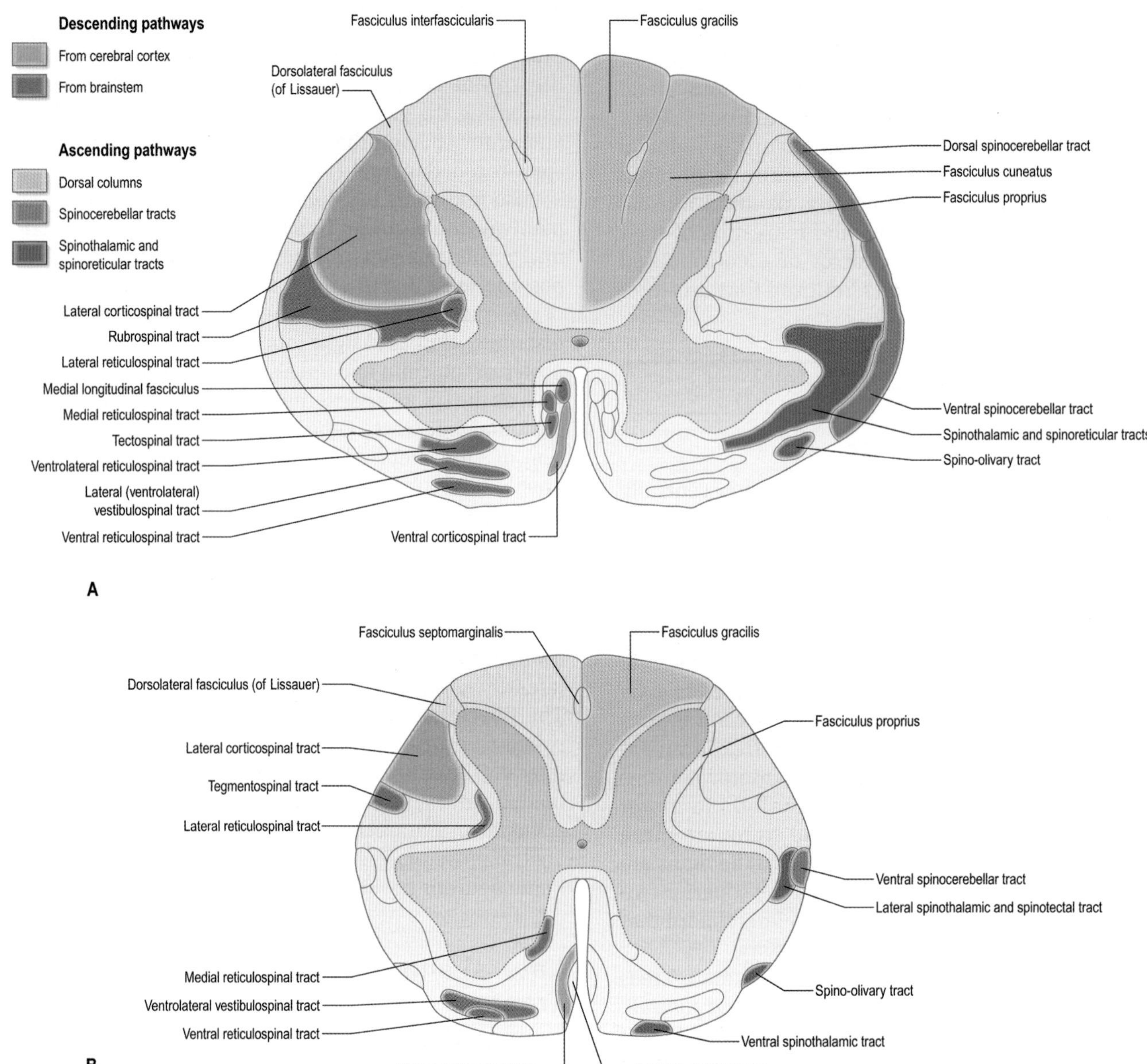

Fig. 1.4 The approximate positions of the ascending and descending white matter tracts of the spinal cord at (A) mid-cervical and (B) lumbar levels. (From Standring S, ed. *Gray's Anatomy*. 42nd ed. Elsevier; 2021 [Fig. 27.7].)

cross the midline via the anterior white commissure, forming the anterior spinothalamic tract.

On the International Standards for Neurological Classification of Spinal Cord Injury examination, the light touch portion of the sensory exam utilizes a wisp of cotton. This light touch sensation is transmitted by the posterior funiculi, the anterior spinothalamic tract, and the spinocervical thalamic tract, so it does not help localize spinal cord lesions.[4] The pinprick portion of the sensory exam assesses the ability to differentiate sharp and dull and is primarily assessing the lateral spinothalamic tract.

The posterior spinocerebellar tract is located in the dorsal aspect of the lateral funiculus. It carries proprioceptive sensory information from receptors located in muscles, tendons, and joints to the cerebellum. These neurons enter the spinal cord, ascend or descend one to two levels in the nucleus gracilis, synapse on the dorsal nucleus of Clarke, and then travel to the medulla. Clinically when this tract is damaged, the effects are typically masked by the damage to the adjacent lateral spinothalamic tract.

Descending Tracts

This section will review key descending tracts of the spinal cord that travel through the lateral and anterior funiculi, including the corticospinal tract, the rubrospinal tract, the

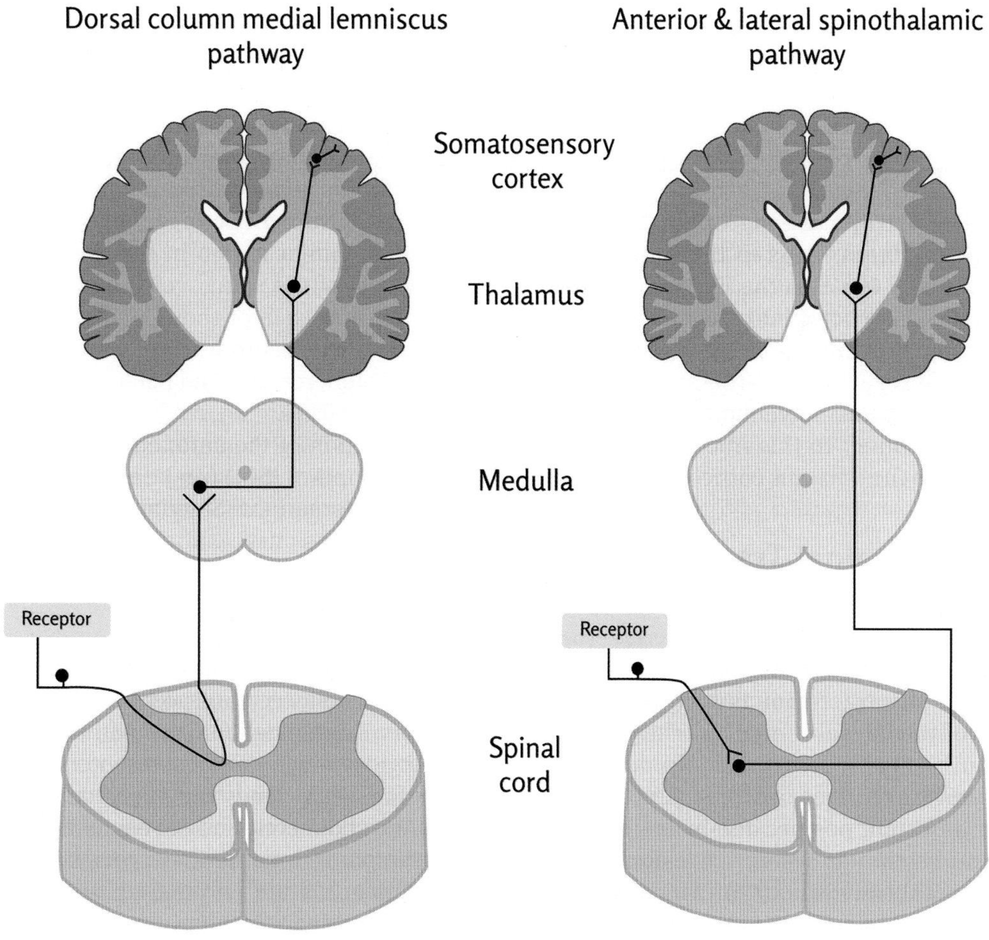

Fig. 1.5 Somatosensory Pathways. The point at which afferent fibers cross to the contralateral side can affect the lateralization patterns of sensory impairments.

lateral vestibulospinal tract, the medial vestibulospinal tract, and the reticulospinal tract (Fig. 1.4).

Corticospinal Tract

The corticospinal tract starts with projections from the primary motor cortex, premotor cortex, and primary sensory cortex, which coalesce in the brainstem. The majority of fibers decussate at the medulla in the pyramidal decussation to form the lateral corticospinal tract found in the lateral funiculus. The remaining uncrossed fibers form the anterior corticospinal tract located in the anterior funiculus of the spinal cord and travel only into the upper thoracic spinal cord to innervate muscles of the upper extremities and neck. The fibers of the anterior corticospinal tract typically cross the midline segmentally. Most corticospinal tract neurons terminate on interneurons, though some terminate on alpha and gamma motor neurons. Functionally, the corticospinal tract contributes greatly to precise movement.

Lesions of the lateral corticospinal tract result in an UMN syndrome. This includes spasticity and increased deep tendon reflexes. Lesions of the alpha motor neurons result in a LMN syndrome, which is observed in cauda equina injuries. This includes loss of reflexes and flaccid paralysis.

Spinal shock is a period of time immediately following injury to the bilateral corticospinal tracts and results in absent and/or depressed spinal reflexes.[5] There is a series of four phases that characterize spinal shock.[5] Phase one, occurring 0 to 1 days post-injury, is characterized by areflexia or hyporeflexia. Phase two, occurring 1 to 3 days after injury, shows initial reflex return. Phase three, occurring 1 to 4 weeks after injury, manifests initial hyperreflexia, and phase four, during 1 to 12 months post-injury, shows final hyperreflexia.[5] The first reflex to reemerge is the delayed plantar response (DPR), typically arising 1 to 6 hours after injury.[5] This is elicited in a similar manner to the Babinski reflex but results in delayed plantar flexion of the great toe and/or other toes. The general pattern of reflex emergence is cutaneous before deep tendon reflexes. The order of reflex emergence after the DPR is sequential: bulbocavernosus, cremasteric, ankle jerk, Babinski sign, and knee jerk.[5]

Rubrospinal Tract

The neurons of the rubrospinal tract originate in the red nucleus of the midbrain, cross in the ventral tegmental decussation, and travel in the lateral funiculus anterior to the lateral corticospinal tract. The fibers terminate in the same gray matter as the corticospinal tract and facilitate flexor motor neuron activity. This tract is quite thin and poorly myelinated in humans, and the effects of any injury to this tract would likely be masked by injury to the adjacent corticospinal tract.[4]

Lateral Vestibulospinal Tract

The lateral vestibulospinal tract neurons originate in the lateral vestibular nucleus located at the junction between the medulla and the pons and travel uncrossed through the tract that is located in the anterior portion of the lateral funiculus. These fibers terminate on both interneurons and alpha motor neurons. This tract activates ipsilateral extensor motor neurons for upright posture and balance based on input from the vestibular system. A lesion to the lateral vestibulospinal tract is not typically observed clinically due to more severe motor deficits from injury to the corticospinal tract.

Reticulospinal Tract

The reticular formation of the brainstem sends projections from the pons and the medulla. Projections from the pons travel ipsilaterally down the medial portion of the anterior funiculus and terminate on interneurons. Projections from the medulla follow a similar course in the anterior portion of the lateral funiculus. Functions of the reticulospinal tract include facilitation or inhibition of voluntary movement and reflex activity, pressor or depressor effects on the circulatory system, and inhibitor effects on sensory transmission.[4]

Neurophysiology of the Autonomic Nervous System

The autonomic nervous system consists of the sympathetic and parasympathetic systems. Lesions of the spinal cord disrupting the autonomic nervous system pathways result in major clinical consequences both acutely after injury and chronically.

Projections, primarily from the hypothalamus, travel through descending autonomic pathways found in the lateral funiculi. The sympathetic preganglionic neurons are found within the lateral horns of the gray matter in the thoracic and superior two lumbar spinal cord segments. They exit the spinal cord via the ventral roots, and most synapse with postganglionic neurons of the sympathetic chain ganglia that are located directly adjacent to the vertebral column. Sympathetic preganglionic neurons synapse directly onto adrenal glands.

The parasympathetic preganglionic neurons can be found in a similar region in the gray matter at the S2 to S4 levels of the spinal cord, but there is no visible lateral horn at each of those levels. The preganglionic parasympathetic neurons travel to the descending colon, sigmoid colon, rectum, and pelvic viscera via the pelvic splanchnic nerves.

The function of the autonomic nervous system after spinal cord injury (SCI) can be evaluated more formally using the International Standards to Document Remaining Autonomic Function after Spinal Cord Injury.

Neurotransmitters

In the sympathetic nervous system, preganglionic neurons are always cholinergic and acetylcholine acts on nicotinic receptors.[1] Postganglionic sympathetic neurons are all adrenergic and act on adrenoreceptors (α1, α2, β1, β2), except for sweat glands and piloerector smooth muscles, which are cholinergic and have muscarinic receptors.

In the parasympathetic nervous system, all preganglionic neurons are cholinergic and act on nicotinic receptors, similar to the sympathetic system. Most of the postganglionic neurons are cholinergic as well with muscarinic receptors.[1]

Sympathetic Physiology

The sympathetic nervous system is known for the "fight or flight" response. Its postganglionic neurons extend to the heart (T1–T5), gastrointestinal tract (T6–T11), kidney (T10–L2), lower urinary tract, reproductive organs (T10–L2), upper body sweat glands (T1–T5), lower body sweat glands (T5–L2), upper body blood vessels (T1–T5), splanchnic blood vessels (T5–L2), and lower body blood vessels (T5–L2).

Parasympathetic Physiology

The parasympathetic nervous system is known for the "rest and digest" response. The vagus nerve (cranial nerve X) controls the heart, respiratory tract, and gastrointestinal tract (proximal to the splenic flexure), so parasympathetic controls to these end organs are not affected in spinal cord injury. The parasympathetic postganglionic neurons are found within ganglia either in the pelvic plexus or within target organs. These provide control to the bladder, lower part of the bowel (beyond the splenic flexure), and reproductive organs.

The autonomic nervous system is covered in further detail in subsequent chapters.

Conclusion

A fundamental knowledge of the neurophysiology of the spinal cord serves to better understand the clinical manifestations of spinal cord injury.

Review Questions

1. A 25-year-old male patient with new T8 American Spinal Injury Association (ASIA) Impairment Scale (AIS) A paraplegia notices that he can no longer feel his cell phone's vibration in his pants pocket. Which mechanoreceptors were most likely involved in transmitting these vibrational alerts to the spinal cord?
   a. Pacinian corpuscles
   b. Merkel receptors
   c. Ruffini corpuscles
   d. Meissner corpuscles
2. A 35-year-old female is referred to you for "new focal weakness." She shows you a screenshot of one slice of her recent cervical spine magnetic resonance imaging (MRI) that reveals a small intramedullary mass suspicious for astrocytoma, anterolaterally in the left anterior horn. There appears to be no compressive effect on the surrounding white matter. The cervical level of the slice is unclear. Based on your knowledge of somatotopic organization of the anterior horn, where would you expect to find muscle weakness on exam?
   a. Distal flexors
   b. Distal extensors
   c. Proximal flexors
   d. Proximal extensors
3. A 64-year-old male underwent an abdominal aortic aneurysm repair and awoke from surgery with flaccid paraplegia. MRI is suggestive of an infarct of the thoracic anterior cord. What sensory modality or modalities would you expect to be intact despite this lesion?
   a. Visceral pain
   b. Crude touch
   c. Somatic pain and temperature
   d. Vibration and proprioception
4. A 54-year-old male sustained a gunshot wound to the abdomen. In the field report, it was mentioned that one of the patient's legs was flaccid. Computed tomography (CT) spine revealed a bullet fragment penetrating the spinal cord in the right posterolateral white matter near the vertebral level T11. The lumbosacral spinal cord appears intact. Assuming the right corticospinal tract was severed at T11, which leg was likely flaccid, and do you expect it to be flaccid or spastic one year after the injury?
   a. Right leg, flaccid
   b. Left leg, flaccid
   c. Right leg, spastic
   d. Left leg, spastic
5. A 32-year-old female with chronic C8 AIS A tetraplegia has a feeling of anxiety and headache and notices her recently replaced suprapubic catheter is kinked and the collection bag is empty. She had used that brand of catheter once before. Her spouse notices that her skin is unusually red through her face, neck, and arms, but her abdomen is normal in color. What is the most likely cause of this change in skin color?
   a. Net postganglionic cholinergic activity
   b. Excessive dilation of the abdominal vascular bed
   c. Hypersensitivity reaction to the new catheter
   d. Excessive stimulation of cardiac β-receptors

REFERENCES

1. Costanzo L. *Physiology*. 6th ed. Philadelphia, PA: Elsevier; 2018.
2. Bear M, Connors B, Paradiso M. *Neuroscience: Exploring the Brain*. 2nd ed. Baltimore: Lippincott Williams & Wilkins; 2001.
3. Wolfe JM, Kluender KR, Levi DM, et al. *Sensation & Perception*. Sunderland, MA: Sinauer; 2006.
4. Kirshblum S, Lin V. *Spinal Cord Medicine*. 3rd ed. New York: Demos Medical Publishing; 2019.
5. Ditunno JF, Little JW, Tessler A, Burns AS. Spinal shock revisited: a four-phase model. *Spinal Cord*. 2004;42(7): 383–395.

CHAPTER 2

Neuroanatomy

Krysten Kasting and Stephanie Cowherd Ryder

OUTLINE

Introduction

This book serves as a board review and will focus on high-yield content. Specifically, this chapter will focus on neuroanatomy, setting a framework for topics to be discussed in greater detail later. This chapter is broken down into six sections: bony anatomy, neuroanatomical organization of gray and white matter, nerve roots and dermatomes, blood supply, spinal meninges, and autonomic nervous system anatomy.

Bony Anatomy

The spinal column provides the structural support for the spinal cord and is made up of 33 vertebrae. The spine is divided into cervical, thoracic, lumbar, and sacral segments. There are 7 cervical, 12 thoracic, 5 lumbar, 5 sacral, and 4 coccygeal vertebrae. The normal structure of the spine from the lateral view is an S curve with cervical and lumbar sections in lordosis and the thoracic section in kyphosis.

Between the bony vertebrae are intervertebral discs, which provide shock absorption, flexibility, and space for spinal nerves to exit. There are 25 discs, each of which provides a shock-absorbing effect that helps distribute forces throughout the spine. Discs are nonvascularized and composed of the central gel-like nucleus pulposus, outer collagenous annulus fibrosis, and the endplates, which provide nutrients through diffusion. Of note, there is no disc between C1, termed the atlas, and C2, the axis, as these form the atlantoaxial joint that serves as the pivot joint of the spine, contributing 50% of overall cervical rotation (Fig. 2.1).[1,2]

Each vertebra is made up of a body, posterior vertebral arch, and seven processes. The vertebral arch forms the posterior portion of each vertebra and consists of a left and right pedicle and lamina. Each pedicle forms one of the lateral sides of the arch, whereas each lamina forms the posterior roof of the arch.[3] The opening between the vertebral body and the arch forms the vertebral foramen in which the spinal cord resides. Spaces between adjacent pedicles form the intervertebral foramen through which spinal nerves exit the vertebral column.

Several processes arise from each arch. The paired transverse processes arise from the junction between the pedicle and lamina and project laterally. A single spinous process projects posteriorly. The spinous and transverse processes act as attachments for muscles of the back.

The last set of processes that arise from each arch are the superior and inferior articular processes. The superior articular process extends upward and pairs with the inferior articular process from the next higher vertebral level to form the facet joints of the spine. The orientation and shape of the articular processes vary depending on the level within the spinal column and are a determinant in the range of motion at that level.

Nerve Roots and Dermatomes

The spinal cord is the extension of the central nervous system that begins after the medulla and typically ends around L1–L2 in most adults. The most terminal end of the spinal cord is termed the *conus medullaris*. Distal to the conus is a collection of nerve roots termed the *cauda equina*. Sprouting from the spinal cord at each level are 31 pairs of spinal nerves. There are 8 sets of cervical, 12 thoracic, 5 lumbar, 5 sacral, and 1 pair of coccygeal nerve roots. The first seven cervical roots exit above the correspondingly numbered vertebra. The C8 nerve roots exit between the C7 and T1 vertebrae. At the thoracic

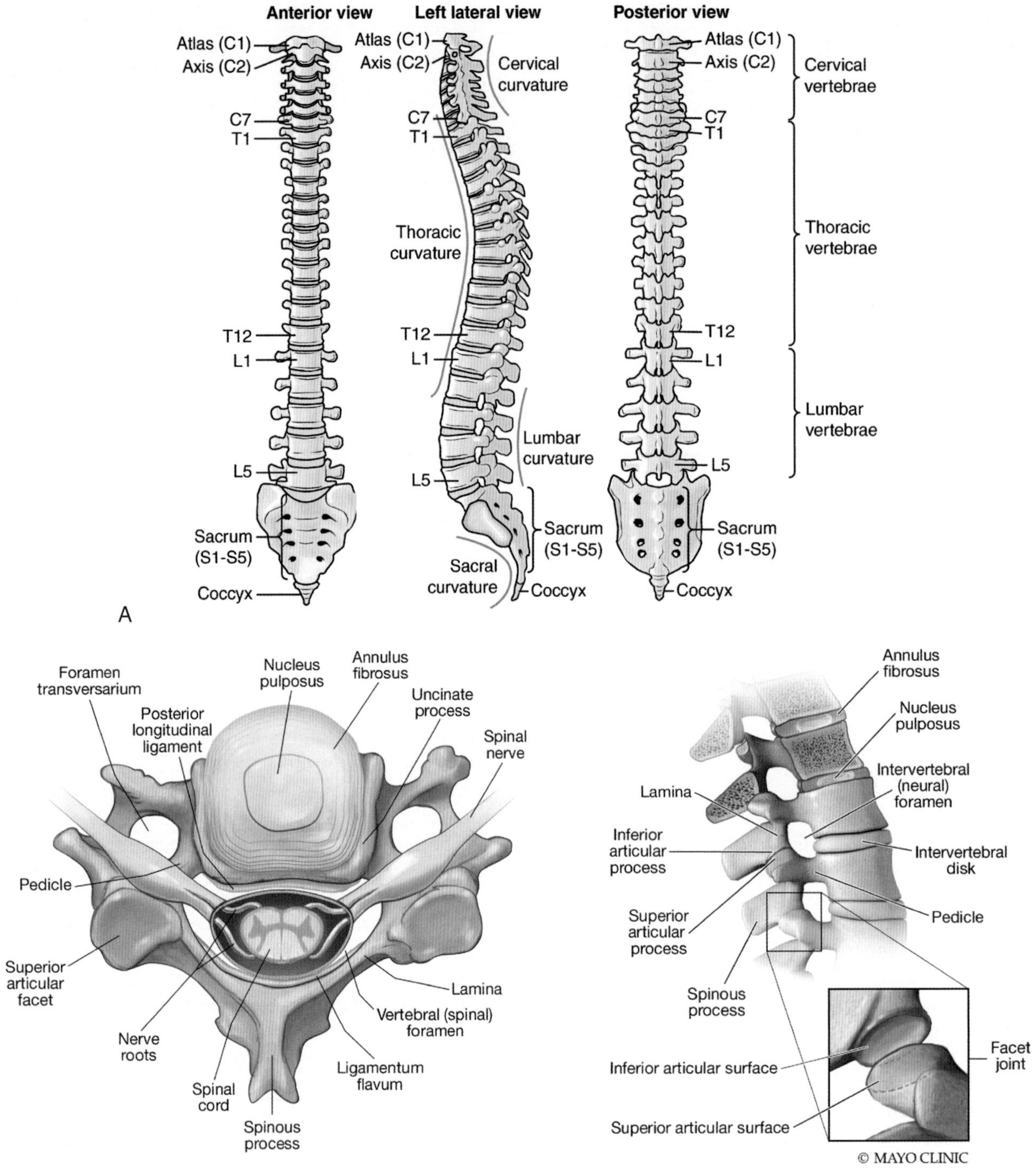

Fig. 2.1 The Spine. (A) The bony anatomy and alignment of the spine. (B) Anatomy of the vertebra and the vertebral column. (A, From Miller MD, Hart JA, MacKnight JM, eds. *Essential Orthopaedics*. Philadelphia: Saunders; 2010:454; B, from Daxon BT, Pasternak JJ. Disorders of the spine and spinal cord. In: Hines RL, Jones SB, eds. *Stoelting's Anesthesia and Co-Existing Disease*. 8th ed. Philadelphia: Elsevier; 2021:309–320 [Fig. 14.1].)

and lumbar levels, each nerve level exits below its corresponding vertebra. In the sacrum the spinal nerves pass through the sacral foramina. The cauda equina is 10 sets of nerve root pairs that arise from the conus and occupy the lumbar cistern until they exit at their respective vertebral level, supplying L2–S5. The function of the spinal nerves is to receive sensory information from the peripheral nervous system to the central nervous system (CNS) as well as deliver motor information from the CNS to the periphery (Fig. 2.2).[5]

Spinal nerves begin as nerve roots that emerge from the level of the spinal cord. At each level of the spinal

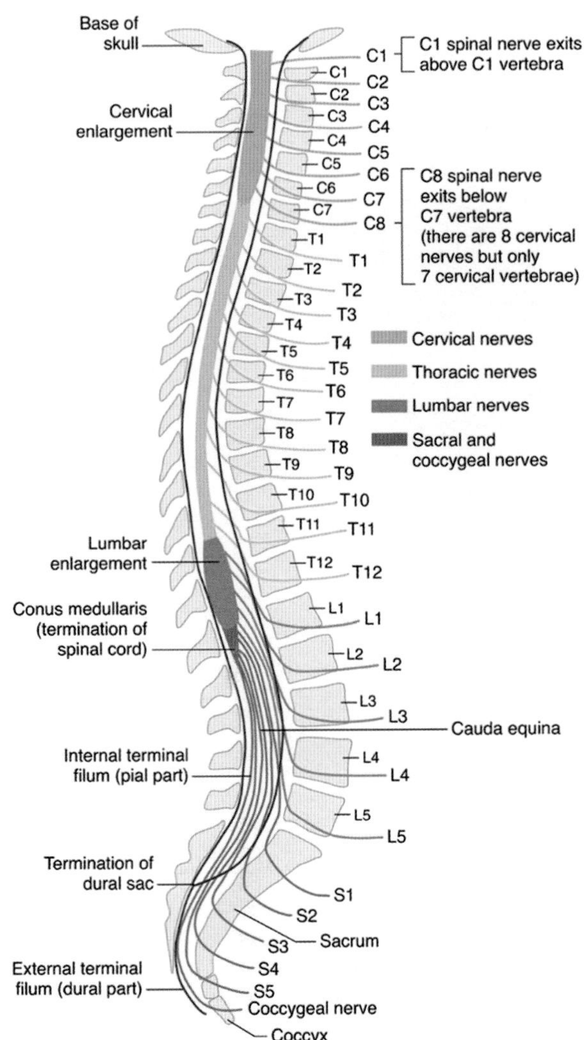

Fig. 2.2 Anatomy of the Spinal Cord With Exiting Spinal Nerves. Note that C1 spinal nerve exits above the C1 vertebra and C8 spinal nerve exits below the C7 vertebra. The remaining spinal nerves exit below the corresponding vertebrae. (From Goldman L, Schafer AI. *Goldman-Cecil Medicine*. 26th ed. Elsevier; 2020.)

cord approximately eight rootlets exit to form the dorsal and ventral roots. The dorsal root contains afferent sensory fibers that transmit information to the CNS. The cell bodies of these fibers are located in the dorsal root ganglion. The ventral root contains efferent motor and preganglionic autonomic fibers that carry information away from the CNS. The cell bodies of the ventral roots are located in the central gray matter of the spinal cord. The dorsal and ventral roots join together to form the spinal nerve proper, which contains sensory, motor, and autonomic fibers (Fig. 2.3).[6]

Dermatomes are defined areas of the skin that are mainly supplied by a single spinal nerve. Dermatomes are useful to help localize neurologic levels of injury. Some important landmarks for dermatomal testing are identified in Fig. 2.4. Myotomes are similar to dermatomes but refer to all the muscles served by a spinal nerve (Fig. 2.4).

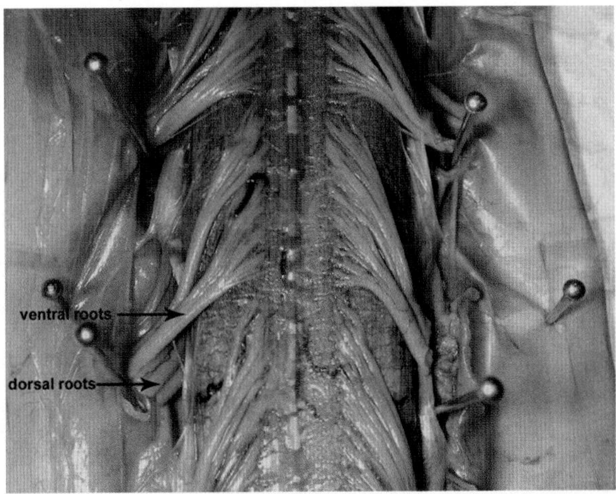

Fig. 2.3 This photograph is a dissection showing the ventral surface of the spinal cord and the ventral and dorsal rootlets. Groups of rootlets form the doral and ventral roots of the spinal nerves. (From Kayalioglu G. The spinal nerves. In: Watson C, Paxinos G, Kayalioglu G, eds. *The Spinal Cord*. Academic Press; 2009:37–56.)

Neuroanatomical Organization of Gray and White Matter

Similar to the brain, the spinal cord is made up of both gray and white matter. The gray matter contains high concentrations of neuronal cell bodies, whereas white matter contains high concentrations of myelin. In the spinal cord, gray matter is central to the cord with white matter on the periphery (Fig. 2.5).[4]

White matter is subdivided into three main columns: dorsal, lateral, and ventral. Ascending tracts carry sensory information, whereas descending tracts carry motor pathways. The dorsal columns contain only sensory pathways, whereas the ventral and lateral columns contain both sensory and motor pathways.[5]

Gray matter is primarily split into the dorsal and ventral horns. The dorsal horn is a sensory zone that receives afferent information, and the ventral horn is a motor zone. The horns are connected by interneurons. In the midline of the gray matter lies the central canal, which is filled with cerebrospinal fluid. The different tracts of the spinal cord are discussed in greater detail in Chapter 1.

The amount of white matter decreases caudally as fewer axons travel to and from the lower regions of the cord. The gray matter shape varies depending on the level of the cord. In the cervical and lumbosacral enlargement of the cord, there is expansion of ventral horn gray matter corresponding to motor function of the arms and legs, whereas the thoracic gray matter in the ventral horn is reduced.

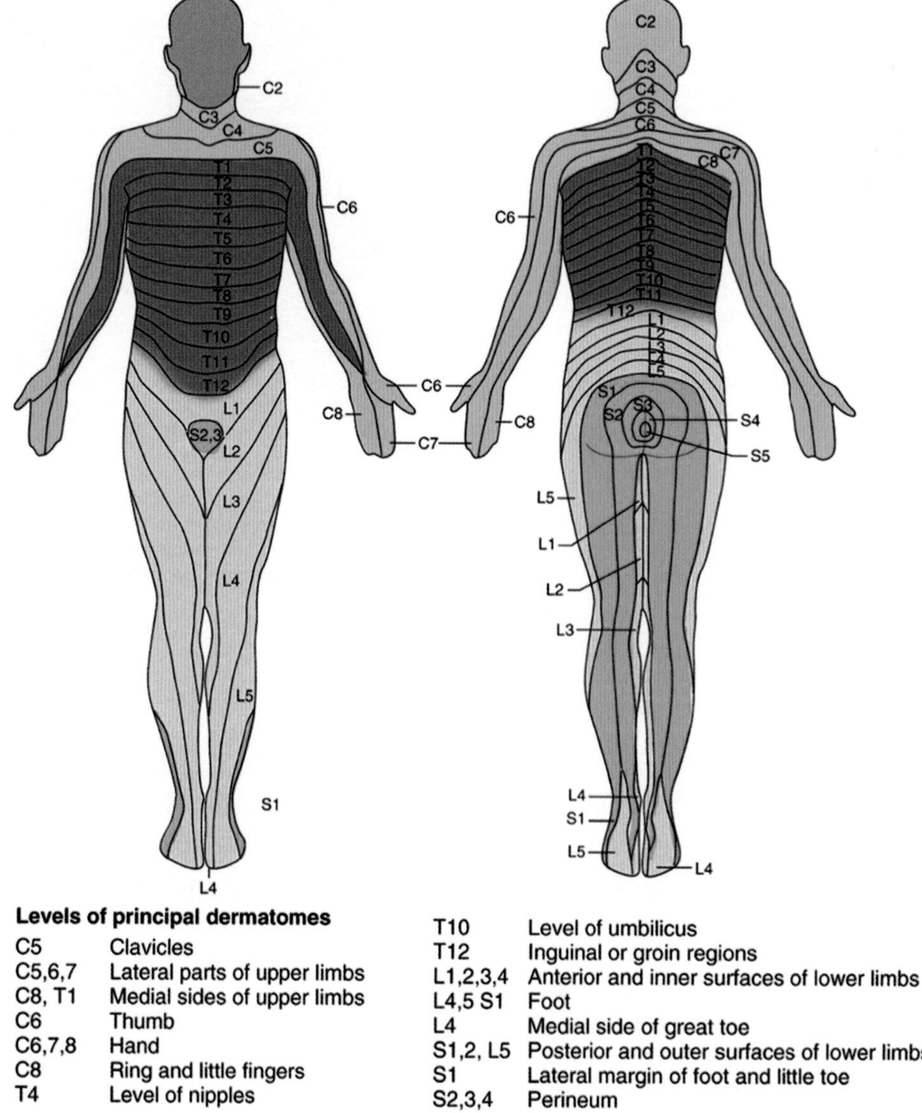

Fig. 2.4 Dermatomes, or the areas of the skin that are mainly supplied by a single spinal nerve, are demarcated by spinal level. (Courtesy of Professor Mete Erturk, Ege University.)

In the thoracic cord there is a lateral protrusion of the gray matter called the lateral horn, also known as the intermediolateral column. These are the preganglionic sympathetic neurons, which will be further discussed later in the chapter. There is a similar group of cells in the sacral gray matter that create the parasympathetic neurons.

Blood Supply

Arterial

Blood supply to the spinal cord comes primarily from the anterior spinal artery (ASA) and the two posterior spinal arteries (PSA). The ASA provides blood flow to the anterior two-thirds of the spinal cord, and the posterior arteries supply blood to the posterior one-third. The ASA is a united branch from each vertebral artery and travels caudally in the anterior sulcus. The origin of the posterior spinal arteries can be more variable, coming from either the posterior inferior cerebellar artery or the preatlantal vertebral arteries.[7] The PSA then travels caudally through the two posterior sulci of the spinal cord (Fig. 2.6).[8]

Both the anterior and posterior arteries are fed throughout their course at each level by segmental spinal arteries. These segmental arteries enter through the intervertebral foramen and then split into posterior and anterior radicular arteries and feed the PSA and ASA, respectively. Along the way, they supply blood to

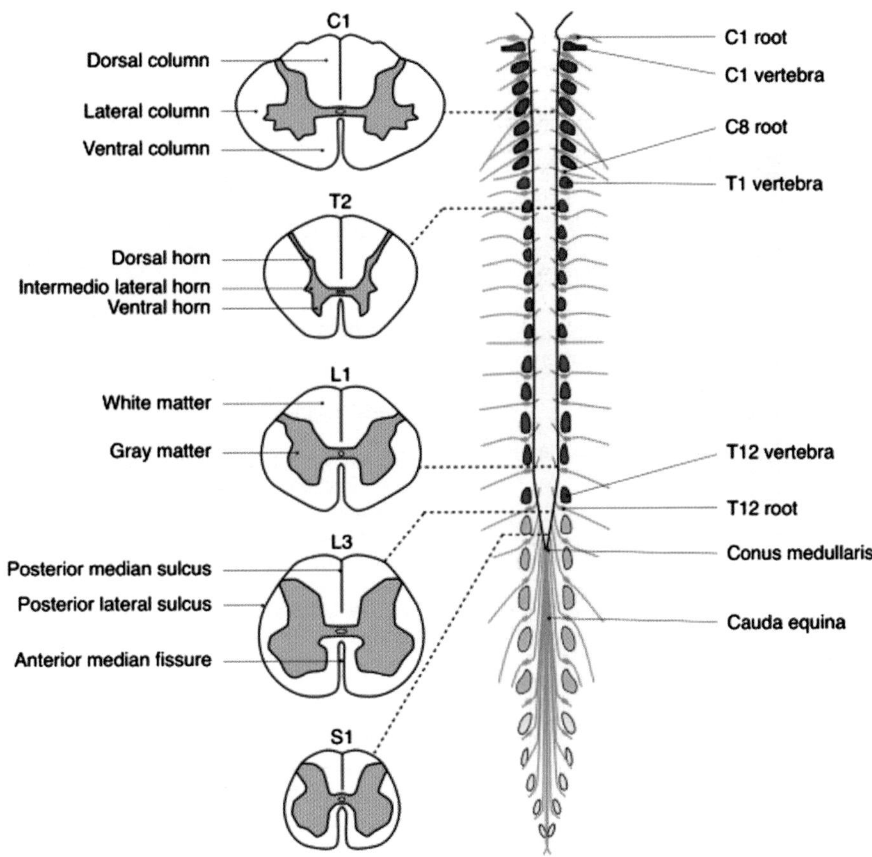

Fig. 2.5 A Schematic View of the Vertebral Levels With Spinal Roots. Axial slices shown on left demonstrate the gray and white matter distribution at various levels. (From Cohen-Adad J, Wheeler-Kingshott CAM, eds. *Quantitative MRI of the Spinal Cord*. Elsevier; 2014.)

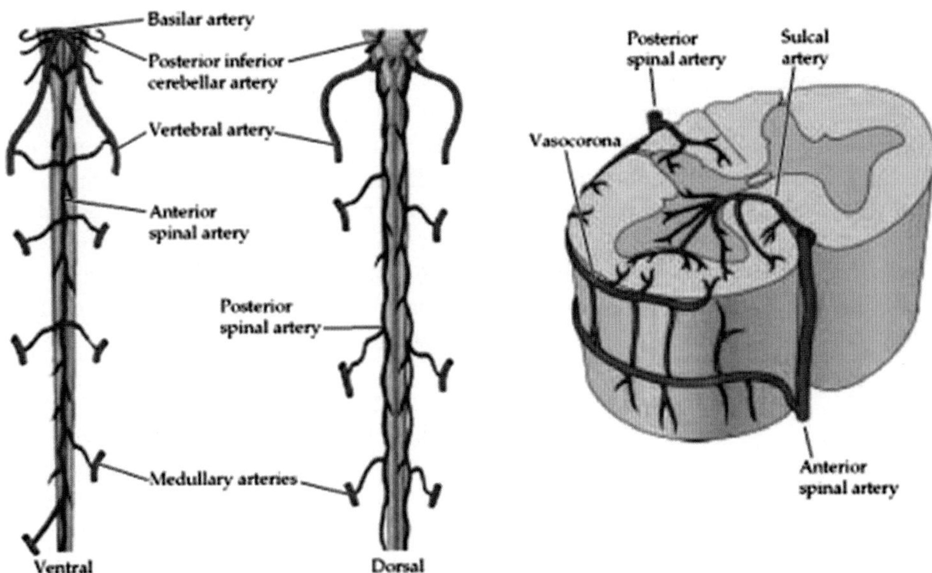

Fig. 2.6 The figure shows the arteries supplying the spinal cord. It is noted that all spinal nerve roots have associated radicular or segmental radiculomedullary arteries as seen in Fig. 2.7.

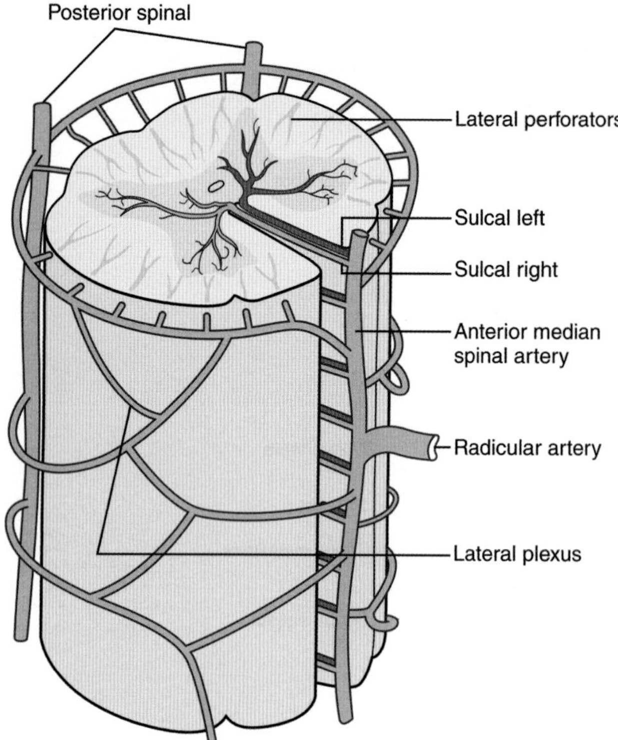

Fig. 2.7 The anterior and posterior spinal arteries are fed at each level by segmental spinal arteries that enter through the intervertebral foramen. (From Goldman L, Schafer AI. *Goldman-Cecil Medicine*. 26th ed. Elsevier; 2020 [Fig. 372.1].)

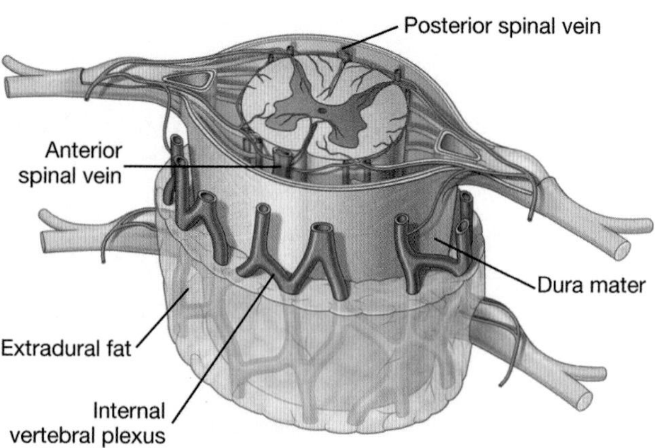

Fig. 2.8 Veins That Drain the Spinal Cord. These longitudinal channels drain into an extensive internal vertebral plexus in the extradural (epidural) space of the vertebral canal, which then drains into segmentally arranged vessels that connect with major systemic veins, such as the azygos system in the thorax. The internal vertebral venous plexus also communicates with intracranial veins. (From Drake RL, Vogl W, Mitchell AWM, eds. *Gray's Basic Anatomy*. 2nd ed. Elsevier; 2018:31–55 [Fig. 2.34].)

the nearby nerve roots. The anterior and posterior spinal arteries are fed at each level by segmental spinal arteries that enter through the interveterbral foramen (Fig. 2.7).[9]

Importantly, the mid-thoracic region of the spinal cord, T3–T7, usually only receives one radiculomedullary artery and consequently is characterized by poor blood supply. The thoracolumbar portion of the cord derives its supply from the artery of Adamkiewicz, which branches off the left side of the descending aorta between T8–L2 and connects to the central side of the spinal cord to supply the ASA. The cauda equina is supplied by one to two branches of the lumbar, iliolumbar, and lateral/median sacral arteries.

Venous Drainage

Venous drainage is accomplished via a complex plexus of veins that travel with the arteries. The plexus consists of veins both inside and outside the vertebral canal called the internal and the external venous plexus.[10] The internal plexus drains into the external plexus, which in turn drains into the azygous venous system, the portal venous system, renal veins, and the superior or inferior vena cava depending on the level (Fig. 2.8).[11]

Spinal Meninges

Like the brain, the spinal cord is also enclosed by three layers of meninges: the dura, arachnoid, and pia mater. The meninges extend from the brain to enclose the brainstem and spinal cord and end as filum terminale (Fig. 2.9).[12]

The epidural space is located between the ligamentum flavum and the dura mater. It contains fat, connective tissue, the internal vertebral venous plexus, and lymphatics. Of note, this space is used for analgesic injections and is a potential space for infection.

The dura mater is the most superficial and strongest of the three meningeal layers. Unlike the cranial dura, in the spinal cord the dura mater only has one layer (the meningeal layer). Extensions of the dura cover the nerve roots as they exit the vertebral canal and continue as the epineurium of spinal nerves. The subdural space between the dura and the arachnoid is only a potential space that is not typically present under normal physiologic conditions.

The arachnoid mater is a loose covering that extends from the foramen magnum and terminates around S2. The main function of the arachnoid mater is to maintain cerebrospinal fluid (CSF) metabolism.

The subarachnoid space is the space between the arachnoid and pia mater and contains CSF. The CSF in this space is made within the brain ventricles and flows downward to fill the subarachnoid space. It provides both protection and nutrients to the spinal cord. Because the conus ends around L2 and the subarachnoid continues to the level of S2, this allows space for lumbar punctures to be performed.

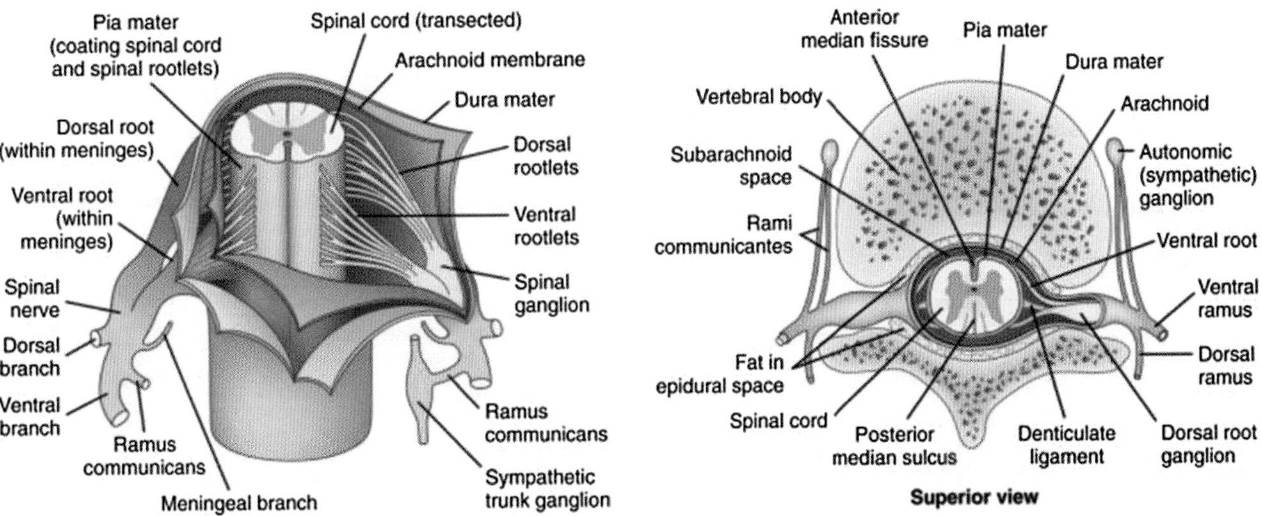

Fig. 2.9 The Spinal Meninges. The dura mater, arachnoid membrane, and pia mater encasing the spinal cord. (From Varthi A, Russo G, Whang P. *Rothman-Simeone and Herkowitz's the Spine*. 7th ed. Elsevier; 2018.)

The pia mater is the deepest layer of meninges and closely attaches to the spinal cord. The pia continues downward after the conus to form the filum terminale, anchoring the spinal cord to the coccyx. The pia also extends into the denticulate ligaments that project outward from the cord midway between the dorsal and ventral roots and act as stabilization for the cord.

Autonomic Nervous System

The autonomic nervous system (ANS) is a division of the nervous system with both central and peripheral nervous system components. Functionally it is divided into sympathetic and parasympathetic components. More discussion will arise in later chapters about the importance of the autonomic nervous system in spinal cord injury (SCI); here we will focus on the anatomy of the ANS.

The sympathetic nervous system originates in the thoracic and lumbar segments of the spinal cord and thus is also called the *thoracolumbar division*. The parasympathetic nervous system originates in the brainstem and sacral segments and is also called the *craniosacral division*.[13] In this section we will discuss the anatomy of the ANS; the pathophysiology and how it applies to SCI will be discussed in further chapters (Fig. 2.10).[14]

Sympathetic Nervous System

The cell bodies of the sympathetic nervous system (SNS) are located in the intermediolateral columns of the thoracic and lumbar spinal cord gray matter. In the thoracic cord the intermediolateral column is also termed the *lateral horn*. The cell bodies of the SNS give rise to the preganglionic fibers, which exit the spinal cord through the anterior roots to synapse with one of the two groups of SNS ganglia, either the paravertebral ganglia or prevertebral ganglia. There are two groups of SNS ganglia, the paravertebral and prevertebral. The paravetebral ganglia run parallel to the vertebral column and link together to form the sympathetic trunk or chain. The prevertebral ganglia form several plexuses around the major branches of the abdominal aorta.

Paravertebral ganglia exist as nodules throughout the length of the sympathetic trunk. Although the number varies, in general there are 3 cervical, 12 thoracic, 4 lumbar, and 5 sacral ganglia. The cervical ganglia are named (the superior, middle, and inferior cervical ganglia), whereas all other ganglia within the sympathetic chain are not. There are four paths an axon can take to reach its final destination once it enters the paravetebral ganglion: synapse in this ganglion, ascend or descend to another paravertebral ganglion level, or descend to a prevertebral ganglion.

Parasympathetic Nervous System

Parasympathetic nervous system (PNS) preganglionic neurons originate in the brainstem and sacral spinal cord, specifically S2–S4. Preganglionic fibers of the PNS are much longer than those of the SNS. The preganglionic fibers synapse with postganglionic neurons in ganglia on or near the target organ. This can be remembered as "para-" means "adjacent to," hence parasympathetic. Short postganglionic axons then relay signals to the organ. Preganglionic fibers that originate at the brainstem level exit through cranial nerves III, VII, IX, and X. PNS fibers originating in the sacral cord travel with the pelvic splanchnic nerves.

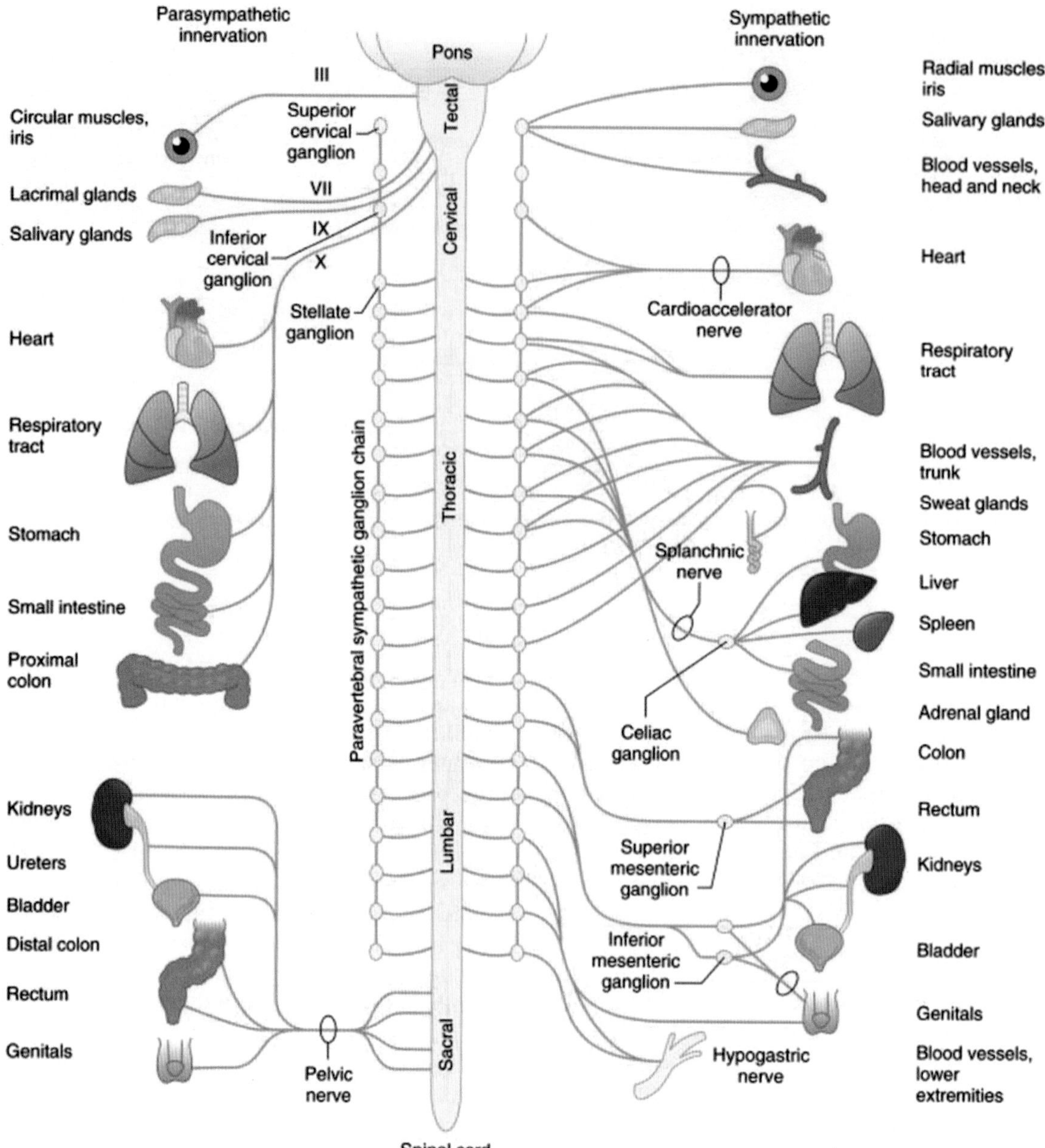

Fig. 2.10 A Visual Representation of the Autonomic Nervous System. The sympathetic nervous system originates in the thoracic and lumbar segments of the spinal cord, whereas the parasympathetic nervous system originates in the brainstem and sacral segments. (From Stein E, Glick D. *Basics of Anesthesia*. Elsevier; 2018 [Fig. 6.1].)

Review Questions

1. A 50-year-old male is admitted to rehabilitation after undergoing C1–C5 posterior spinal fusion. The atlantoaxial joint provides what percentage of cervical rotation?
   a. 25%
   b. 40%
   c. 50%
   d. 75%
2. The intermediolateral column in the thoracolumbar spinal cord contains the cell bodies of which neurons?
   a. Preganglionic sympathetic neurons
   b. Motor neurons
   c. Preganglionic parasympathetic neurons
   d. Second-order neurons for the spinothalamic pathway
3. A 35-year-old female is involved in a rollover motor vehicle collision. She sustains a C7–T1 fracture with dislocation and bilateral locked facets. What nerve root would be damaged as it exits the C7–T1 foramen?
   a. C6
   b. C7
   c. C8
   d. T1

4. A patient underwent bilateral L2–L3 transforaminal steroid injection for radicular pain and within minutes, developed flaccid paraplegia. What is the most likely cause of this presentation?
   a. Transverse myelitis
   b. Occlusion of the artery of Adamkiewicz
   c. Bilateral posterior spinal artery occlusion
   d. Allergic reaction to steroid
5. The filum terminale anchors the spinal cord to the coccyx and is formed by:
   a. Pia mater
   b. Dura mater
   c. Arachnoid mater
   d. Ligamentum flavum

REFERENCES

1. Miller MD, Hart JA, MacKnight JM, eds. *Essential Orthopaedics*. Philadelphia: Saunders; 2010:454.
2. Daxon BT, Pasternak JJ. Disorders of the spine and spinal cord. In: Hines RL, Jones SB, eds. *Stoelting's Anesthesia and Co-Existing Disease*. 8th ed. Philadelphia: Elsevier; 2021: 309–320.
3. O'Rahilly R, Muller F. *Basic Human Anatomy: A Regional Study of Human Structure*. Philadelphia: Saunders; 1983. mouth. edu/%7Ehumananatomy/part_7/index.html.
4. Cohen-Adad J, Wheeler-Kingshott CAM, eds. *Quantitative MRI of the Spinal Cord*. Elsevier; 2014.
5. Goldman L, Schafer AI. *Goldman-Cecil Medicine*. 26th ed Elsevier; 2020.
6. Kayalioglu G. The spinal nerves. In: Watson C, Paxinos G, Kayalioglu G, eds. *The Spinal Cord*. Academic Press; 2009: 37–56.
7. Berg EJ, Ashurst J. *Anatomy, back, cauda equina. Stat Pears*. StatPearls Publishing; 2020.
8. Purves D, Augustine GJ, Fitzpatrick D, et al. *Neuroscience*. 2nd ed. Sunderland, MA: Sinauer Associates; 2001.
9. Lazorthes G, Gouaze A, Zadeh JO, et al. Arterial vascularization of the spinal cord: recent studies of the anastomotic substitution pathways. *J Neurosurg*. 1971;35:253–262.
10. Griessenauer CJ, Raborn J, Foreman P, Shoja MM, Loukas M, Tubbs RS. Venous drainage of the spine and spinal cord: a comprehensive review of its history, embryology, anatomy, physiology, and pathology. *Clinical Anatomy*. 2015;28:75–87.
11. Drake RL, Vogl W, Mitchell AWM, eds. *Gray's Basic Anatomy*. 2nd ed. Elsevier; 2018:31–55.
12. Varthi A, Russo G, Whang P. *Rothman-Simeone and Herkowitz's the Spine*. 7th ed. Elsevier; 2018.
13. Waxenbaum J, Reddy V, Varacallo M. *Anatomy, autonomic nervous system. [Updated 2021 Jul 29]*. StatPearls Publishing; Aug. 2020. https://www.ncbi.nlm.nih.gov/books/NBK539845/.
14. Stein E, Glick D. *Basics of Anesthesia*. Elsevier; 2018.

CHAPTER 3

Epidemiology, Risk Factors, and Genetics

Scott Schubert and Christina Draganich

OUTLINE

Introduction

Spinal cord injury (SCI) is one of the most devastating injuries that an individual can sustain and substantially impacts all aspects of an individual's life, including their social, medical, emotional, and economic well-being. This chapter aims to provide an overview of the demographic, injury-related, and health characteristics of individuals with SCI as well as the economic impact to both these individuals and society at large. A greater understanding of the trends in the epidemiology and risk factors underlying SCI can provide the necessary information to assist in policy development to aid this population.

Incidence

Since the 1970s, a variety of state registries and nationwide administrative databases have been used to estimate the incidence of SCI, with estimates ranging between 25 cases per million and 83 cases per million.[1–10] The annual incidence of SCI in the United States is currently estimated to be **54 cases per million individuals**, or approximately **17,810 new SCI cases per year**.[1,5,11]

- The estimates may be explained by differences in regional population characteristics and research methodology.
- Limitations of these reports include that emergency room physicians' definitions of acute SCI diagnosis vary between providers and that most studies did not include individuals who died at the site of injury.
- The incidence of SCI-related deaths prior to hospitalization has been reported in only a few studies and ranges between 4 and 21 cases per million.[7,9,10,12]
- Children were included in the initial state-developed reports but not in the more recent nationwide studies.[5]
- The estimated annual incidence of SCI in children 0 to 19 years is **10 to 25 new cases per million**, indicating a lower risk of SCI in children compared to adults.[3,4,8–10,13,14]

Risk Factors

Age

- The average age at injury has increased from 29 years during the 1970s to 43 years since 2015.[11]
- Incidence of SCI varies by age:
  - lowest for the pediatric group (defined as age younger than 16 years),[5]
  - highest for individuals in their late teens and 20s,[5]
  - increasing for individuals older than 65 years of age.[1,8,15]
- Etiology of injury varies by age:[11,16]
  - Violent etiologies decline with advancing age.
  - SCIs resulting from falls and medical or surgical complications increase with advancing age.
  - Recreational sports injuries are most common among individuals younger than 15 years.

Gender

- Approximately 78% of new SCI cases are male.[1,11]
- The percentage of females with SCI has increased from 18.2% in the 1970s to 22% in 2015–2017.[1,8]

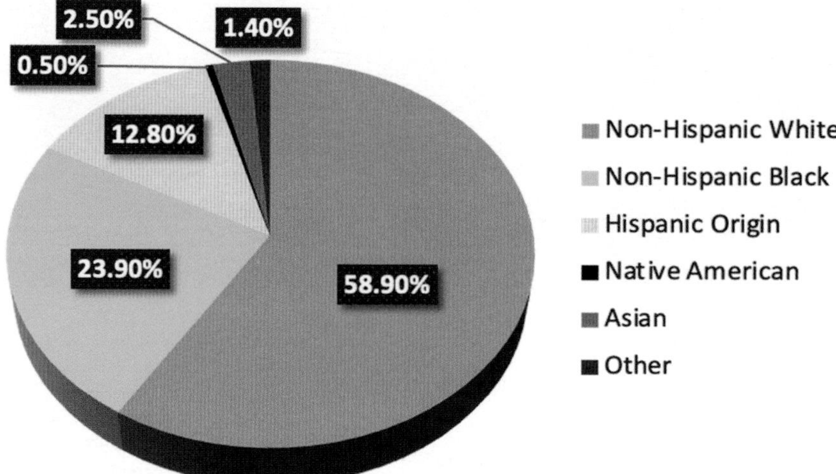

Fig. 3.1 Race/Ethnicity Since 2015. (Data from National Spinal Cord Injury Statistical Center. Annual Statistical Reports for the Spinal Cord Injury Model Systems. Published online 2017.)

Race/Ethnicity

- Non-Hispanic Whites have the highest incidence of SCI (Fig. 3.1), followed by non-Hispanic Blacks and individuals of Hispanic origin.[11,17]
- Twenty-four percent of injuries occur in non-Hispanic Blacks, which is higher than the proportion of non-Hispanic Blacks in the general population (13%).[6,12,14,15]
- There has been an increasing incidence of SCI within the Hispanic population, doubling from 6% to 12.8% in the last five decades, which is in line with growth of the Hispanic population.[18]

Other Risk Factors

- **Alcohol:** Between 22% and 50% of patients presenting with new SCI report using alcohol or have a positive blood alcohol at the time of injury.[3,4,9,10,19]
- **Time of week:** The incidence of SCI is higher on weekends, with the exception of SCIs resulting from medical or surgical complications.[8,20] SCIs resulting from medical/surgical complications occur more commonly on Mondays and Tuesdays.[16]
- **Time of year:** The incidence of SCI increases during warm-weather months, with the fewest SCIs in February (6.3%) and the most SCIs during July (10.9%).[16]

Prevalence and Demographics

The number of people with SCI living in the United States is approximately **294,000 persons**, with estimates ranging from 250,000 to 368,000 individuals.[11,21,22]

Age

- The average age of all persons living with SCI in the United States (including new and existing cases) is estimated to be 45 years.

Gender

- The male-to-female prevalence ratio is lower than the male-to-female incidence ratio (2.6 vs. 4.0), which can be explained by women having a longer life expectancy than men.[23]

Race/Ethnicity

- The White-to-non-White prevalence ratio is approximately 1.5, which is similar to the White-to-non-White incidence ratio.[23,24]

Education

- The percentage of people with a college degree or higher at the time of injury has increased from 7.0% to 24.0% over the last five decades.[25]
- Since 2015, approximately 24% of individuals with SCI have a college degree at the time of injury compared with 45% of individuals who have survived 40 years of injury (Table 3.1).[11]

Occupational Status

- Since 2015, there has been an increase in the percentage of working responders over the postinjury years.
    - 18% of individuals with SCI are employed at 1 year postinjury
    - 32% are employed at 40 years postinjury (Table 3.2 and Fig. 3.2)[11]
- The percentage employed is only slightly higher for those with paraplegia than those with tetraplegia.[11]

Marital Status

- Since 2015, the percentage of married individuals is relatively consistent up to 40 years postinjury, with

Table 3.1 Education Status After Injury (%)

Education	At Injury	Year 1	Year 10	Year 20	Year 30	Year 40
High School Only	51.6	52.1	50.4	46.6	41.3	34.0
College or Higher	24.0	26.4	27.6	26.3	34.9	45.3

Table 3.2 Employment Status After Injury (%)

Employment Status	At Injury	Year 1	Year 10	Year 20	Year 30	Year 40
Employed	67.3	18.0	23.8	29.2	31.2	32.1
Student	8.1	7.3	2.8	0.9	0.4	0

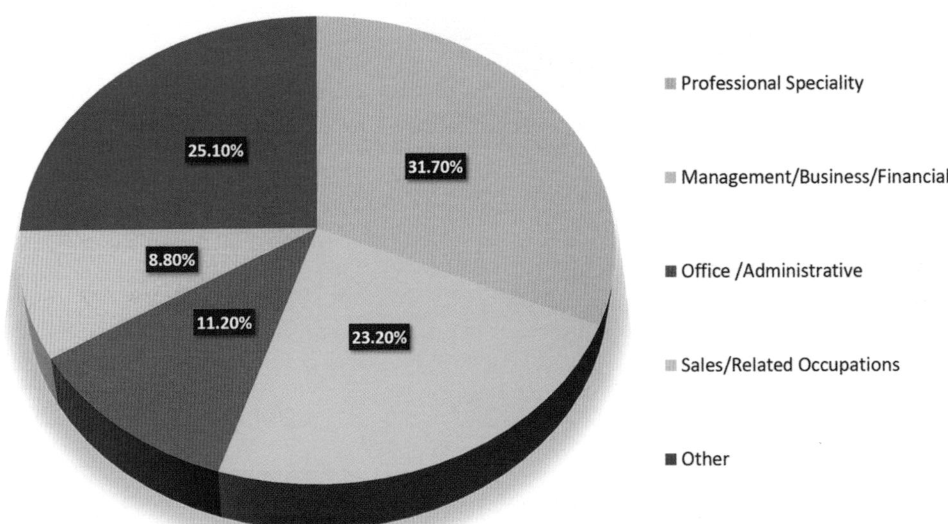

Fig. 3.2 Most Common Job Types After Spinal Cord Injury. (Data from National Spinal Cord Injury Statistical Center. Annual Statistical Reports for the Spinal Cord Injury Model Systems. Published online 2017.)

Table 3.3 Marital Status After Injury (%)

Status	At Injury	Year 1	Year 10	Year 20	Year 30	Year 40
Single	44.6	43.1	37.1	38.1	33.5	24.7
Married	37.4	36.4	34.7	33.6	36.2	44.2
Divorced	8.6	10.8	20.1	19.7	21.3	21.6

the percentage of single/never married individuals decreasing and the percentage of divorced individuals increasing (Table 3.3).[11]

- The marriage rate is lower in the SCI population than in the general population.[26,27]
- Marriage is associated with favorable psychosocial outcomes for individuals with SCI.[26,27]

Injury Characteristics

Causes of Injury

Motor vehicle accidents are the leading cause of injury, followed by falls (Fig. 3.3). Acts of violence (primarily gunshot wounds) and sports/recreation activities are also relatively common etiologies (Fig. 3.4).[11,16]

Trends in Causes of Injury[28]

- The percentage of SCIs due to motor vehicle accidents has decreased.
- The percentage of SCIs due to falls has increased, especially among individuals 45 years or older.
- The percentage of SCIs due to violence peaked in the 1990s and has since decreased.
- The percentage of SCIs due to sports has declined since the 1970s.

Trends in Sports-Related Injuries[29]

- There has been a shift in sports-related etiologies of injury since the 1970s.
- SCIs due to diving, football, and trampoline injuries have declined.
- SCIs due to skiing, winter sports, and surfing have increased.

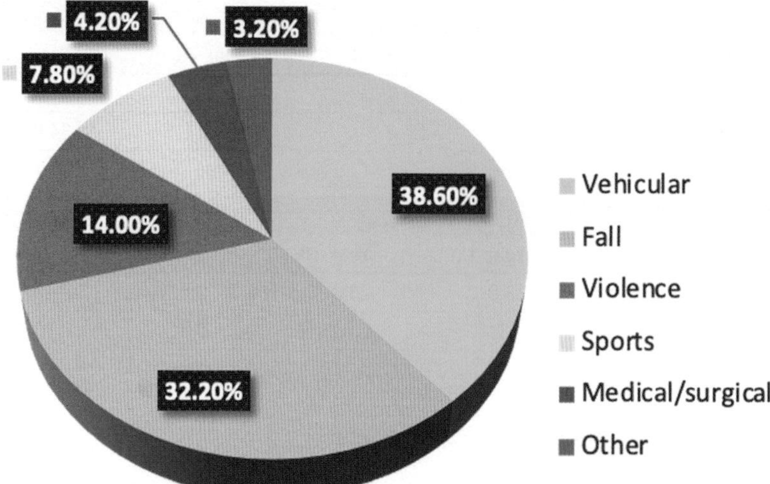

Fig. 3.3 Etiology of Injury. (Data from National Spinal Cord Injury Statistical Center. Annual Statistical Reports for the Spinal Cord Injury Model Systems. Published online 2017.)

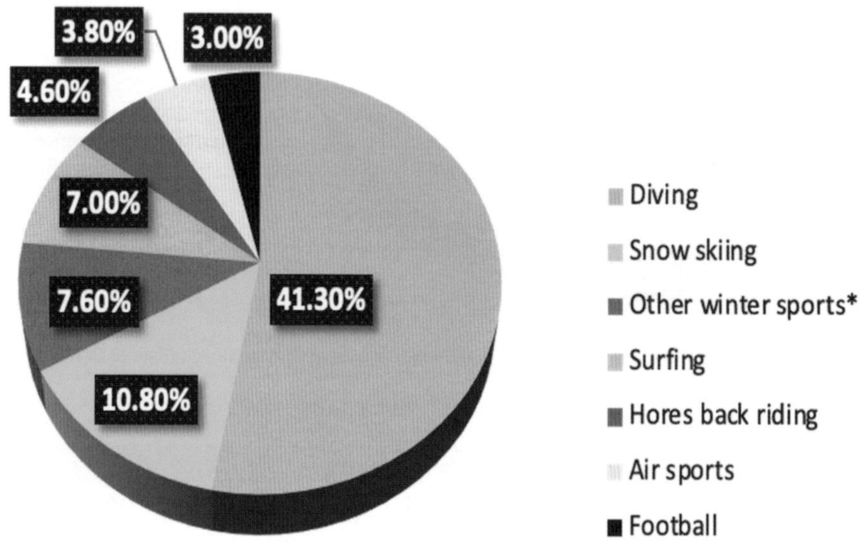

Fig 3.4 Etiology of Sports Related Injuries. (Data from National Spinal Cord Injury Statistical Center. Annual Statistical Reports for the Spinal Cord Injury Model Systems. Published online 2017.)

Injury Level and Severity

- Incomplete tetraplegia is the most common neurologic category (Fig. 3.5).[11]
- The frequency of incomplete and complete paraplegia is approximately the same.[11]
- Complete tetraplegia is the least common neurologic category.[11]
- Level and completeness of injury varies by etiology of injury:
  - Firearm-related injuries are more likely to result in complete paraplegia.[16]
  - Diving-related injuries are more likely to result in complete tetraplegia.[16]
  - High falls (from buildings and ladders) are more likely to result in complete paraplegia.[30]
  - Low falls (same level and stairs) are more likely to result in incomplete tetraplegia.

Trends in Injury Level and Severity[17,28]

- The percentage of high cervical injuries has increased over the last five decades, while the percentage of low cervical injuries has decreased, and percentage of thoracic, lumbar, and sacral injuries has remained constant.
- The percentage of incomplete injuries has increased over the last five decades compared to the percentage of complete injuries.

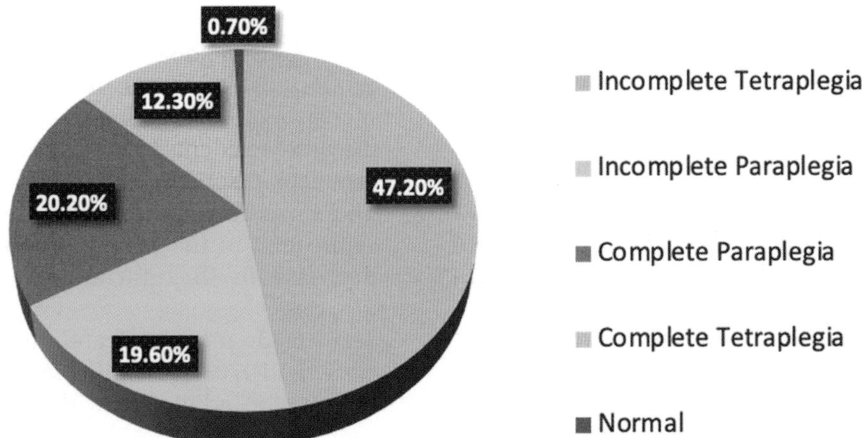

Fig. 3.5 Neurologic Category, Since 2015. (Data from National Spinal Cord Injury Statistical Center. Annual Statistical Reports for the Spinal Cord Injury Model Systems. Published online 2017.)

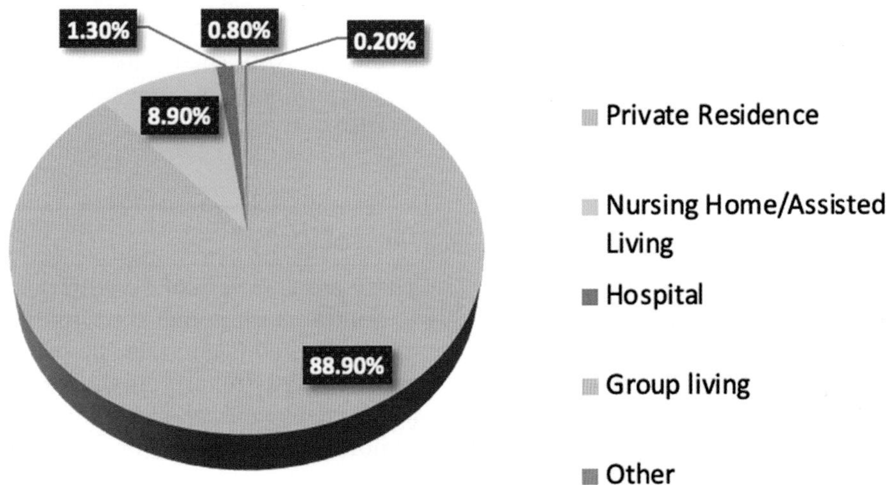

Fig. 3.6 Discharge Placement. (Data from National Spinal Cord Injury Statistical Center. Annual Statistical Reports for the Spinal Cord Injury Model Systems. Published online 2017.)

- Less than 1% of individuals have complete neurologic recovery by the time of hospital discharge.

Associated Injuries

- Approximately 36% of individuals have one or more concomitant injuries along with SCI.[11,15,31]
- Comorbid traumatic brain injury (TBI) has been reported with a frequency ranging from 16% to 74% and is most common among SCIs resulting from motor vehicle crashes and falls.[11,32]
- Vertebral injury has been documented in approximately 80.4% of individuals with acute SCI.[11,31]
- The associated spinal surgery rate is 82.5% and is more common in SCIs caused by vehicular crashes, sports-related injuries, and falls but less frequently performed for SCIs caused by acts of violence and penetrating injuries.[33]

Length of Stay

- Length of stay (LOS) in acute care units has declined from 24 days in the 1970s to 11 days since 2015.[11]
- Rehabilitation LOS has also declined from 98 days in the 1970s to 31 days since 2015.[11]
- A variety of factors account for this decrease in acute and rehabilitation LOS, including the implementation of managed care and other cost-containment measures.[34–36]

Outcomes

Discharge Placement

- Approximately 90% of individuals with SCI are discharged back to the community, either to a private residence or group living situation (Fig. 3.6).[11,37]

- As inpatient rehabilitation LOS has decreased, more individuals are discharged to another hospital, nursing home, or assisted-living community.[11,37]

Rehospitalization

- Since 2015, approximately 30% of individuals with SCI are rehospitalized at least once after their initial hospitalization for SCI.[11]
- Among individuals with SCI who are rehospitalized, the average LOS is approximately 18 days.[11]
- The most common cause of rehospitalization is diseases of the genitourinary system, followed by diseases of the skin, respiratory, digestive, circulatory, and musculoskeletal disease.[11]

Mortality

- Approximately 5.7% to 8.0% of individuals with SCI die prior to acute hospital discharge.[1,8,15,38]
- Risk of in-hospital mortality is associated with[1,8,15]
  - advancing age (≥65 years),
  - motor vehicle crash,
  - high cervical injury,
  - polytrauma,
  - multiple comorbidities,
  - complications, such as venous thromboembolism and TBI.
- The average life expectancy for individuals with SCI remains significantly below the life expectancy for individuals without SCI and has not improved since the 1980s.[11,39]
- Mortality rates are significantly higher during the first year after injury than in later years.[11,40]
- Life expectancy decreases with age, decreases with decreasing level of injury, decreases with increasing completeness of injury, and decreases with ventilator use (Table 3.4).[41–44]

Cause of Death

- The leading causes of death have historically been respiratory diseases, primarily pneumonia, followed by infectious and parasitic diseases, which are usually cases of septicemia (Fig. 3.7).[11]
- In the past 45 years, mortality rates have been declining for cancer, heart disease, stroke, arterial diseases, pulmonary embolus, urinary diseases, digestive diseases, and suicide.[11]
- In the past 45 years, mortality rates have been increasing for endocrine, metabolic, and nutritional diseases, accidents, nervous system diseases, musculoskeletal disorders, and mental disorders.[11]
- There has been no change in the mortality rate for septicemia in the past 45 years and only a slight decrease in the mortality rate for respiratory diseases.[11]
- The suicide mortality rate after SCI has decreased since the 1970s but is still approximately three times the rate for individuals without SCI.[45]

Cost

- The average yearly expenses, including health care and living expenses (Table 3.5), and estimated lifetime costs directly attributable to SCI (Table 3.6) vary based on neurological impairment, preinjury employment history, and education.[11,24,46–49]
- Indirect costs, such as losses in wages, fringe benefits, and productivity, are estimated to average $77,701 per year.[11]

Genetics

There are a variety of hereditary conditions that lead to nontraumatic spinal cord injury, which include but are not limited to multiple sclerosis, amyotrophic lateral sclerosis, Friedreich's ataxia, hereditary spastic paraplegia, spinal muscular atrophy, and spinal cord–related tumors.

Summary

- The annual incidence of SCI in the United States is approximately 54 cases per million or 17,810 new SCI cases per year.
- The estimated prevalence of SCI in the United States is approximately 294,000 persons.
- The average age at injury has increased from 29 years in the 1970s to 43 years since 2015.
- Approximately 78% of new SCI cases are male.

Table 3.4 Survival After Spinal Cord Injury

		Survival at Least 1 Year Postinjury				
Age at Injury	**No SCI**	**AIS D (Any level)**	**Para**	**Low Tetra (C5–C8)**	**High Tetra (C1–C4)**	**Ventilator Dependent (Any level)**
20.0	0.6	52.3	45.1	40.0	33.6	16.9
40.0	0.4	35.1	29.9	25.4	21.7	13.1
60.0	0.2	19.4	16.4	16.4	12.4	7.9

AIS, American Spinal Injury Association (ASIA) Impairment Scale; *SCI*, spinal cord injury.

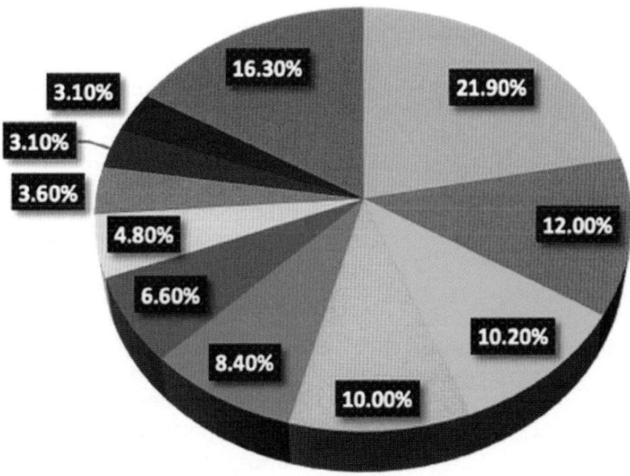

Fig. 3.7 Causes of Mortality. (From Chen Y, Tang Y, Vogel LC, et al. National Spinal Cord Injury Statistical Center. Annual Statistical Reports for the Spinal Cord Injury Model Systems; 2017. https://www.nscisc.uab.edu/Public_Pages/ReportsStats.)

Table 3.5 Average Yearly Expenses After Spinal Cord Injury

	Average Yearly Expenses (2019)	
Severity of Injury	**First Year ($)**	**Each Subsequent Year ($)**
High Tetraplegia (C1–C4) AIS ABC	1,149,629	199,637
Low Tetraplegia (C1–C8) AIS ABC	830,708	122,468
Paraplegia AIS ABC	560,287	74,221
AIS D Any Level	375, 196	45,572

AIS, American Spinal Injury Association (ASIA) Impairment Scale.

Table 3.6 Estimated Lifetime Costs After Spinal Cord Injury

Severity	**Estimated Lifetime Costs ($)**	
	25 years	**50 years**
High Tetraplegia (C1–C4) AIS ABC	5,100,941	2,803,391
Low Tetraplegia (C5–C8) AIS ABC	3,727,066	2,292,479
Paraplegia AIS ABC	2,494,338	1,636,959
AIS D Any Level	1,704,144	1,202,832

AIS, American Spinal Injury Association (ASIA) Impairment Scale.

- Non-Hispanic Whites have the highest incidence of SCI, followed by non-Hispanic Blacks and individuals of Hispanic origin.
- Motor vehicle accidents are the leading cause of injury followed by falls and then violence.
- Length of stay in the acute hospital and in rehabilitation have declined to 11 days and 31 days, respectively.
- Incomplete tetraplegia is the most frequent neurologic category, while complete tetraplegia is the least frequent neurologic category.
- Approximately 25% of individuals with SCI have a college degree at the time of injury, compared with 45% who survive 40 years of injury.
- The percentage of individuals who are married is relatively consistent up to 40 years postinjury, with single/never married status decreasing and divorced status increasing.
- At 1 year postinjury 18% of individuals with SCI are employed, which increases to 32% at 40 years postinjury.
- Thirty percent of individuals with SCI are rehospitalized one or more times following injury.
- The average yearly expenses directly attributable to SCI vary based on neurologic impairment.
- The average life expectancy for an individual with SCI has not improved since the 1980s and remains

significantly below life expectancies of individuals without SCI.

- Mortality rates are significantly higher in the first year postinjury.
- The leading causes of death after SCI are respiratory disorders, primarily pneumonia, and infections, primarily septicemia.

Review Questions

1. Which of the following is **not** a risk factor for developing a SCI?
   a. Age
   b. Alcohol use
   c. Smoking
   d. Race/ethnicity
2. What is the approximate annual incidence of SCI in the United States?
   a. 7,000
   b. 17,000
   c. 27,000
   d. 37,000
3. Which of the following is **not** one of the top three causes of SCI?
   a. Violence
   b. Falls
   c. Sports
   d. Motor vehicle accidents
4. What is the **least** most common neurologic category of injury?
   a. Complete paraplegia
   b. Complete tetraplegia
   c. Incomplete paraplegia
   d. Incomplete tetraplegia
5. What is the leading cause of death among individuals with SCI?
   a. Infection
   b. Respiratory diseases
   c. Cancer
   d. Heart disease

REFERENCES

1. Jain NB, Ayers GD, Peterson EN, et al. Traumatic spinal cord injury in the United States, 1993–2012. *JAMA*. 2015;313(22):2236.
2. Harrison CL, Dijkers M. Spinal cord injury surveillance in the United States: an overview. *Spinal Cord*. 1991;29(4):233–246.
3. Woodruff B, Baron R. A description of nonfatal spinal cord injury using a hospital-based registry. *Am J Preventive Med*. 1994;10(1):10–14.
4. Warren S, Moore M, Johnson M. Traumatic head and spinal cord injuries in Alaska (1991–1993). *Alaksa Med*. 1995;37 (1):11–19.
5. Kirshblum S, Lin VW. *Spinal Cord Medicine*. 3rd ed. Springer Publishing; 2019.
6. Burke D, Linden R, Zhang Y, Maiste A, Shields C. Incidence rates and populations at risk for spinal cord injury: a regional study. *Spinal Cord*. 2001;39(5):274–278.
7. Griffin MR, Opitz JL, Kurland LT, Ebersold MJ, O'Fallon WM. Traumatic spinal cord injury in Olmsted County, Minnesota, 1935–1981. *Am J Epidemiol*. 1985;121(6):884–895.
8. Selvarajah S, Hammond ER, Haider AH, et al. The burden of acute traumatic spinal cord injury among adults in the United States: an update. *J Neurotrauma*. 2014;31(3):228–238.
9. Thurman DJ, Burnett CL, Jeppson L, Beaudoin DE, Sniezek JE. Surveillance of spinal cord injuries in Utah, USA. *Spinal Cord*. 1994;32(10):665–669.
10. Surkin J, Gilbert BJC, Harkey HL, Sniezek J, Currier M. Spinal cord injury in Mississippi: findings and evaluation, 1992–1994. *Spine*. 2000;25(6):716–721.
11. National Spinal Cord Injury Statistical Center. Annual Statistical Reports for the Spinal Cord Injury Model Systems. 2017. https://www.nscisc.uab.edu/Public_Pages/ReportsStats
12. Kraus JF, Franti CE, Riggins RS, Richards D, Borhani NO. Incidence of traumatic spinal cord lesions. *J Chronic Dis*. 1975;28(9):471–492.
13. Vitale MG, Goss JM, Matsumoto H, Roye DP. Epidemiology of pediatric spinal cord injury in the United States: years 1997 and 2000. *J Pediatric Orthop*. 2006;26(6):745–749.
14. Bracken MB, Freeman DH, Hellenbrand K. Incidence of acute traumatic hospitalized spinal cord injury in the United States, 1970–1977. *Am J Epidemiol*. 1981;113(6):615–622.
15. Selassie AW, Varma A, Saunders LL, Welldaregay W. Determinants of in-hospital death after acute spinal cord injury: a population-based study. *Spinal Cord*. 2013;51(1):48–54.
16. Chen Y, Tang Y, Vogel L, DeVivo M. Causes of spinal cord injury. *Top Spinal Cord Injury Rehabilitation*. 2013;19(1):1–8.
17. NSCISC. Recent Trends in Causes of Spinal Cord Injury. Published online 2019. https://www.nscisc.uab.edu/Public/2019%20Annual%20Report%20-%20Complete%20Public%20Version.pdf
18. Williams DR, Wyatt R. Racial bias in health care and health: challenges and opportunities. *JAMA*. 2015;314(6):555.
19. Garrison A, Clifford K, Gleason S, Tun CG, Brown R, Garshick E. Alcohol use associated with cervical spinal cord injury. *J Spinal Cord Med*. 2004;27(2):111–115.
20. Chen Y, Tang Y, Allen V, DeVivo MJ. Aging and spinal cord injury: external causes of injury and implications for prevention. *Top Spinal Cord Injury Rehabilitation*. 2015;21(3): 218–226.
21. Lasfargues J, Custis D, Morrone F, Carswell J, Ngyuen T. A model for estimating spinal cord injury prevalence in the United States. *Int Med Soc Paraplegia*. 1995;33:62–68.
22. Harvey C, Rothschild B, Asmann A, Stripling T. New estimates of traumatic SCI prevalence: a survey-based approach. *Paraplegia*. 1990;28:537–544.
23. Berkowitz M, Harvey C, Greene C. *The Economic Consequences of Traumatic Spinal Cord Injury*. New York, NY: Demos Publications; 1992.
24. DeVivo MJ, Chen Y. Trends in new injuries, prevalent cases, and aging with spinal cord injury. *Arch Phys Med Rehabilitation*. 2011;92(3):332–338.
25. Frieden L, Winnegar AJ. Opportunities for research to improve employment for people with spinal cord injuries. *Spinal Cord*. 2012;50(5):379–381.
26. Cao Y, Krause JS, Saunders LL, Clark JMR. Impact of marital status on 20-year subjective well-being trajectories. *Top Spinal Cord Injury Rehabilitation*. 2015;21(3):208–217.
27. Kalpakjian CZ, Houlihan B, Meade MA, et al. Marital status, marital transitions, well-being, and spinal cord injury: an

examination of the effects of sex and time. *Arch Phys Med Rehabilitation.* 2011;92(3):433–440.
28. Chen Y, He Y, DeVivo MJ. Changing demographics and injury profile of new traumatic spinal cord injuries in the United States, 1972–2014. *Arch Phys Med Rehabilitation.* 2016;97(10):1610–1619.
29. National Spinal Cord Injury Statistical Center. *Recent Trends in Causes of Spinal Cord Injury*. Birmingham, AL: University of Alabama at Birmingham; 2018.
30. Chen Y, Tang Y, Allen V, DeVivo MJ. Fall-induced spinal cord injury: external causes and implications for prevention. *J Spinal Cord Med.* 2016;39(1):24–31.
31. Biering-Sørensen F, DeVivo MJ, Charlifue S, et al. International Spinal Cord Injury Core Data Set (version 2.0)—including standardization of reporting. *Spinal Cord.* 2017;55(8):759–764.
32. Macciocchi S, Seel RT, Thompson N, Byams R, Bowman B. Spinal cord injury and co-occurring traumatic brain injury: assessment and incidence. *Arch Phys Med Rehabilitation.* 2008;89(7):1350–1357.
33. Roach MJ, Chen Y, Kelly ML. Comparing blunt and penetrating trauma in spinal cord injury: analysis of long-term functional and neurological outcomes. *Top Spinal Cord Injury Rehabilitation.* 2018;24(2):121–132.
34. Eastwood EA, Hagglund KJ, Ragnarsson KT, Gordon WA, Marino RJ. Medical rehabilitation length of stay and outcomes for persons with traumatic spinal cord injury—1990–1997. *Arch Phys Med Rehabilitation.* 1999;80(11):1457–1463.
35. Fiedler IG, Laud PW, Maiman DJ, Apple DF. Economics of managed care in spinal cord injury. *Arch Phys Med Rehabilitation.* 1999;80(11):1441–1449.
36. Craven BC, Kurban D, Farahani F, et al. Predicting rehabilitation length of stay in Canada: it's not just about impairment. *J Spinal Cord Med.* 2017;40(6):676–686.
37. DeVivo MJ. Discharge disposition from model spinal cord injury care system rehabilitation programs. *Arch Phys Med Rehabilitation.* 1999;80(7):785–790.
38. Macias CA, Rosengart MR, Puyana J-C, et al. The effects of trauma center care, admission volume, and surgical volume on paralysis after traumatic spinal cord injury. *Ann Surg.* 2009;249(1):10–17.
39. Shavelle RM, DeVivo MJ, Brooks JC, Strauss DJ, Paculdo DR. Improvements in long-term survival after spinal cord injury? *Arch Phys Med Rehabilitation.* 2015;96(4): 645–651.
40. Strauss DJ, DeVivo MJ, Paculdo DR, Shavelle RM. Trends in life expectancy after spinal cord injury. *Arch Phys Med Rehabilitation.* 2006;87(8):1079–1085.
41. De Vivo MJ, Krause JS, Lammertse DP. Recent trends in mortality and causes of death among persons with spinal cord injury. *Arch Phys Med Rehabilitation.* 1999;80(11):1411–1419.
42. Cao Y, Selassie AW, Krause JS. Risk of death after hospital discharge with traumatic spinal cord injury: a population-based analysis, 1998–2009. *Arch Phys Med Rehabilitation.* 2013;94(6):1054–1061.
43. Krause JS, Saunders LL, DeVivo MJ. Income and risk of mortality after spinal cord injury. *Arch Phys Med Rehabilitation.* 2011;92(3):339–345.
44. Savic G, DeVivo MJ, Frankel HL, Jamous MA, Soni BM, Charlifue S. Long-term survival after traumatic spinal cord injury: a 70-year British study. *Spinal Cord.* 2017;55(7):651–658.
45. Cao Y, Massaro JF, Krause JS, Chen Y, Devivo MJ. Suicide mortality after spinal cord injury in the United States: injury cohorts analysis. *Arch Phys Med Rehabilitation.* 2014;95(2):230–235.
46. Cao Y, Chen Y, DeVivo M. Lifetime direct costs after spinal cord injury. *Top Spinal Cord Injury Rehabilitation.* 2011;16(4):10–16.
47. Berkowitz M, O'Leary P, Kruse D. *Spinal Cord Injury: An Analysis of Medical and Social Costs.* New York, NY: Demos Medical Publishing, Inc.; 1998.
48. DeVivo MJ. Causes and costs of spinal cord injury in the United States. *Spinal Cord.* 1997;35(12):809–813.
49. Merritt CH, Taylor MA, Yelton CJ, Ray SK. Economic impact of traumatic spinal cord injuries in the United States. *Neuroimmunol Neuroinflammation.* 2019;6:9.

CHAPTER 4

Prevention of Spinal Cord Injury

Jacob Jeffers and David Coons

OUTLINE

Introduction

The annual incidence of acute traumatic spinal cord injury (SCI) is 54 cases per one million people in the United States or approximately 17,810 people yearly.[1] Expenses directly related to SCI vary greatly depending on neurological impairment, education, premorbid work history, and many other factors. Average yearly expenses the first year after injury range from $375,196 to $1,149,629 and $45,572 to $199,637 each year thereafter, with high tetraplegia at the upper end of the range.[2,3] This does not include indirect costs such as lost wages. Employment rates are approximately 18% to 32% in those with SCI and depend on time since injury.[2] Given the significant disability, cost, and lack of cure, prevention is a worthwhile endeavor.

Types of Prevention

- Primary: Prevention of the onset of disease or future incidence of a problem. This can be done by intervening before health effects occur (e.g., measures such as vaccinations or altering risky behaviors).
- Secondary: Early identification of a disease/injury and limiting or reversing the initial damage.
- Tertiary: Focuses on people who are already affected by a disease. The goal is to improve quality of life by reducing disability, limiting or delaying complications, and restoring function.

Primary Prevention

Road Traffic Accident Prevention

Vehicle crashes are the leading cause of SCI at 38.6%.[2] The basis of reducing traumatic SCI secondary to road traffic accidents relies on reducing accidents and protecting those involved when they occur. The following are some strategies for improving road safety:

- Required use of seatbelts and age-appropriate child restraints[4,5] with additional use of seatbelt reminder systems.[6]
- Required use of motorcycle and bicycle helmets meeting safety standards.[4,5]
- Laws to prevent drinking and driving with support of mass media campaigns.[4,5]
- Inclusion of safety features in cars including frontal[7] and side[8] curtain airbags and assessment of vehicles with crash testing programs to ensure safety standards are met.[4,5]
- Safety standards for roads including lighting, advisory signs, speed limits, separate paths and lanes for pedestrians and cyclists, adequate lane sizing and delineation.[4,5]

Fall Prevention

Falls are the second most common cause of SCI at 32.2%.[2] Etiology varies with high falls predominantly in a younger population, rural or semiurban developing countries, or occupational in nature. Low falls are more prevalent in the elderly. The following are strategies to reduce falls in each given cohort.

- Falls in the elderly:
  - supervised programs for stretching, balance, coordination, and strengthening exercise,[9]
  - tapering of psychotropic medications,[10]
  - environmental modifications including removal of trip hazards such as rugs, installation of adequate lighting, and installation of railings and grab bars.[11]
- Falls in children[12]:
  - household modifications including use of window guards, guard rails, and gates;
  - evaluating the safety of playground equipment and use of protective surfaces such as wood chips, sand, or rubber.

- High falls, particularly those at the workplace[13]:
  - inspection of safety equipment including but not limited to ropes, harnesses, ladders, scaffolding, and others prior to use;
  - having an additional support person available on the ground;
  - adequate training for personnel.

Sports Specific Prevention

Most of the prevention strategies focus on education, equipment, and changes in regulation. The following are some sport-specific strategies to reduce the incidence of traumatic SCI.

- Diving[14,15]:
  - avoidance of diving into shallow water;
  - education about diving safety and discouraging risky behaviors such as alcohol use and pushing others into bodies of water;
  - securing pools with fences when not in use, marking depths, and having lifeguards available.
- Rugby:
  - Educational programs and regulation changes on scrums (method of restarting play where players are close together and have their heads down while attempting to gain possession of the ball).[16,17]
- American football:
  - Regulation change penalizing spearing (using the crown of the helmet to initiate contact).[18,19]
- Ice hockey:
  - Education and implementation of rules against body checking from behind.[20–22]

Nontraumatic SCI (NTSCI)

- 400 μg daily of folic acid can help prevent neural tube defects such as spina bifida.[23–25]
- Improved nutrition in high-risk population can limit NTSCI such as subacute combined degeneration secondary to vitamin B12 deficiency.[23]
- Access to adequate medical care including vaccines (i.e., polio), diagnostic testing, and treatment are important for prevention of infections and tumors leading to NTSCI.[26]
- Use of insect repellent and methods for mosquito control can help prevent West Nile virus–related myelitis.[27]
- Degenerative conditions remain one of the most common causes of NTSCI; however, there are limited data to support when conservative management vs. surgery is most appropriate.

Secondary Prevention

- There is a lack of evidence to support the use of pharmacologic agents for neuroprotection in populations after acute traumatic SCI.[28,29]
- Early surgical decompression (within first 24 hours) is safe and improves neurologic outcomes for patients with a traumatic cervical spine injury.[30]

Author, Year, Study Design	Measure	Early, ≤24 Hours	Late, >24 Hours	Effect Size
Fehlings, 2012 Prospective cohort study	AIS Improvement at 6 months ≥1 grade improvement ≥2 grade improvement	n = 131 74 (56.5) 26 (19.8)	n = 91 45 (49.5) 8 (8.8)	OR_{adj}: 1.37 (95% CI = 0.80 to 2.57), P = .31 2.83 (95% CI = 1.10 to 7.28), P = .03

- Early avoidance of hypotension to promote tissue perfusion has reported favorable outcome.

Table 4.1 Summary of the National Acute Spinal Cord Injury Study (NASCIS) I–III Trials

Study	Arms	Results
NASCIS I	1. 100 mg bolus methylprednisolone followed by 25 mg every 6 h for 10 days 2. 1000 mg bolus methylprednisolone followed by 250 mg every 6 h for 10 days	No observable difference in benefit between the observed treatment groups. Increased wound infections in high-dose treatment group.
NASCIS II	1. 30 mg/kg bolus methylprednisolone followed by 5.4 mg/kg per h for 23 h 2. 5.4 mg/kg bolus naloxone followed by 4.0 mg/kg per h for 23 h 3. Placebo	Potential benefit of steroid if given within 8 hours of injury, but otherwise no observable differences.
NASCIS III	All patients received methylprednisolone 30 mg/kg bolus followed by: 1. 5.4 mg/kg per h methylprednisolone for 24 h 2. 5.4 mg/kg per h methylprednisolone for 48 h 3. 2.5 mg/kg tirilazad every 6 h for 48 h	No difference in primary endpoints. Possible benefit with longer treatment duration if steroid initiated 3–8 h postinjury. Increased risk of severe sepsis and pneumonia with prolonged steroid use.

Maintaining MAP of 85 mmHG for a minimum of 7 days is recommended.[28]

- Transferring a patient to a center with a hyperbaric unit is necessary to manage and prevent further injury for patients with decompression sickness (e.g., scuba diver).[28]
- There is a lack of evidence to support the clinical use of hypothermia following acute SCI.[28]
- Methylprednisolone is not recommended as standard of care due to concern of potential insignificant functional improvements and increased adverse events in the steroid-treated populations.[29] Table 4.1 includes a summary of the National Acute Spinal Cord Injury Study (NASCIS) I to III trials.

Review Questions

1. Which of the following is not a primary prevention strategy proven to reduce falls in the elderly?
   a. Placing rugs in a hallway
   b. Tapering of psychotropic medications
   c. Addition of grab bars in the bathroom
   d. Supervised exercise programs
2. A woman presents to clinic and has a child with a history of spina bifida. She is considering trying for a second child. What medication would you recommend?
   a. Folic acid 400 μg daily
   b. Folic acid 800 μg daily
   c. Folic acid 4000 μg daily
   d. Folic acid 8000 μg daily
   e. None of the above
3. Which of the following is an example of tertiary prevention in SCI?
   a. Placement of a cervical collar on a patient by emergency medical services at the accident site
   b. Wearing a seatbelt when driving
   c. Treatment of neuropathic pain
   d. Marking pool depths and diving zones

REFERENCES

1. Jain NB, Ayers GD, Peterson EN, et al. Traumatic spinal cord injury in the United States, 1993–2012. *JAMA.* 2015;313(22):2236–2243.
2. National Spinal Cord Injury Statistical Center. *Facts and Figures at a Glance*. Birmingham, AL: University of Alabama at Birmingham; 2020. https://www.nscisc.uab.edu/Public/Facts%20and%20Figures%202020.pdf.
3. Cao Y, Chen Y, DeVivo MJ. Lifetime direct cost after spinal cord injury. *Top Spinal Cord Inj Rehabil.* 2011;16:10–16.
4. Peden M, Scurfield R, Sleet D, et al. *World Report on Road Traffic Prevention.* Geneva: World Health Organization; 2004.
5. World Health Organization. *Global Status Report on Road Safety 2013: Supporting a Decade of Action.* Geneva: World Health Organization; 2013.
6. Lie A, Krafft M, Kullgren A, Tingvall C. Intelligent seat belt reminders – do they change driver seat belt use in Europe? *Traffic Inj Prev.* 2008;9(5):446–449.
7. Fitzharris M, Fildes B, Newstead S, Logan D. *Crash-Based Evaluation of Adr69; Past Success and Future Directions.* Canberra: Australian Transport Safety Bureau; 2006.
8. Fitzharris M, Stephan K. *Assessment of the Need for, and the Likely Benefits of, Enhanced Side Impact Protection in the Form of a Pole Side Impact Global Technical Regulation.* Clayton: Monash University; 2013.
9. Means KM, Rodell DE, O'Sullivan PS. Balance, mobility, and falls among community-dwelling elderly persons: effects of a rehabilitation exercise program. *Am J Phys Med Rehabil.* 2005;84(4):238–250.
10. Campbell AJ, Robertson MC, Gardner MM, Norton RN, Buchner DM. Psychotropic medication withdrawal and home-based exercise program to prevent falls: a randomized, controlled trial. *J Am Geriatr Soc.* 1999;47:850–853.
11. World Health Organization. WHO Global Report on Falls Prevention in Older Age, 2007. https://www.who.int/ageing/publications/Falls_prevention7March.pdf.
12. Chhabra HS, Sachdev G, Sharawat R. Prevention of spinal cord injury due to falls. In: Chhabra HS, ed. *ISCoS Textbook on Comprehensive Management of Spinal Cord Injuries.* New Delhi, India: Wolters Kluwer; 2015.
13. Government of Western Australia, Department of Mines, Industry Regulation and Safety. Code of Practice: Prevention of Falls From Height at Workplaces. Commission for Occupational Safety and Health; 2020. https://www.commerce.wa.gov.au/sites/default/files/atoms/files/preventionoffalls_2020-10.pdf.
14. Bellon K, Kolakowsky-Hayner SA, Chen D, McDowell S, Bitterman B, Klass SJ. Evidence-based practice in primary prevention of spinal cord injury. *Top Spinal Cord Inj Rehabil.* 2013;19(1):25–30.
15. Krassioukov A, Eng JJ, Chan C, Tator C. Prevention of spinal cord injury due to sports activity. In: Chhabra HS, ed. *ISCoS Textbook on Comprehensive Management of Spinal Cord Injuries.* New Delhi, India: Wolters Kluwer; 2015.
16. Bohu Y, Julia M, Bagate C, et al. Declining incidence of catastrophic cervical spine injuries in French rugby: 1996–2006. *Am J Sports Med.* 2009;37(2):319–323.
17. Reboursiere E, Bohu Y, Retière D, et al. Impact of the national prevention policy and scrum law changes on the incidence of rugby-related catastrophic cervical spine injuries in French Rugby Union. *Br J Sports Med.* 2018;52(10):674–677.
18. Chao S, Pacella MJ, Torg JS. The pathomechanics, pathophysiology and prevention of cervical spinal cord and brachial plexus injuries in athletics. *Sports Med.* 2010;40(1):59–75.
19. Torg JS, Vesgo JJ, Sennett B, Das M. The national football head and neck injury registry. 14-year report on cervical quadriplegia, 1971 through 1984. *JAMA.* 1985;254(24):3439–3443.
20. Tator CH, Provvidenza C, Lapczak L, Carson J, Raymond D. Spinal injuries in Canadian ice hockey: documentation of injuries sustained from 1943–1999. *Can J Neurol Sci.* 2004;31:461–466.
21. Tator CH, Provvidenza C, Cassidy JD. Spinal injuries in Canadian ice hockey: an update to 2005. *Clin J Sports Med.* 2009;19(6):451–456.
22. Tator CH, Provvidenza C, Cassidy JD. Update and overview of spinal injuries in Canadian ice hockey, 1943 to 2011: the continuing need for injury prevention and education. *Clin J Sports Med.* 2016;26(3):232–238.

23. Reynolds E. Vitamin B12, folic acid, and the nervous system. *Lancet Neurol.* 2006;5(11):949–960.
24. MRC Vitamin Study Group. Prevention of neural tube defects: results of the Medical Research Council Vitamin Study. *Lancet.* 1991;338:131–137.
25. Czeizel AE, Dudas I. Prevention of the first occurrence of neural tube defects by peri-conceptional vitamin supplementation. *N Engl J Med.* 1992;327:1832–1835.
26. New P, Reeves R, Marshall R. Prevention of nontraumatic spinal cord injury. In: Chhabra HS, ed. *ISCoS Textbook on Comprehensive Management of Spinal Cord Injuries.* New Delhi, India: Wolters Kluwer; 2015.
27. Petersen LR, Brault AC, Nasci RS. West Nile Virus: review of the literature. *JAMA.* 2013;310(3):308–315.
28. Consortium for Spinal Cord Medicine. Early acute management in adults with spinal cord injury: a clinical practice guideline for health-care professionals. *J Spinal Cord Med.* 2008;31(4):403–479.
29. Cheung V, Hoshide R, Bansal V, Kasper E, Chen CC. Methylprednisolone in the management of spinal cord injuries: lessons from randomized, controlled trials. *Surg Neurol Int.* 2015;6:142.
30. Fehlings MG, Vaccaro A, Wilson JR, Singh A, Cadotte DW, Harrop JS, et al. Early versus delayed decompression for traumatic cervical spinal cord injury: results of the Surgical Timing in Acute Spinal Cord Injury Study (STASCIS). *PLoS One.* 2012;7(2):e32037.

CHAPTER 5

Clinical and Basic Research

Jed E. Olson and Jennifer Wahl

OUTLINE

Research and Statistical Methods

Quantitative research study designs commonly used in spinal cord injury (SCI) research include cohort/observational trials and randomized controlled trials. These designs emphasize objective numerical outcomes for participants in trials and the statistical and mathematical analysis of data collected. Quantitative research creates the ability to generalize the outcomes across a group of people with similar characteristics.[1,2]

Cohort/Observational Trials

Cohort/observational comparison research is designed to measure outcomes for a large group of people with similar characteristics. For example, this type of research might compare functional outcomes in two groups: patients with cervical level 6 (C6) complete tetraplegia who received a specific treatment modality, with a similar number of age-matched patients with C6 complete tetraplegia who did **not** get that treatment. This type of study may identify measurable differences in outcomes, depending on differences in the intervention that the two groups received.

Randomized Controlled Trials

Randomized controlled trials (RTCs) are generally prospective, assigning participants into an experimental group receiving a certain intervention and a control group that receives either no intervention or a different intervention—a "positive control." The outcomes expected to be impacted by the intervention are preferably specified ahead of time. Randomization ideally allows the only measured difference between study groups to be the outcome variable being studied.[1,2]

Statistical Methods

Statistical methods utilized for cohort comparisons or randomized control trials include logistic regression, linear regression, and mixed models/repeated measures. Although randomized controlled trials are more statistically robust and much more expensive to conduct that cohort/observational trials, the statistical methods in cohort trials are often much more complex; this is because they need to control for a large number of variables in the observed groups, which can be sources of bias. RTCs are superior in measuring *causation*—for example, if a medication *causes* improvement in health; cohort or observational studies often can only robustly prove *correlation*.

Important therapeutic human clinical trials in SCI research include (1) neuroprotective and (2) neuroregenerative approaches. Neuroprotective approaches are based on the clinical pathophysiology of SCI and modulating tissue injury and recovery utilizing surgical and pharmacological therapies.[3] Neuroprotective studies have included trials of methylprednisolone, GM-1 ganglioside, excitatory neurotransmitter agonists, erythropoietin, calcium channel blockers, potassium channel blockers, minocycline, and hypothermia. Neuroregenerative trials attempt to enhance the endogenous regeneration process and healing of injured spinal cord tissue. Neuroregenerative trial outcomes include remyelination, healing of neural and axonal injuries, cell replacement including stem cells, and alteration of the microenvironment in the spinal cord. No gold standard for SCI clinical trials currently exists, although cell therapy has shown promising outcomes.[3]

Contrary to quantitative research with objective measurements and numerical data, qualitative research methods use social science approaches, and the individual's perspective as compared to others with 'like' life perspectives.[1,2] Measurements in this type of research include descriptive outcomes and theme analysis, focusing on individual outcomes as compared to group outcomes; these may be used to analyze how individuals perceive worldly experiences.

Neural Injury

Neural injury is an injury of or relating to a nerve or the nervous system.[4] Injury to the peripheral nervous system (PNS) damages neurons connecting the brain and spinal cord to the other parts of the body. These nerves convey signals to and from the brain or spinal cord to other areas. Damage to these nerves creates a disconnect in the body's ability to convey messages to and from the body organs and muscles to the central nervous system.[5,6]

Nerve or neuronal damage may occur when pressure, swelling, bleeding, laceration, contusion, or inflammation disrupt peripheral nerves, spinal cord nerve roots, neuronal tracts within the spinal cord, or the entire cord itself. Nerves contain nerve cell bodies, their axons and dendrites, supporting cells, and synapses; these may be prone to damage even with small physical insults. Neural damage may result in temporary, permanent, complete or incomplete loss of sensation, movement, or visceral organ function. Spinal cord damage may result in multisystem complications, with the majority of damage occurring during the acute phase of injury. During the acute phase of neural injury, special attention must be given to respiratory, cardiovascular, and gastrointestinal compromise.[7]

Primary neural injury refers to the initial mechanical damage to the nerves.[8] Mechanical trauma creates direct compression of neural elements and blood vessels by fractured and displaced bone fragments or disc material. Secondary neural injury includes a cascade of biochemical and cellular processes such as electrolyte abnormalities, formation free radicals, vascular ischemia, edema, posttraumatic inflammatory reaction, apoptosis, and programmed cell death.

Nerve Injury Classification

A complete SCI is an injury resulting in loss of spine-mediated neurologic function below the level of the injury. An incomplete SCI injury allows some function or sensation below the level of injury. Sacral root sparing is an indication that the injury is incomplete, indicating a better prognosis for recovery of some degree of neurologic function.[9]

Tetraplegia refers to impairments from damage to the cervical spinal cord, in which upper and lower extremities are impacted; paraplegia refers to damage to neural elements within the thoracic, lumbar, or sacral spinal canal, in which the lower extremities are affected.[10]

Regarded as the gold-standard impairment scale for SCI impairment evaluation, The American Spinal Cord Injury Association Impairment Scale (AIS) is used for evaluating sensation and motor function in patients with SCI. The nerve roots at each level of the spinal cord are tested at their sensory dermatomes and motor myotomes to determine a clinical level of sensation and motor function. Upper and lower extremities and right and left sides are tested individually. Certain syndromes such as central cord syndrome or Brown-Séquard syndrome may cause "skip" patterns or have unilateral asymmetric deficits.[7]

An SCI may cause lost motor control and/or sensation below the injury level completely or in part, designating a complete or incomplete SCI according to the AIS impairment scale. A complete SCI indicates no spine-mediated neurologic function below the level of the injury, including sacral roots distal to the injury. This type of injury does not always reflect a complete laceration, with injury due to compression or lost/impaired blood flow at the affected level of cord being possible. These complete injuries receive a Grade A on the AIS.[9]

Incomplete injuries are defined as those with some degree of retained motor or sensory function below the level of injury. These types of injuries are graded B through E on the AIS scale. Incomplete SCIs retain some sensory function with or without some motor function and are the most common type of SCI. AIS Grade C injuries have a motor grade **less than 3** below the neurologic level of injury, while AIS Grade D injuries have a motor grade of **at least 3** below the injury level. Patients with Grade E injuries have normal motor and sensory examinations but display delayed or abnormal reflexes or other neurologic symptoms.[9]

Neurologic levels signify the relationship of segmental spinal nerve roots to numbered vertebra in the bony spinal column and can be identified by performing a clinical exam using the AIS scale and identifying the area of skin innervated by the sensory nerves and the function of muscles innervated by motor nerves.[11] Usually, an injury at a given spinal level will create deficits at all levels below the injury.

Preclinical Research and Regeneration

Spinal Cord Injury Research: Preclinical Studies

Preclinical research in the field of spinal cord injury simply refers to basic science investigation: studies of cells and substances in biochemical assays, cells cultured in the laboratory, and studies in nonhuman animals. Basic science research is particularly important and fascinating in the field of SCI. Some vertebrates can reconnect a completely transected spinal cord, offering important clues for clinical researchers and potential methods for harnessing biological processes to treat patients.[12,13] Several important themes in basic spinal cord injury research will be explored in more detail below.

Despite decades of intense study, the prospect of regenerating working spinal cord tissue in humans is still years away from being widely deployed for SCI patients. There remains much to be done in the laboratory and in animal models. Given that treatments, particularly invasive ones, carry significant risks, new treatment modalities must be thoroughly tested in animals for both safety and clinical effectiveness.

Regeneration of Injured Spinal Cord: Introduction

Urgent treatment of acute SCI and mitigation of neural tissue damage in the immediate and subacute phases are crucial for reducing the severity of SCI-related neurologic deficits and disability. However, these interventions themselves are often insufficient. Early surgical stabilization, aggressive inpatient management, and postinjury rehabilitation cannot completely halt the loss of nerve pathways and neuron cell death that occur in the injured spine. Irreversible damage to neurons following SCI begins within minutes, and can continue to progress for months to years after the initial insult.[14] While many individuals undergo spontaneous or therapy-related recovery, neurologic recovery is rarely complete; most patients are left with some degree of motor, sensory, and end-organ dysfunction after SCI.[15] Finally, improved outcomes related to initial treatments for SCI (such as halting nervous system inflammation, cell death, and scar formation) are of little benefit to the majority of the SCI population: those who have reached recovery plateau, and who have been living with neurologic disability for years.

With the aging of the population in general, and increased life expectancy of individuals who have survived spinal cord injury in particular, the number of patients living with SCI-related disability has increased over time.[16] These patients may not benefit from new surgical techniques or novel medications for acute and subacute SCI; therefore, the science of neural regeneration to restore lost spinal cord connectivity holds the greatest promise. Indeed, this may be the most rapidly changing, complex, and technically difficult field in SCI research, with a wide variety of modalities and approaches (Table 5.1). This section will focus on cellular approaches.

Table 5.1 Treatment Approaches to Facilitating Spinal Cord Regeneration

Strategy	Regenerative Goal
Early surgical stabilization	Prevent vertebral instability, relieve cord compression
Intensive physical therapy; stimulation of muscle groups	Stimulate spinal cord tracts to promote healing/plasticity; promote development of novel neuronal relay pathways
Aggressive inhibition of inflammation	Reduce immune system infiltration, pressure, and scarring
Electrical stimulation of neuronal tracts	Prevent atrophy/dieback of damaged axons and tracts
Pharmacologic and hormonal medications	Reduce cell death, promote trophic factors/transcription factors
Surgical implantation of new cells	Replace destroyed/degenerating neurons, axons, and support cells
Surgical implantation of bridging tissue scaffolds	Guide recovering or replaced axons across injury gap toward synapse

Spinal Cord Injury and the Goals of Regeneration

In acute and subacute SCI phase of recovery, there is a complex interaction of glial cells, fibroblasts, blood products, axon fragments, proteins, and inflammatory cytokines. The blood–spinal cord barrier is disrupted, leading to influx of immune cells that promote inflammation, swelling, and necrosis. There follows increased astrocyte activity, Wallerian degeneration of axons, dispersal of myelin proteins and amino acids, cell death, and infiltration of fibroblasts.[17] The result is a dense fibrous scar in the injured cord, surrounding a fluid-filled cavitation. This scar and fluid cavity present a mechanical barrier to the growth, regeneration, and elongation of axons by neurons attempting to bridge the gap of the injury. The scar and fluid cavity contain few viable neurons or synapses, and biochemically they present an unfavorable milieu for differentiation of new cells, axon growth, and the remyelination of axons by oligodendrocytes.[14,18] The cavity space fills with cerebrospinal fluid, and axon terminals reaching this area cannot extend across to their targets or form synapses with dendrites. Entire tracts can be permanently lost, leading to symptoms seen in affected persons with SCI: paralysis, sensation loss, paraplegia and tetraplegia, loss of normal smooth muscle function, and dysfunction of the autonomic nervous system.

The goal of regenerative treatments is not only to replace lost cells and neural connections. It is of critical importance that these cells and connections can reestablish organized tracts capable of restoring sensory, motor, and autonomic function. Moreover, restoration must be of sufficient magnitude to provide clinically meaningful improvements in symptom relief and function for patients with SCI. Overcoming the pathology of the SCI scar thus involves a number of distinct steps for regenerative researchers. We must also keep in mind that in vivo regeneration research studies often use uniform injury mechanisms in particular animal models of SCI. By contrast, real-world human spinal cord injuries are heterogeneous in extent, mechanism, and outcome, and they occur in a wide range of people with respect to age and health status.

Challenges to Neuronal Regeneration

Historically, disrupted neurons and critically damaged neuronal tracts in the central nervous system (CNS) were regarded as permanently lost. However, the CNS is now recognized as having remarkable cellular plasticity, reorganization, and repair capabilities. Although myelinated axons in the CNS, once severed or injured, do not typically grow back correctly, myelinated axons and nerves within the peripheral nervous system (PNS) are known to do so.[19,20] In animals, this has led to successful implantation, myelination, and neurologic function of PNS tissue implanted into damaged spinal cord, restoring some lost CNS functionality.[21] As a result, there is tremendous interest in identifying and implanting various nerve cells, growth factors, and regeneration-promoting support materials in animal models and in humans. Each of these approaches has had limited success in some studies, and each faces current and future challenges as regeneration techniques are refined (Table 5.2).

Table 5.2 Regeneration Strategies Under Research

Regeneration Modality	Challenges to Success
Disruption of astroglial scar by injecting enzymes or cell inhibitors	Scar extracellular matrix has factors important for preservation of existing neurons; glial scar protects adjacent cord from inflammation and helps preserve blood–spinal cord barrier
Inhibition or enzymatic degradation of axon growth inhibitors	Complex variety and activity of growth-inhibiting proteins and molecules, which act on receptors. Receptors may need to be blocked as well
Implantation of stem cells into injured area	Few implanted stem cells engraft and grow successfully; stem cells can be tumorigenic; hamartomas are common in animal models
Implantation of biomaterial gel/scaffold into injured area	May need complex engineering to guide axon terminals, yet ideally must also be biodegradable and flexible
Injection of neuronal growth factors	Growing neurons need appropriate structural support to guide them toward synapses along the appropriate pathway; erroneous connections can lead to undesired gain of function such as increased neuropathic pain
Injection of myelin growth factors	There is complexity of timing so that regenerating axons can simultaneously be ensheathed by myelin

The variety of regeneration strategies under investigation is broad and continually evolving. The following section will provide a review of promising cellular and molecular strategies that are likely to be used in human clinical trials. These methods have the same ultimate goal: to restore or replace neuronal connections across the injury site following SCI, thereby promoting clinically meaningful neurologic recovery.

Regeneration of Spinal Cord Cells: Strategies

Reversing the Mechanical Barrier of the Fibroglial Scar

Most SCIs leave an impermeable glial scar around the margins of the injury site, and neuron cell death within results in cavitation. As discussed earlier, the scar is dense and inhibits axon growth, and the fluid cavity cannot be bridged by recovering nerve fibers.[16] Early strategies for cellular regeneration in the subacute phase after SCI were designed to prevent formation of the fibroglial scar.

However, it is now recognized that astrocyte-fibroblast scar formation, known as gliosis, is to some degree protective.[22,23] The mechanical barrier provided by the gliosis process contains the area of inflammation and cell death, preventing it from affecting rostral and caudal cord levels, and it helps preserve the blood–spinal cord barrier. In addition, there are growth factors and transcription products in the scar that enhance neuronal preservation and regeneration of at least some of the axons.[23] Some strategies to reduce the barrier of the fibroglial scar without reducing its protective effects have included reducing neutrophil migration into spinal cord lesions and promoting the conversion of M1 (reactive) macrophages to M2 (resolution-phase) macrophages by manipulating cytokine levels.[24,25] The goal of these strategies is to limit the extent of fibroblast activity so that the spinal cord scar is more permeable, allowing axons to regrow across the injured area.

Removing or Blocking Growth-Inhibiting Proteins

A number of proteins within the fibroglial scar inhibit regeneration of neurons and extension of axons across the injury. These proteins themselves are by-products of tissue destruction. They include:

- Free amino acids liberated by cell destruction.
- Nogo inhibitors, or myelin-associated proteins, which become active when myelin is destroyed and inhibit neurite outgrowth.
- Chondroitin sulfate proteoglycans (CSPGs), which inhibit axonal growth and interact with receptors thought to arrest growth of axon terminals.

Human anti-Nogo antibodies have been employed in a phase 1 clinical trial; it was subsequently found that Nogo inhibitors act via receptors that are also activated by CSPGs, and that regeneration was inhibited even in the presence of anti-Nogo antibodies.[18]

CSPGs appear to be the most important regeneration-inhibiting protein, and they impede growing axons more powerfully at increasing concentrations. They are abundant at the margins of spinal cord scar tissue, forming a mechanical barrier to growing axon terminals (known as growth cones). In addition, CSPGs have activity at distinct receptors on axon growth cones, where they impede growth and inhibit synapse formation.[16,26] CSPGs are therefore an important target in regeneration therapies. CSPG removal has been accomplished in studies by injecting the enzyme chondroitinase ABC (ChABC), which cleaves side chains from CSPGs. This enzyme has been shown to increase the success of implanted nervous system tissues when these two regeneration modalities are used together. Injured CNS tissues treated with ChABC demonstrate regrowth of axons and reinnervation of injured nerves and their functional targets.[27] Importantly, this has been shown to occur even in animal models of chronic spinal cord injury, in which a scar has been present for years. Future clinical trials using other techniques, such as implanted biomaterials or progenitor cells, are likely to incorporate ChABC to enhance graft success.

Injection of Growth Factors to Promote Axonal Regeneration

The ability of some vertebrates to regenerate completely transected spinal cord tissue has led to intense interest in growth factors and transcription factors as therapeutic modalities for spinal cord regeneration.[12,20] In preclinical trials, growth factors have been infused locally into injured spinal cord in order to promote growth of neurons and supportive glial cells. Notable growth factors tested with this technique include nerve growth factor, brain-derived neurotrophic factor, and glial cell-derived neurotrophic factor.[18]

Intra-injury injection of trophic growth factors is probably not sufficient to regrow axons across the injury site. Axon terminals, even when growing briskly, cannot elude or penetrate the barrier of fibrosis or the growth-inhibitory activity of CSPGs and other extracellular matrix proteins. A future role for growth factors will likely involve their use to support the health of implanted progenitor cells, or in spinal cord injury areas that have been pretreated with an enzyme such as ChABC to make the glial scar more conducive to nerve growth.[18]

Implantation of Stem Cells to Regrow Damaged Cord Cells

Stem cells present an attractive prospect in the field of SCI regeneration because of their potential to replace lost neurons and regrow interrupted nervous system pathways. The biology of stem cells is extremely complex, but there are several main ways they have been deployed (Table 5.3).

Table 5.3 Selected Stem/Progenitor Cells Promising for Spinal Cord Regeneration

Cell Type	Issues
Embryonic stem cells	Ethical concerns as these come from fetal tissue
Neural stem cells	Most turn into glial cells with few axons
Oligodendrocyte precursor cells	May turn into neurons, astrocytes, or oligodendrocytes
Induced pluripotent stem cells	May have unwanted growth/ tumorigenesis

Alternatives to embryonic stem cells have been sought due to ethical concerns about the source of these cells. In addition, the majority (80%–90%) of embryonic stem cells undergo programmed cell death when implanted into spinal cord tissue.[15,28] Neural stem cells may be sourced from human patients themselves, although this is an invasive procedure and expanding cell samples is a challenge. Oligodendrocyte precursor cells and induced pluripotent stem cells (iPSCs) can also be generated in autologous fashion, presumably reducing the need for immunosuppression when used to treat patients. Of note, iPSCs may differentiate into undesired tissues and form tumors; this challenge has been addressed in animal studies by deploying growth factors that condition iPSCs to expand into desired nervous system cell lines.[18,29]

Implantation of Gels and Scaffolds to Support Axon Growth

Many surviving spinal cord neurons attempt to grow axons in rostral and caudal directions during the healing process after SCI. In normal spinal cord, growing axons are guided both by trophic growth factors and a perineuronal net of extracellular matrix and supporting glial cells. However, this structured guiding support for axon growth is lost when injured spinal cord forms a glial scar and cavitation.

To address this, another treatment modality for regeneration is injecting a supportive matrix into the injured area, to form a "bridge" to guide and support axon growth. A wide variety of materials have been used to accomplish this; what they have in common is that they are conformable so that they may be injected into spinal cord and can expand across the scar cavity. Inert materials such as polyethylene glycol have been used successfully in animal models, as well as hydrogels and collagen.[16] Scaffolds of collagen with axon channels arrayed in linear fashion that are implanted, rather than injected, have also had some success.[15,30] Finally, a number of microtubule-containing gel suspensions have been developed, some of which may be oriented in the direction of desired axon growth via external magnetic fields. Any of these bridging materials may also be impregnated with appropriate growth factors and have been studied with stem and progenitor cells suspended in the supportive material.[18]

Restoring Myelination

A challenge to therapies that aim to replace or regrow functional neurons after SCI is that these neurons must be remyelinated by oligodendrocytes in order to function properly. There appears to be some endogenous proliferation of oligodendrocytes after injury, and these extend toward injured axons.[31] In some vertebrates such as axolotl salamanders and zebrafish, these glial cells remyelinate injured neurons and guide them toward functional synapses, thus healing spinal cord injury.[12,20] In humans, however, the new oligodendrocytes do not form functional myelin sheaths. The use of oligodendrocyte precursor cells alone or combined with neural stem cells is a potential solution.[32] Injectable supports containing neural stem cells, oligodendrocyte precursors to provide myelination, trophic factors to encourage the appropriate differentiation, and growth of multiple cell types have already shown promise in animal models of subacute as well as chronic SCI.

Review Questions

1. Which of the following best characterizes preclinical research in SCI?
   a. Research on SCI patients who are still in the hospital
   b. Research in the laboratory and in animal models that may lead to advances in SCI treatment
   c. Observational research on SCI patient populations
   d. Epidemiology of SCI
2. Which of the following is a problem with aggressive inhibition of scar formation after SCI?
   a. It can lead to disfiguring surgical scars after surgical stabilization
   b. It can delay surgery
   c. It stimulates fibroblasts
   d. It inhibits glial cell containment of the injured area and preservation of the blood–spinal cord barrier
3. Which protein in injured spinal cord inhibits the outgrowth of axon terminals?
   a. Brain derived growth factor
   b. Collagen
   c. Chondroitin sulfate proteoglycans (CSPGs)
   d. Chondroitinase ABC (ChABC)
4. Which cells make the myelin sheath to protect regenerating axons after SCI?
   a. Oligodendrocytes
   b. Astrocytes
   c. Fibroblasts
   d. Schwann cells

REFERENCES

1. Otani T. What is qualitative research? *Yakugaku zasshi: J Pharm Soc Jpn*. 2017;137(6):653–658.
2. Sawatsky AP, Ratelle JT, Beckman TJ. Qualitative research methods in medical education. *Anesthesiology*. 2019;131(1):14–22.
3. Kim YH, Ha KY, Kim SI. Spinal cord injury and related clinical trials. *ClOrthopedic Surg*. 2017;9(1):1.
4. Merriam Webster (2021). Retrieved from www.merriam-webster.com/dictionary/neural.
5. Ambrozaitis KV, Kontautas E, Spakauskas B, Vaitkaitis D. Pathophysiology of acute spinal cord injury. *Medicina (Kaunas, Lithuania)*. 2006;42(3):255–261.
6. Lee SK, Wolfe SW. Peripheral nerve injury and repair. *JAAOS-Journal Am Acad Orthopaedic Surg*. 2000 Jul 1; 8(4):243–252.
7. Eckert MJ, Martin MJ. Trauma: Spinal cord injury. *Surgical Clin*. 2017;97(5):1031–1045.
8. Rogers WK, Todd M. Acute spinal cord injury. *Best Pract & Res Clin Anaesthesiology*. 2016;30(1):27–39.
9. Roberts TT, Leonard GR, Cepela DJ. Classifications in brief: American Spinal Injury Association (ASIA) impairment scale. *Clin Orthop Relat Res*. 2017;475(5):1499–1504.
10. Encyclopedia Britannica. Peripheral Nervous System. Retrieved from https://www.britannica.com/science/human-nervous-system/The-peripheral-nervous-system.
11. Chhabra A, Ahlawat S, Belzberg A, Andreseik G. Peripheral nerve injury grading simplified on MR neurography: as referenced to Seddon and Sunderland classifications. *Indian J Radiology & Imaging*. 2014;24(3):217.
12. Ghosh S, Hui SP. Axonal regeneration in zebrafish spinal cord. *Regen Oxf Engl*. 2018;5(1):43–60.
13. Tazaki A, Tanaka EM, Fei J-F. Salamander spinal cord regeneration: the ultimate positive control in vertebrate spinal cord regeneration. *Dev Biol*. 2017;432(1):63–71.
14. Profyris C, Cheema SS, Zang D, Azari MF, Boyle K, Petratos S. Degenerative and regenerative mechanisms governing spinal cord injury. *Neurobiol Dis*. 2004;15(3):415–436.
15. Katoh H, Yokota K, Fehlings MG. Regeneration of spinal cord connectivity through stem cell transplantation and biomaterial scaffolds. *Front Cell Neurosci*. 2019;13:248.
16. Tran AP, Warren PM, Silver J. The biology of regeneration failure and success after spinal cord injury. *Physiol Rev*. 2018;98(2):881–917.
17. Grossman SD, Rosenberg LJ, Wrathall JR. Temporal–spatial pattern of acute neuronal and glial loss after spinal cord contusion. *Exp Neurol*. 2001;168(2):273–282.
18. Ashammakhi N, Kim H-J, Ehsanipour A, Bierman RD, Kaarela O, Xue C, et al. Regenerative therapies for spinal cord injury. *Tissue Eng Part B Rev*. 2019;25(6):471–491.
19. Ahuja CS, Nori S, Tetreault L, et al. Traumatic spinal cord injury-repair and regeneration. *Neurosurgery*. 2017;80(3S): S9–22.
20. Vajn K, Plunkett JA, Tapanes-Castillo A, Oudega M. Axonal regeneration after spinal cord injury in zebrafish and mammals: Differences, similarities, translation. *Neurosci Bull*. 2013;29(4):402–410.
21. Steward O, Willenberg R. Rodent spinal cord injury models for studies of axon regeneration. *Exp Neurol*. 2017;287(Pt 3): 374–383.

22. Anderson MA, Burda JE, Ren Y, et al. Astrocyte scar formation aids central nervous system axon regeneration. *Nature.* 2016;532(7598):195–200.
23. Rust R, Kaiser J. Insights into the dual role of inflammation after spinal cord injury. *J Neurosci.* 2017;37(18):4658–4660.
24. Shechter R, London A, Varol C, et al. Infiltrating blood-derived macrophages are vital cells playing an anti-inflammatory role in recovery from spinal cord injury in mice. *PLoS Med.* 2009;6(7):e1000113.
25. Trivedi A, Olivas AD, Noble-Haeusslein LJ. Inflammation and spinal cord injury: infiltrating leukocytes as determinants of injury and repair processes. *Clin Neurosci Res.* 2006;6(5):283–292.
26. Tran AP, Sundar S, Yu M, Lang BT, Silver J. Modulation of receptor protein tyrosine phosphatase sigma increases chondroitin sulfate proteoglycan degradation through cathepsin B secretion to enhance axon outgrowth. *J Neurosci J Soc Neurosci.* 2018;38(23):5399–5414.
27. Suzuki H, Ahuja CS, Salewski RP, et al. Neural stem cell mediated recovery is enhanced by chondroitinase ABC pretreatment in chronic cervical spinal cord injury. *PLoS One.* 2017;12(8):e0182339.
28. Mothe AJ, Tator CH. Review of transplantation of neural stem/progenitor cells for spinal cord injury. *Int J Dev Neurosci.* 2013;31(7):701–713.
29. Deng J, Zhang Y, Xie Y, Zhang L, Tang P. Cell transplantation for spinal cord injury: tumorigenicity of induced pluripotent stem cell-derived neural stem/progenitor cells. *Stem Cells Int.* 2018;2018:5653787.
30. Li X, Xiao Z, Han J, et al. Promotion of neuronal differentiation of neural progenitor cells by using EGFR antibody functionalized collagen scaffolds for spinal cord injury repair. *Biomaterials.* 2013;34(21):5107–5116.
31. Zai LJ, Wrathall JR. Cell proliferation and replacement following contusive spinal cord injury. *Glia.* 2005;50(3):247–257.
32. Zhang YW, Denham J, Thies RS. Oligodendrocyte progenitor cells derived from human embryonic stem cells express neurotrophic factors. *Stem Cells Dev.* 2006;15(6):943–952.

CHAPTER 6

Prehospital Evaluation and Management

Allison Kessler and Stephanie Hendrick

OUTLINE

Primary Survey

Management of the patient with spinal cord injury (SCI) begins immediately on the scene with the trauma primary survey[1–4]:

- Airway management with use of manual in-line stabilization of the cervical spine if intubation is necessary.
- Breathing and ventilation assessment with initial inspection for tracheal position, chest wounds, flail chest, and paradoxical or asymmetric chest wall movement. Diminished or absent breath sounds can be signs of pneumothorax or hemothorax. Supplemental oxygen should be administered in all trauma patients.
- Circulatory management with hemorrhage control through use of direct pressure or application of tourniquets, establishment of large-bore intravenous access, and fluid resuscitation.
- Disability assessment of the patient's neurological status utilizing the Glasgow coma scale (GCS). The GCS assesses an individual's eye-opening response, verbal response, and motor response. The maximum score is 15 and the minimum score is 3. If the patient is intubated, their score is followed by a T.
- Exposure and environmental control involve completely undressing the individual to assess for any concomitant injuries followed by application of warming blankets to prevent or limit risks of hypothermia. Heat loss may be exacerbated by general anesthesia or vasodilation from higher lesions, therefore heated fluids, blankets, or other temperature-regulating measures should be employed to maintain body temperature.

Secondary Survey

Following completion of the primary survey, a brief secondary survey is performed to aid in identification of injuries in the prehospital setting. This evaluation should be done with the assumption that the individual has a SCI and thus full spinal immobilization should be maintained.

Evaluating for SCI includes[2]:

- a brief motor assessment with hand grip and ankle dorsiflexion
- gross sensory assessment
- response to pain
- rectal exam to assess for the presence of sphincter tone

Additional findings suggestive of a SCI include[5]:

- paradoxical breathing
- bowel or bladder incontinence
- priapism
- bradycardia
- hypotension
- warm or flushed skin

In the setting of polytrauma, identification of concomitant injuries includes evaluating for traumatic brain injury, facial fractures, trauma to the chest, intraabdominal injuries, extremity fractures, pelvic fractures, vascular injuries, and penetrating injuries.

Immobilization

Immobilization is recommended in trauma patients with a potential SCI. The following five criteria should be utilized to determine the risk of SCI and need for immobilization[6]:

- spinal pain or tenderness
- altered mental status
- intoxication
- presence of neurological deficits
- distracting injuries

The use of a rigid cervical collar, blocks on a backboard and straps or taping keeps the spine in a neutral position and limits spinal motion. The patient's age and presence of abnormal spinal curvature or deformity should be considered for adjustment of positioning to prevent excessive neck flexion or neck extension. For example, in children less than 8 years of age, backboards with occipital cutouts are utilized to avoid excessive neck flexion due to their relatively large heads. Alternatively, padding under the shoulders and chest can be used.[7,8]

Transportation

Following proper immobilization, the patient should be transferred to a level 1 trauma center or center with SCI specialists. The patient should remain immobilized until definitive treatment. In the event a patient needs to be transferred or repositioned, emergency personnel should utilize the logroll technique to maintain spinal alignment.

Emergency Department Triage and Management

Respiratory Management and Airway Stabilization

All cervical SCI patients should be monitored closely for respiratory failure. Virtually all complete injuries above C5 will require intubation and mechanical ventilation. Careful intubation without hyperextension of the neck is indicated to prevent further injury, and controlled intubation should be considered prior to an emergency situation. If not intubated, supplemental oxygen should be considered to prevent hypoxemia and subsequent secondary spinal cord ischemia. For those who are not intubated immediately, baseline respiratory parameters should be obtained with frequent respiratory monitoring. Monitoring may include vital capacity, tidal volume, forced expiratory volume in the first second (FEV1), and negative inspiratory force (NIF). Pulse oximetry should not be relied on exclusively, and arterial blood gas or capnography should be monitored to look for a significant increase in partial pressure of carbon dioxide (pCO_2). Frequent monitoring should continue for at least 72 hours as approximately 90% of individuals who develop respiratory failure will do so within this timeframe.[9–11]

Early tracheostomy (<7 days) has been associated with fewer ventilatory days, shorter ICU says, decreased laryngotracheal complications, and earlier decannulation when compared to prolonged intubation. A tracheostomy may also assist in secretion management. Airway clearance is an essential part of early respiratory management in order to help prevent ventilator-associated pneumonia and assist in ventilator weaning. Airway clearance includes manually assisted coughing, mechanical insufflation-exsufflation, and suctioning.[11–13]

Circulatory and Hemodynamic Instability Management

Circulatory shock is common after traumatic SCI and includes neurogenic, cardiogenic, septic, and hypovolemic shock. Spinal shock is not a circulatory shock syndrome and should be considered separately. Spinal shock refers to the temporary loss of spinal reflexes below the level of injury.

Table 6.1 shows normal patterns of shock. Neurogenic shock classically presents with hypotension and bradycardia. It is more commonly seen in complete injuries and injury levels T6 or above that result in a loss of thoracic sympathetic innervation (T1–T5). This causes a loss of sympathetic tone and an unopposed parasympathetic response, which leads to vasodilation with inappropriate bradycardia. In injuries above T1, there may be profound bradycardia due to unopposed parasympathetic vagal activity. Up to 77% of cervical injuries will have bradycardia with a heart rate of less than 60 beats per minute. In some circumstances, transcutaneous pacing or administration of atropine may be indicated to treat profound or symptomatic bradycardia. In cases of trauma, it is important to avoid attributing hypotension solely to neurogenic shock and evaluate for other causes such as blood loss, which may be masked by bradycardia.[14,15]

During the acute setting, mean arterial pressure (MAP) should be kept below 85 to 90 mmHg for spinal cord perfusion for at least 7 days post SCI. Methods to maintain perfusion include fluids, transfusions, and pharmacologic vasopressors or inotropes depending on the patient's age as well as mechanism and level of injury.[16–20] For injuries above T1, phenylephrine (pure alpha-1 agonist) may worsen bradycardia, therefore other agents such as norepinephrine (alpha and beta) should be used.[16,21–23] An indwelling catheter should be placed in order to obtain accurate urine output for blood pressure monitoring and to treat urinary retention until hemodynamically stable.

Table 6.1 Patterns of Shock

Type of Shock:	Cardiac Output	Heart Rate	Systemic Vascular Resistance	Skin
Hypovolemic	Decreased	Increased	Increased	Cool, pale
Cardiogenic	Decreased	Increased	Increased	Cool, pale
Septic	Decreased	Increased	Decreased	Warm, flushed
Neurogenic	Decreased	Decreased	Decreased	Warm, Dry

Concomitant Injuries

The number one cause of SCI is motor-vehicle accidents. Falls, sports injuries, and violence are also common causes of SCI.[24] Given these mechanisms, concomitant injuries with SCI are not uncommon. Initial evaluation in the emergency department (ED) should focus not only on evaluation of the spinal cord but also on careful evaluation of insensate areas, as additional injuries may be missed.

The Focused Assessment with Sonography in Trauma (FAST) is a quick and noninvasive exam used to identify hemoperitoneum or hemopericardium in trauma patients. The FAST has largely replaced diagnostic peritoneal lavage with sensitivities between 85% to 96% and specificities exceeding 98%. It should be used in all blunt and/or penetrating abdominal or thoracic trauma as well as undifferentiated shock or hypotension in the ED as part of the Rapid Ultrasound for Shock and Hypotension (RUSH) exam. Computed tomography (CT) is the gold standard for detecting intraabdominal bleeding; however, it is more time consuming and may delay resuscitation.[25] Cervical SCIs should also be evaluated with CT angiography (CTA) or magnetic resonance angiography (MRA) to evaluate the neck vasculature.

Radiological Assessment of the Spine

The national emergency X-radiography utilization study (NEXUS) and Canadian C-spine rule (CCR) are two equally effective (90% sensitivity) guidelines for neck imaging in the ED.[26] Initial three-view radiographs can be obtained quickly, but cervicothoracic and craniocervical junction injuries may be missed. CT has better detection for bony spinal column injuries and should be used in all high-risk individuals for spinal injury (such as high-speed motor vehicle accidents) even if the initial plain radiographs are negative. MR imaging (MRI) is more sensitive for soft tissue and spinal cord injuries but is more time intensive, may not be available for unstable patients, and may delay surgery. It is also not suitable for unstable patients. Rarely, individuals may have a neurological exam consistent with a spinal cord injury but without radiographic abnormality.

Canadian C-spine rule for imaging[27]:

- age ≥65 years
- paresthesias in extremities
- dangerous mechanism of injury:
    - fall from an elevation ≥3 ft or 5 stairs
    - axial load to the head (e.g., diving)
    - motor vehicle collision at high speed (>100 km/h) or with rollover or ejection
    - bicycle collision
    - collision involving a motorized recreational vehicle.

NEXUS criteria: image if one of the following is present[28]:

- focal neurologic deficit
- midline spinal tenderness
- altered level of consciousness
- intoxication
- distracting injury.

(See Chapter 10 on Neuroimaging for further details of additional imaging modalities.)

Surgical Intervention

The optimal timing of surgical intervention for decompression of the spinal cord is unknown, but currently most recommend decompression within 24 hours. Recent studies have shown improved neurological outcomes, decreased complications, and shorter hospital stays with earlier decompression. Some studies show potential for better outcomes with intervention within 8 hours, though this may not be possible for all individuals given time to presentation and concomitant injuries. In addition, patients with central cord syndrome may be one subset of patients who do not have the same improvement in outcomes with early decompression.[29–37] The decision to proceed to surgery involves patient stability, comorbidities, and type of injury with assessment of spinal stability. While historically Denis' three-column model of the spine was used to assess spinal stability, newer classification systems such as the AOSpine Trauma Classification are now used.[38]

Neurological Exam

Proper baseline neurological assessment is essential for both treatment and prognostication of persons with traumatic SCI. The International Standards for Neurological Classification of Spinal Cord Injury (ISNCSCI) exam should be performed within 72 hours of initial injury for classification of neurological level of injury and completeness of injury. Further discussion of the ISNCSCI exam is available in Chapter 8. The rates of concomitant traumatic brain injury (TBI) may be as high as 60% in individuals with cervical spinal cord injury; therefore, it is essential to evaluate for TBI in all SCI patients as early as possible.[39–42] Please see Chapter 34 for an in depth discussion of the TBI evaluation and management.

Neuroprotection

Multiple agents either have been investigated or are currently undergoing investigation for neuroprotection after SCI. Although early data were promising, currently there is not enough evidence to support steroids for all acute traumatic SCI due to unclear benefit and demonstrated increase in complications such as pneumonia and hyperglycemia. Some studies have suggested improvement with use of steroids if given within 8 hours of injury and stopped within 24 hours, but there are not enough data to support routine use given the known complications, as other studies have failed to show the same improvement.[43–47]

Other interventions that have been or are undergoing investigation include but are not limited to hypothermia, riluzole, minocycline, glyburide, hepatocyte growth factor, granulocyte colony stimulating factor, basic fibroblast growth factor, stem cells, and cellular scaffolding. Various biomarkers are also under investigation to identify SCI.

Secondary Prevention

Pressure Injuries (PI)

- PIs are common and can develop within 4 to 6 hours.[48] Positioning, frequent turning, and offloading should be started as soon as possible.

Gastrointestinal (GI) Ulcer

- Acute GI ulceration is common in critically ill patients, and GI hemorrhage is estimated to occur in between 5% to 22% of SCI patients. Prophylaxis with an H2 blocker or proton-pump inhibitor should be initiated in the acute care setting.[49]

Venous Thromboembolism (VTE) Prevention in the Acute Care Setting

- VTE is a common and potentially life-threatening complication after SCI, with an estimated 49% to 100% of SCI patients developing VTE within 12 weeks of injury without chemoprophylaxis.[50,51]
- VTE chemoprophylaxis should be initiated within 72 hours. Risk of VTE prior to 72 hours is lower,[50] but the risk of VTE is highest during the first 2 weeks following injury.[50,52]
- Chemoprophylaxis should be initiated for all adults as soon as no active bleeding is confirmed.[52]

Review Questions

1. Venous thromboembolism is a common complication of SCI. In the emergency room chemoprophylaxis may need to be deferred due to active bleeding or imminent surgery; however, chemoprophylaxis should ideally be initiated within:
   a. 24 hours
   b. 48 hours
   c. 72 hours
   d. 96 hours
2. Which of the following patterns of shock would you most likely see in an individual with a complete spinal cord injury above T6?
   a. Hypotension, decreased cardiac output, decreased heart rate, decreased systemic vascular resistance
   b. Hypotension, increased cardiac output, decreased heart rate, decreased systemic vascular resistance
   c. Hypotension, decreased cardiac output, increased heart rate, decreased systemic vascular resistance
   d. Hypotension, increased cardiac output, decreased heart rate, increased systemic vascular resistance
3. What is the current recommendation for maintenance of spinal perfusion in the acute care setting?
   a. A MAP of >85–90 for 14 days
   b. A MAP of >90–95 for 14 days
   c. A MAP of >85–90 for 7 days
   d. A MAP of >90–95 for 7 days
4. Which of the following is not part of the NEXUS criteria for imaging?
   a. Altered mental status
   b. High speed motor vehicle accident
   c. Distracting injury
   d. Cervical spine pain or tenderness
5. A 28-year-old male is a restrained driver involved in a head-on motor vehicle collision. Emergency medical services are activated, and upon arrival the patient has altered mental status with a GCS of 7. What is the next step in the acute management of this patient?
   a. Establish an airway with intubation using manual in-line stabilization of his cervical spine
   b. Early treatment of hypotension with fluid resuscitation
   c. Evaluate for concomitant injuries by undressing the patient
   d. Assess ventilation and breathing by inspecting for open chest wounds and paradoxical breathing.
6. Which of the following should be initiated as soon as possible in order to prevent secondary complications after an acute spinal cord injury?
   a. Insertion of an IVC filter to prevent pulmonary embolism
   b. High dose steroids
   c. Pressure injury prevention strategies
   d. NPO status to ensure no GI ulceration

REFERENCES

1. Planas JH, Waseem M, Sigmon DF. Trauma primary survey. [Updated 2021 Feb 10]. In: StatPearls [Internet]. Treasure Island (FL): StatPearls Publishing; 2021 Jan-. https://www.ncbi.nlm.nih.gov/books/NBK430800/.
2. Whetstone W. Prehospital management of spinal cord injury. In: Kirshblum S, Lin VW, eds. *Spinal Cord Medicine*. New York: Springer Publishing Company; 2019:166–171.
3. American College of Surgeons. *Advanced Trauma Life support*. Chicago, IL; 2008.
4. Fox A. Management of trauma patients with complex injuries. In: Kirshblum S, Lin VW, eds. *Spinal Cord Medicine*. New York: Springer Publishing Company; 2019:172–176.

5. Sabharwal S. *Prehospital management of spinal cord injury*. In: *Essentials of Spinal Cord Medicine*. New York: Demos Medical; 2013:35–40.
6. Domeier RM. Indications for prehospital spinal immobilization. National Association of EMS Physicians Standards and Clinical Practice Committee. *Prehosp Emerg Care*. 1999 Jul-Sep;3(3):251–253.
7. Lemley K, Bauer P. Pediatric spinal cord injury: recognition of injury and initial resuscitation, in hospital management, and coordination of care. *J Pediatr Intensive Care*. 2015;4(1):27–34.
8. Nypaver M, Treloar D. Neutral cervical spine positioning in children. *Ann Emerg Med*. 1994 Feb;23(2):208–211.
9. Velmahos GC, Toutouzas K, Chan L, et al. Intubation after cervical spinal cord injury: to be done selectively or routinely? *American Surgeon*. 2003;69(10):891–894.
10. Galeiras Vázquez R, Rascado Sedes P, Mourelo Fariña M, Montoto Marqués A, Ferreiro Velasco ME. Respiratory management in the patient with spinal cord injury. *Biomed Res Int*. 2013;2013:168757.
11. Ganuza JR, Forcada AG, Gambarrutta C, et al. Effect of technique and timing of tracheostomy in patients with acute traumatic spinal cord injury undergoing mechanical ventilation. *J Spinal Cord Med*. 2011;34(1):76–84.
12. Leelapattana P, Fleming JC, Gurr KR, Bailey SI, Parry N, Bailey CS. Predicting the need for tracheostomy in patients with cervical spinal cord injury. *J Trauma Acute Care Surg*. 2012;73(4):880–884.
13. Dave S, Cho JJ. Neurogenic shock. [Updated 2021 Feb 9]. In: StatPearls [Internet]. Treasure Island (FL): StatPearls Publishing; 2021 Jan-. https://www.ncbi.nlm.nih.gov/books/NBK459361/.
14. Biering-Sørensen F, Biering-Sørensen T, Liu N, Malmqvist L, Wecht JM, Krassioukov A. Alterations in cardiac autonomic control in spinal cord injury. *Auton Neurosci*. 2018 Jan;209:4–18.
15. Levi L, Wolf A, Belzberg H. Hemodynamic parameters in patients with acute cervical cord trauma: description, intervention, and prediction of outcome. *Neurosurgery*. 1993 Dec; 33(6):1007–1016. discussion 1016-1017.
16. Vale FL, Burns J, Jackson AB, Hadley MN. Combined medical and surgical treatment after acute spinal cord injury: results of a prospective pilot study to assess the merits of aggressive medical resuscitation and blood pressure management. *J Neurosurg*. 1997 Aug;87(2):239–246.
17. Yue JK, Tsolinas RE, Burke JF, et al. Vasopressor support in managing acute spinal cord injury: current knowledge. *J Neurosurg Sci*. 2019 Jun;63(3):308–317.
18. Furlan JC, Fehlings MG. Cardiovascular complications after acute spinal cord injury: pathophysiology, diagnosis, and management. *Neurosurg Focus*. 2008;25(5):E13.
19. Krassioukov AV, Karlsson AK, Wecht JM, Wuermser LA, Mathias CJ, Marino RJ. Joint Committee of American Spinal Injury Association and International Spinal Cord Society. Assessment of autonomic dysfunction following spinal cord injury: rationale for additions to International Standards for Neurological Assessment. *J Rehabil Res Dev*. 2007;44(1): 103–112.
20. Hadley MN, Walters BC, Grabb PA, et al. Blood pressure management after acute spinal cord injury. *Neurosurgery*. 2002 Mar;50(3 Suppl):S58–S62.
21. Catapano JS, John Hawryluk GW, Whetstone W, et al. Higher mean arterial pressure values correlate with neurologic improvement in patients with initially complete spinal cord injuries. *World Neurosurg*. 2016 Dec;96:72–79.
22. Saadeh YS, Smith BW, Joseph JR, et al. The impact of blood pressure management after spinal cord injury: a systematic review of the literature. *Neurosurgical Focus FOC*. 2017 Nov;43(5):E20.
23. National Spinal Cord Injury Statistical Center. *Facts and Figures at a Glance*. Birmingham, AL: University of Alabama at Birmingham; 2020.
24. Bloom BA, Gibbons RC. Focused assessment with sonography for trauma. [Updated 2020 Jul 31]. In: StatPearls [Internet]. Treasure Island (FL): StatPearls Publishing; 2020 Jan-.
25. Ala A, Shams Vahdati S, Ghaffarzad A, Mousavi H, Mirza-Aghazadeh-Attari M. National emergency X-radiography utilization study guidelines versus Canadian C-Spine guidelines on trauma patients, a prospective analytical study. *PLoS One*. 2018;13(11):e0206283.
26. Stiell IG, Wells GA, Vandemheen KL, et al. The Canadian C-spine rule for radiography in alert and stable trauma patients. *JAMA*. 2001 Oct 17;286(15):1841–1848.
27. Hoffman JR, Wolfson AB, Todd K, Mower WR. Selective cervical spine radiography in blunt trauma: methodology of the National Emergency X-Radiography Utilization Study (NEXUS). *Ann Emerg Med*. 1998 Oct;32(4):461–469.
28. Liu Y, Shi CG, Wang XW, et al. Timing of surgical decompression for traumatic cervical spinal cord injury. *Int Orthop*. 2015;39:2457–2463.
29. Du JP, Fan Y, Zhang JN, Liu JJ, Meng YB, Hao DJ. Early versus delayed decompression for traumatic cervical spinal cord injury: application of the AOSpine subaxial cervical spinal injury classification system to guide surgical timing. *Eur Spine J*. 2019;28(8):1855–1863.
30. Badhiwala JH, Ahuja CS, Fehlings MG. Time is spine: a review of translational advances in spinal cord injury. *J. Neurosurg. Spine SPI*. 2019;30(1):1–18.
31. van Middendorp JJ, Hosman AJ, Doi SA. The effects of the timing of spinal surgery after traumatic spinal cord injury: a systematic review and meta-analysis. *J Neurotrauma*. 2013;30:1781–1794.
32. Wilson JR, Tetreault LA, Kwon BK, Arnold PM, Mroz TE, Shaffrey C. Timing of decompression in patients with acute spinal cord injury: a systematic review. *Global Spine J*. 2017;7(3 Suppl):95S–115S.
33. Fehlings MG, Vaccaro A, Wilson JR, et al. Early versus delayed decompression for traumatic cervical spinal cord injury: results of the Surgical Timing in Acute Spinal Cord Injury Study (STASCIS). *PLoS One*. 2012;7(2):e32037.
34. Fehlings MG, Tetreault LA, Wilson JR, Aarabi B, Anderson P, Arnold PM. A clinical practice guideline for the management of patients with acute spinal cord injury and central cord syndrome: recommendations on the timing (≤24 hours versus >24 hours) of decompressive surgery. *Global Spine J*. 2017;7(3 Suppl):195S–202S.
35. Furlan JC, Noonan V, Cadotte DW, Fehlings MG. Timing of decompressive surgery of spinal cord after traumatic spinal cord injury: an evidence-based examination of pre-clinical and clinical studies. *J Neurotrauma*. 2011;28:1371–1399.
36. Jug M, Kejžar N, Vesel M, Al Mawed S, Dobravec M, Herman S. Neurological recovery after traumatic cervical spinal cord

injury is superior if surgical decompression and instrumented fusion are performed within 8 hours versus 8 to 24 hours after injury: a single center experience. *J Neurotrauma.* 2015;32:1385–1392.

37. Divi SN, Schroeder GD, Oner FC, et al. AOSpine-Spine Trauma Classification System: the value of modifiers: a narrative review with commentary on evolving descriptive principles. *Global Spine J.* 2019;9(1 Suppl):77S–88S.
38. Hagen EM, Eide GE, Rekand T, Gilhus NE, Gronning M. Traumatic spinal cord injury and concomitant brain injury: a cohort study. *Acta Neurol Scand Suppl.* 2010(190):51–57.
39. Macciocchi S, Seel RT, Thompson N, Byams R, Bowman B. Spinal cord injury and co-occurring traumatic brain injury: assessment and incidence. *Arch Phys Med Rehabil.* 2008 Jul;89(7):1350–1357.
40. Kushner DS, Alvarez G. Dual diagnosis: traumatic brain injury with spinal cord injury. *Phys Med Rehabil Clin N Am.* 2014 Aug;25(3):681–696. ix-x.
41. Pandrich MJ, Demetriades AK. Prevalence of concomitant traumatic cranio-spinal injury: a systematic review and meta-analysis. *Neurosurg Rev.* 2020;43:69–77.
42. Bracken MB. Steroids for acute spinal cord injury. *Cochrane Database Syst Rev.* 2012 Jan 18;1:CD001046.
43. Bracken MB, Shepard MJ, Collins WF, Jr., et al. Methylprednisolone or naloxone treatment after acute spinal cord injury: 1-year follow-up data. Results of the second National Acute Spinal Cord Injury Study. *J. Neurosurg.* 1992;76(1): 23–31.
44. Tsutsumi S, Ueta T, Shiba K, Yamamoto S, Takagishi K. Effects of the Second National Acute Spinal Cord Injury Study of high-dose methylprednisolone therapy on acute cervical spinal cord injury-results in spinal injuries center. *Spine (Phila Pa 1976).* 2006;31(26):2992–2996.
45. Bracken MB, Shepard MJ, Holford TR, et al. Administration of methylprednisolone for 24 or 48 hours or tirilazad mesylate for 48 hours in the treatment of acute spinal cord injury. Results of the third national acute spinal cord injury randomized controlled trial. *National acute spinal cord injury study. JAMA.* 1997;277(20):1597–1604.
46. Sultan I, Lamba N, Liew A, et al. The safety and efficacy of steroid treatment for acute spinal cord injury: a systematic review and meta-analysis. *Heliyon.* 2020 Feb 19;6(2):e03414.
47. Gefen A. How much time does it take to get a pressure ulcer? Integrated evidence from human, animal, and in vitro studies. *Ostomy Wound Manage.* 2008 Oct;54(10):26–28, 30–35.
48. Anwar F, Al-Khayer A, El-Mahrouki H, Purcell M. Gastrointestinal bleeding in spinal injuries patient: is prophylaxis essential? *BJMP.* 2013;6(1):a607.
49. Merli GJ, Crabbe S, Paluzzi RG, Fritz D. Etiology incidence and prevention of deep vein thrombosis in acute spinal cord injury. *Arch Phys Med Rehabit.* 1993;74:1199–1205.
50. Piran S, Schulman S. Incidence and risk factors for venous thromboembolism in patients with acute spinal cord injury: a retrospective study. *Thromb Res.* 2016;147:97–101.
51. Green D, Lee MY, Lim AC, et al. Prevention of thromboembolism after spinal cord injury using low-molecular-weight heparin. *Ann Intern Med.* 1990;113:571–574.
52. Consortium for Spinal Cord Medicine. Prevention of venous thromboembolism in individuals with spinal cord injury: Clinical practice guidelines for health care providers, 3rd ed. Consortium for Spinal Cord Medicine. *Top Spinal Cord Inj Rehabil.* 2016;22(3):209–240.

Neurological Assessment and Classification

CHAPTER 7

Andrea T. Aguirre and Venessa A. Lee

OUTLINE

Overview

The International Standards for Neurological Classification of Spinal Cord Injuries (ISNSCI) is the gold standard for neurological assessment and classification of spinal cord injuries (SCI). The assessment published by the American Spinal Injury Association (ASIA) classifies a SCI based off of level of injury as well as the completeness of the SCI via the AISA Impairment Scale (AIS).[1] This exam replaced the Frankel scale, which did not specify the spinal level of injury.[2] The ASIA examination includes both sensory and motor components that are used to determine a patient's motor, sensory, and neurologic levels, the overall completeness of the injury, and the AIS.[1] The assessment also includes a rectal exam that tests for both voluntary anal contraction (VAC) as well as deep anal pressure (DAP) and contributes to the determination of the AIS. For the examination, the patient is in the supine position with the exception of the rectal exam, which is performed in the side-lying position.[1] The assessment is best performed within 72 hours to 1 week of injury.[3]

Neurologic Assessment

Sensory Exam

The sensory exam involves testing 28 dermatomes on each side of the body. The dermatomes known as "key sensory points" (Table 7.1) are tested for both light touch and pinprick in comparison to sensation of the face, which is used as a control. Both of these modalities are scored based on the presence, impairment, or absence of sensation in comparison to the face. This is scored using a three-point grading scale from 0–2:

- 0: absent, no appreciation of tested sensation
- 1: abnormal sensation including hypo- and hyperesthesia
- 2: intact, same sensation as the face.

For light touch, a soft cotton tip is lightly stroked 1 cm across the skin along the 28 key sensory points. A clean safety pin is used for the pinprick portion of the sensory exam. Of note, for the pinprick exam, in order to score a "1," the patient must be able to differentiate between sharp and dull. If unable to differentiate, the dermatome is scored as a "0." In both examinations of sensation, the patient's eyes are closed.

The sensory examination also includes testing sensation at the S4–S5 dermatomes as well as testing DAP. S4–S5 are included together as one of the 28 key sensory points, which is located less than 1 cm lateral to the mucocutaneous junction of the anus. DAP involves a rectal examination in which a lubricated gloved finger is inserted into the anus. Scoring of DAP is either "Yes" if the patient can appreciate pressure or "No" if pressure is not appreciated.[4]

Motor Exam

The motor exam consists of both the testing of the bilateral upper and lower extremity muscles as well as VAC. The 10 key muscle groups (Table 7.2) are scored via a six-point scale (0–5) based on the Manual Muscle Testing grading scale. Before beginning muscle strength testing, the range of motion of the joint the muscle crosses should first be assessed. Additionally, each muscle is first tested in the grade 3 testing position.[5] Similar to the sensory exam, the patient is in the supine position for motor testing.[4]

Manual Muscle Testing[6]:

- 0: no observable or palpable muscle contraction
- 1: palpable or visible contraction
- 2: full range of motion with gravity eliminated
- 3: full range of motion against gravity
- 4: full range of motion against gravity, meets some resistance
- 5: full range of motion against gravity, meets full resistance.

Table 7.1 Key Sensory Points

Root Level	Location
C2	1 cm lateral to occipital protuberance
C3	Supraclavicular fossa at midclavicular line
C4	Acromioclavicular joint
C5	Lateral antecubital fossa
C6	Dorsal surface of proximal phalanx of thumb
C7	Dorsal surface of proximal phalanx of middle finger
C8	Dorsal surface of proximal phalanx of little finger
T1	Medial antecubital fossa
T2	Apex of axilla
T3	3rd intercostal space at midclavicular line
T4	4th intercostal space at midclavicular line (nipple line)
T5	5th intercostal space at midclavicular line
T6	6th intercostal space at midclavicular line (level of xiphoid)
T7	7th intercostal space at midclavicular line
T8	8th intercostal space at midclavicular line
T9	9th intercostal space at midclavicular line
T10	10th intercostal space at midclavicular line (level of umbilicus)
T11	11th intercostal space at midclavicular line
T12	Midpoint of inguinal ligament
L1	Midway between key sensory point for T12 and L2
L2	Midpoint of T12 key sensory point and medial femoral condyle
L3	Medial femoral condyle
L4	Medial malleolus
L5	Dorsal third metatarsal phalangeal joint
S1	Lateral calcaneus
S2	Midpoint of popliteal fossa
S3	Ischial tuberosity
S4–S5	1 cm lateral to the mucocutaneous junction of the anus

From Kirshblum SC, Burns SP, Biering-Sorensen F, et al. International standards for neurological classification of spinal cord injury (Revised 2011). *J Spinal Cord Med.* 2011;34(6):535–546.

Of note, only whole numbers are used for muscle grading, and pluses and minuses are excluded from official scoring. If a muscle is tested and graded as below a 5 in setting of pain, deconditioning, or another condition that would otherwise score the muscle as a 5, the muscle can be graded with an asterisk (*) to indicate that a non-SCI condition is present. However, if a muscle is unable to be tested for reasons such as spasticity, cognitive status, or fracture, the muscle should be graded as not tested or NT.

Table 7.2 Key Muscle Groups

Root Level	Movement
C5	Elbow flexion
C6	Wrist extensors
C7	Elbow extensors
C8	Finger flexors
T1	Finger abductors
L2	Hip flexors
L3	Knee extensors
L4	Ankle dorsiflexors
L5	Long toe extensors
S1	Ankle plantar flexors

From Kirshblum SC, Burns SP, Biering-Sorensen F, et al. International standards for neurological classification of spinal cord injury (Revised 2011). *J Spinal Cord Med.* 2011;34(6):535–546.

Similar to the DAP portion of the sensory exam, VAC is tested by inserting a lubricated, gloved finger into the anus. The patient is asked to "hold back a bowel movement" by squeezing. If contraction is present, VAC is scored as a "Yes" and as a "No" if absent.[4]

Neurologic Classification

Sensory Level

A patient's sensory level is defined as the most caudal level in which both light touch and pinprick sensation are graded as a 2 or normal. Additionally, all levels above this level must also have a grade of 2. If sensation at C2 is abnormal, the sensory level is designated as C1.

Motor Level

The lowest key muscle that has a grade of 3 on the manual muscle test is used to determine the motor level. However, all muscles above this level must have a grade of 5. If a myotome is not able to be tested (C1–C4, T2–L1, and S2–S5), they are assumed to be a 5 on the manual muscle test if the corresponding sensation to light touch and pinprick is intact.

Neurologic Level of Injury

The neurologic level of injury is the highest level from both the left and right side that has both normal sensation and motor function. A patient is given one neurologic level of injury.[4]

Table 7.3 American Spinal Association Impairment Scale (AIS) Grades

AIS	Degree of Impairment	Definition
A	Complete	No sensory or motor function is preserved in S4–S5.
B	Sensory Incomplete	Sensory but not motor function is preserved below the neurological level and includes the sacral segments S4–S5 and no motor function is preserved more than three levels below the motor level on either side of the body.
C	Motor Incomplete	Motor function is preserved in voluntary anal contraction, or sensory function preserved at S4–S5 by light touch, pinprick, or deep anal pressure. Plus, some sparing of motor function more than three levels below the ipsilateral motor level on either side of the body. For AIS C, more than half of key muscle functions below the single neurologic level of injury have a muscle grade <3.
D	Motor Incomplete	Motor incomplete status as defined above, with at least half of key muscle functions below the single neurologic level of injury having a muscle grade ≥ 3.
E	Normal	If sensation and motor function are graded as normal in all segments, and the patient had prior deficits, then the AIS grade is E. Someone without an initial SCI does not receive an AIS grade.

From Kirshblum SC, Burns SP, Biering-Sorensen F, et al. International standards for neurological classification of spinal cord injury (Revised 2011). *J Spinal Cord Med.* 2011;34(6):535–546.

Zone of Partial Preservation

The zone of partial preservation (ZPP) is determined for complete injuries as well as incomplete injuries in which there is no VAC, DAP, or sensation of segments S4–S5, including light touch or pinprick. The ZPP refers to the most caudal segments with any motor or sensory function.[1]

American Spinal Injury Association Impairment Scale Grade

Once the sensory, motor, and neurologic levels are determined, the American Spinal Association Impairment Scale (AIS) Grade is calculated as outlined in Table 7.3.

Of note, the testing of nonkey muscles can be helpful in distinguishing between an AIS grade of B or C.[4]

Review Questions

1. A patient has no sensation including pinprick and light touch sensation in the S4–S5 dermatomes as well as no deep anal pressure or voluntary anal contraction. What American Spinal Injury Association (ASIA) Impairment Scale (AIS) grade is the patient?
   a. AIS A
   b. AIS B
   c. AIS C
   d. AIS D
2. When performing an ASIA exam on a patient, you note that a patient has a motor level of C6 bilaterally with sensation to light touch and pinprick intact to C7. Additionally, you note voluntary anal contraction on the rectal exam. On further review of the exam, half of the key muscles below the neurologic level of injury have a grade of ≥ 3. What is the patient's AIS grade?
   a. C7 AIS C
   b. C7 AIS D
   c. C6 AIS C
   d. C6 AIS D
3. What is the significance of nonkey muscles in regard to the ASIA exam?
   a. They are used to determine the motor level.
   b. They are used to differentiate between AIS B and AIS C.
   c. They are used to determine the zone of partial preservation.
   d. They are used to differentiate between AIS C and AIS D.
4. The following are the manual muscle testing results from your ASIA exam:
   a. C5 – Right 5, Left 5
   b. C6 – Right 5, Left 5
   c. C7 – Right 5, Left 3
   d. C8 – Right 4, Left 3
   What is the overall motor level for this patient?
   e. C5
   f. C6
   g. C7
   h. C8
5. When performing an ASIA exam on a patient, you determine that a patient's neurologic level of injury is T8. Voluntary anal contraction is absent. However, the patient reports intact sensation at S4–S5. There is no motor activity noted at L2–S1. What is the patient's AIS grade?
   a. T8 AIS A
   b. T8 AIS B
   c. T8 AIS C
   d. T8 AIS D

6. What is the earliest reliable standard time frame for completing the ASIA exam for an acute spinal cord injury?
   a. <24 hours after injury
   b. 24–48 hours after injury
   c. 48–72 hours after injury
   d. 72 hours after injury

REFERENCES

1. American Spinal Injury Association *International Standards of Neurological Classification of Spinal Cord Injury*. Richmond: American Spinal Injury Association; 2019.
2. Roberts TT, Leonard GR, Cepela DJ. Classifications in brief: American Spinal Injury Association (ASIA) Impairment Scale. *Clin Orthop Relat Res*. 2017;475(5):1499–1504.
3. Kirshblum SC, O'Connor KC. Predicting neurologic recovery in traumatic spinal cord injury. *Arch Phys Med Rehabil*. 1998;79:1456–1466.
4. Kirshblum S, Solinksy R. Neurological assessment and classification of spinal cord injury. In: Kirshblum S, Lin VW, eds. *Spinal Cord Medicine*. 3rd ed. New York: DemosMedical; 2019:63–76.
5. Bryce TN. Spinal cord injury. In: Cifu DX, ed. *Braddom's Physical Medicine & Rehabilitation*. 5th ed. Philadelphia: Elsevier; 2016:1095–1136.
6. Ciesla N, Dinglas V, Fan E, Kho M, Kuramoto J, Needham D. Manual muscle testing: a method of measuring extremity muscle strength applied to critically ill patients. *J Vis Exp*. 2011;50(2632):1–5.

CHAPTER

8 Neuroimaging

Heather Asthagiri and Justin Tu

OUTLINE

Advancements in imaging technology have allowed for the diagnosis of spinal cord injury and neuropathology to be improved significantly, allowing more accurate and timely management. Choosing the most appropriate imaging modality for a patient with suspected spinal cord injury, and appropriately determining the findings, is imperative.

Advanced Imaging Basics

Computed Tomography

Computed tomography (CT) scanners emit ionizing radiation from a motorized X-ray source that circles the patient in a gantry, with digital X-ray detectors positioned just opposite the source. These data are transmitted to the CT computer, which creates cross-sectional images or slices. With the advent of multidetector computed tomography (MDCT), two-dimensional detector elements allow for very rapid acquisition of submillimeter section data (volume data instead of individual slice data), resulting in high spatial resolution, which makes it ideal for CT angiography.[1,2] Although CT is the superior modality to visualize bony anatomy, fractures, and spinal canal dimensions, CT imaging does not adequately image the spinal cord.

Magnetic Resonance Imaging

Magnetic resonance imaging (MRI) employs a high-strength main magnetic field, magnetic field gradients, radio waves, and a computer, which detects change in the rotational axis of hydrogen protons to the magnetic fields and radiofrequency currents at different intervals to generate images. Protons in water and protons in fat molecules have different relaxation times, or changes in proton alignment. The most common MRI sequences used to measure this are T1-weighted and T2-weighted images. On T1-weighted images, fat has a high-signal intensity (white) and water or fluid has a low-signal intensity (black), whereas on T2-weighted images, fluid has high-signal intensity (white). Administering IV gadolinium during T1-weighted imaging increases the speed at which protons realign with the magnetic field, producing brighter (white) fluid. With short tau inversion recovery (STIR) imaging, fluid is bright, with suppressed fat signals. A technique that can highlight the presence of hemorrhage by increasing the conspicuity of signal loss includes susceptibility-weighted imaging.[3,4] Other MRI sequences are shown in Table 8.1. Of note, on conventional MRI sequences, adequate visualization of the spinal cord and characterization of intramedullary lesions can be challenging; some advanced sequences can provide a better depiction of spinal cord anatomy[5] (Table 8.2).

Traumatic Spinal Cord Injury

Although it is classically the standard imaging modality for fracture evaluation, plain radiography can miss a large percentage of spine fractures, particularly in the cervical spine. In the setting of suspected spine trauma, use of CT for screening has largely replaced plain films.[6–11]

MRI is the modality of choice for imaging spinal cord compression and spinal cord pathology, and thus the preferred modality for assessment of the spinal cord in the area of suspected injury after CT.[3,12,13] MRI can evaluate for spinal cord edema or hemorrhage, spinal cord compression from traumatic disc herniations or bony fragments, epidural/subdural hemorrhage, prevertebral edema, and ligamentous injury.[5,11,14]

Although the initial physical exam is the single best predictor of neurological outcome, T2 sagittal imaging findings of parenchymal hemorrhage, transection, and longer length of injury within the spinal cord correlate with a poorer neurologic recovery, whereas no spinal cord abnormality on MRI is associated with favorable outcomes.[12,15]

In the setting of cervical fractures sustained during high-velocity injuries, imaging of the entire spine is recommended given the strong association between cervical spine fractures and thoracolumbar fractures.[16,17] Further,

■ MRI findings with a less favorable neurologic outcome:

- parenchymal hemorrhage
- transection
- longer lesion length

Table 8.1 Selected Magnetic Resonance Imaging (MRI) Sequences

MRI Sequence	Property	Clinical Application
T1	Fat bright, water dark	Good visualization of anatomy • Subacute hemorrhage is hyperintense
T2	Water bright Fat: appearance depends on whether the image is fat-saturated (dark) or not fat-saturated (bright)	Good visualization of spinal cord pathology, such as: • Spinal cord edema • Demyelination • Infarction
T1 with gadolinium (Gad)	Gad: fluid very bright	Detect lesions (tumor/metastasis, abscess) Inflammation (e.g., MS, HSV encephalitis) Imaging of vessels/vascular pathology (MR angiography)
STIR	Suppresses fat (dark), fluid bright	High signal with edema, such as bone marrow edema
FLAIR (T2)	T2 with selective suppression of CSF signal (nullifies signal from fluids)	Shows edema, demyelination, infarction High signal with white matter abnormalities, such as in MS, SAH, and meningitis
DWI & ADC *Difficult to evaluate spinal cord due to its small size, breathing artifact, and CSF pulsations	Motion of protons	Shows cytotoxic edema and inflammation Detects axon integrity, myelin disruption, and axon swelling Helps distinguish *acute ischemia* (abnormal diffusion) vs chronic ischemia and contents of abscess (abnormal diffusion) vs necrosis in a tumor
DTI	Measures rate of water diffusion between cells	Tractography: maps of white matter tracts Used for presurgical planning of spinal tumors

ADC, Apparent diffusion coefficient; *CSF*, cerebrospinal fluid; *DTI*, diffusion tensor imaging; *DWI*, diffusion-weighted imaging; FLAIR, fluid-attenuated inversion recovery; *HSV*, herpes simplex virus; *MS*, multiple sclerosis; *SAH*, subarachnoid hemorrhage; *STIR*, short tau inversion recovery.

for cervical spine fractures with high suspicion of vertebral artery injury, such as fractures involving the transverse foramen or in the setting of facet dislocations, CT angiography can be performed[18] (Figs. 8.1–8.3; Table 8.3).

Table 8.2 Comparison of Computed Tomography Versus Magnetic Resonance Imaging

Imaging Modality	Pros	Cons
CT	Fast Excellent for fracture detection and bony alignment Higher sensitivity for acute hemorrhage	Radiation exposure Need myelography to visualize the spinal cord outline (CT myelogram may be used if MRI contraindicated) Misses syrinxes and other intramedullary pathology
MRI	Excellent soft tissue contrast, essential for detecting spinal ligamentous injury **No radiation**	Much longer acquisition time than CT, may require sedation Susceptible to motion artifact Contraindications to MRI: • Some cardiac pacemakers, medication pumps, and other implanted electronic devices • Cochlear implants • Some vascular clips • Intraocular metallic foreign bodies • Bullets or shrapnel • Unstable patient Administration of IV gadolinium can cause adverse reactions, such as bronchospasms, anaphylactic reactions, or nephrogenic systemic fibrosis in setting of renal insufficiency

CT, Computed tomography; *IV*, intravenous; *MRI*, magnetic resonance imaging.

Vascular Pathology: Hematomas, Infarctions

Spinal Hematomas and Hemorrhages

There are four types of spinal hematomas identified by location: epidural (Fig. 8.4), subdural, subarachnoid, and intramedullary (Fig. 8.5). As with intracranial hemorrhages, age of hemorrhage can be divided into five stages based on MRI findings that evolve over time (Table 8.4).[4]

Spinal Cord Infarctions

Similar to spinal cord hemorrhages, MRI findings in spinal cord ischemia evolve over time. Although MRIs most often appear normal in the acute phase after spinal cord infarction, after 1 to 2 days focal spinal cord enlargement with T2 and STIR hyperintensity is typically seen (Fig. 8.6), followed later by gadolinium enhancement.[19,20] Although diffusion-weighted imaging (DWI) is an extremely sensitive MRI sequence for detection of acute stroke on brain MRI, use of DWI in the

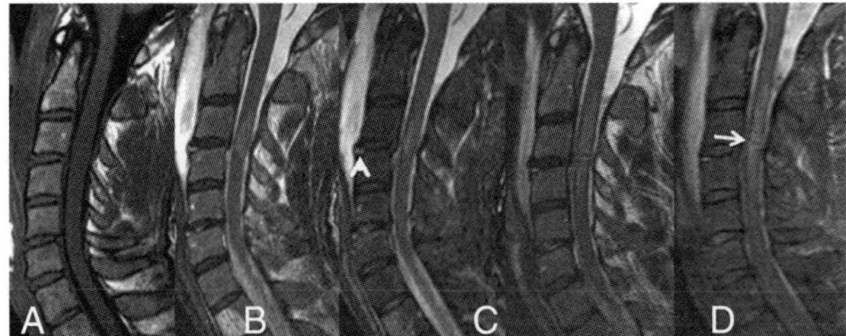

Fig. 8.1 Spinal Cord Injury in a 47-Year-Old Male. At presentation, patient was categorized as AIS grade C. (A) Initial outside hospital T1-weighted magnetic resonance imaging, (B) T2-weighted, and (C) short tau inversion recovery (STIR) imaging shows prevertebral edema from C1 to C4–C5, with mild widening of anterior C3–C4 disc space and focal disc T2 signal abnormality *(arrowhead)*. There is spinal cord edema spanning the C3 level. There is interspinous edema extending from C2 to C5. A 32-hour follow-up (D) T2-weighted, and (E) STIR magnetic resonance imaging show progression of cord edema with a new focus of T2 hypointensity *(arrow)* within the cord at C3–C4, indicating progression to hemorrhagic contusion. Adapted from: Talekar K, Poplawski M, Hegde R, Cox M, Flanders A. Imaging of spinal cord injury: acute cervical spinal cord injury, cervical spondylotic myelopathy, and cord herniation. *Semin Ultrasound CT MR*. 2016;37(5):431–447.

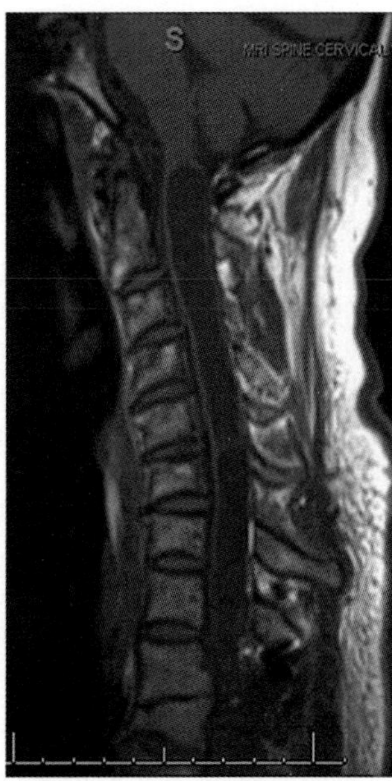

Fig. 8.3 Syringomyelia. Male in his 60s who was involved in a car accident sustaining T3 fracture and paraplegia 43 years earlier. T1-weighted magnetic resonance imaging shows a holocord syrinx extending from C1 past the fracture and constriction to the conus. Adapted From: Karam Y, Hitchon PW, Mhanna NE, He W, Noeller J. Post-traumatic syringomyelia: outcome predictors. *Clin Neurol Neurosurg*. 2014;124:44–50.

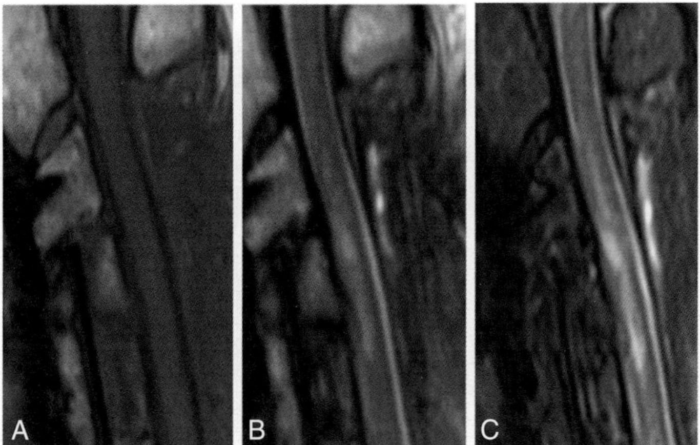

Fig. 8.2 Myelomalacia. (A) Sagittal T1-weighted image in a patient with cervical decompression and anterior/posterior spinal fusion. (B) Sagittal T2 and (C) sagittal short tau inversion recovery (STIR) images demonstrate noncystic T2 hyperintensity in the spinal cord between C3 and C5 with cord thinning, compatible with myelomalacia. There is no corresponding signal abnormality in the cord on the T1-weighted image, unlike in the posttraumatic cyst shown in Figure 3. Adapted from: Zohrabian VM, Flanders AE. Imaging of trauma of the spine. *Handb Clin Neurol*. 2016;136:747–767.

spine is limited by the small size of the spinal cord, cardiorespiratory motion, and physiologic cerebral spinal fluid (CSF) flow-induced artifact; however, DWI utilization for assessment of the spinal cord has been increasingly utilized.[4]

In addition, depending on the affected artery, differing patterns of spinal cord ischemia can be seen. The single anterior spinal artery supplies the anterior horns bilaterally and the adjacent white matter, or the anterior two-thirds of the spinal cord, and infarction results in anterior cord syndrome. On MRI, involvement of the anterior horn cells, which are particularly vulnerable to ischemia, can be seen on T2-weighted sequences as pencil-like high intensity signals spanning multiple levels on sagittal views and an “owl’s eye sign” on axial images (Fig. 8.6). In addition, anterior spinal artery infarction

Table 8.3 Time Course of Spinal Cord Injury After Trauma and Its Associated Imaging Findings

Acute period after traumatic SCI (see Fig. 8.1)	Spinal cord swelling: enlargement of the cord contour Spinal cord edema: high signal on T2-weighted images Intramedullary hemorrhage: central focus of hypointensity surrounded by a thick rim of hyperintensity on T2-weighted images
Subacute period after traumatic SCI	Myelomalacia: findings similar to edema, with T2 hyperintensity and T1 signal in between cord and CSF (see Fig. 8.2) Subacute intramedullary hemorrhage as T1 hyperintensity
Chronic	Syringomyelia/syrinx: expanded cord with dilated or beaded cystic cavity and surrounding gliosis/myelomalacia, seen in 25% of SCI (see Fig. 8.3) Spinal cord atrophy: anterior-posterior (A–P) dimensions of 7 mm or less in the cervical cord or 6 mm or less in the thoracic cord

CSF, Cerebrospinal fluid; *SCI,* spinal cord injury.
From Ellingson BM, Salamon N, Holly LT. Imaging techniques in spinal cord injury. *World Neurosurg.* 2014;82(6):1351–1358; Freund P, Curt A, Friston K, Thompson A. Tracking changes following spinal cord injury insights from neuroimaging. *Neuroscientist.* 2013;19(2):116–128; Potter K, Saifuddin A. Pictorial review: MRI of chronic spinal cord injury. *Br J Radiol.* 2003;76(905):347–352.

can be associated with vertebral body infarction in adults, with high signal and enhancement of the adjacent disk, owing to the common vascularization of the vertebral body, disk, and spinal cord. Hemorrhagic transformation may occur. The uncommon posterior spinal artery infarction manifests clinically as posterior cord syndrome, is typically unilateral due to the paired posterior spinal arteries, and limited to the posterior columns.[21]

Review Questions

1. The imaging modality of choice to detect spine fractures in a trauma patient with suspected spinal cord injury is:
   a. Magnetic resonance imaging (MRI)
   b. Computed tomography (CT)
   c. Plain radiography
   d. Digital subtraction angiography (DSA)
2. Which of the following is the MRI sequence that best detects acute ischemia in the brain and spinal cord, but has had limited use in spinal cord imaging until recent advances?
   a. T2-weighted
   b. T1-weighted
   c. STIR
   d. DWI

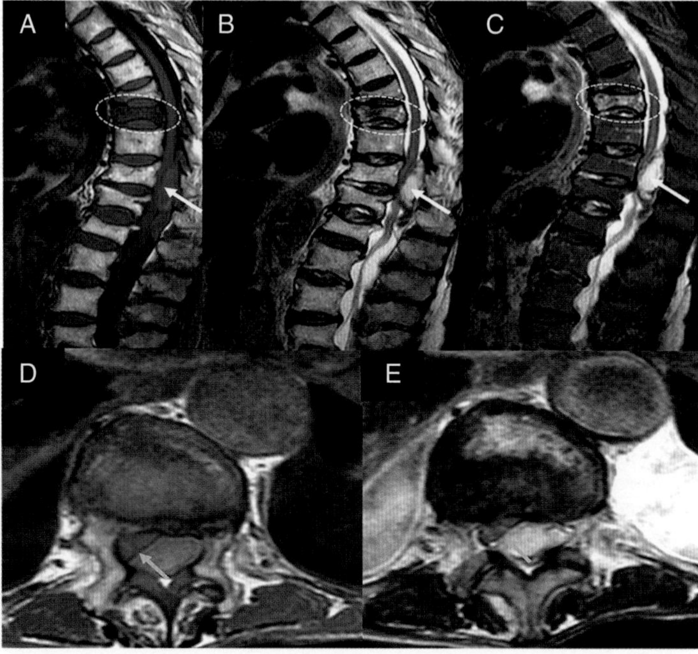

Fig. 8.4 Epidural Hematoma. Sagittal T1 (A), T2 (B), short tau inversion recovery (STIR) (C) magnetic resonance images showing multiple thoracic vertebral fractures and a posterior epidural fluid collection *(arrow)* extending from T9 to T11. Axial T1 (D) and T2 (E) weighted magnetic resonance images further illustrate this, with anterolateral displacement of spinal cord *(orange arrow)*. The T7 vertebra *(dotted circle)* is characterized by diffuse bone edema, suggesting recent fracture. Adapted from: Romano N, Castaldi A. What's around the spinal cord? Imaging features of extramedullary diseases. *Clin Imaging.* 2020;60(1):109–122.

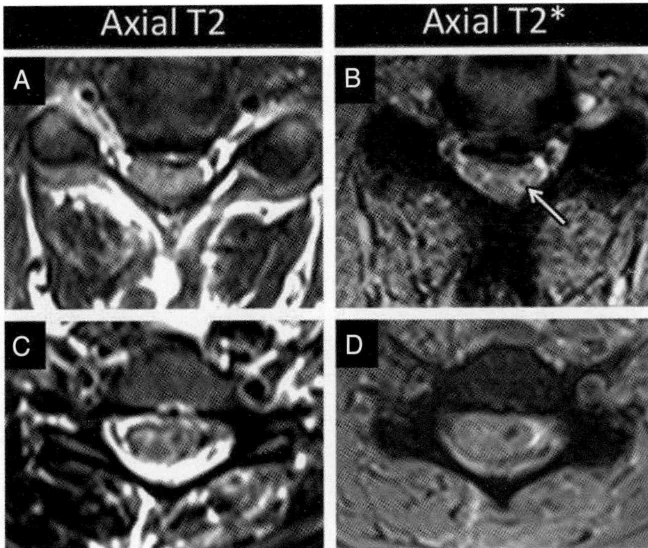

Fig. 8.5 T2-Weighted (T2W) and T2*-Weighted (T2*W) Imaging for Hemorrhage Detection. (A) Axial T2W image at epicenter of acute spinal cord injury shows subtle centromedullary T2 hyperintensity and no hypointense hemorrhage. Axial T2*W image at the same axial level (B) shows a punctate hypointense focus of hemorrhage in the left lateral cord (*white arrow*). This was not seen on the axial T2W image. (C) Axial T2W and (D) axial T2*W images from a different patient both demonstrate hypointense hemorrhage within the left frontal horn of the spinal cord, although hemorrhage is more conspicuous in the T2*W image (D). Adapted from: Talbott JF, Huie JR, Ferguson AR, Bresnahan JC, Beattie MS, Dhall SS. MR imaging for assessing injury severity and prognosis in acute traumatic spinal cord injury. *Radiol Clin North Am*. 2019;57(2):319–339.

Table 8.4 Magnetic Resonance Imaging Appearance of Hemorrhage

Stage	Age	T1 Signal Intensity	T2 Signal Intensity
Hyper-acute	<1 day	Isointense	Slightly hyperintense
Acute	1–3 days	Slightly hypointense	Hypointense
Early subacute	3–7 days	Hyperintense	Hypointense
Late subacute	7–14 days	Hyperintense	Hyperintense
Chronic	>14 days	Slightly hypointense	Hypointense

From Romano N, Castaldi A. What's around the spinal cord? Imaging features of extramedullary diseases. *Clin Imaging.* 2020;60(1):109–122; Pierce JL, Donahue JH, Nacey NC, Quirk CR, Perry MT, Faulconer N, et al. Spinal hematomas: what a radiologist needs to know. *Radiographics.* 2018;38(5):1516–1535.

3. Which of the following is hyperintense on T1-weighted MRI?
   a. Subacute early spinal cord hemorrhage
   b. Syringomyelia
   c. Spinal cord edema
   d. Demyelination
4. What can give the “owl eye sign” on T2-weighted axial imaging?
   a. Posterior column demyelination
   b. Spinal cord swelling
   c. Anterior spinal artery infarction
   d. Subdural hemorrhage
5. Which of the following MRI findings on T2 sagittal images have been associated with poor outcomes after traumatic spinal cord injury?
   a. Intramedullary hemorrhage
   b. Longer lesion length
   c. Cord transection
   d. All of the above

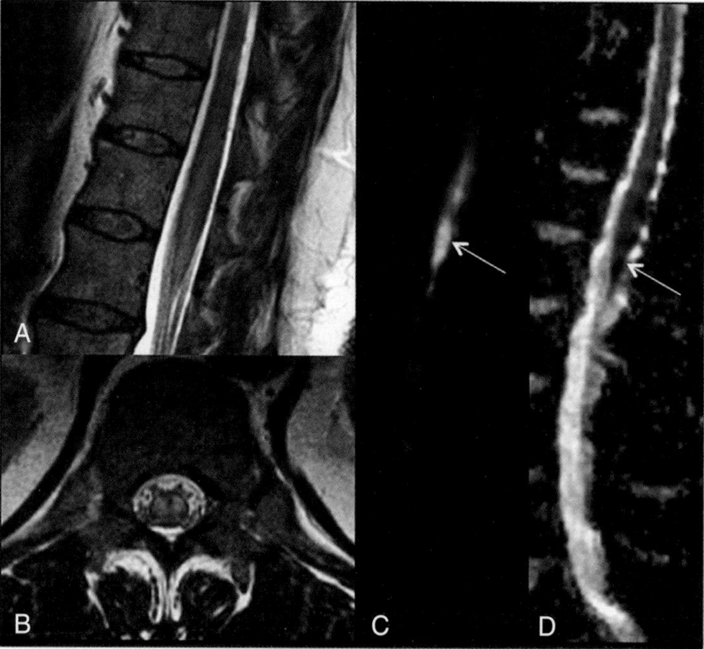

Fig. 8.6 Spinal Cord Infarction. Sudden paraparesis in a patient after aortic intervention. Sagittal and axial T2WI (A,B), sagittal diffusion-weighted imaging (C) and apparent diffusion coefficient map (D) show a slightly hyperintense area (A,B) with diffusion-restriction *(arrows)*, involving the anterior columns of the conus medullaris, consistent with spinal cord ischemia. Note the "owl's eye sign" (B) with infarction of the anterior gray horns. Adapted from: Sarbu N, Lolli V, Smirniotopoulos JG. Magnetic resonance imaging in myelopathy: a pictorial review. *Clin Imaging*. 2019;57:56–68.

REFERENCES

1. Sliker CW. Blunt cerebrovascular injuries: imaging with multidetector CT angiography. *Radiographics*. 2008;28(6):1689–1708, discussion 1709-1710.
2. Crim JR, Tripp D. Multidetector CT of the spine. *Semin Ultrasound CT MR*. 2004;25(1):55–66.
3. Ellingson BM, Salamon N, Holly LT. Imaging techniques in spinal cord injury. *World Neurosurg*. 2014;82(6):1351–1358.
4. Goldberg AL, Kershah SM. Advances in imaging of vertebral and spinal cord injury. *J Spinal Cord Med*. 2010;33(2):105–116.
5. Vargas MI, Delattre BMA, Boto J, et al. Advanced magnetic resonance imaging (MRI) techniques of the spine and spinal cord in children and adults. *Insights Imaging*. 2018;9(4):549–557.
6. Nuñez Jr. DB, Quencer RM. The role of helical CT in the assessment of cervical spine injuries. *AJR Am J Roentgenol*. 1998;171(4):951–957.
7. Mann FA, Cohen WA, Linnau KF, Hallam DK, Blackmore CC. Evidence-based approach to using CT in spinal trauma. *Eur J Radiol*. 2003;48(1):39–48.
8. Crim JR, Moore K, Brodke D. Clearance of the cervical spine in multitrauma patients: the role of advanced imaging. *Semin Ultrasound CT MR*. 2001;22(4):283–305.
9. Pinto A, Berritto D, Russo A, Riccitiello F, Caruso M, Belfiore MP, et al. Traumatic fractures in adults: missed diagnosis on plain radiographs in the Emergency Department. *Acta Biomed*. 2018;89(1-S):111–123.
10. Dreizin D, Letzing M, Sliker CW, Chokshi FH, Bodanapally U, Mirvis SE, et al. Multidetector CT of blunt cervical spine trauma in adults. *Radiographics*. 2014;34(7):1842–1865.
11. Parizel PM, van der Zijden T, Gaudino S, et al. Trauma of the spine and spinal cord: imaging strategies. *Eur Spine J*. 2010;19(Suppl 1):S8–S17.
12. Bozzo A, Marcoux J, Radhakrishna M, Pelletier J, Goulet B. The role of magnetic resonance imaging in the management of acute spinal cord injury. *J Neurotrauma*. 2011;28(8):1401–1411.
13. Fehlings MG, Martin AR, Tetreault LA, et al. A clinical practice guideline for the management of patients with acute spinal cord injury: recommendations on the role of baseline magnetic resonance imaging in clinical decision making and outcome prediction. *Global Spine J*. 2017;7(3 Suppl):221S–230S.
14. Utz M, Khan S, O'Connor D, Meyers S. MDCT and MRI evaluation of cervical spine trauma. *Insights Imaging*. 2014;5(1):67–75.
15. Lammertse D, Dungan D, Dreisbach J, Falci S, Flanders A, Marino R, et al. Neuroimaging in traumatic spinal cord injury: an evidence-based review for clinical practice and research. *J Spinal Cord Med*. 2007;30(3):205–214.
16. Winslow 3rd JE, Hensberry R, Bozeman WP, Hill KD, Miller PR. Risk of thoracolumbar fractures doubled in victims of motor vehicle collisions with cervical spine fractures. *J Trauma*. 2006;61(3):686–687.
17. Consortium for Spinal Cord Medicine Early acute management in adults with spinal cord injury: a clinical practice guideline for health-care professionals. *J Spinal Cord Med*. 2008;31(4):403–479.
18. Mueller CA, Peters I, Podlogar M, et al. Vertebral artery injuries following cervical spine trauma: a prospective observational study. *Eur Spine J*. 2011;20(12):2202–2209.
19. Alblas CL, Bouvy WH, Lycklama ANGJ, Boiten J. Acute spinal-cord ischemia: evolution of MRI findings. *J Clin Neurol*. 2012;8(3):218–223.
20. Grassner L, Klausner F, Wagner M, et al. Acute and chronic evolution of MRI findings in a case of posterior spinal cord ischemia. *Spinal Cord*. 2014;52(Suppl 1):S23–S24.
21. Vargas MI, Gariani J, Sztajzel R, et al. Spinal cord ischemia: practical imaging tips, pearls, and pitfalls. *AJNR Am J Neuroradiol*. 2015;36(5):825–830.

CHAPTER 9

Electrodiagnostics in Spinal Cord Injury

Lindsay A. Smith, Derek Bui, David R. Schulze, Ryan A. Smith, and Anne Nastasi

OUTLINE

Introduction

Spinal cord injury (SCI) assessment is best performed using physical examination and radiological findings (radiography, computed tomography [CT], magnetic resonance imaging [MRI]). Physical examination and imaging modalities can assess the level and extent of SCI. Electrodiagnostics (EDX) is not a commonly used clinical tool in SCI due to the lack of standardized use and reporting of electrodiagnostic data.[1] Adding electrodiagnostics to the SCI workup, particularly in clinical research, may provide additional information regarding the type and degree of SCI and aid in estimating neural recovery and prognosis.[2–4] However, there are certain clinical scenarios in which the utility of electrodiagnostic studies is appreciated and affects the clinical care of patients.

This chapter will highlight important electrodiagnostic information related to SCI:

- Differentiating brachial plexopathy from cervical root avulsions in SCI patients
- Importance of EDX in confirming motor neuron disease and differentiating motor neuron disease from central stenosis with myelopathy
- Situations in which somatosensory evoked potentials (SSEPs) can aid in diagnosis and prognostication
- Use of EDX to evaluate for appropriateness of diaphragmatic pacing in SCI
- Use of EDX to help diagnose and specify urinary dysfunction type in SCI patients

Electrodiagnostics Background

An understanding of spinal cord anatomy and the peripheral nervous system is essential to the use of electrodiagnostics in SCI evaluations.[5] Spinal cord gray matter consists of densely concentrated neuronal cell bodies and is surrounded by heavily myelinated white matter.[6]

Motor Signaling

The ventral (anterior) spinal cord contains alpha motor neurons and anterior horn cells (AHCs), whose axons transmit signals for voluntary movement from the brain to the muscles.[5]

- AHC cell bodies are located *inside* the spinal cord in the gray matter.[6]
- A motor unit is made up of an AHC body, axon, and terminal branches and the muscle fibers they innervate.[5]
- The neuromuscular junction (NMJ) is a specialized synapse between the terminal branch of an AHC axon and its corresponding muscle fiber's motor endplate.[7]
- A single AHC may innervate around 200 to over 1600 muscle fibers.
- When an AHC fires, all affiliated NMJs *simultaneously* depolarize, causing muscle contraction.

Sensory Signaling

The dorsal (posterior) spinal cord contains fibers that transmit sensory signals to the brain.

- The cell bodies of peripheral sensory fibers are located in the dorsal root ganglion (DRG) *outside* the spinal cord.[6]
- The DRG's location outside the spinal cord facilitates faster signaling from the peripheral sensory nerves.

At each spinal cord segment, somatic motor and sensory axons exit the spinal cord in a spinal nerve root.[5]

- A myotome is the distribution of muscles innervated by the motor axons of a single spinal cord segment.
- A dermatome is the distribution of skin innervated by the sensory axons of a single spinal cord segment.
- Myotomes and dermatomes are fundamental to performing and interpreting electrodiagnostic tests.

Electrodiagnostic Fundamentals

- Given the wide range of SCI etiologies, injury patterns, and presentations, there are no pathognomonic EDX findings for diagnosing SCI.
- EDX is primarily useful for excluding other neuropathologies, particularly radiculopathies, plexopathies, and peripheral neuropathies.

Common Electrodiagnostics Studies

- Nerve conduction studies (NCS)[5]
  - NCS assess spinal nerve root and peripheral nerve integrity by measuring *conduction velocity*, *distal latency*, and *amplitude* of a peripheral motor, sensory, or mixed nerve action potential.
  - Conduction velocity and distal latency are particularly useful to evaluate a peripheral nerve's myelination.
  - Amplitude indicates the number of axons that can be stimulated and the range of conduction velocities among axons.
  - Motor NCS:
    - A motor nerve is stimulated with an electrical impulse to the skin at two points along its course.
    - Compound muscle action potential (CMAP) amplitude is recorded in millivolts (mV).
    - Low CMAP amplitudes are caused by peripheral nerve pathology and nonneurologic etiologies (muscle fiber or NMJ disease).
  - Sensory NCS:
    - A sensory nerve is stimulated with an electrical impulse to the skin at one point along its course.
    - Sensory nerve action potential (SNAP) amplitude is recorded in microvolts (μV).
    - Low SNAP amplitudes are caused only by peripheral nervous system pathology (peripheral nerve fibers, DRG pathology).
  - Special tests, including F-wave and H-reflex testing:
    - H-reflex is a spinal monosynaptic reflex in response to increasingly stronger stimulations of a mixed nerve. In adults with spasticity and in young children, H-waves are elicitable from many peripheral nerves. In neurologically healthy adults, H-waves are only obtainable in a select few limb muscles.[5]
    - F-wave is a variation of NCS that assesses only motor axons and their AHC within the spinal cord. It excludes sensory portions of the peripheral nervous system.[5]
- Needle Electromyography
  - Needle electromyography (EMG), also called needle electrode examination, is performed using needle stimulation of skeletal (voluntary) limb and paraspinal muscles. EMG complements the motor and sensory NCS.
  - Three phases of muscle activation are observed to assess the entire motor unit (AHCs to muscle fibers).[5]
    - Insertion Phase: While the muscle is at rest, a needle recording electrode is advanced into the muscle, and insertional (electrical) activity is observed. Myotonic discharges suggest myopathy.
    - Rest Phase: While the muscle is at rest and the needle is already inserted, electrical activity is observed.
      - *Fibrillation potentials* ("fibs") are small, abnormal potentials produced by a single denervated muscle fiber, suggestive of upper motor neuron (UMN), lower motor neuron (LMN), myopathic, or NMJ pathology.
      - *Fasciculation potentials* are larger abnormal potentials produced by partial or entire motor units. These are often caused by focal chronic demyelination.
        - Fasciculation and fibrillation potentials demonstrate that although the motor unit is irritated, it remains intact.
      - *Complex repetitive discharges* (CRDs) are abnormal potentials produced by repetitive firing of a muscle fiber group with primary and secondary pacemakers. Etiologies include neurologic or myopathic disorders present for 6+ months.
    - Motor unit action potential (MUAP) Phase: While the needle is inserted, the patient voluntarily contracts (activates) the muscle being investigated. MUAPs are examined for firing frequency, stability on repeat firing, amplitude, duration, and internal configuration (shape) such as polyphasicity and serrations.
      - The presence of fewer MUAPs and a faster firing rate (>10 Hz) due to reduced MUAP recruitment is pathognomonic for LMN injury (AHC body, or axon destruction, or demyelinating conduction block).
      - The presence of fewer MUAPs and a slow-to-moderate firing rate (<10 Hz) is

suggestive of UMN lesions, pain-limited recruitment, or malingering (voluntary incomplete activation).
- Polyphasic and serrated MUAPs suggest chronic neurogenic changes with reinnervation.

Electrodiagnostic Findings in Spinal Cord Injury:[5]

- EDX findings superior to the neurologic level of injury (NLI): normal
- EDX findings at the NLI:
  - AHC or primary motor root destruction results in lower CMAP amplitudes on motor NCS and unelicitable F-waves and H-reflexes, consistent with a LMN injury pattern *at that level.*
  - The duration of the lesion matters. Initially, after SCI, CMAP amplitudes will be low. Chronically, axons of surviving AHC may reinnervate denervated muscle fibers, which can restore CMAP amplitudes to normal range.
  - Needle EMG performed a few months after SCI may demonstrate reduced MUAP recruitment and polyphasics suggestive of reinnervation by axonal sprouting.
  - Unless the DRG (recall that this is outside the spinal cord) or distal nerve is damaged, the sensory NCS for nerves derived from the spinal level will be normal.
- EDX findings inferior to the NLI:
  - AHCs below the NLI demonstrate an UMN injury pattern.
  - Sensory NCS is normal.
  - Motor NCS demonstrates low CMAP amplitudes in small muscles but normal CMAP amplitudes in large muscles (deltoid, quadriceps, tibialis anterior).
  - Needle EMG shows incomplete MUAP activation, which is observed as absent or few MUAPs with decreased firing rate.

Somatosensory Evoked Potentials

Another electrodiagnostic method that is used to clinically monitor neurologic function is SSEPs. SSEPs are action potentials of afferent peripheral nerves that are generated by tactile or electrical stimuli. SSEPs are primarily useful for localizing a neurologic lesion along somatosensory dorsal column pathways. SSEPs have a wide range of recording locations from distal dermatomes to proximal peripheral nerves, the spinal cord, and brain.

In traumatic cervical spine injuries, intact sensory levels have been localized using segmental SSEPs.[8] In the acute period after a traumatic SCI, it may be difficult to determine the relative completeness of the injury with SSEP alone. SSEP scalp recordings following a complete SCI will have an absent signal below the NLI. However, even with incomplete lesions it may not be possible to measure cortical response to stimulation below the NLI.[9] Despite this, SSEPs may offer some prognostic value following SCI. If responses are preserved below the NLI, this indicates an incomplete lesion, which has more favorable long-term functional outcomes.[9–12]

While potentially beneficial for prognosis, studies comparing SSEP and the standardized American Spinal Injury Association examination have shown comparable accuracy at predicting outcomes after SCI. However, in the following situations, SSEP evaluation may offer an advantage in the acute period after injury:

- If the patient is unable to participate in the physical exam (e.g., unresponsive, agitated), using SSEP measurements may provide useful information about the extent of the injury and expected recovery.[3,13]
- During the spinal shock phase, SSEP measurements are unlikely to be affected, unlike the physical examination.[11]

Evaluating for Comorbid Brachial Plexopathy

Polytrauma patients who suffer from traumatic SCI may concurrently injure the brachial plexus and have a brachial plexopathy or cervical root avulsion. While the physical exam and MRI findings may help differentiate these conditions, electrodiagnostics can confirm the diagnosis and provide additional information to help guide important management.

Understanding the physical examination and radiological findings can help guide which specific nerves and muscles to test in the EDX study. As a result, the physician can then localize the lesion in the brachial plexus.

- Sensory NCS is useful for determining whether a lesion is preganglionic or postganglionic (proximal or distal to the DRG). All sensory nerve fibers in the brachial plexus are postganglionic. Motor NCS is therefore less useful than sensory NCS in distinguishing between brachial plexopathy, radiculopathy, and SCI.[14,15]
  - Brachial plexus lesions result in a decreased SNAP in the corresponding nerves affected by the trunk or cord lesion.
  - The contralateral side can be tested if the symptomatic side's SNAPs are slightly decreased or normal; greater than 50% side-to-side amplitude difference indicates an abnormal value.
  - Motor NCS are helpful to exclude multiple entrapment neuropathies that can mimic a brachial plexopathy.

  - The CMAP may be decreased in the corresponding nerve that is distal to the trunk or cord lesion.
- EMG can evaluate the severity of the lesion.[14,15]
  - At the minimum, a physician should sample at least one muscle from the peripheral nerve distribution and muscles innervated by the same nerve but different root.[14,15]
  - Proximal muscles must be tested to determine root or preganglionic lesions. Muscles such as the paraspinals, rhomboid, and serratus anterior receive innervation from the roots; therefore they will exhibit abnormal EMG findings if the root is affected.
  - Surgical consultation should be considered if there is absence of CMAP, lack of MUAP during recruitment, or presence of profuse denervation.

Evaluating for Motor Neuron Disease Versus Cervical Myelopathy

EDX is a key tool for diagnosing amyotrophic lateral sclerosis (ALS), the most common motor neuron disease. Also known as Lou Gehrig's Disease, ALS is a progressive, sporadic, degenerative disorder that affects both UMN and LMN function. While ALS is the most well-known motor neuron disease and carries with it one of the worst prognoses, it is not the only one. Thus, it is key to find ways to correctly differentiate ALS from other motor neuron diseases. This is where EDX studies shine. They are key tools to help exclude other conditions, many of which are possibly treatable, that can appear like ALS. Yet, the electrodiagnostic study alone is not enough to diagnose ALS. The diagnosis is still one made clinically but supported by the EDX exam.

ALS typically affects patients in their late 50s and tends to affect males more than females. It is a progressive disorder that is somewhat specific for the motor system, with it being uncommon to see sensory findings or complaints on examination.[14,15] The initial signs of ALS include muscle cramps, atrophy, weakness, and fasciculations. Patients may also present with hyperreflexia, positive Babinski sign, slow movement, and stiffness. This disease frequently starts in one segment of the body and progresses to additional myotomes, often beginning with weakness in one limb. To diagnose ALS, both UMN and LMN signs must be seen in two regions of the body. For a definitive diagnosis of ALS, positive signs must be seen in three or more body regions: craniobulbar, cervical, thoracic, and lumbosacral.

Motor neuron diseases may be divided into several categories based on their suspected origin.[14,15]

- Genetic: familial amyotrophic lateral sclerosis, Kugelberg-Welander syndrome, Kennedy disease, distal spinal muscular atrophy, and hexosaminidase A deficiency
- Infectious: poliomyelitis, postpolio syndrome, retroviral-associated syndromes, and West Nile encephalitis
- Idiopathic: monomelic amyotrophy and amyotrophic lateral sclerosis (and its known variants), progressive bulbar palsy, primary lateral sclerosis, and progressive muscular atrophy

Several other conditions can mimic motor neuron disease, including cervical and lumbar lesions, lead poisoning, postirradiation syndromes, lymphoma, and immune-mediated demyelinating motor neuropathies.

Cervical and lumbar stenosis often lead to myelopathy, which can present similarly to motor neuron disease. Degenerative disease of the neck and the back are more common in older populations. When cervical and lumbar spondylosis occur simultaneously, the presentation may mimic ALS. For example, Cervical cord compression classically causes gait disturbance and can present with LMN dysfunction in the upper extremities and UMN dysfunction in the lower extremities. If spinal compression occurs above C5, UMN signs may be seen in the upper extremities. These findings, combined with lumbar stenosis, can present with LMN signs in the lumbosacral myotome. When viewed together, this presentation resembles ALS. In such cases, EMG can be very helpful to evaluate the bulbar and thoracic paraspinals, which should not be abnormal in lesions restricted to the cervical or the lumbar spine.[14,15]

Diaphragmatic Pacing

Patients with cervical SCI may suffer from pulmonary compromise and require noninvasive or invasive ventilation. Diaphragmatic pacing with artificial phrenic nerve stimulation can prevent or liberate patients from mechanical ventilation.[16]

- A diaphragmatic pacer is implanted via surgical procedure. Stimulation sites include the neck, chest, or diaphragm.
- A patient must have an intact phrenic nerve to be considered for pacing. Thus, electrodiagnostic evaluation is integral to evaluating a patient's candidacy.
- Contraindications to consider include external pacemaker, internal jugular catheter, implanted cardiac pacemaker, and nearby cardioverter-defibrillator.
- Diaphragmatic pacers are not MRI compatible.

The phrenic nerve nucleus is located in the anterior spinal cord and receives innervation from C3, C4, and C5. Patients with a high-level cervical SCI (above C3) will likely have an intact phrenic nerve and therefore be eligible for diaphragmatic pacing.

- Phrenic NCS under fluoroscopy assesses for phrenic nerve integrity. During the study, the phrenic nerve is stimulated.

- Presence of a CMAP response suggests an intact phrenic nerve.[17] The CMAP amplitude may be low in cases of damage to the nerve nucleus or axon, depending on the level or location of injury.[18]
- If there is no CMAP response, EMG detection of MUAPs may suggest a functioning phrenic nerve, which may or may not respond to pacing.[19,20]

Urodynamic Studies

Most incomplete and all complete SCI patients require assistance with bladder function.[21] Depending on the level of injury, the disrupted interaction between the central and peripheral nervous systems causes specific patterns of urinary dysfunction. Specifically, a lesion located between the pontine micturition center and sacral spinal cord can result in simultaneous external urethral sphincter contraction and detrusor contraction.[22] This condition, known as detrusor sphincter dyssynergia (DSD), can increase bladder pressure and vesicoureteral reflux, resulting in urinary tract infections, kidney injury, and autonomic dysreflexia.

DSD is typically diagnosed by clinical history of a known or potential UMN lesion and abnormal voiding phase during urodynamic studies.[23] Such studies can include voiding cystourethrogram, urethral profile pressure, and electromyography.[24]

DSD on EMG demonstrates increased detrusor muscle action potential activity in the absence of Valsalva and Credé maneuvers. In addition to the diagnosis, EMG can further characterize DSD subtypes to help guide treatment:[22]

- Type 1: Progressive increase in external urethral sphincter contraction that peaks at maximal detrusor contraction, followed by sudden relaxation of the external urethral sphincter as the detrusor pressure declines to allow urination
- Type 2: Clonic contractions of the external urethral sphincter that occur intermittently during detrusor contraction, causing an intermittent urinary stream
- Type 3: Continuous external urethral sphincter contraction throughout detrusor contraction, resulting in urinary obstruction

Other types of neurogenic bladder include bladder flaccidity, detrusor hyperactivity, and sphincter hyperactivity.

Review Questions

1. A 44-year-old right-handed male is referred for electrodiagnostic evaluation. The patient reports pain and paresthesias in the right upper extremity that started after a motorcycle accident 4 months ago. He localizes the symptoms to the medial forearm but also associates hand weakness. You perform the physical exam and begin to suspect a lower trunk brachial plexopathy. Muscles innervated by which of the following peripheral nerves would you expect to show abnormalities on EMG?
   a. Median
   b. Ulnar
   c. Radial
   d. All of the above
2. For the patient above, NCS demonstrates that SNAP and CMAP amplitudes are very low in the C8–T1 distribution. Additionally, EMG demonstrates fibrillations and sharps in muscles innervated by C8–T1. The cervical paraspinals demonstrate sharps and fibrillations. What is the most likely diagnosis?
   a. Cervical radiculopathy
   b. Cervical radiculopathy with carpal tunnel and cubital tunnel syndrome
   c. C8–T1 cervical root avulsion
   d. Lower trunk brachial plexopathy
3. Which of the following is a motor neuron disease with a significant genetic component?
   a. West Nile encephalitis
   b. Distal spinal muscular atrophy
   c. Monomelic amyotrophy
   d. Progressive bulbar palsy
4. Which of the following is true of electrodiagnostic studies in SCI patients?
   a. EMG study can be useful in determining the extent of intraspinal injury because voluntary muscle contraction is not required.
   b. Electrodiagnostic studies are important for patient selection and stratification for clinical trials.
   c. Electrodiagnostics are very commonly used clinically for prognosis because it is an objective extension of the physical exam.
   d. EMG can be used to accurately localize a thoracic spinal level injury and is low risk.
5. Which spinal levels can be fully examined with EMG?
   a. C3–S2
   b. C4–C8 and L2–S1
   c. C2–L5
   d. C5–T1 and L3–S1 (because these innervate limb muscles)
6. Which of the following statements about electrodiagnostic studies is FALSE?
   a. Compound motor action potential (CMAP) amplitude indicates the number of axons that can be stimulated and the range of conduction velocities among axons.
   b. The cell bodies of peripheral sensory fibers are located in the dorsal root ganglion (DRG) outside the spinal cord.
   c. A single anterior horn cell innervates a single muscle fiber.
   d. Complex repetitive discharges (CRDs) are abnormal EMG potentials produced by neurologic or myopathic disorders present for 6+ months.

REFERENCES

1. Korupolu R, Stampas A, Singh M, Zhou P, Francisco G. Electrophysiological outcome measures in spinal cord injury clinical trials: a systematic review. *Top Spinal Cord Inj Rehabil.* 2019;25(4):340–354. Fall.
2. Zakrasek EC, Jaramillo JP, Lateva ZC, Punj V, Kiratli BJ, McGill KC. Quantitative electrodiagnostic patterns of damage and recovery after spinal cord injury: a pilot study. *Spinal Cord Ser Cases.* 2019 Dec 12;5:101.
3. Curt A, Dietz V. Electrophysiological recordings in patients with spinal cord injury: significance for predicting outcome. *Spinal Cord.* 1999 Mar;37(3):157–165.
4. Hubli M, Kramer JLK, Jutzeler CR, et al. Application of electrophysiological measures in spinal cord injury clinical trials: a narrative review. *Spinal Cord.* 2019 Nov;57(11): 909–923.
5. Wilbourn AJ, Shields Jr. RW. The electrodiagnostic examination in spinal cord disorders. In: Lin VW, ed. *Spinal Cord Medicine Principles and Practice.* 2nd ed. New York: Demos Medical Publishing; 2010.
6. Mercadante AA, Tadi P. Neuroanatomy, gray matter. [Updated 2020 Jul 31]. In: *StatPearls [Internet].* Treasure Island (FL): StatPearls Publishing; 2021 Jan. https://www.ncbi.nlm.nih.gov/books/NBK553239/.
7. Omar A, Marwaha K, Bollu PC. Physiology, neuromuscular junction. [Updated 2021 May 9]. In: *StatPearls [Internet].* Treasure Island (FL): StatPearls Publishing; 2021 Jan. https://www.ncbi.nlm.nih.gov/books/NBK470413/.
8. Louis AA, Gupta P, Perkash I. Localization of sensory levels in traumatic quadriplegia by segmental somatosensory evoked potentials. *Electroencephalogr Clin Neurophysiol.* 1985 Jul;62(4):313–316.
9. Cruccu G, Aminoff MJ, Curio G, et al. Recommendations for the clinical use of somatosensory-evoked potentials. *Clin Neurophysiol.* 2008 Aug;119(8):1705–1719.
10. Jacobs SR, Yeaney NK, Herbison GJ, Ditunno Jr. JF. Future ambulation prognosis as predicted by somatosensory evoked potentials in motor complete and incomplete quadriplegia. *Arch Phys Med Rehabil.* 1995 Jul;76(7):635–641.
11. Kirshblum SC, O'Connor KC. Predicting neurologic recovery in traumatic cervical spinal cord injury. *Arch Phys Med Rehabil.* 1998 Nov;79(11):1456–1466.
12. Sedgwick EM, el-Negamy E, Frankel H. Spinal cord potentials in traumatic paraplegia and quadriplegia. *J Neurol Neurosurg Psychiatry.* 1980 Sep;43(9):823–830.
13. Li C, Houlden DA, Rowed DW. Somatosensory evoked potentials and neurological grades as predictors of outcome in acute spinal cord injury. *J Neurosurg.* 1990 Apr;72(4):600–609.
14. Preston DC, Shapiro BE. *Electromyography and Neuromuscular Disorders Clinical-Electrophysiologic Correlations.* 2nd ed. Philadelphia: Butterworth-Heinemann; 2005:138–139.
15. Preston DC, Shapiro BE. *Electromyography and Neuromuscular Disorders.* 2nd ed. Elsevier; 2020.
16. Elefteriades JA, Quin JA, Hogan JF, et al. Long-term follow-up of pacing of the conditioned diaphragm in quadriplegia. *Pacing Clin Electrophysiol.* 2002 Jun;25(6):897–906.
17. Alshekhlee A, Onders RP, Syed TU, Elmo M, Katirji B. Phrenic nerve conduction studies in spinal cord injury: applications for diaphragmatic pacing. *Muscle Nerve.* 2008 Dec;38(6):1546–1552.
18. Dalal K, DiMarco AF. Diaphragmatic pacing in spinal cord injury. *Phys Med Rehabil Clin N Am.* 2014 Aug;25(3):619–629, viii.
19. Strakowski JA, Pease WS, Johnson EW. Phrenic nerve stimulation in the evaluation of ventilator-dependent individuals with C4- and C5-level spinal cord injury. *Am J Phys Med Rehabil.* 2007 Feb;86(2):153–157.
20. Skalsky AJ, Lesser DJ, McDonald CM. Evaluation of phrenic nerve and diaphragm function with peripheral nerve stimulation and M-mode ultrasonography in potential pediatric phrenic nerve or diaphragm pacing candidates. *Phys Med Rehabil Clin N Am.* 2015 Feb;26(1):133–143.
21. McKinley WO, Jackson AB, Cardenas DD, DeVivo MJ. Long-term medical complications after traumatic spinal cord injury: a regional model systems analysis. *Arch Phys Med Rehabil.* 1999 Nov;80(11):1402–1410.
22. Bacsu CD, Chan L, Tse V. Diagnosing detrusor sphincter dyssynergia in the neurological patient. *BJU Int.* 2012 Apr;109(Suppl 3):31–34.
23. Spettel S, Kalorin C, De E. Combined diagnostic modalities improve detection of detrusor external sphincter dyssynergia. *ISRN Obstet Gynecol.* 2011;2011:323421.
24. Stoffel JT. Detrusor sphincter dyssynergia: a review of physiology, diagnosis, and treatment strategies. *Transl Androl Urol.* 2016 Feb;5(1):127–135.

CHAPTER

10 Functional Assessments

Justin Foley, Nicholas Gavern, Justin Provo, Elizabeth York, Andrea T. Aguirre, and Venessa A. Lee

OUTLINE

Overview

Functional assessments are tools used in both clinical practice and research to quantify how much a person's function deviates from normal. For these assessments "normal" can be considered a patient's preinjury status or the level of functioning that would be expected for patients without disabilities. In regard to spinal cord injury (SCI), they help determine the degree of difficulty in performing day-to-day activities that may be due to physical, cognitive, or emotional impairments. Additionally, they help set functional goals for a patient and monitor a patient's progress throughout rehabilitation.[1]

Functional Independence Measure

The functional independence measure (FIM) is a widely popular tool that quantifies a patient's physical, psychological, and social function as it focuses on the burden of care. The two primary categories are motor (13 items) and cognitive–communication (7 items). All items are measured on a 7-point scale (1 = total assist; 7 = complete independence) with higher scores indicating greater independence (Fig. 10.1). The FIM is used during inpatient rehabilitation to track progress from admission to discharge.[2,3]

- Cognitive–communication items are rarely utilized and FIM is primarily used to quantify gross motor ability rather than burden of care.[4]
- Motor subscale is most relevant for SCI patients, but FIM does not capture improvement in high-level tetraplegic patients due to the way the motor category is scored. Overall, it is insensitive for the SCI population.[4,5]
- Spinal cord independence measure (SCIM), quadriplegia index of function, and tetraplegia hand activity questionnaire are likely better choices more specific to higher-level SCI patients.[3–5]

Functional Independence Measure–Locomotor

The functional independence measure–locomotor (FIM-L) is a subset of the FIM and is primarily helpful in populations with significantly impaired ambulation. The FIM-L investigates the burden of care in the patient's primary mode of locomotion (walking or wheelchair). Scored by a trained observer, values are based on a combination of assistive device use, distance traveled, and assistance provided by others. Similar to the FIM, the FIM-L is scored on a 7-point scale (1 = total assist; 7 = independent without equipment) with higher scores indicating greater independence. Traditionally, the FIM-L is the most applicable portion of the FIM for SCI patients.

- FIM-L scores have been shown to be insensitive and inaccurate in predicting outcomes and tracking rehabilitation progress in SCI patients.
- The test is useful when assessing assistance needed to ambulate, but not overall ambulatory capacity.[6,7]
- The 10-minute walk test, walking index for SCI, and 6-minute walk test are more useful tools in evaluating overall ambulation following SCI.[7]

Functional Independence Measure Instrument

LEVELS		
	Independence 7—Complete independence (no helper, no setup, no device) 6—Modified independence (device, extra time, safety)	NO HELPER
	Modified Dependence 5—Supervision (standby assist, setup) 4—Minimal assist (patient = 75%+) 3—Moderate assist (patient = 50% to 74%)	HELPER NEEDED
	Complete Dependence 2—Maximal assist (patient = 25% to 49%) 1—Total assist (patient = less than 25%)	

DOMAINS	
	Self-Care Eating Grooming *Bathing Dressing: upper body Dressing: lower body Toileting
	Sphincter Control Bladder management Bowel management
	Transfers Bed, chair, wheelchair Toilet Tub, shower
	Locomotion Walk/wheelchair Stairs
	Motor Subtotal Rating **Communication** Comprehension Expression
	Social Cognition Social interaction Problem solving Memory ***Cognitive Subtotal Rating***

Fig. 10.1 Functional Independence Measure Instrument. (From Annaswamy TM, Houtrow A, Deepthi S, Yang W. Quality and outcome measures for medical rehabilitation. In: Cifu DX. *Braddom's Physical Medicine & Rehabilitation*. 5th ed. Philadelphia: Elsevier; 2016:121.)

Activity Outcome Measurement for Postacute Care

The activity outcome measurement for postacute care (AM-PAC) is designed as a conceptually grounded system for comprehensive outcome assessment across postacute care settings. Outcome measures were based on the activity domains of the international classification of functioning, and developed into a three-dimensional model of functional activity: the applied cognition, personal care & instrumental, and physical & movement. It can be completed by a trained therapist or by patient survey.

In the inpatient rehabilitation setting, therapists typically use the "6 Click" shortened version. Each domain has six activities where therapists rank how much difficulty a patient has performing each task; unable, a lot of difficulty, a little difficulty, and no difficulty. These correspond to an assigned point system, 1–4 respectively, with a total score ranging from 6–24.[8]

Walking Index for Spinal Cord Injury

The walking index for spinal cord injury (WISCI/WISCI II) measure is a standardized functional capacity assessment of improvements in walking in patients with acute and chronic SCI. It was developed as a research tool in clinical trials to assess improvement in walking by 24 SCI experts in walking function from eight countries, who established and agreed on a hierarchical ranking of 20 items. The WISCI II has not been assessed for validity and reliability in patients under the age of 18.

The WISCI takes into consideration the level of assistance needed in walking, as well as use of assistive devices and braces, in ambulation of a standard 10-m distance. Assistive devices are arranged in a hierarchy that correlates with the overall score, from parallel bars to use of a cane. Scores range from 0–20, with 0 being unable to stand or participate in assistive walking, and 20 being ambulation without any assistance or assistive devices.[9]

Spinal Cord Independence Measure

The spinal cord independence measure (SCIM) is a comprehensive functional rating scale developed to enhance the sensitivity of functional assessments in patients with tetra- and paraplegia. In addition to assessing ability, SCIM defines quantitative goals for functional restoration of primary daily activities. SCIM items are scored by observing the patient performing a task and choosing the score most compatible with the patient's performance from those listed in the SCIM evaluation sheet next to the scoring criterion definition.[10]

The SCIM covers 19 activities of daily living tasks, which are divided into three areas of function.[11]

- The self-care domain is scored from 0–20, and includes feeding, bathing, dressing, and grooming.
- The respiration and sphincter management domain is scored from 0–40, and includes respiration, bowel, bladder, and use of toilet.
- The mobility domain is also scored from 0–40, and assesses bed mobility, transfers from bed to wheelchair, and transfers from wheelchair to toilet/tub.

The domains of each subscale were determined by a consensus of experienced professionals to enable unidimensionality of SCIM subdivisions.[12] Each area is scored according to its proportional weight in these patients' general activity, and range from 0–100.

Spinal Cord Injury–Functional Index

The spinal cord injury-functional index (SCI-FI) is a series of patient-reported outcome measures designed specifically for SCI patients with a goal to better assess SCI specific function. It was developed across seven SCI model system centers, item banks generated by literature review, clinician focus groups, and patient input. The initial study group utilized applied factor analysis and item response theory to generate five functional domains.[13] These domains help assess an individual's functional level with more sensitivity than traditional generic functional assessments.[14] Testing utilizes computerized adaptive testing or paper in both short and long form, with versions for both tetraplegic and paraplegic individuals to help alleviate measurement challenges typically found in the SCI patient population[15] (Table 10.1).

International Standards of Neurological Classification of Spinal Cord Injury

The international standards of neurological classification of spinal cord injury (ISNCSCI) is a measure that uses key motor and sensory exam components to determine the neurologic level of injury and severity of injury as described by the American Spinal Injury Association (ASIA) impairment scale (AIS). This measure is the gold standard for diagnosis and prognosis of spinal cord injuries.[16–18]

- Widely used tool that is highly recommended by SCI evaluation database to guide effectiveness (EDGE) task force and other systematic reviews.[17,18]
- Results are used by rehabilitation teams to set functional goals for patients.[18]

Table 10.1 Spinal Cord Injury–Functional Index (SCI-FI)

SCI-FI Domain	Measurement
Basic Mobility	54-item bank assessing body positioning, transfers, carrying objects, and mobility in different locations.
Self-Care	90-item bank assessing bathing, grooming, bowel and bladder management, UE and LE dressing and feeding.
Fine Motor	36-item bank assessing tasks requiring fine motor control.
Ambulation	39-item bank assessing ability to perform walking activities at varying speeds, surfaces (level, uneven, stairs), and other conditions.
Wheelchair Mobility	56-item bank assessing ability to operate manual or power wheelchair in a variety of situations/conditions.

Upper Extremity
Lower Extremity

Spinal Cord Ability Ruler

The spinal cord ability ruler (SCAR) is a new measure focused on "volitional performance," which is defined as "voluntary task-specific physical actions contributing to independence in [activities of daily living] ADLs." This assessment combines select items from ISNCSCI and SCIM assessments with a new scoring system that utilizes a standardization formula (Rasch analysis). The measure is recorded as 0–100 points for each item (100 = fully achieved/independence; 0 = not achieved/dependent) and helps measure severity of SCI from initial injury until 1 year post injury.[19,20]

- The SCAR assessment is not fully clinically validated, but is a promising new tool.[20,21]
- It can be used retrospectively if ISNCSCI and SCIM were previously recorded.
- It does not work well for patients with central cord syndromes.[19]

Tetraplegia Hand Activity Questionnaire

The tetraplegia hand activity questionnaire (THAQ) is designed to assess arm and hand function in persons with tetraplegia using a questionnaire with 153 items related to nine groups of activities (self-care, dressing, continence, mobility, eating/drinking, work, leisure, household tasks, and miscellaneous).

Scoring is on a 2–3 point scale and is based on the respondent's ratings. Lower scores indicate greater independence.[22]

- Ability to perform the activity: 0 = without difficulty to 3 = help from others needed.
- Importance of performing the activity independently: 0 = not important to 2 = very important.
- Use of an aid: 0 = never to 3 = always.

Some experts (SCI EDGE Task Force) state that the THAQ is not recommended to be used in the inpatient setting as exposure to out of facility activities is required.[23,24] Additionally, there are no reliability studies in the SCI population. However, an expert panel found activities in the tool to be relevant and useful in tracking functional progress.[24]

Quadriplegia Index of Function

The quadriplegia index of function (QIF) is a functional assessment specifically designed to assess patients with tetraplegia. It was originally developed by the authors in 1980 because the popular Barthel index was deemed too insensitive to document the small but significant functional gains made by tetraplegics during medical rehabilitation. It assesses 10 activities of daily living, including transfers, grooming, bathing, dressing, feeding, mobility, bed activities, bowel program, bladder program, and understanding of personal care. Each category score is weighted to contribute a different percentage to the final score. Functional categories are scored from 0–180, and personal care from 0–20. The final score is then divided by 2 for a final score on a 100-point scale.[25]

Physical Activity Recall Assessment for People With Spinal Cord Injury

The physical activity recall assessment for people with spinal cord injury (PARA-SCI) was developed to measure the type, frequency, duration, and intensity of physical activity performed by persons with SCI who use a wheelchair as their primary mode of mobility. It can be used among people with paraplegia or tetraplegia, and is designed to capture three categories of physical activity: leisure time physical activity, lifestyle activity (activities that are part of one's daily routine), and cumulative activity. It aims to facilitate collection of epidemiologic data to develop health-promoting physical activity guidelines and interventions for patients with SCI.

Information is obtained from the patient in a 3-day-recall format, with each day divided into eight periods: morning routine, breakfast, morning, lunch, afternoon, dinner, evening, and evening routine. The morning and evening routines are further subdivided into transferring, bowel and bladder management, bathing, personal hygiene, and dressing. Participants also self-classify the intensity of activities into mild, moderate, or heavy classification.[26]

Other Assessments

Berg Balance Scale

- The Berg balance scale (BBS) is a 14-item inventory that assesses a patient's risk of falling. Each item is scored on a scale of 0–4, with the highest possible score being 56. The higher the score, the better the balance. Tasks range from sitting in a chair to standing on one leg.[27] This scale was initially created for elderly individuals, and is best utilized in individuals with incomplete SCI who are somewhat ambulatory.[28]

Graded Redefined Assessment of Strength Sensibility and Prehension

- Graded redefined assessment of strength sensibility and prehension (GRASSP) is a multidimensional assessment developed to detect change in upper extremity ability in individuals with tetraplegia. This assessment includes measurements of strength, sensation, and both qualitative and quantitative prehension.[29]

Jebsen-Taylor Hand Function Test

- The Jebsen-Taylor hand function test is a scale utilized to objectively measure hand functions that are commonly utilized during activities of daily living (ADLs). It assesses hand dexterity by using seven timed subtests, including writing, stacking, moving both light and heavy objects, and simulated feeding.[30]

Van Lieshout Test of Hand Function

- The Van Lieshout hand function test (VLT) is a 19-item assessment utilized in individuals with tetraplegia to measure the quality of hand and arm functioning in ADLs. This test provides information about how upper extremity tasks are carried out, which is helpful in the establishment of treatment goals.[31]

Ten-Meter Walk Test

- The 10-meter walk test assesses walking speed in meters per second over a short duration. It has been shown to be highly valid and reliable in detecting changes in walking speed in incomplete spinal cord injury patients who are less than 6 months postinjury.[32]

Timed Up and Go Test

- The timed up and go (TUG) test is an assessment of functional gait that measures the time (in seconds) for a patient to stand from a seated position, ambulate 3 meters, and return to and sit down in the chair.[33]

Barthel Index

- The Barthel index (BI) is a 10-item performance measure that assesses properties of ADLs and functional mobility in order to predict the ability of an individual to care for oneself. Items that are measured include feeding, grooming, bathing, dressing, bowel/bladder control, toileting, ambulation, and transfers.[34]

Needs Assessment Checklist

- The needs assessment checklist (NAC) is an assessment tool that addresses the rehabilitation needs of patients, taking into consideration a variety of factors ranging from bowel protocol, bladder management, skin care, psychological sequelae, and discharge coordination. The biopsychosocial framework through which this checklist addresses patient needs has rendered this checklist both an efficient and effective patient-centered tool for guiding SCI rehabilitation.[35]

Continuity Assessment Record and Evaluation

- The continuity assessment record and evaluation (CARE) is standardized patient assessment data set, including functional status at admission and discharge, and clinical data encompassing a variety of ADLs.[36]

Wheelchair Skills Test

- The wheelchair skills test (WST) is a 32-item instrument that is utilized for a comprehensive evaluation of manual wheelchair skills, measuring both safety and performance.[37]

Craig Handicap Assessment and Reporting Technique

- The Craig handicap assessment and reporting technique (CHART) aims to comprehensively measure handicap and assess for community integration by evaluating domains of physical independence, mobility, occupation, social integration, and economic self-sufficiency.[38]

Community Integration Questionnaire

- The community integration questionnaire (CIQ) is a 15-item measure that is utilized for assessing home integration, community integration, and productivity.[39]

Reintegration to Normal Living Index

- The reintegration to normal living (RNL) index measures daily activities as well as the patient's perception of self and relationships.[40]

Impact on Autonomy and Participation

- The impact on autonomy and participation (IPA) is a 32-item questionnaire that has five subscales to identify limitations to participation and autonomy. The subscales are: autonomy indoors, autonomy outdoors, social life, work/education, and role of family.[41]

Quality of Well-Being Scale

- The quality of well-being scale measures four domains (mobility, social activities, physical activities, and problematic symptoms) to assess health status and general well-being.[42]

Euro-Quality of Life

- The Euro-quality of life dimension is an instrument that aims to assess the quality of life for rehabilitation patients. It is a five-dimensional scale, that evaluates mobility, self-care, ADLs, pain, and mental health.[43]

Review Questions

1. As a physiatrist working in inpatient rehabilitation you need to track a spinal cord injury patient's progress from admission to discharge. Which functional assessment tool would be most beneficial for this task?
   a. Spinal cord injury–functional index (SCI-FI)
   b. Functional independence measure (FIM)
   c. Spinal cord ability ruler (SCAR)
   d. Functional independence measure–locomotor (FIM-L)
2. You are assessing the ambulation of a patient with a chronic spinal cord injury in your outpatient clinic. Which functional assessment would best quantify improvements in your patient's walking?
   a. Walking index for spinal cord injury (WISCI)
   b. Spinal cord ability ruler (SCAR)
   c. Functional independence measure–locomotor (FIM-L)
   d. Spinal cord independence measure (SCIM)
3. As part of a physiatry consult service, you are called to evaluate a patient with an acute spinal cord injury. Which functional assessment is the gold standard for diagnosis and prognosis of spinal cord injuries?
   a. Functional independence measure (FIM)
   b. Spinal cord injury–functional index (SCI-FI)
   c. International standards of neurological classification of SCI (ISNCSCI)
   d. Spinal cord independence measure (SCIM)
4. A patient with acute SCI is working on completing activities of daily living such as feeding, bathing, bed mobility, and bowel management. Which functional assessment scale can help set goals for functional restoration of primary daily activities?
   a. Spinal cord injury–functional index (SCI-FI)
   b. Spinal cord ability ruler (SCAR)
   c. Functional independence measure (FIM)
   d. Spinal cord independence measure (SCIM)
5. Your clinic patient with chronic SCI is hoping to improve their physical fitness. They use a wheelchair for mobility and are unsure if they are reaching

physical activity guidelines. Which functional assessment scale would best measure their physical activity?

a. Spinal cord ability ruler (SCAR)
b. Physical activity recall assessment for people with spinal cord injury (PARA-SCI)
c. Spinal cord injury–functional index (SCI-FI)
d. Functional independence measure–locomotor (FIM-L)

REFERENCES

1. Dijkers MPJ, Zanca JM. Functional assessment in spinal cord injury. In: Kirshblum S, Lin VW, eds. *Spinal Cord Medicine*. 3rd ed. New York: demosMedical; 2019:130–148.
2. Velstra IM, Ballert CS, Cieza A. A systematic literature review of outcome measures for upper extremity function using the international classification of functioning, disability, and health as reference. *PM&R*. 2011;3(9):846–860.
3. Rehabilitation Measures. Shirley Ryan AbilityLab. https://www.sralab.org/rehabilitation-measures/fimr-instrument-fim-fimr-trademark-uniform-data-system-fro-medical.
4. Anderson K, Aito S, Atkins M, et al. Functional recovery measures for spinal cord injury: an evidence-based review for clinical practice and research. *J Spinal Cord Medicine*. 2008;31(2):133–144.
5. Dawson J, Shamley D, Jamous MA. A structured review of outcome measures used for the assessment of rehabilitation interventions for spinal cord injury. *Spinal Cord*. 2008;46(12):768–780.
6. Jackson A, Carnel C, Ditunno J, et al. Outcome measures for gait and ambulation in the spinal cord injury population. *J Spinal Cord Medicine*. 2008;31(5):487–499.
7. Lam T, Noonan VK, Eng JJ. A systematic review of functional ambulation outcome measures in spinal cord injury. *Spinal Cord*. 2007;46(4):246–254.
8. Haley SM, Coster WJ, Andres PL, et al. Activity outcome measurement for postacute care. *Med Care*. 2004 Jan;42(1 Suppl):I49–I61.
9. Ditunno JF, Ditunno PL, Graziani V, et al. Walking index for spinal cord injury (WISCI): an international multicenter validity and reliability study. *Spinal Cord*. 2000;38(4):234–243.
10. Catz A, Itzkovich M. Spinal cord independence measure: comprehensive ability rating scale for the spinal cord lesion patient. *J Rehabil Res Dev*. 2007;44(1):65–68.
11. Catz A, Itzkovich M, Agranov E, Ring H, Tamir A. SCIM–spinal cord independence measure: a new disability scale for patients with spinal cord lesions. *Spinal Cord*. 1997 Dec;35(12):850–856.
12. Itzkovich M, Tripolski M, Zeilig G, et al. Rasch analysis of the Catz-Itzkovich spinal cord independence measure. *Spinal Cord*. 2002;40(8):396–407.
13. Jette AM, Slavin MD, Ni P, et al. Development and initial evaluation of the SCI-FI/AT. *J Spinal Cord Med*. 2015 May;38(3):409–418.
14. Tulsky DS, Jette AM, Kisala PA, et al. Spinal cord injury-functional index: item banks to measure physical functioning in individuals with spinal cord injury. *Arch Phys Med Rehabil*. 2012;93(10):1722–1732.
15. Fyffe D, Kalpakjian CZ, Slavin M, et al. Clinical interpretation of the Spinal Cord Injury Functional Index (SCI-FI). *J Spinal Cord Med*. 2016;39(5):527–534.
16. Furlan JC, Noonan V, Singh A, Fehlings MG. Assessment of impairment in patients with acute traumatic spinal cord injury: a systematic review of the literature. *J Neurotrauma*. 2011;28(8):1445–1477.
17. Rehabilitation Measures. Shirley Ryan AbilityLab. https://www.sralab.org/rehabilitation-measures/international-standards-neurological-classification-spinal-cord-injury-asia.
18. van Middendorp JJ, Goss B, Urquhart S, Atresh S, Williams RP, Schuetz M. Diagnosis and prognosis of traumatic spinal cord injury. *Global Spine J*. 2011;1(1):1–8. https://doi.org/10.1055/s-0031-1296049.
19. Reed R, Mehra M, Kirshblum S, et al. Spinal cord ability ruler: an interval scale to measure volitional performance after spinal cord injury. *Spinal Cord*. 2017 Aug;55(8):730–738.
20. Harvey LA. The spinal cord ability ruler (SCAR): combining aspects of two widely-used outcome measures into one. *Spinal Cord*. 2018;56(5):413.
21. Bach Jønsson A, Møller Thygesen M, Krogh S, Kasch H. Feasibility of predicting improvements in motor function following SCI using the SCAR outcome measure: a retrospective study. *Spinal Cord*. 2019;57(11):966–971.
22. Land NE, Odding E, Duivenvoorden HJ, Bergen MP, Stam HJ. Tetraplegia hand activity questionnaire (THAQ): the development, assessment of arm-hand function-related activities in tetraplegic patients with a spinal cord injury. *Spinal Cord*. 2004 May;42(5):294–301.
23. Kahn JH, Tappan R, Newman CP, et al. Outcome measure recommendations from the Spinal Cord Injury EDGE Task Force. *Phys Ther*. 2016;96(11):1832–1842.
24. Rehabilitation Measures. Shirley Ryan AbilityLab. https://www.sralab.org/rehabilitation-measures/tetraplegia-hand-activity-questionnaire.
25. Gresham GE, Labi ML, Dittmar SS, Hicks JT, Joyce SZ, Stehlik MA. The quadriplegia index of function (QIF): sensitivity and reliability demonstrated in a study of thirty quadriplegic patients. *Paraplegia*. 1986 Feb;24(1):38–44.
26. Ginis KA, Latimer AE, Hicks AL, Craven BC. Development and evaluation of an activity measure for people with spinal cord injury. *Med Sci Sports Exerc*. 2005 Jul;37(7):1099–1111.
27. Downs S. The Berg balance scale. *J Physiother*. 2015;61(1):46.
28. Wirz M, Müller R, Bastiaenen C. Falls in persons with spinal cord injury: validity and reliability of the Berg balance scale. *Neurorehabil Neural Repair*. 2010;24(1):70–77.
29. Marino RJ, Sinko R, Bryden A, et al. Comparison of responsiveness and minimal clinically important difference of the capabilities of upper extremity test (CUE-T) and the graded redefined assessment of strength, sensibility and prehension (GRASSP). *Top Spinal Cord Inj Rehabil*. 2018;24(3):227–238. Summer.
30. Panuccio F, Galeoto G, Marquez MA, et al. Internal consistency and validity of the Italian version of the Jebsen-Taylor hand function test (JTHFT-IT) in people with tetraplegia. *Spinal Cord*. 2021 Mar;59(3):266–273.
31. Berardi A, Biondillo A, Màrquez MA, et al. Validation of the short version of the Van Lieshout Test in an Italian population with cervical spinal cord injuries: a cross-sectional study. *Spinal Cord*. 2019;57(4):339–345.
32. Kahn J, Tefertiller C. Measurement characteristics and clinical utility of the 10-meter walk test among individuals with spinal cord injury. *Arch Phys Med Rehabil*. 2014;95(5):1011–1012.

33. van Hedel HJ, Wirz M, Dietz V. Assessing walking ability in subjects with spinal cord injury: validity and reliability of 3 walking tests. *Arch Phys Med Rehabil.* 2005;86(2): 190–196.
34. Barthel Index. Shirley Ryan AbilityLab. https://www.sralab.org/rehabilitation-measures/barthel-index.
35. Kennedy P, Smithson EF, Blakey LC. Planning and structuring spinal cord injury rehabilitation: the needs assessment checklist. *Top Spinal Cord Inj Rehabil.* 2012;18(2):135–137. Spring.
36. Deutsch A, Kline T, Kelleher C, et al. *Analysis of crosscutting Medicare functional status quality metrics using the continuity and assessment record and evaluation (CARE) item set.* ASPE, U.S. Dept. of Health and Human Services; 2012. https://aspe.hhs.gov/basic-report/analysis-crosscutting-medicare-functional-status-quality-metrics-using-continuity-and-assessment-record-and-evaluation-care-item-set.
37. Wheelchair Skills Test 4.1. Shirley Ryan AbilityLab. https://www.sralab.org/rehabilitation-measures/wheelchair-skills-test-41.
38. Hall K, Dijkers M, Whiteneck G, Brooks CA, Krause JS. The Craig handicap assessment and reporting technique (CHART): metric properties and scoring. *Top Spinal Cord Inj Rehabil.* 1998;4(1):16–30.
39. Kratz AL, Chadd E, Jensen MP, Kehn M, Kroll T. An examination of the psychometric properties of the community integration questionnaire (CIQ) in spinal cord injury. *J Spinal Cord Med.* 2015;38(4):446–455.
40. Hitzig SL, Romero Escobar EM, Noreau L, Craven BC. Validation of the reintegration to normal living index for community-dwelling persons with chronic spinal cord injury. *Arch Phys Med Rehabil.* 2012;93(1):108–114.
41. Piatt JA, Van Puymbroeck M, Zahl M, Rosenbluth JP, Wells MS. Examining how the perception of health can impact participation and autonomy among adults with spinal cord injury. *Top Spinal Cord Inj Rehabil.* 2016;22(3):165–172. Summer.
42. Quality of Well Being and Self-Administered Version. Shirley Ryan AbilityLab. https://www.sralab.org/rehabilitation-measures/quality-well-being-and-self-administered-version.
43. Balestroni G, Bertolotti G. EuroQol-5D (EQ-5D): an instrument for measuring quality of life. *Monaldi Arch Chest Dis.* 2012;78(3):155–159.

Outcomes After Traumatic Spinal Cord Injury

CHAPTER 11

Brittany Snider, Einat Engel-Haber, and Steven Kirshblum

OUTLINE

After traumatic spinal cord injury (SCI), an understanding of a person's anticipated neurological and functional recovery is essential, as this information often guides management decisions, discussions of prognosis, goal setting, and the formulation of individualized rehabilitation programs. Researchers must also consider expected natural recovery when designing an SCI clinical trial (i.e., determination of inclusion/exclusion criteria and outcome measures) and evaluating the effectiveness of a treatment or intervention.

Neurological Recovery

Prognostication of neurological outcomes following traumatic SCI depends on successful utilization of the International Standards for Neurological Classification of Spinal Cord Injury (ISNCSCI), in conjunction with the American Spinal Injury Association (ASIA) Impairment Scale (AIS). A large amount of data has been collected on longitudinal neurological recovery, and the most recent analyses have focused on studies published after 1992,[1] as this is when injury completeness was redefined based on the presence or absence of sacral sparing. The timing of the ISNCSCI examination may influence its predictive capabilities. In general, the literature has shown that the most reliable exams are performed from the 24-hour to 1 week post-injury period.[2] While the timing of the initial exam varies by study, most of the papers referenced below used a baseline exam within 30 days of injury (unless otherwise specified).

Conversion from a complete to incomplete injury is one of the most significant neurological outcomes. Between 20-30% of persons who are classified as having a complete (AIS A) injury on baseline exam will convert to incomplete status by 1 year.[2–6] Of these individuals, approximately 50% will become sensory incomplete (AIS B), and 50% will become motor incomplete (AIS C or D).[2–6] In general, persons with initial complete tetraplegia have a greater likelihood of converting to incomplete status than those with initial complete paraplegia.[2,3,7] Neurological recovery is observed most rapidly during the first 3 months after injury, and conversion after 1 year is less likely.[2] Conversion can occur in a small percentage of patients after 1 year.[8]

Between 20-40% of persons with AIS B grade (all levels) on initial exam will remain AIS B, approximately 10% will convert to AIS A, and up to 68% will improve to motor incomplete status by 1 year.[2,4–6,9] Between 65-85% of persons with initial AIS C will improve to AIS D/E, 10-20% remain AIS C, and a smaller percentage (~8%) regress to motor complete status by 1 year.[4–6,10] For those with initial AIS D SCI, roughly 100% will remain AIS D or improve to AIS E at 1 year.[6,10]

For individuals with initial AIS A tetraplegia, average motor score gains are approximately 8-12 points by 1 year.[2,3,10–16] Most of these gains are due to improvements in the upper extremity motor score (UEMS), although small improvements in the lower extremity motor score (LEMS) may also be seen (average 2-3 point improvement in LEMS by 6-12 months).[7,14] Approximately 60-70% of persons with initial complete tetraplegia will gain at least 1 motor level, and up to 30% will gain at least 2 motor levels.[14] Motor recovery is relatively limited in persons with complete paraplegia, most especially if above the level of T9, in part due to the lack of clinically testable myotomes in the thoracic region.[2,7,16-19] Lumbar level injuries have the greatest potential for motor recovery, while upper thoracic injuries have the lowest.[16,17,19–21] Most persons with initial complete thoracic level injuries have a motor score improvement of <5 points, with the greatest recovery in those with lesions at T10-12.[20]

There is variability in reported motor recovery for individuals with initial AIS B SCI,[2] with a mean motor score change ranging from 20-38 points for those with AIS B tetraplegia, and an average LEMS improvement of 13-23 points for persons with AIS B paraplegia, from initial assessment to follow up exam (6 months to 2 years after injury).[3,10,22] In general, persons with motor incomplete injuries have a greater prognosis for motor recovery than persons with motor complete lesions.[2] Mean improvement in motor scores for persons with motor incomplete tetraplegia is between 22-52 points from baseline exam to 1 year after injury.[2,3,7,10,11,14] For persons with initial motor incomplete paraplegia, mean change in LEMS ranges from 9-34 points in the first post-injury year.[2,3,7,10,11,14]

A number of studies have evaluated the effects of age on neurological recovery.[2] Various ages (i.e. >30 years,[7,23] >50 years,[24] >60 years,[25] and >65 years[26,27]) have been reported as negative predictors of recovery, although there continues to be debate about the best age cutoff. The literature is mixed, as results of several other studies failed to show significant differences in neurological outcomes, including AIS grade change and motor score improvement, between younger and older age groups.[28-30]

Penetrating injuries are more likely to result in complete injuries than blunt trauma.[10,31,32] There is evidence that persons with initial complete lesions caused by a penetrating injury have a lower likelihood of conversion to incomplete status than those with a complete injury caused by blunt trauma.[2]

Functional Recovery

Establishing functional goals is a key aspect of rehabilitation. This process should be individualized and include participation of the patient, caregivers, and interdisciplinary rehabilitation team. It is also important to differentiate between short- and long-term goals, set realistic timelines, and identify potential barriers to achieving functional independence. Functional progress is continually reviewed, and goals are updated throughout the patient's rehabilitation course.

Numerous factors may influence functional recovery following SCI. These include concomitant injuries, medical comorbidities/secondary complications, cognitive abilities, age, psychosocial factors, access to care and resources, and injury-specific characteristics. Motor level, injury completeness, and AIS grade are most useful in predicting functional outcomes. Tables 11.1 and 11.2 show expected functional outcomes (under optimal conditions) based on motor level at 1 year post-injury for persons with motor complete SCI.[33,34]

Upper Extremity Function

Among individuals with tetraplegia, regaining arm and hand function is the primary priority.[35,36] Beginning in the 1950s, estimation of functional capacity was based on injury level and severity.[37,38] Functional outcome tables (see example in Table 11.1) are commonly used to describe the expected functional outcomes (including eating, dressing, grooming, etc.) of individuals with motor complete SCI at various injury levels.[37] In addition to the AIS grade[39,40] and NLI,[37,41,42] several other components of the ISNCSCI have been utilized in prognostication of upper extremity function in tetraplegia, including motor level,[43,44] UEMS[40,43-45] and LEMS.[45] Both the UEMS and motor level have a superior correlation to self-care function in individuals with motor-complete tetraplegia, compared to NLI.[43] Additionally, a 2-motor level recovery in the upper extremity (over the course of a year) results in significantly improved Spinal Cord Independence Measure (SCIM) self-care scores compared with those recovering 1 or no motor levels.[46]

The Graded and Redefined Assessment of Strength, Sensibility, and Prehension (GRASSP) was developed as a quantitative outcome measure, specifically for upper limb function in tetraplegia.[35] Manual muscle testing and Semmes and Weinstein monofilament (SWM, tactile cutaneous sensation) are two of its subsets. Performance of these tests (and the manual muscle testing component in particular) at 16 – 40 days post injury has been found to accurately predict self-care and upper limb outcomes at 1 year, using the SCIM self-care subcategory and Quantitative Grasping (QtG), respectively.[47] The latter is another GRASSP subtest, used to measure performance of 6 task-oriented prehension skills.[47] The same group had also shown that a combination of muscle scores of the flexor digitorum profundus and anterior deltoid had the best prediction accuracy for prehension tasks (QtG), while a combination of elbow flexors, wrist extensors, extensor digitorum communis and flexor pollicis longus best predicted SCIM self-care outcomes.[44]

Ambulation

Regaining the ability to walk is a common and important functional goal for individuals with SCI.[48–50] Patients often ask their rehabilitation providers, "Will I walk again?" It is the responsibility of the SCI medicine specialist to predict a person's likelihood of achieving ambulation as well as to utilize this information when disclosing prognosis and helping to establish realistic functional goals. Prognosis for ambulation also has a significant role in rehabilitation, equipment, and discharge planning. Ambulation training during inpatient rehabilitation has benefits if an individual has a high likelihood of achieving ambulation at discharge.[51] However, for those who are unlikely to be functional ambulators at 1 year postinjury, ambulation training during inpatient rehabilitation has been associated with potential disadvantages, such as less training dedicated to transfers and wheelchair mobility and worse Craig handicap assessment and reporting technique (CHART) scores in the domains of physical independence, mobility, and occupation.[52]

With the exception of persons with lower level injuries (particularly L2 and below), those with an initial AIS A injury have a poor prognosis for ambulation recovery (~3%).[31] Individuals who remain neurologically complete and gain some walking function typically have low thoracic or lumbar level injuries and often require orthoses and gait aids.[31] A small percentage of individuals who convert to incomplete status may achieve functional recovery in the lower extremities.[5] The percentages of individuals with initial AIS grades B-D who regain walking ability at 1 year vary within

Table 11.1 Expected Functional Outcomes at 1 Year Postinjury for Persons With Motor Complete Tetraplegia[33,34]

Activity	C1–C4	C5	C6	C7	C8
Respiration	Dependent on ventilator (C4 > C3 may be able to breathe independently)	Reduced vital capacity and endurance; may require some assistance for secretion clearance			
Feeding	Dependent	Dependent for set-up, then independent with adaptive equipment	Dependent for cutting; independent with/without adaptive equipment after set-up	Independent with/without adaptive equipment	Independent
Grooming	Dependent	Dependent for set-up, then minimal assistance (with adaptive equipment)	Independent with adaptive equipment to some assistance	Independent with or without adaptive equipment	Independent
Upper body dressing	Dependent	Moderate assistance to dependent	Independent with adaptive equipment	Independent	Independent
Lower body dressing	Dependent	Dependent	Some assistance to independent with adaptive equipment	Independent with adaptive equipment	Independent with adaptive equipment
Bathing	Dependent	Dependent	Independent with upper body; some assistance to dependent with lower body	Independent with upper body; some assistance to independent with adaptive equipment for lower body	Independent with adaptive equipment
Bladder management	Dependent	Dependent	Moderate to maximal assistance	Independent to some assistance	Independent
Bowel management	Dependent	Dependent	Some assistance or dependent for set-up; independent with adaptive equipment for suppository insertion/digital stimulation	Some assistance or dependent for set-up; independent with adaptive equipment for suppository insertion/digital stimulation	Independent
Bed mobility	Dependent	Some assistance	Independent to some assistance	Independent to some assistance	Independent
Transfers	Dependent	Maximal assistance to dependent	Independent to some assistance for level transfers; some assistance to dependent for uneven transfers	Independent with or without transfer board for level transfers; independent to some assistance for uneven transfers	Independent with or without transfer board
Weight shifts	Dependent; independent with power wheelchair	Dependent; independent with power wheelchair	Independent with or without equipment	Independent	Independent
Wheelchair propulsion	Manual: dependent; Power: independent	Manual: independent with adaptations (i.e., push rims) on level surfaces; Power/power assist: independent	Manual: independent on level surfaces; Power and power assist: Independent	Manual: independent on level surfaces	Manual: independent
Transportation	Dependent	Independent with adapted van	Independent with adapted van	Independent with adapted van or car with hand controls	Independent with adapted van or car with hand controls

Table 11.2 Expected Functional Outcomes at 1 Year Postinjury for Persons With Motor Complete Paraplegia[33]

Activity	T1–T9	T10–L1	L2–S5
Feeding, grooming, dressing, bathing	Independent	Independent	Independent
Bladder/bowel management	Independent	Independent	Independent
Transfers	Independent with/without transfer board	Independent with/without transfer board	Independent
Wheelchair propulsion	Independent	Independent	Independent
Standing	Independent with standing frame	Independent with standing frame	Independent with/without standing frame
Ambulation	Not functional; for exercise with HKAFO/KAFO and walker/forearm crutches	Household ambulation, independent to some assistance with KAFO and forearm crutches/walker	Community ambulation, independent to some assistance with KAFO/AFO and forearm crutches/cane
Transportation	Independent with hand controls	Independent with hand controls	Independent with hand controls

Table modified from Paralyzed Veterans of America (PVA) Clinical Practice Guidelines for Health-Care Professionals, Outcomes Following Traumatic Spinal Cord Injury 1999. https://pva.org/research-resources/publications/clinical-practice-guidelines/.
AFO, ankle foot orthosis, *HKAFO*, Hip, knee, ankle, foot orthotic; *KAFO*, knee, ankle, foot orthotic.

the literature and depend on a variety of factors, including sensory preservation and age. Functional ambulation is achieved in up to 50% of persons with initial AIS B grade, 75% of individuals with initial AIS C injuries, and 95% of persons with initial AIS D grade.[33]

Due to the heterogeneity of SCI and the many factors that may influence walking ability (i.e., injury level and severity, demographic factors, comorbidities, medical complications, and access to healthcare/rehabilitation), determining a person's prognosis for ambulation can be challenging. A few algorithms have been created to predict recovery of ambulation.[53–55]

The most widely used model was published by van Middendorp et al.[54] and was developed using prospectively collected data from the European Multicenter Study about Spinal Cord Injury (EM-SCI). This prediction rule uses the patient's age and components of the ISNCSCI examination (completed within 15 days of injury) to determine the probability of independent indoor ambulation at 1 year. Independent indoor ambulation is defined by scores 4–8 on item 12 (ability to walk <10 m) on the SCIM. The prediction variables included in the final model are age (<65 years vs. ≥ 65 years), L3 motor score, S1 motor score, L3 light touch (LT) score, and S1 LT score. The highest motor and LT scores between the right and left sides are applied. This model was found to have high discriminatory ability and has been externally validated with several other datasets.[38–40] Hicks and colleagues[55] developed a simplified, 3-variable prediction model using age at injury (<65 years vs. ≥65 years), L3 motor score, and S1 LT score to predict the probability of ambulation at 1 year. This simplified model was also found to have high discriminatory ability.[55] These algorithms are associated with several challenges and limitations. For example, they do not incorporate some important clinical variables, such as medical comorbidities/secondary complications, body habitus, and psychosocial factors that may influence a person's potential for recovery. Dichotomization of age is another potential oversimplification. Additionally, the algorithm by van Middendorp et al.[54] and the 3-variable algorithm by Hicks et al.[55] were found to have lower predictive capabilities for individual AIS grades compared to a single cohort that combines all grades. Furthermore, there is lower predictive accuracy for AIS B + C subgroups compared to the AIS A + D subgroup.[56]

REFERENCE

1. American Spinal Injury Association. International Standards for Neurological and Functional Classification of Spinal Cord Injury. Chicago, IL: American Spinal Injury Association; 1992.
2. Kirshblum S, Snider B, Eren F, Guest J. Characterizing Natural Recovery after Traumatic Spinal Cord Injury. *J Neurotrauma [Internet]*. 2021;38(9):1267–1284. [cited 2022 Jun 19] Available from: https://pubmed.ncbi.nlm.nih.gov/33339474/.
3. Fawcett JW, Curt A, Steeves JD, Coleman WP, Tuszynski MH, Lammertse D, et al. Guidelines for the conduct of clinical trials for spinal cord injury as developed by the ICCP panel: Spontaneous recovery after spinal cord injury and statistical power needed for therapeutic clinical trials. *Spinal Cord.* 2007;45(3):190–205.
4. Spiess MR, Müller RM, Rupp R, Schuld C, Van Hedel HJA. Conversion in ASIA impairment scale during the first year after traumatic spinal cord injury. *J Neurotrauma [Internet]*. 2009;26(11):2027–2036. [cited 2022 Jun 26] Available from. https://pubmed.ncbi.nlm.nih.gov/19456213/.
5. Van Middendorp JJ, Hosman AJF, Pouw MH, Van De Meent H. ASIA impairment scale conversion in traumatic SCI: Is it related with the ability to walk? A descriptive comparison with functional ambulation outcome measures in 273 patients. *Spinal Cord.* 2009;47(7):555–560.
6. Kirshblum SC, Botticello AL, Dyson-Hudson TA, Byrne R, Marino RJ, Lammertse DP. Patterns of Sacral Sparing Components on Neurologic Recovery in Newly Injured Persons With Traumatic Spinal Cord Injury. *Arch Phys Med Rehabil.* 2016;97(10):1647–1655.

7. Coleman WP, Geisler FH. Injury severity as primary predictor of outcome in acute spinal cord injury: retrospective results from a large multicenter clinical trial. *Spine J [Internet]*. 2004;4(4):373–378. [cited 2022 Jun 19] Available from: https://pubmed.ncbi.nlm.nih.gov/15246294/.
8. Kirshblum S, Millis S, McKinley W, Tulsky D. Late neurologic recovery after traumatic spinal cord injury. *Arch Phys Med Rehabil [Internet]*. 2004 Nov [cited 2022 Jun 26];85(11):1811–1817. Available from: https://pubmed.ncbi.nlm.nih.gov/15520976/
9. Burns AS, Lee BS, Ditunno JF, Tessler A. Patient selection for clinical trials: the reliability of the early spinal cord injury examination. *J Neurotrauma [Internet]*. 2003;20(5):477–482. [cited 2022 Jun 26] Available from: https://pubmed.ncbi.nlm.nih.gov/12803979/.
10. Marino RJ, Ditunno JF, Donovan WH, Maynard F. Neurologic recovery after traumatic spinal cord injury: Data from the Model Spinal Cord Injury Systems. *Arch Phys Med Rehabil.* 1999;80:1391–1396.
11. Curt A, Van Hedel HJA, Klaus D, Dietz V. Recovery from a spinal cord injury: significance of compensation, neural plasticity, and repair. *J Neurotrauma [Internet]*. 2008;25(6):677–685. [cited 2022 Jun 26] Available from: https://pubmed.ncbi.nlm.nih.gov/18578636/.
12. Steeves JD, Kramer JK, Fawcett JW, Cragg J, Lammertse DP, Blight AR, et al. Extent of spontaneous motor recovery after traumatic cervical sensorimotor complete spinal cord injury. *Spinal Cord [Internet]*. 2011;49(2):257–265. [cited 2022 Jun 26] Available from: https://pubmed.ncbi.nlm.nih.gov/20714334/.
13. Waters RL, Adkins RH, Yakura JS, Sie I. Motor and sensory recovery following complete tetraplegia. *Arch Phys Med Rehabil [Internet]*. 1993;74(3):242–247. [cited 2022 Jun 26] Available from: https://pubmed.ncbi.nlm.nih.gov/8439249/.
14. Marino RJ, Burns S, Graves DE, Leiby BE, Kirshblum S, Lammertse DP. Upper- and Lower-Extremity Motor Recovery After Traumatic Cervical Spinal Cord Injury: An Update From the National Spinal Cord Injury Database. *Arch Phys Med Rehabil [Internet]*. 2011;92(3):369–375. [cited 2022 Jun 26] Available from: http://www.archives-pmr.org/article/S0003999310008208/fulltext.
15. Evaniew N, Sharifi B, Waheed Z, Fallah N, Ailon T, Dea N, et al. The influence of neurological examination timing within hours after acute traumatic spinal cord injuries: an observational study. *Spinal Cord [Internet]*. 2020;58(2):247–254. [cited 2022 Jun 26] Available from: https://pubmed.ncbi.nlm.nih.gov/31595042/.
16. Zariffa J, Kramer JLK, Fawcett JW, Lammertse DP, Blight AR, Guest J, et al. Characterization of neurological recovery following traumatic sensorimotor complete thoracic spinal cord injury. *Spinal Cord [Internet]*. 2011;49(3):463–471. [cited 2022 Jun 26] Available from: https://pubmed.ncbi.nlm.nih.gov/20938451/.
17. Lee BA, Leiby BE, Marino RJ. Neurological and functional recovery after thoracic spinal cord injury. *J Spinal Cord Med [Internet]*. 2016;39(1):67 [cited 2022 Jun 19] Available from: /pmc/articles/PMC4725794/.
18. Fisher CG, Noonan VK, Smith DE, Wing PC, Dvorak MF, Kwon B. Motor recovery, functional status, and health-related quality of life in patients with complete spinal cord injuries. *Spine (Phila Pa 1976) [Internet]*. 2005;30(19):2200–2207. [cited 2022 Jun 19] Available from: https://journals.lww.com/spinejournal/Fulltext/2005/10010/Motor_Recovery,_Functional_Status,_and.13.aspx.
19. Waters RL, Yakura JS, Adkins RH, Sie I. Recovery following complete paraplegia. *Arch Phys Med Rehabil.* 1992;73:784–789.
20. Aimetti AA, Kirshblum S, Curt A, Mobley J, Grossman RG, Guest JD. Natural history of neurological improvement following complete (AIS A) thoracic spinal cord injury across three registries to guide acute clinical trial design and interpretation. *Spinal Cord.* 2019;57(9):753–762.
21. Khorasanizadeh MH, Yousefifard M, Eskian M, Lu Y, Chalangari M, Harrop JS, et al. Neurological recovery following traumatic spinal cord injury: a systematic review and meta-analysis. *J Neurosurg Spine [Internet]*. 2019;30(5):683–699. [cited 2022 Jun 20] Available from: https://thejns.org/spine/view/journals/j-neurosurg-spine/30/5/article-p683.xml.
22. Kirshblum S, Botticello A, Benedetto J, Eren F, Donovan J, Marino R. Characterizing Natural Recovery of People With Initial Motor Complete Tetraplegia. *Arch Phys Med Rehabil [Internet]*. 2022;103(4):649–656. Available from: https://doi.org/10.1016/j.apmr.2021.09.018.
23. Bravo P, Labarta C, Alcaraz MA, Mendoza J, Verdú A. An assessment of factors affecting neurological recovery after spinal cord injury with vertebral fracture. *Paraplegia [Internet]*. 1996;34(3):164–166. [cited 2022 Jun 19] Available from: https://pubmed.ncbi.nlm.nih.gov/8668357/.
24. Scivoletto G, Morganti B, Molinari M. Neurologic recovery of spinal cord injury patients in Italy. *Arch Phys Med Rehabil [Internet]*. 2004 Mar 1 [cited 2022 Jun 19];85(3):485–489. Available from: http://www.archives-pmr.org/article/S0003999303007664/fulltext.
25. Dai LY. Acute central cervical cord injury: the effect of age upon prognosis. *Injury [Internet]*. 2001 Apr 1 [cited 2022 Jun 19];32(3):195–199. Available from: http://www.injuryjournal.com/article/S0020138300001765/fulltext.
26. Cifu DX, Seel RT, Kreutzer JS, McKinley WO. A multicenter investigation of age-related differences in lengths of stay, hospitalization charges, and outcomes for a matched tetraplegia sample. *Arch Phys Med Rehabil.* 1999;80(7):733–740.
27. Aito S, D'Andrea M, Werhagen L, Farsetti L, Cappelli S, Bandini B, et al. Neurological and functional outcome in traumatic central cord syndrome. *Spinal Cord.* 2007;45(4):292–297.
28. Harrop JS, Naroji S, Maltenfort MG, Ratliff JK, Tjoumakaris SI, Frank B, et al. Neurologic improvement after thoracic, thoracolumbar, and lumbar spinal cord (conus medullaris) injuries. *Spine (Phila Pa 1976) [Internet]*. 2011;36(1):21–25. [cited 2022 Jun 19] Available from: https://journals.lww.com/spinejournal/Fulltext/2011/01010/Neurologic_Improvement_After_Thoracic,.5.aspx.
29. Seel RT, Huang ME, Cifu DX, Kolakowsky-Hayner SA, McKinley WO. Age-Related Differences In Length Of Stays, Hospitalization Costs, And Outcomes For An Injury-Matched Sample Of Adults With Paraplegia. https://doi-org.proxy.libraries.rutgers.edu/101080/107902682001117535 81 *[Internet]*. 2016 [cited 2022 Jun 19];24(4):241–50. Available from: https://www-tandfonline-com.proxy.libraries.rutgers.edu/doi/abs/10.1080/10790268.2001.11753581.
30. Jakob W, Wirz M, Van Hedel HJA, Dietz V. Difficulty of elderly SCI subjects to translate motor recovery-"body function"-into daily living activities. *J Neurotrauma.* 2009;26(11):2037–2044.
31. Khorasanizadeh M, Yousefifard M, Eskian M, Lu Y, Chalangari M, Harrop JS, et al. Neurological recovery following traumatic spinal cord injury: a systematic review and

meta-analysis. *J Neurosurg Spine [Internet]*. 2019 Feb 15 [cited 2022 Jun 19];30(5):1–17. Available from: http://www.ncbi.nlm.nih.gov/pubmed/30771786.

32. Roach MJ, Chen Y, Kelly ML. Comparing Blunt and Penetrating Trauma in Spinal Cord Injury: Analysis of Long-Term Functional and Neurological Outcomes. *Top Spinal Cord Inj Rehabil [Internet]*. 2018 Mar [cited 2022 Jun 20];24(2):121–132. Available from: https://pubmed.ncbi.nlm.nih.gov/29706756.
33. Paralyzed Veterans of America (PVA) Clinical Practice Guidelines for Health-Care Professionals, Outcomes Following Traumatic Spinal Cord Injury 1999. https://pva.org/research-resources/publications/clinical-wpractice-guidelines/
34. Donovan J., Kirshblum S., Didesch M., McNiece M. Spinal cord medicine. In: Kirshblum S, Lin VW, eds. Spinal Cord Rehabilitation. 3rd ed. 2018;690-708.
35. Anderson KD. Targeting recovery: priorities of the spinal cord-injured population. *J Neurotrauma.* 2004;21(10):1371–1383.
36. Snoek GJ, Ijzerman MJ, Hermens HJ, Maxwell D, Biering-Sorensen F. Survey of the needs of patients with spinal cord injury: impact and priority for improvement in hand function in tetraplegics. *Spinal Cord [Internet]*. 2004;42(9):526–532. [cited 2022 Jun 25] Available from: https://pubmed.ncbi.nlm.nih.gov/15224087/.
37. Outcomes following traumatic spinal cord injury: Clinical practice guidelines for health-care professionals.
38. Long C, Lawton E. Functional significance of spinal cord lesion level. *Arch Phys Med Rehabil.* 1955;36(4):245–255.
39. Kalsi-Ryan S, Beaton D, Curt A, Popovic MR, Verrier MC, Fehlings MG. Outcome of the upper limb in cervical spinal cord injury: Profiles of recovery and insights for clinical studies. *J Spinal Cord Med [Internet]*. 2014;37(5):503 [cited 2022 Jun 25] Available from: /pmc/articles/PMC4166185/.
40. Carrasco-López C, Jimenez S, Mosqueda-Pozon MC, Pérez-Borrego YA, Alcobendas-Maestro M, Gallego-Izquierdo T, et al. New Insights from Clinical Assessment of Upper Extremities in Cervical Traumatic Spinal Cord Injury. *J Neurotrauma [Internet]*. 2016;33(18):1724–1727. [cited 2022 Jun 25] Available from: https://pubmed.ncbi.nlm.nih.gov/26936413/.
41. Welch R, Lobley S, O'Sullivan S, Freed M. Functional independence in quadriplegia: critical levels. *Arch Phys Med Rehabil.* 1986;67(4):235–240.
42. Zafonte RD, Demangone DA, Herbison GJ, Ditunno JF. Daily Self-Care in Quadriplegic Subjects. *Neuro Rehabilitation.* 1991;1(4):17–24.
43. Marino RJ, Ditunno JF, Foster DR, Maissel G. Superiority of motor level over single neurological level in categorizing tetraplegia. *Spinal Cord.* 1995;33(9):510–513. 339 *[Internet]*. 1995 [cited 2022 Jun 25]; Available from: https://www.nature.com/articles/sc1995111.
44. Velstra IM, Bolliger M, Krebs J, Rietman JS, Curt A. Predictive Value of Upper Limb Muscles and Grasp Patterns on Functional Outcome in Cervical Spinal Cord Injury. *Neurorehabil Neural Repair [Internet.* 2016;30(4):295–306. [cited 2022 Jun 25] Available from: https://pubmed.ncbi.nlm.nih.gov/26156192/.
45. Hayashi T, Kawano O, Sakai H, Ideta R, Ueta T, Maeda T, et al. The potential for functional recovery of upper extremity function following cervical spinal cord injury without major bone injury. *Spinal Cord [Internet]*. 2013;51(11):819–822. [cited 2022 Jun 25] Available from: https://pubmed.ncbi.nlm.nih.gov/24042986/.
46. Kramer JLK, Lammertse DP, Schubert M, Curt A, Steeves JD. Relationship between motor recovery and independence after sensorimotor-complete cervical spinal cord injury. *Neurorehabil Neural Repair [Internet]*. 2012;26(9):1064–1071. [cited 2022 Jun 25] Available from: https://journals.sagepub.com/doi/10.1177/1545968312447306?url_ver=Z39.88-2003&rfr_id=ori%3Arid%3Acrossref.org&rfr_dat=cr_pub++0pubmed.
47. Velstra IM, Bolliger M, Tanadini LG, Baumberger M, Abel R, Rietman JS, et al. Prediction and stratification of upper limb function and self-care in acute cervical spinal cord injury with the graded redefined assessment of strength, sensibility, and prehension (GRASSP). *Neurorehabil Neural Repair [Internet]*. 2014;28(7):632–642. [cited 2022 Jun 25] Available from: https://journals.sagepub.com/doi/10.1177/1545968314521695?url_ver=Z39.88-2003&rfr_id=ori%3Arid%3Acrossref.org&rfr_dat=cr_pub++0pubmed.
48. Simpson LA, Eng JJ, Hsieh JT. Wolfe and the Spinal Cord Injury Rehabilitation Evidence (SCIRE) research team DL. The health and life priorities of individuals with spinal cord injury: a systematic review. *J Neurotrauma.* 2012;29(8):1548–1555.
49. Scivoletto G, Tamburella F, Laurenza L, Torre M, Molinari M. Who is going to walk? A review of the factors influencing walking recovery after spinal cord injury. *Front Hum Neurosci.* 2014;8(MAR):1–11.
50. Ditunno PL, Patrick M, Stineman M, Ditunno JF. Who wants to walk? Preferences for recovery after SCI: a longitudinal and cross-sectional study. *Spinal Cord [Internet]*. 2008;46(7):500–506. [cited 2022 Jun 21] Available from: https://pubmed.ncbi.nlm.nih.gov/18209742/.
51. Donovan J, Snider B, Miller A, Kirshblum S. Walking after spinal cord injury: Current clinical approaches and future directions. *Proc EBC Congr.* 2020;8:149–158.
52. Rigot S, Worobey L, Boninger ML. Gait Training in Acute Spinal Cord Injury Rehabilitation—Utilization and Outcomes Among Nonambulatory Individuals: Findings From the SCIRehab Project. *Arch Phys Med Rehabil [Internet]*. 2018;99(8):1591–1598. [cited 2022 Jun 21] Available from: http://www.archives-pmr.org/article/S0003999318301515/fulltext.
53. Zorner B, Blanckenhorn WU, Dietz V, et al. Clinical algorithm for improved prediction of ambulation and patient stratification after incomplete spinal cord injury. *J Neurotrauma.* 2010;27:241–252.
54. van Middendorp JJ, Hosman AJ, Donders AR, et al. A clinical prediction rule for ambulation outcomes after traumatic spinal cord injury: a longitudinal cohort study. *Lancet.* 2011;377:1004–1010.
55. Hicks KE, Zhao Y, Fallah N, Rivers CS, Noonan VK, Plashkes T, et al. . A simplified clinical prediction rule for prognosticating independent walking after spinal cord injury: a prospective study from a Canadian multicenter spinal cord injury registry. *Spine J.* 2017;17(10):1383–1392.
56. Phan P, Budhram B, Zhang Q, Rivers CS, Noonan VK, Plashkes T, et al. Highlighting discrepancies in walking prediction accuracy for patients with traumatic spinal cord injury: an evaluation of validated prediction models using a Canadian Multicenter Spinal Cord Injury Registry. *Spine J [Internet]*. 2019;19(4):703–710. [cited 2022 Jun 22] Available from: https://pubmed.ncbi.nlm.nih.gov/30179672/.

CHAPTER 12

Cardiovascular Issues in Spinal Cord Injury: Neurogenic Shock, Spinal Shock, and Orthostatic Hypotension

William Carter

OUTLINE

Neurogenic shock, spinal shock, and orthostatic hypotension all have symptoms that begin around the onset of an acute spinal cord injury (SCI). The appropriate and timely diagnosis and treatment of these conditions are essential to acute care and rehabilitation plans, and are specifically needed to prevent complications and maximize assessment and functional outcomes.

Neurogenic Shock

Neurogenic or vasogenic shock, which occurs after acute SCI, is caused by hypotension from vasodilation and bradycardia, and is defined by a systolic blood pressure less than 100 mmHg with a heart rate less than 80 beats per minute.[1] It is caused by unopposed, cranial-based parasympathetic activity without the compensatory mechanisms from thoracic-derived, sympathetic output. Neurogenic shock classically occurs in injuries T6 and above, resulting from vasodilation of the large venous volume in the splanchnic vessels innervated by the mid-thoracic cord. In isolated traumatic SCI, 20% of those with cervical and 7% with thoracic or lumbar injuries present to the emergency room with neurogenic shock. The incidence for total hospital stay related to neurogenic shock may be as high as 50% in cervical injuries[2,3] and it typically lasts 1–3 weeks but can last as long as 6 weeks.[3,4]

Other perfusion-related types of shock include cardiogenic shock (due to heart problems), hypovolemic shock (caused by low blood volume), anaphylactic shock (caused by allergic reaction), and septic shock (due to infections). When investigating for perfusion-related shock, neurogenic shock is a diagnosis of exclusion and other types of shock must be ruled out first, especially in the setting of polytraumatic injuries. The initial management for neurogenic shock focuses on excluding hypovolemic shock through hemodynamic stabilization. Hypotension should be treated with intravenous fluid resuscitation to establish euvolemia and reduce the risk of secondary hypoperfusion injury. After euvolemia, if hypotension persists, vasopressors and inotropes can be considered.

When considering vasopressors, no single agent is superior, and caution must be taken regarding vasoconstrictive properties and the risk for secondary injury. It is recommended that mean arterial pressure (MAP) be kept at 85–90 mmHg for the first 7 days to improve spinal cord perfusion.[5–7] Phenylephrine is commonly used because of its pure alpha-1 agonist causing peripheral vasoconstriction; however, the lack of beta activity can lead to reflex bradycardia, which augments the already unopposed vagal tone. Norepinephrine has both alpha and beta activity, aiding both hypotension and bradycardia, thus it is often the preferred agent. Epinephrine has been cited for refractory cases of hypotension and is rarely needed.

Treatment for bradycardia includes atropine and glycopyrrolate to oppose vagal tone, especially before suctioning. Isoproterenol is considered for a pure chronotropic effect. Theophylline and aminophylline have been cited for refractory cases of bradycardia.[4]

Spinal Shock

Spinal shock is not defined by perfusion and should be separated from other shocks. It is defined as a temporary loss or depression of all or most spinal reflex activity below the level of the lesion and applies to all phenomena surrounding transection of the spinal cord. These phenomena include not only muscle spindle reflexes but also ejaculatory, vasomotor, sweating, bowel, and bladder. The suppression of these reflexes impacts rehabilitative management strategies, most notably for bowel and bladder. A proposed mechanism for spinal shock is presynaptic inhibition due to hyperpolarization of neurons, which effectively blocks monosynaptic and polysynaptic reflex arcs throughout the spinal cord.[8] In general, the more severe and acute the SCI, the more profound the state of spinal shock.[9,10] Thus it is less likely to be seen in slowly progressive compression or incomplete injuries, such as from cervical stenosis without major trauma.

Spinal shock may be delayed up to several hours after the onset of injury[9] and can persist for days to weeks. Prolongation may occur due to toxic or septic conditions, such as urinary tract infections or pressure sores. Muscle spindle reflexes always return and typically are caudal to cephalad. The end of the complete spinal shock phase is signaled by the return of elicitable abnormal cutaneospinal or muscle spindle reflex arcs.[10] Due to its caudal nature, the bulbocavernosus reflex is an early clinical sign for reemergence of reflexes. The result is always spasticity or hyperactive reflexes with abnormal spread to adjacent isolated spinal cord segments. Because autonomic function involves second-order neurons located in ganglia outside the spinal cord, the return of vasomotor tone, ejaculation, and sweating can be variable. The return of muscle spindle reflex activity and progression to spasticity are not indicators of the spinal shock "wearing off" but are hypothesized to be an active reorganization of receptors involving mechanisms of upregulation, enhanced sensitivity, increased number of receptors, or any combination of these (Table 12.1).[10]

Table 12.1 Comparison of Neurogenic and Spinal Shock

	Neurogenic Shock	Spinal Shock
Defined as	Systolic blood pressure less than 100 mmHg with a heart rate less than 80 beats per minute[1]	A state of transient physiologic (rather than anatomic) reflex depression of cord function below the level of injury, with associated loss of sensorimotor functions[19]
Caused by	Autonomic dysregulation[1]	Presynaptic inhibition from hyperpolarized neurons
Spinal cord injury level	Above T6	Any
Timing	Anytime from the onset of injury	Several hours after injury onset
Character	Systemic hypotension and bradycardia Respiratory insufficiency and pulmonary dysfunction Temperature dysregulation hypothermia; flushed, warm skin	Flaccid paralysis Anesthesia Areflexia or hyporeflexia
Duration	1–6 weeks[4]	Days to months
Managed by	Administering fluids and vasopressors with appropriate temperature monitoring[20]	Most often resolves on its own

Orthostatic Hypotension

Orthostatic hypotension (OH) is defined as a decrease in systolic blood pressure of more than 20 mmHg or decrease in diastolic blood pressure of more than 10 mmHg with upright posture. Symptoms may include weakness, dizziness, lightheadedness, blurred vision, syncope, dyspnea, and nausea.

In normal human physiology, upright posture creates pooling of blood in the lower extremities, which reduces blood return to the heart. Decreased blood return reduces cardiac output and lowers blood pressure, which results in the aortic and carotid sinus baroreceptors activating a sympathetic response from the rostral ventral medulla. This sympathetic response results in vasoconstriction and parasympathetic inhibition.[11]

With SCI, the excitatory descending sympathetic signals from the rostral ventral medulla cannot reach their peripheral targets. This results in failed vasoconstriction, impaired venous return to the heart, low resting blood pressure, and loss of blood pressure autoregulation. More proximal and complete SCIs are more likely to have OH.[12]

Several studies have documented the presence of OH following SCI,[13,14] which, unlike neurogenic and spinal shock, can persist years after the injury.[15,16] Standard mobilization during rehabilitation is reported to trigger blood pressure decreases that are diagnostic of OH in 74% of SCI patients, and cause symptoms of OH (e.g., lightheadedness or dizziness) in 59% of SCI individuals.[12] Thus, OH may discourage individuals with SCI from participating in rehabilitation. Management of OH consists of pharmacological and nonpharmacological interventions.

Unlike neurogenic and spinal shock, OH is not purely an SCI-mediated phenomenon and thus can be exacerbated and treated by other mechanisms (Table 12.2). Fluid status, prolonged time supine, hormones, prandial status, infection, medications, and other factors with impacting vasoconstrictive or cardiac chronicity may contribute to OH. Thus, etiology can be multifactorial, with clinical selection of treatments depending upon

Table 12.2 Factors Predisposing to Orthostatic Hypotension Following Spinal Cord Injury (SCI)[18,21–24]

Loss of sympathetic control
Altered baroreceptor sensitivity
Lack of skeletal muscle pumps
Cardiovascular deconditioning/ bedrest
Altered salt and water balance
Hyponatremia
High SCI lesion
Traumatic > nontraumatic SCI
Low plasma volume

Table 12.3 Pharmacologic and Nonpharmacologic Management of Orthostatic Hypotension

Pharmacologic	Nonpharmacologic
Midodrine	Prandial timing
Fludrocortisone	Compression stocking
Dihydroergotamine	Abdominal binder
Ephedrine	Whole body vibration[25]
L-threo-3,4-dihydroxyphe-nylserine	Functional electrical stimulation
Nitro-L-arginine methyl ester	Upright training (treadmill, standing frame)
Increase fluids	Physical activity
Increase salt intake	Head of bed elevation 10–20 degrees

context and risk/benefit ratios, few of which have been rigorously studied in SCI.[17] Midodrine has strong evidence supporting its use.[18] Other interventions, such as increases in fluid intake and a diet high in salt/sodium, have strong support for usage in idiopathic OH without SCI.[16] Elastic stocking and abdominal binders may improve cardiovascular responses during submaximal arm exercise.[18] Many other strategies (Table 12.3) may also be employed that are of anecdotal benefit.

Review Questions

1. A 42-year-old male patient is admitted with a SCI. The patient is experiencing severe hypotension and bradycardia. The patient is diagnosed with neurogenic shock. Why is hypotension occurring in this patient with neurogenic shock?
   a. The patient has an increased systemic vascular resistance. This increases preload and decreases afterload, which will cause severe hypotension.
   b. The patient's autonomic nervous system has lost the ability to regulate the diameter of the blood vessels, and vasodilation is occurring.
   c. The patient's parasympathetic nervous system is being unopposed by the sympathetic nervous system, which leads to severe hypotension.
   d. The increase in capillary permeability has depleted the fluid volume in the intravascular system, which has led to severe hypotension.
2. You receive a patient in the emergency room who has sustained a cervical SCI. You know this patient is at risk for neurogenic shock. What hallmark signs and symptoms, if experienced by this patient, would indicate the patient is experiencing neurogenic shock? Select all that apply:
   a. Blood pressure 69/38
   b. Heart rate 170 beats per minute
   c. Blood pressure 250/120
   d. Heart rate 29 beats per minute
   e. Warm and dry extremities
   f. Cool and clammy extremities
   g. Temperature 40 Celcius
   h. Temperature 35 Celcius
3. In neurogenic shock, a patient will experience a decrease in tissue perfusion. This deprives the cells that make up the tissues and organs of oxygen. Select all the mechanisms, in regard to pathophysiology, of why this is occurring:
   a. Loss of vasomotor tone
   b. Increase systemic vascular resistance
   c. Decrease in cardiac preload
   d. Increase in cardiac afterload
   e. Decrease in venous blood return to the heart
   f. Venous blood pooling in the extremities
4. A patient with neurogenic shock is experiencing a heart rate of 30 beats per minute. What medication needs to be ordered by the physician STAT? (See Question 8 for STAT example.)
   a. Adenosine
   b. Warfarin
   c. Atropine
   d. Norepinephrine
5. A 25-year-old male with trauma to the cervical spine presents to the emergency room with heart rate 40 and blood pressure (BP) 60/40. After a brief trauma assessment, what is your first intervention in treating these vital signs?
   a. Fluid resuscitation
   b. IV Norepinephrine
   c. IV Dopamine
   d. IV Epinephrine
   e. Abdominal binder & compression stockings
   f. Transcutaneous pacing
6. The cardiovascular consequences of neurogenic shock include:
   a. Hypertension, tachycardia, and hyperthermia
   b. Hypotension, bradycardia, and hypothermia
   c. Hypotension, tachycardia, and hyperthermia
   d. Hypertension, bradycardia, and hyperthermia

7. A person with complete thoracic SCI developed the following symptoms immediately after going from supine to sitting in bed: dizziness; fatigue; sweating; nausea; blurred vision; palpitations; headache; dyspnea; chest, neck, and shoulder pain; cognitive impairment; and syncope. How will you manage him?
   a. If the individual is supine, immediately make the patient sit.
   b. Make the patient lie down and check the BP; start intravenous fluids if necessary.
   c. Check for precipitating factors and start on oral hypotensives.
   d. Take electrocardiogram and get a cardiologist's opinion.
8. A 37-year-old IT consultant was involved in a bike vs. vehicle traffic accident. He was flung from his bike and landed 20 feet away. He was conscious and oriented but had severe pain in his upper back and abdomen. He was brought to hospital on a spine board. Evaluation revealed:
   - Pulse: 120 beats per minute, tongue dry
   - BP: 89/59 mmHg
   - Bulbocavernosus reflex was positive
   - Noted to be American Spinal Injury Association impairment scale A on neurological exam

   A computed tomography (CT) scan was done on the spine, which showed fracture dislocation at T3–T4 level. Hemoglobin was 9.6 g/dL and hematocrit was 34%. What is the most appropriate initial management?
   a. The patient should be managed for neurogenic shock, as this is common in injuries above T4 due to sympathetic disruption and unopposed vagal activity.
   b. A CT of the abdomen and chest should be done, and other causes of hypovolemic shock should be ruled out.
   c. Intravenous colloids should be started, as volume replacement is important.
   d. The patient should be closely observed, as neurogenic shock is transient and pulse and BP will gradually return to normal with time.
9. What is the definition of spinal shock?
   a. Injury to the spinal cord with associated autonomic dysregulation
   b. Temporary loss or depression of all or most spinal reflex activity below the level of the injury
   c. Loss of all reflexes and motor function with hypertension and tachycardia
   d. Severe drop in BP that results in highly abnormal problems with how cells work and produce energy
10. For better neurological outcome after an SCI, MAP should be maintained at what level for the first 7 days:
   a. 65–70 mmHg
   b. 75–80 mmHg
   c. 85–90 mmHg
   d. 90–95 mmHg

REFERENCES

1. Dave S, Cho JJ. Neurogenic shock. *In: StatPearls*. [Updated 2022 Feb 10]. StatPearls Publishing; 2021. https://www.ncbi.nlm.nih.gov/books/NBK459361/.
2. Guly HR, Bouamra O, Lecky FE. Trauma Audit and Research Network. The incidence of neurogenic shock in patients with isolated spinal cord injury in the emergency department. *Resuscitation*. 2008;76(1):57–62.
3. Fink MP, Newman MF, Fleisher LA. *Perioperative Medicine: Managing for Outcome*. Elsevier Health Sciences; 2007.
4. Casha S, Christie S. A systematic review of intensive cardiopulmonary management after spinal cord injury. *J Neurotrauma*. 2011;28(8):1479–1495.
5. Vale FL, Burns J, Jackson AB, Hadley MN. Combined medical and surgical treatment after acute spinal cord injury: results of a prospective pilot study to assess the merits of aggressive medical resuscitation and blood pressure management. *J Neurosurg*. 1997;87(2):239–246.
6. Yue JK, Tsolinas RE, Burke JF, et al. Vasopressor support in managing acute spinal cord injury: current knowledge. *J Neurosurg Sci*. 2019;63(3):308–317.
7. Furlan JC, Fehlings MG. Cardiovascular complications after acute spinal cord injury: pathophysiology, diagnosis, and management. *Neurosurg Focus*. 2008;25(5):E13.
8. Aisen ML, Brown W, Rubin M. Electrophysiologic changes in lumbar spinal cord after cervical cord injury. *Neurology*. 1992;42(3 Pt 1):623–626.
9. Christensen PB, Wermuth L, Hinge HH, Bømers K. Clinical course and long-term prognosis of acute transverse myelopathy. *Acta Neurol Scand*. 1990;81(5):431–435.
10. Atkinson PP, Atkinson JLD. Spinal shock. *Mayo Clinic Proceedings*. 1996;71(4):384–389.
11. Bravo G, Guízar-Sahagún G, Ibarra A, Centurión D, Villalón CM. Cardiovascular alterations after spinal cord injury: an overview. *Curr Med Chem Cardiovasc Hematol Agents*. 2004;2(2):133–148.
12. Illman A, Stiller K, Williams M. The prevalence of orthostatic hypotension during physiotherapy treatment in patients with an acute spinal cord injury. *Spinal Cord*. 2000;38(12):741–747.
13. Cariga P, Catley M, Nowicky AV, Savic G, Ellaway PH, Davey NJ. Segmental recording of cortical motor evoked potentials from thoracic paravertebral myotomes in complete spinal cord injury. *Spine (Phila Pa 1976)*. 2002;27(13):1438–1443.
14. Chelvarajah R, Knight SL, Craggs MD, Middleton FR. Orthostatic hypotension following spinal cord injury: impact on the use of standing apparatus. *NeuroRehabilitation*. 2009;24(3):237–242.
15. Sidorov EV, Townson AF, Dvorak MF, Kwon BK, Steeves J, Krassioukov A. Orthostatic hypotension in the first month following acute spinal cord injury. *Spinal Cord*. 2008;46(1):65–69.
16. Claydon VE, Steeves JD, Krassioukov A. Orthostatic hypotension following spinal cord injury: understanding clinical pathophysiology. *Spinal Cord*. 2006;44(6):341–351.
17. Krassioukov A, Eng JJ, Warburton DE, Teasell R. A systematic review of the management of orthostatic hypotension following spinal cord injury. *Arch Phys Med Rehabil*. 2009;90(5):876–885.
18. Krassioukov A, Wecht JM, Teasell RW, Eng JJ. Orthostatic hypotension following spinal cord injury. In: Eng JJ, Teasell

RW, Miller WC, eds. *Spinal Cord Injury Rehabilitation Evidence.* Version 6.0. Vancouver; 2018:1–31.

19. Volski A, Ackerman DJ. Neurogenic Shock. In: Stawicki SP, Swaroop M, eds. *Clinical Management of Shock - The Science and Art of Physiological Restoration.* [Internet]. London: IntechOpen; 2019. https://www.intechopen.com/chapters/69817.
20. Flanagan EP, Pittock SJ. Diagnosis and management of spinal cord emergencies. In: Wijdicks EFM, Kramer AH, eds. *Handbook of Clinical Neurology.* Vol 140 Critical Care Neurology Part I. Elsevier; 2017:319–335.
21. Wecht JM, De Meersman RE, Weir JP, Spungen AM, Bauman WA. Cardiac autonomic responses to progressive head-up tilt in individuals with paraplegia. *Clin Auton Res.* 2003;13(6):433–438.
22. Raymond J, Davis GM, van der Plas M. Cardiovascular responses during submaximal electrical stimulation-induced leg cycling in individuals with paraplegia. *Clin Physiol Funct Imaging.* 2002;22(2):92–98.
23. Hopman MTE, Groothuis JT, Flendrie M, Gerrits KHL, Houtman S. Increased vascular resistance in paralyzed legs after spinal cord injury is reversible by training. *J Appl Physiol (1985).* 2002;93(6):1966–1972.
24. Houtman S, Colier WN, Oeseburg B, Hopman MT. Systemic circulation and cerebral oxygenation during head-up tilt in spinal cord injured individuals. *Spinal Cord.* 2000;38(3):158–163.
25. Yarar-Fisher C, Pascoe DD, Gladden LB, Quindry JC, Hudson J, Sefton J. Acute physiological effects of whole body vibration (WBV) on central hemodynamics, muscle oxygenation and oxygen consumption in individuals with chronic spinal cord injury. *Disabil Rehabil.* 2014;36(2):136–145.

CHAPTER 13

Autonomic Dysreflexia

William McKinley

OUTLINE

Definition

Autonomic dysreflexia (AD) is a symptom complex characterized by a sudden exaggerated increase in blood pressure (systolic ≥20 mmHg above baseline), and often reflex bradycardia, triggered by somatosensory input below the level of spinal cord injury (SCI).[1,2] AD is considered a medical emergency. It can develop suddenly in individuals with SCI at neurological levels T6 and above and, if not treated promptly, can lead to serious complications (e.g., seizures, stroke, death).

Incidence

AD has been documented in 48%–90% of individuals with SCI above T6, and is typically more severe in individuals with higher levels of injury, more complete levels of injury, and with chronic SCI.

Pathophysiology

AD represents a reflex sympathetic hyperactivity brought on by underlying noxious stimuli that is compounded by a loss of supraspinal inhibition (modulation) of these reflex responses below the SCI level.[3–8] Though sympathetic nervous system (SNS) outflow occurs from T1–L2 spinal cord levels from the intermediolateral cell column, the major splanchnic outflow of the SNS occurs from T5–L2. Alpha-adrenoceptor SNS stimulation leads to vasoconstriction manifested clinically as hypertension, urinary retention, pallor, piloerection, and sudomotor sweating. The inability to modulate this area, through inhibition by supraspinal centers, results in prolonged vasoconstriction, to this vast blood flow area, and hypertension.

Other factors thought to be involved include denervation hypersensitivity of sympathetic alpha-1 receptors and the formation of abnormal synaptic connections due to axonal sprouting.[9–16] High blood pressure can lead to a baroreceptor reflex response and a parasympathetic-induced bradycardia (via the vagus nerve). During AD, supraspinal inhibition above the level of SCI leads to vasodilation with flushing of face, neck, upper chest, and upper arms; profuse sweating; increased cutaneous temperature; and nasal congestion. Headaches are common, due to dilation of pain-sensitive intracranial arteries. The profuse sweating above the level of the SCI is a consequence of sympathetic cholinergic hyperactivity.

Clinical Presentation

Symptoms[17–20]

- Hypertension: increase in systolic blood pressure (SBP) of >20 mmHg above baseline
  - Be aware that individuals with an SCI are likely to have lower baseline SBP
- Bradycardia, dysrhythmias
- Headache
- Sweating and/or flushing of the skin above the level of injury
- Piloerection or goose bumps
- Blurred vision, nasal congestion second sympathetic inhibition above the level of injury
- Anxiety, chest tightness, nausea, or trouble breathing

Below the SCI	Above the SCI

• Cold, dry skin, piloerection (alpha-1 hyperstimulation)
• Sweating: alpha-1 hyperstimulation vs sweating limited to apocrine sweat glands)
	• Compensatory vasodilation response to hypertension (HTN)
	  • Flushing, nasal congestion, headache (stretch-r)
	  • Hyperhidrosis: increased blood flow leads to increased temperature
	• Hypertensive encephalopathy: headache, papilledema, change in vision, change in mental status, seizure, cerebrovascular accident

"Silent" AD: Be aware that AD may appear with no symptoms other than a significantly elevated BP.[21]

Complications

Severe, but rare, complications have been associated with the severe hypertension of AD, including[22–24]:

- Neurologic disorders such as seizures; retinal or cerebral hemorrhage
- Cardiac disorders such as atrial fibrillation, myocardial infarction

The potential long-term consequences of repeated episodes of severe AD are unknown.

Evaluation

AD begins with a noxious stimulus originating below the level of SCI. This most commonly arises from the bladder but can also occur due to bowel impaction, an ingrown toenail, a pressure sore, or an acute abdominal emergency. A list of reported stimuli and conditions associated with the development of AD follows.[25]

Urinary System

- Bladder distention
- Bladder or kidney stones
- Blocked catheter
- Detrusor sphincter dyssynergia
- Urinary tract infection

Gastrointestinal System

- Bowel impaction
- Appendicitis
- Gallstones
- Gastrointestinal ulcers or gastritis
- Hemorrhoids, anal fissures

Integumentary System

- Constrictive clothing
- Blisters
- Burns
- Ingrown toenail
- Bites
- Pressure injuries
- Sunburn

Reproductive System

- Sexual activity
- Sexually transmitted disease
- High sexual arousal

Male

- Ejaculation
- Epididymitis
- Priapism
- Prostatitis
- Testicular torsion
- Scrotal compression

Female

- Lactation, breastfeeding, mastitis
- Menstruation
- Painful intercourse
- Labor and delivery
- Vaginitis

Other Systemic Causes

- Deep vein thrombosis, pulmonary embolism
- Excessive alcohol, caffeine, or other diuretic intake, substance abuse, stimulants
- Fractures or other trauma below the level of the injury
- Functional electrical stimulation
- Heterotopic bone
- Syringomyelia
  - Surgical or invasive diagnostic procedures
- Boosting (see later)

Treatment[26–30]

Acute Treatment

1. Sit patient upright, which will orthostatically decrease HTN
2. Loosen restrictive clothing/devices; remove noxious stimuli
3. Monitor BP and pulse every 5 min until stabilized
4. Evaluate for noxious stimuli. The identification and removal of the possible trigger and subsequent decrease of afferent stimulation to the spinal cord is the most effective prevention strategy in clinical practice. Consider bladder, the most common trigger:
   a. If Foley catheter in place, flush and check for kinks/obstructions (if so, gently irrigate bladder with 10–15 mL saline)
   b. If the catheter is blocked, remove and replace it (use lidocaine jelly)
   c. If no Foley catheter, catheterize using lidocaine jelly
   d. Send urine for urinalysis and culture
5. Consider fecal impaction (check rectum for stool using lidocaine jelly)
6. Consider less common AD triggers: inflammatory processes, infection, erection, hemorrhoids, ingrown nail, thrombosis, pregnancy, drugs, intentional "boosting"
7. If SBP ≥150 mmHg, use rapid-onset/short-duration antihypertensive: Nitrates (clinical consensus,

especially nitropaste), then oral or sublingual (SL) Nifedipine, intravenous (IV) Nitroprusside, SL Captopril, IV Hydralazine, IV Labetalol

8. Continue to monitor BP at least 2 h after HTN resolves
9. Consider emergency room referral or hospital admission if poor response to medications, cause unidentified, or suspicion of obstetrical complication
10. If successful identification of the trigger and treatment, monitor for symptomatic hypotension

Chronic (Prophylactic) Treatment

- Avoid idiosyncratic AD trigger stimuli and use prophylactic bladder and bowel programs
- Alpha-1-r antagonists (Prazosin, best supporting evidence)
- Prostaglandin E2 agonists
- Bladder detrusor or sphincter ablation/denervation (Botox, surgery)

Monitoring Treatment Efficacy

- The underlying cause has been identified
- BP and pulse are restored, no signs or symptoms
- An education plan has been reviewed with the individual with SCI and their family
- Follow-up monitoring and care has been arranged

Additional Autonomic Dysreflexia–Related Issues

Boosting

Boosting, or voluntarily induced AD, is a practice that is illegal in competition and unique to athletes with an SCI above T6, which is sometimes used to improve exercise performance by inducing high blood pressure, heart rate, and oxygen utilization. Various methods include sitting on scrotum, clamping Foley catheter, tightening leg straps, or breaking a toe.[31,32]

Hyperhidrosis

The estimated prevalence of excessive sweating has been reported to be about 25% with an identifiable cause noted in about one-third (e.g., infections, dyspepsia, AD). Sweating is present both above and below the level of the SCI. Sweating is a normal mechanism of thermal regulation aimed at cooling the body. Abnormal stimulation and hyperactivity of the eccrine sweat glands (with postganglionic SNS acetylcholine release) is thought to be responsible for hyperhidrosis.

Autonomic Dysreflexia During Pregnancy, Delivery, and Postpartum

AD occurs during labor in approximately two-thirds of pregnant women with SCI above T6.[33–36]

Adequate anesthesia (spinal or epidural anesthesia) is needed with labor, vaginal delivery, cesarean delivery, or instrumental delivery in order to prevent AD by blocking stimuli that arise from pelvic organs. An antepartum consultation with an anesthesiologist and a plan for induction of epidural or spinal anesthesia at the onset of labor is recommended. Careful and frequent fetal monitoring is recommended, especially during labor and delivery. AD must be differentiated from preeclampsia during labor to ensure appropriate treatment. AD can also occur during postpartum breastfeeding, with breast engorgement, or with mastitis.

Thermodysregulation

Individuals with SCI at or above T6 are at risk for hyperthermia or hypothermia.[37–41] Core body temperature is regulated by the hypothalamus via several mechanisms, including heat production and release. Under high temperatures, heat is released by increased skin blood flow and sweating.[7] SCI above T6 can lead to interruptions to appropriate cutaneous vasodilation or vasoconstriction and inappropriate sweating, which can lead to hyper- or hypothermia even at mild, ambient temperature.[7] In hot environments, patients with cervical SCI cannot sweat, thus causing a rapid elevation in their body temperature compared with healthy subjects.[8]

- Hypothermia (core temperature <35.0°C) prevention includes temperature regulation with warm clothing, blankets, fluids, heating devices (with caution), and avoidance of alcohol (causes vasodilation and heat loss). Certain medications may disrupt temperature regulation (alpha-agonists, narcotics, oxybutynin, gabapentin, and norepinephrine and serotonin-reuptake inhibitors).
- Hyperthermia (core temperature >37.8°C) management includes removal from hot environment, wearing lightweight and light-colored clothing, maintaining a proper temperature-controlled room (air-conditioning, fan), hydration, and cold fluids. During exercise, individuals with SCI at or above T6 should be monitored for hyperthermia. In hospitalized cases, the differential diagnosis of hyperthermia include diseases that cause temperature elevation—infectious and noninfectious diseases (such as drug fever, deep vein thrombosis, heterotopic ossification, or thyroid storm).

Review Questions

1. The pathophysiology of AD includes all of the following, EXCEPT:
   a. Sympathetic hyperactivity
   b. Prolonged vasoconstriction
   c. Parasympathetic hyperactivity
   d. T6 and above levels of SCI
   e. Inadequate descending inhibition through the spinal cord
2. Clinical presentation of AD includes all of the following, EXCEPT:
   a. Hypertension: increase in SBP (>20 mmHg above baseline)
   b. Tachycardia
   c. Sweating below the level of injury
   d. Anxiety
   e. Headache
3. Complications associated with AD include all of the following, EXCEPT:
   a. Seizures
   b. Cerebral hemorrhage
   c. Retinal hemorrhage
   d. Atrial fibrillation
   e. Orthostatic hypotension
4. Evaluation and management of AD include all of the following, EXCEPT:
   a. Placing patient in the supine position
   b. Evaluation of bladder catheterization patency
   c. Frequent BP monitoring
   d. Loosening restrictive clothing
   e. Utilization of antihypertensive medications

REFERENCES

1. Consortium for Spinal Cord Medicine. *Evaluation and Management of Autonomic Dysreflexia and other Autonomic Dysfunctions*. Washington, DC: Paralyzed Veterans of America; 2020.
2. Consortium for Spinal Cord Medicine. *Early Acute Management in Adults With Spinal Cord Injury: Clinical Practice Guidelines for Health-Care Professionals*. Washington, DC: Paralyzed Veterans of America; 2008.
3. Mathias CJ, Frankel HL. Cardiovascular control in spinal man. *Ann Rev Physiol*. 1988;50:577–592.
4. Mathias CJ, Frankel HL. The cardiovascular system in tetraplegia and paraplegia. In: Frankel HL, ed. *Handbook of Clinical Neurology*. Philadelphia: Elsevier Science; 1992:435–456.
5. Karlsson AK. Autonomic dysreflexia. *Spinal Cord*. 1999;37:383–391.
6. Teasell RW, Arnold JM, Krassioukov A, Delaney GA. Cardiovascular consequences of loss of supraspinal control of the sympathetic nervous system following spinal cord injuries. *Arch Phys Med Rehabil*. 2000;81:506–516.
7. Krassioukov AV, Furlan JC, Fehlings MG. Autonomic dysreflexia in acute spinal cord injury: an under-recognized clinical entity. *J Neurotrauma*. 2003;20:707–716.
8. Curt A, Rodic B, Schurch B, Dietz V. Assessment of autonomic dysreflexia in patients with spinal cord injury. *J Neurol Neurosurg Psychiatry*. 1997 May;62(5):473–477.
9. Arnold JM, Feng QP, Delaney GA, Teasell RW. Autonomic dysreflexia in tetraplegic patients: evidence for alpha-adrenoceptor hyper-responsiveness. *Clin Auton Res*. 1995;5:267–270.
10. Erickson RP. Autonomic hyperreflexia: pathophysiology and medical management. *Arch Phys Med Rehabil*. 1980;61:431–440.
11. Furlan JC, Fehlings MG, Shannon P, Norenberg MD, Krassioukov AV. Descending vasomotor pathways in humans: correlation between axonal preservation and cardiovascular dysfunction after spinal cord injury. *J Neurotrauma*. 2003;20:1351–1363.
12. Krassioukov AV, Bunge RP, Ruckett WR, Bygrave MA. The changes in human spinal cord sympathetic preganglionic neurons after spinal cord injury. *Spinal Cord*. 1999;37:6–13.
13. Lehmann KG, Lane JG, Piepmeier JM, Batsford WP. Cardiovascular abnormalities accompanying acute spinal cord injury in humans: incidence, time course and severity. *J Am Coli Cardiol*. 1987;10:46–52.
14. Mathias CJ, Christensen NJ, Frankel HL, et al. Cardiovascular control in recently injured tetraplegics in spinal shock. *Q J Med*. Apr 1979;48(190):273–287.
15. Piepmeier JM, Lehmann KB, Lane JG. Cardiovascular instability following acute cervical spinal cord trauma. *Cent Nerv Syst Trauma*. 1985;2(3):153–160.
16. Young W, DeCrescito V, Tomasula JJ, et al. The role of the sympathetic nervous system in pressor responses induced by spinal injury. *J Neurosurg*. Apr 1980;52(4):473–481.
17. Forrest GP. Atrial fibrillation associated with autonomic dysreflexia in patients with tetraplegia. *Arch Phys Med Rehabil*. 1991;72(8):592–594.
18. Ho CP, Krassioukov AV. Autonomic dysreflexia and myocardial ischemia. *Spinal Cord*. 2010;48:714–715.
19. Liu N, Zhou M, Biering-Sørensen F, Krassioukov AV. Iatrogenic urological triggers of autonomic dysreflexia: a systematic review. *Spinal Cord*. 2015 Jul 1;53(7):500–509.
20. Mathias CJ, Frankel HL. Clinical manifestations of malfunctioning sympathetic mechanisms in tetraplegia. *J Auton Nerv Syst*. 1983;7(3–4):303–312.
21. Ekland M, Krassioukov A, McBride KE, Elliott SL. Incidence of autonomic dysreflexia and silent autonomic dysreflexia in men with SCI undergoing sperm retrieval: implications for clinical practice. *J Spinal Cord Med*. 2008;30:43–50.
22. Eltorai I, Kim R, Vulpe M, Kasravi H, Ho W. Fatal cerebral hemorrhage due to autonomic dysreflexia in a tetraplegic patient: case report and review. *Paraplegia*. 1992;30:355–360.
23. Vallès M, Benito J, Portell E, Vidal J. Cerebral hemorrhage due to autonomic dysreflexia in a spinal cord injury patient. *Spinal Cord*. 2005;43:738–740.
24. Yarkony GM, Katz RT, Wu Y. Seizures secondary to autonomic dysreflexia. *Arch Phys Med Rehabil*. 1986;67:834–835.
25. Krassioukov A, Claydon VE. The clinical problems in cardiovascular control following spinal cord injury: an overview. *Prog Brain Res*. 2006;152:223–229.
26. Braddom RL, Rocco JF. Autonomic dysreflexia. A survey of current treatment. *Am J Phys Med Rehabil*. 1991;70:234–241.
27. Krassioukov A, Warburton DE, Teasell R, Eng JJ. A systematic review of the management of autonomic dysreflexia after spinal cord injury. *Arch Phys Med Rehabil*. 2009;90:682–695.
28. Naftchi NE, Richardson JS. Autonomic dysreflexia: pharmacological management of hypertensive crises in spinal cord injured patients. *J Spinal Cord Med*. 1997;20:355–360.

29. Waites KB, Canupp KC, DeVivo MJ. Epidemiology and risk factors for urinary tract infection following spinal cord injury. *Arch Phys Med Rehabil.* 1993;74:691–695.
30. Coggrave MJ, Ingram RM, Gardner BP, Norton CS. The impact of stoma for bowel management after spinal cord injury. *Spinal Cord.* 2012;50:848–852.
31. Gee CM, West CR, Krassioukov AV. Boosting in elite athletes with spinal cord injury: a critical review of physiology and testing procedures. *Sports Med.* 2015;45(8):1133–1142.
32. Mazzeo F, Santamaria S, Iavarone A. Boosting in Paralympic athletes with spinal cord injury: doping without drugs. *Funct Neurol.* 2015 Apr–Jun;30(2):91–98.
33. American College of Obstetrics and Gynecology. ACOG committee opinion. Obstetric management of patients with spinal cord injuries. Number 275, September 2002. Committee on Obstetric Practice. American College of Obstetrics and Gynecology. *Int J Gynaecol Obstet.* 2002;79:189–191.
34. Cross LL, Meythaler JM, Tuel SM, Cross LA. Pregnancy, labor and delivery post spinal cord injury. *Paraplegia.* 1992;30:890–902.
35. Hughes SJ, Short DJ, Usherwood MM, Tebbutt H. Management of the pregnant woman with spinal cord injuries. *Br J Obstet Gynaecol.* 1991;98:513–518.
36. Lambert DH, Deane RS, Mazuzan JE. Anesthesia and the control of blood pressure in patients with spinal cord injury. *Anesth Analg.* 1982;61:344–348.
37. Attia M, Engel P. Thermoregulatory set point in patients with spinal cord injuries (spinal man). *Paraplegia.* 1983;21:233–248.
38. Colachis 3rd SC, Otis SM. Occurrence of fever associated with thermoregulatory dysfunction after acute traumatic spinal cord injury. *Am J Phys Med Rehabil.* 1995;74(2):114–119.
39. Downey JA, Huckaba CE, Myers SJ, Darling RC. Thermoregulation in the spinal man. *J Appl Physiol.* 1973;34(6): 790–794.
40. Khan S, Plummer M, Martinez-Arizala A, Banovac K. Hypothermia in patients with chronic spinal cord injury. *J Spinal Cord Med.* 2007;30(1):27–30.
41. Price MJ, Campbell IG. Effects of spinal cord lesion level upon thermoregulation during exercise in the heat. *Med Sci Sports Exerc.* 2003;35(7):1100–1107.

Pulmonary Issues After Spinal Cord Injury

CHAPTER 14

Teodoro Castillo

OUTLINE

Introduction

Physiologic changes in respiratory function after acute spinal cord injury (SCI) increase the risk for pulmonary complications, including atelectasis, bronchitis, pneumonia, sleep-disordered breathing, and respiratory failure. These respiratory complications are the main causes of morbidity and mortality following acute SCI and can occur after 36% to 83% of all injuries, with approximately two-thirds of individuals experiencing complications requiring mechanical ventilation.[1,2] Prospective data from five SCI Model System of Care sites revealed that 67% of new injuries experienced severe respiratory complications within the first several days after the injury. These difficulties included atelectasis (36.4%), pneumonia (31.4%), and respiratory failure (22.6%), which occurred an average of 17.7, 24.5, and 4.5 days postinjury, respectively.[3] Data from the National SCI Database demonstrates that complete tetraplegia had the highest rate of atelectasis, pneumonia, and aspiration. These were commonly observed in those over 60 years of age.[4] Despite improvements in acute management and 2-year survival, pulmonary complications still pose the greatest risk.[5,6] There is limited evidence-based literature on respiratory management in acute SCI, with most management principles based on expert panel opinion and the clinical expertise of the clinician. Systemic aggressive pulmonary management has been shown to significantly reduce pulmonary related morbidity and mortality after SCI.[7] This chapter serves as a guide for an interdisciplinary treatment approach of the implementation of treatment strategies to prevent and manage respiratory complications during the acute and chronic care of individuals with SCI.

Respiratory Physiology in Individuals Without Spinal Cord Injury

Muscles of Inspiration

Lung inspiration is an active process that is the result of contraction of the diaphragm, external intercostals, and accessory muscles (scalene, sternocleidomastoid, trapezius, and pectoralis). The diaphragm, innervated by the phrenic nerve that arises from cervical nerve roots C3–C5, is the primary muscle responsible for normal tidal, or quiet, breathing and for two-thirds of normal inspiratory capacity.[8–10] During inspiration, the diaphragm muscle shortens, descends, increases the thoracic cavity, displaces abdominal contents caudally, and elevates the lower rib cage,[11] which creates a negative intrathoracic pressure, drawing air into the lungs.

The external intercostals and the parasternal component of the internal intercostals of the upper rib cage are innervated by T1–T6 levels. During inspiration, they have a synergistic action with the diaphragm,[12] elevating the ribs,[13,14] and expanding and stabilizing the chest wall.[8]

Accessory muscles of inspiration, which include the sternocleidomastoid (innervated by cranial nerve [CN] XI), scalene (innervated at C2–C7), and upper trapezius (innervated by CN XI) muscles, function to elevate the upper ribs and sternum.[15] Together with the external intercostals, the accessory muscles elevate and stabilize the chest wall to its greatest diameter, improving the efficacy of diaphragmatic breathing as it descends.

Muscles of Expiration

Normal tidal or quiet lung expiration is a passive process that is the result of the elastic recoil of the lungs and chest wall. The muscles active in forced or active expiration or cough include the abdominal, the interosseous part of the internal intercostals, triangularis sterni, serratus posterior inferior, latissimus dorsi, and quadratus lumborum muscles. The rectus abdominis and internal/external oblique muscles, which are innervated by T5–L1 and lower six intercostal and subcostal nerves, respectively, compress both the rib cage and the abdomen. The interosseous internal intercostals are innervated by T2–T12, and lower the rib cage. Accessory muscles are the clavicular portion of the pectoralis major and latissimus dorsi and are innervated by C5–C7 and C6–C8, respectively.[16]

Respiratory Function After Spinal Cord Injury

Individuals with a SCI neurologic level above T12 have varying degrees of inspiratory and expiratory muscle paralysis, depending on the neurologic level and completeness of SCI. The higher the level, the weaker the muscles of respiration. Individuals with high tetraplegia (C1–C3) will have some accessory muscles to assist in breathing but will likely have weak or absent diaphragm function. Typically, the accessory muscles will be unable to sustain respiratory independence, and there will be a requirement of mechanical ventilation.[17] Individuals with mid and lower cervical (C4–C8) level and high paraplegia (T1–T5) level injuries, may be able to breathe independently but will have a weak cough due to the loss of abdominal and intercostal muscles, which elevates their risk for respiratory complications. Individuals with T6–T12 levels of injury will have progressive losses of normally innervated musculature that correspond to their level of injury, and this will correspondingly affect their forced expiratory muscles.

Respiratory Muscle Weakness

Decreased Inspiration

In individuals with complete SCI, the accessory muscles (sternocleidomastoid and scalene) play a significant role in inspiration. In injuries above C5, paralysis of the diaphragm results in reduced tidal volume (TV) and vital capacity (VC).[18] The neurologic level of injury correlates inversely with a reduction in VC.[18,19] Ventilatory restriction is described by decreased forced vital capacity (FVC), 1-second forced expiratory volume (FEV1), inspiratory capacity, total lung capacity, and increased residual volume.[20,21] Pulmonary hyperventilation or even a single large breath stimulates pulmonary surfactant production, which decreases surface tension between gaseous–aqueous interphase in the lungs and prevents alveolar collapse that can affect perfusion. The decreased inspiratory capacity seen after cervical and thoracic SCI leads to decreased surfactant production that results in hypoxia and increased risk for atelectasis.

Decreased Expiration

Since expiration is passive, ventilation depends on the recoil of the diaphragm, which is impaired after some cervical injuries. In complete tetraplegia injuries, the medial part of the pectoralis major becomes important for "active" expiration.[15] A weakened cough results from paralysis of the abdominal musculature. Additionally, an effective cough requires deep inspiration, which is impaired after cervical SCI.[22–24] The clavicular portion of the pectoralis major plays an important role in effective coughing after tetraplegia.[15,25] Training of the pectoralis major can improve the strength of cough.[21] Impaired cough can cause retained secretions and subsequent respiratory tract infections, which are the leading acute cause of death in patients with chronic SCI.[26]

Autonomic Dysfunction

Increased Bronchial Secretions

In acute cervical and high thoracic SCI, patients develop excessive production of bronchial secretions, bronchoconstriction, and decreased tone caused by unopposed vagal activity from the loss of peripheral sympathetic nervous system tone.[27–29] This results in accumulation and retention of secretions that predispose the patient to atelectasis, pneumonia, and potential respiratory failure.[30]

Bronchial Reactivity and Bronchoconstriction

Bronchial spasm, increased vascular congestion, and decreased mucociliary activity result from parasympathetic predominance, which increases airway resistance and the work of breathing in individuals with SCI who already have limited respiratory muscles.[20,31,32] With poor cough, secretions will accumulate and cause the patient to "drown" in their own secretions, increasing the risk for respiratory complications such as mucus plugging, atelectasis, and pneumonia. If not addressed, these will lead to respiratory muscle fatigue and potential respiratory failure.

Change in Chest and Abdominal Wall Dynamics

Flaccid Chest, Abdominal, and Pelvic Walls

Spinal shock occurs immediately following acute traumatic SCI and is characterized by flaccid paralysis and areflexia below the level of injury.[33] This loss of muscle tone increases compliance of the lung, chest, abdomen, and pelvic wall muscles that can affect the work of breathing. This tone loss prevents protrusion of abdominal contents into the pelvis as the diaphragm descends, thus decreasing the VC even with an intact diaphragm and accessory respiratory muscles. Loss of muscle tone also decreases the ability to recoil, or elasticity, of the chest, abdominal, and pelvic walls, which reduces passive expiration. Patients with complete tetraplegia who have preserved diaphragm function present with a paradoxical breathing pattern, where the upper rib cage retracts inward, and the abdomen protrudes outward with each inspiration due to paralysis of the intercostal muscles. This pattern of breathing reduces the efficiency of ventilation by lowering TV for a given diaphragmatic excursion.[1,34] Decreased efficiency of breathing leads to increased work of breathing, respiratory muscle fatigue, and respiratory failure.

Position

In SCI, VC is influenced by the position of the patient. The resting position of the diaphragm is affected by the pressure exerted by the abdominal viscera. In a supine position, the diaphragm is at a higher position in the rib cage, allowing greater excursion than in an upright position. This results in greater VC and improves ease of breathing in the supine position.[17,35] In sitting, VC decreases when the diaphragm tends to flatten and remain partially collapsed due to the effect of gravity and loss of abdominal support. Thus, individuals with SCI typically feel more breathless when upright than supine. Use of a fitted abdominal binder increases abdominal pressure support by positioning the diaphragm in a higher, more optimal point on its length-tension curve, improving forced VC, FEV1, peak expiratory flow, and maximal inspiratory pressure in people with tetraplegia.[36]

Respiratory Muscle Fatigue

SCI results in a restrictive respiratory dysfunction with greater compromise to expiratory as compared with inspiratory muscle function. This combination of restrictive ventilation, weak cough, bronchoconstriction, and hypersecretion are all risk factors for atelectasis, poor secretion clearance, and pulmonary infections. Although clinicians may apply principles of respiratory management for able-bodied populations, adjustments are needed for the unique changes seen after SCI. Therefore the approach to pulmonary management should focus on providing adequate ventilation, aggressive secretion management, and protecting the diaphragm function. Benefits of this approach include decreasing the work of breathing, allowing the diaphragm to rest, improving perfusion (oxygen saturation), helping to wean off oxygen supplement, decreasing carbon dioxide (CO_2), and preventing atelectasis, which will decrease complications and optimize success of ventilator weaning.

Acute Respiratory Assessment After Spinal Cord Injury

Since patients with cervical and high thoracic SCI have a risk of respiratory complications, the SCI specialist should be consulted at the time of hospital admission. Their initial evaluation, including history, physical, and American Spinal Injury Association (ASIA) and ASIA Impairment Scale (AIS) assessments in the first 24–48 hours postinjury, will identify the sensory and motor completeness of SCI injury and help determine the degree of respiratory muscle impairment. Greater respiratory compromise is associated with higher spinal level and complete motor injuries. Initial evaluation should also include evaluation of other comorbidities that can affect respiration, such as smoking history, chronic obstructive pulmonary disease, sleep-disordered breathing, aspiration risks, associated chest trauma, and concomitant brain injury.

Respiratory Assessment

Respiratory assessment should include the patient's breathing pattern, ability to cough, and diaphragm function.

Bedside Assessment

Careful assessment of the patient's breathing pattern should be done by identifying signs of ventilatory insufficiency that include shortness of breath, tachypnea, hypophonia (or weakening voice, as speech is a function of expiration), prominent use of accessory muscles, nasal flaring, cyanosis, flushing, oxygen desaturation, paradoxical breathing, and respiratory distress. All these signs and symptoms can serve as red flags, suggesting respiratory muscle fatigue and impending respiratory failure.

Cough Strength Evaluation

A good cough to mobilize secretions requires a large inspiratory effort followed by a quick and forceful expiration. One can observe the quality of the cough or consider measuring the peak cough flow meter. This can be done at bedside but may not be helpful for higher levels of injury with very weak or absent expiratory muscles. However, the reliability of these devices remains poor.[37]

Diaphragm Function

Since the diaphragm is the main muscle of inspiration, monitoring its function is essential in preventing respiratory complications in a patient with cervical SCI. SCI causes a restrictive ventilatory deficit,[10] and this loss of expiratory muscles causes a loss of expiratory reserve volume making VC the same as the inspiratory capacity.[7,38–41] Thus, VC can be used as a good indicator of diaphragm muscle strength.[7,10,42] Once spinal shock resolves, intercostal and abdominal muscle tone will return and increase the efficiency of diaphragm action.[10,43,44] Although values can vary in tetraplegia with a similar level of injury, VC averages 40%–60% of predicted value at 3–6 months post injury.[10,44] In addition to VC, maximal inspiratory pressure (MIP) and sniff nasal inspiratory pressure are also good measures of functional respiratory muscle strength. These can be easily measured at bedside,[45] so VC should be monitored as frequently as every nursing shift for the first several days.[46] VC in C5 and C6 SCI can be reduced from 30% to 50% within the first week.[10,47,48] Close observation of the breathing pattern and serial measurements of VC, MIP, nasal inspiratory pressure, oxygen (O_2), and CO_2 will alert the team to the patient's level of fatigue and the impending need for intubation. Serial chest X-rays should be done to monitor for atelectasis, pulmonary edema, effusion, or pneumonia. A reduction in VC to below 15 mL/kg, a MIP below −20 cmH_2O, and an increase in partial pressure CO_2 (pCO_2) confirm respiratory muscle fatigue, impending respiratory failure, and the need for immediate intubation.[30]

Intubation Assessment

Parameters After Spinal Cord Injury

The neurologic level and completeness of SCI help predict who will need to be intubated. Patients with tetraplegia must be assessed with respect to their need for mechanical ventilation during the acute phase. In acute tetraplegia, up to 80% of all individuals will require ventilatory support, and even in those with levels of injury caudal to C4 will do so.[49,50] Sixty-five percent of individuals with injuries at levels from T1 to T12 may have severe respiratory complications.[30] Edema or hematoma in the spinal cord may cause a loss of up to one ASIA level, which has significant consequences to respiratory function. With C5–C6 injuries, a 30%–50% reduction of VC is described in the first week after an injury. In patients with tetraplegia, respiratory failure can occur 4–6 days after injury. Berlly recommended that VC and arterial blood gases be measured at regular intervals until the patient is stable.[30] In one study, 90% of individuals with traumatic SCI who required ventilation did so in the first 3 days after injury. This showed that early aggressive secretion management can decrease the number of patients needing mechanical ventilation.[51]

Noninvasive Ventilation

Uncomplicated SCI can be managed with noninvasive ventilatory support[52,53] in units with significant SCI and noninvasive ventilation expertise. This alternative option requires that the patient be conscious and cooperative, since the preferred method is delivered through a mouthpiece for the period of ventilation during the day and a mask (nasal or custom molded oral seal) at night. However, this is not available in most intensive care units, so patients with high cervical and complete SCI will need to be placed on invasive ventilatory support.[50]

Invasive Ventilation

Neurologic level and completeness of injury are specific risk factors for intubation. Velmahos found 74% of patients with complete C5 injuries and above required intubation.[49] The majority of patients with acute traumatic SCI will require intubation for surgical stabilization of the spine. Lack of awareness of the respiratory impairment associated with acute SCI can lead to failed extubation, requiring reintubation. Como recommended semielective intubation in complete cervical spine injuries, especially C5 and above, when the first sign of respiratory distress is documented.[54] Close monitoring of diaphragm, FVC, MIP, oximetry partial pressure of oxygen (pO_2), and pCO_2 can determine the need for ventilatory support. This can prevent emergent intubation, which can increase the risk of neurological damage due to improper manipulation of the neck or by hypoxia. Criteria for intubation include declining VCs below 15 mL/kg ideal body weight (IBW), increasing oxygen requirements, increasing respiratory rate with low tidal volumes, rising pCO_2, and diminishing breath sounds in the lung fields. Tracheostomy is recommended early on for patients who are very likely to be dependent on long-term mechanical ventilation or slow weaning.[30]

Tracheostomy Assessment

Tracheostomy is commonly performed in complete cervical or high thoracic level of injury. Most of these patients, if not all, will require mechanical ventilation. These patients have limited respiratory muscle strength and are at risk for respiratory muscle fatigue, which can lead to respiratory failure. One way to prevent this is to get VC in postoperative patients; if is less than 15 mL/kg of IBW, these patients will require a slow wean and elective tracheostomy should be considered. One case series showed tracheostomy done before 7 days reduced the duration of mechanical ventilation and intensive care unit length of stay.[55] Several studies have found that there was no increase in wound or implant infection if tracheostomy was done within the first 10 days of anterior cervical spine fixation.[56,57] Tracheostomy can be safely done surgically or percutaneously in the intensive care unit. Ganuza found no differences in complications between surgical and percutaneous tracheostomy.[58] Percutaneous tracheostomy can be easily and more safely performed due to the availability of anatomic landmarks without neck extension.[57–60] This minimizes the risk of injury to the adjacent neck structures and has fewer late infections of the stoma.[61] There is limited evidence on the best time to perform, but it has been reported that surgical site infection can be minimized if done within 1–2 weeks postsurgery.[57,62,63]

Despite requiring surgery, tracheostomy is more comfortable compared with nasotracheal and endotracheal intubation. It has multiple benefits, including most importantly that it is easier to suction and perform pulmonary hygiene, which facilitates perfusion and ventilation by decreasing airway resistance. Inflated cuffs will not allow communication, but once deflated, the use of a Passy Muir Valve will allow vocalization. Cuff deflation should be explored as soon as possible. If deflation is not feasible, then at least tracheostomy allows communication with staff by "lip reading," which is not possible with endotracheal intubation. Tracheostomy does carry the risk of bleeding, infection, and tracheal injury. Other negative aspects of tracheostomy include increased secretion production, bacterial colonization, and risk of infections. Despite the risks, early tracheostomy should be recommended if the need for tracheostomy is inevitable.[56,58]

Ventilatory Management After Spinal Cord Injury

Patients with SCI rely almost exclusively on the function of the diaphragm for inspiration, which is responsible for providing 90% of the TV.[64] Since expiration relies on the recoil of the diaphragm in normal breathing, ventilation is dependent on inspiration. In addition, weak cough from the loss of expiratory muscles, increased production of secretions, and bronchoconstriction secondary to autonomic dysfunction result in accumulation of secretions that can lead to atelectasis.[32,65] All these can increase the work of breathing and diaphragm fatigue, which makes SCI patients more vulnerable to diaphragm fatigue and respiratory failure. The pillars of early treatment of respiratory dysfunction in SCI are lung expansion by providing adequate ventilation (expansion of lungs) and intensive management of secretions and atelectasis (clearing of secretions).

High Tidal Volume Ventilation

Despite the controversy regarding low-volume and high-volume ventilation, current clinical practice guidelines recommend high tidal volumes of 10–15 mL/kg IBW and optimization of minute ventilation as tolerated for individuals with spinal cord injury.[66] Lower TVs used for the able-bodied population increases risk for atelectasis and mucous plugging, and decreases surfactant production in individuals with SCI. The Rocky Mountain Regional Spinal Injury System established a protocol that supports high TV from 15–20 mL/kg IBW, by increasing TV by 100 mL and ventilator flow rate by 10 L/min at periodic intervals.[67] High volume and flow rates can bring down pCO_2 below 28, so dead space between ventilator and tracheostomy can be added as needed. High volumes achieve the goal of avoiding or treating atelectasis, improving the production of surfactant, preventing the collapse of the airway, and promoting recruitment.[32,64,65,68] Fenton found no significant difference in the time to wean, incidence of ventilator acquired pneumonia, or occurrence of adverse events in patients with tetraplegia ventilated with TV of 10 vs. 20 mL/kg IBW. Mechanical ventilation with higher TV was not associated with any episodes of acute respiratory distress syndrome or barotrauma.[69]

Supplemental Oxygen

Most individuals with SCI on mechanical ventilation are admitted on supplemental oxygen. If the patient does not have any cardiac or lung/chest wall pathology, the most common cause of hypoxia on room air (oxygen levels <94%) is due to inadequate ventilatory support (low TV) and ineffective airway secretion management. Instead of increasing ventilation (TV), clinicians often (inappropriately) provide supplemental O_2, which can be detrimental to the patient, as it can exacerbate hypercapnia, cause CO_2 narcosis, and decrease respiratory drive that can lead to respiratory failure. Instead, high TV should be used to facilitate improved perfusion (oxygenation), weaning off oxygen supplementation, decreasing CO_2 (increased ventilation), maintaining the compliance and elasticity of the chest wall, and suppressing the sense of "air hunger" (dyspnea), improving vocalization.[70]

Positive End-Expiratory Pressure

There is limited evidence to support the use of positive end-expiratory pressure (PEEP) in treating atelectasis in acute SCI. By gradually increasing TVs, the risk of barotrauma remains low because peak pressures only increase slightly. The amount of PEEP to use in ventilated patients with SCI has not been well studied. Too much PEEP can flatten the diaphragm due to high abdominal compliance, causing a mechanical disadvantage of the diaphragm during inspiration. Too little PEEP may cause atelectasis, particularly in the dependent portions of the lungs and left lower lobe. Ventilation strategies using high TV generally use low or no PEEP[68,71] and rely on the high TV to prevent atelectasis.

Ventilatory Weaning

The best predictors for survival in ventilator-dependent patients with SCI are age, level, completeness of injury, and time since injury. The life expectancy of a ventilator-dependent patient (at any level) who survives the first 24 hours and 1 year post-SCI is increased if weaned off the ventilator successfully (Table 14.1).

Table 14.1 Life Expectancy in Years Post Spinal Cord Injury

Age at Injury	No SCI	Life Expectancy (years) for Postinjury by Severity of Injury and Age at Injury									
		For Persons Who Survive the First 24 Hours					For Persons Surviving at Least 1 Year Postinjury				
		AIS D: Motor Functional at any Level	Para	Low Tetra (C5–C8)	High Tetra (C1–C4)	Ventilator Dependent any Level	AIS D: Motor Functional at any Level	Para	Low Tetra (C5–C8)	High Tetra (C1–C4)	Ventilator Dependent any Level
20	60.6	52.6	45.5	40.1	33.7	11.2	53.0	46.0	40.9	34.9	18.7
40	41.7	35.0	29.6	24.8	20.8	8.8	35.3	30.0	25.5	21.9	13.3
60	24.1	19.3	15.9	13.1	11.1	3.7	19.5	16.4	13.8	12.4	7.9

AIS, American Spinal Injury Association (ASIA) Impairment Scale; *SCI*, spinal cord injury.

Once the patient's spine is stabilized and the patient is medically stable, they should be transferred to a SCI center where concerted efforts can be made to wean patients off mechanical ventilation during the initial hospitalization. These interdisciplinary efforts will reduce the financial and emotional burden of care and improve life expectancy and quality of life. A weaning program requires a comprehensive approach with an experienced team of professionals, including physicians, respiratory therapists, nurses, speech, physical, and occupational therapists working with patients and family caregivers.[72] There are three modalities used for weaning: synchronized intermittent mandatory ventilation (SIMV), pressure support ventilation, and progressive ventilator-free breathing (PVFB).[72] PVFB has been shown to have the highest success rates for ventilator weaning in SCI.[73]

Synchronized Intermittent Mandatory Ventilation

SIMV has been the standard method of weaning off the ventilator in non-SCI populations. This modality allows the patient to trigger pressure-supported breaths above the set back-up rate of intermittent positive pressure breaths. Back-up rate and pressure support levels are then gradually reduced so patients will need to increase spontaneous respirations between assisted breaths. Non-SCI patients tolerate this modality well, since all their respiratory muscles remain intact; however, patients with high cervical and thoracic SCI with limited respiratory muscles are at an increased risk for muscle fatigue. This approach does not allow the muscles to rest and exercise. If not discontinued in time, SIMV can lead to respiratory muscle fatigue, tachypnea, hypercapnia, O_2 desaturation, and respiratory failure that can stop the weaning process. This modality takes longer and does not improve the success rate of weaning and thus is not recommended for SCI.[74,75]

Progressive Ventilator-Free Breathing

PVFB is the recommended modality for individuals with SCI and ventilator dependency. With this approach, the patient is taken off the ventilator for a few minutes a day (e.g., 15 minutes 2 × day) to build up the individual's muscle strength and tolerance. Supplemental oxygen can be used as needed when off the ventilator. T (period of time) off the ventilator is gradually increased as tolerated and team monitors for any respiratory muscle fatigue after each trial. Peterson compared the two modes of weaning and found PVFB was twice as effective as SIMV for ventilator-dependent tetraplegia, with a weaning success rate of 67.7% compared with 34.6%.[73] PVFB allows the diaphragm and accessory muscles to rest in between weaning trials to prevent muscle fatigue. The main objective is to preserve diaphragm function while on mechanical ventilation. Diaphragmatic dysfunction from fatigue is a common cause of weaning failure.[76] High-volume ventilation and PVFB help the weak muscles gain strength, prevent respiratory complications, improve endurance, and improve the chance of successfully weaning off the ventilator.

Criteria for Weaning[30]

- Afebrile with vital signs stable
- Manageable secretions
- Medically stable for at least 24 hours
- Chest X-ray clear
- Psychologically willing and ready to participate
- VC at least 15 mL/kg IBW
- Inspiratory force >24 cmH_2O
- Respiratory stable for at least 24 hours
- pO_2 >75
- pCO_2 = 35–45
- pH = 7.35–7.45
- No PEEP
- Fraction of inspired oxygen no more than 25%

Secretion Management/Respiratory Support

Glossopharyngeal Breathing

This is a long-established technique of breath stacking to improve cough and maintain ventilation. Speech therapists are principally involved in training. The patient inspires air to total lung capacity, then uses mouth and throat muscles to repeatedly gulp or piston air into the lungs as many times as possible, thus exceeding total lung capacity. This is followed by passive exhalation. Glossopharyngeal breathing improves VC and peak cough flow with possible improvement in lung compliance and vocal quality.[16,17] These exercises can be done independently, require no equipment, and have no contraindications.

Postural Drainage

Postural drainage and passive positioning techniques using gravity can facilitate the movement of secretions from the most peripheral regions of the lungs to the main airway. This allows secretions to be removed using coughing or other methods of aspiration. Depending on the affected lung area, the patient can be positioned in several ways to allow gravity to help in the drainage. Trendelenburg, supine, prone, and left and right lateral positions should be held for at least 5–10 minutes, depending on tolerance. Postural drainage can be enhanced by external manipulations like percussion and vibration.

Percussion and Vibration

Percussion and vibration are external manipulations of the chest that can help mobilize secretions. Percussion consists of rhythmically tapping on different areas of the chest with a cupped hand. The intensity and duration of the percussion should be adjusted to the patient's comfort level. Vibration can be administered using the hands, a hand held device, or a vest to the chest wall and soft tissues to help loosen secretions for expectoration. Both may be combined with postural drainage.

Manually Assisted Coughing

Due to weak cough after SCI, manually assisted coughing or the "quad cough" is a maneuver used where a care provider performs an abdominal thrust and squeeze over the chest wall that is coordinated with the patient's spontaneous breath. Without using any devices, this maneuver can greatly increase coughing to help clear secretions in the upper airways. Contraindications to quad coughing include an unstable spine in traction, internal abdominal complications, chest trauma such as fractured ribs, recently placed vena cava filter, and pregnancy. It can be performed safely; however, repetitive quad coughing may pose a potential risk for injuries for staff members performing this maneuver given the strenuous nature of the technique.

Mechanical Insufflation–Exsufflation Device

Mechanical insufflation–exsufflation devices use is a highly effective therapy that can be used for both acute and chronic SCI. It promotes clearance of secretions and augments VC. Cough is simulated by gradually applying a positive pressure to the airway and rapidly shifting to negative pressure producing a high expiratory flow. This can be applied through tracheostomy, facemask, or mouthpiece, and it is more effective than manually assisted cough. It reduces the need for deep endotracheal suctioning, making it less irritating for the lungs and more comfortable for the patient. It effectively clears retained bronchial secretions, reducing the risk of respiratory complications. The use of an insufflation–exsufflation device during intensive and post intensive care may reduce the number of bronchoscopies, respiratory complications, and the weaning time.[77] Use should be avoided in patients with pneumothorax, pneumomediastinum, and bullous emphysema.

Respiratory Muscle Training

As with other muscle training programs, the goal of respiratory muscle training (RMT) is to increase strength and endurance. To be effective, training sessions should have a set repetition and frequency over a specified duration of time. RMT can be inspiratory, expiratory, or both depending on the neurologic level of injury. RMT is safely used in patients with acute tetraplegia with increased VC, maximal inspiratory and expiratory pressures, and endurance during the training period.[78–80] Mueller reported on a randomized, controlled clinical trial comparing various RMT methods in tetraplegic patients and concluded that training the inspiratory force is more beneficial than training the respiratory muscle resistance in improving respiratory function, voice, chest mobility, and quality of life in patients with tetraplegia during the first year of the injury.[81] RMT is relatively safe and inexpensive training that may be of benefit in tetraplegia.[82] This training modality can be used during the ventilator weaning phase, but only when the patient is able to tolerate periods of spontaneous respiration. Initially, the resistance is set to 7–10 cmH_2O for a maximum of 1 minute, twice a day. The resistance, frequency, and duration are gradually increased as the inspiratory force improves. For chronic SCI patients, RMT can be used on a maintenance exercise program. Precautions include avoiding use in the setting of unstable asthma, pneumothorax, or other barotrauma.

Inspiratory Muscle Training

Inspiratory muscle training uses resistance during inspiration to improve the strength and resistance of the inspiratory musculature. The devices have spring-loaded valves that allow for expiration and offer resistance to inspiration. It can be connected to the tracheostomy tube or to a mouthpiece. Incentive spirometers or weights placed on the abdomen offer resistance to inspiration.

Expiratory Muscle Training

Strengthening of the pectoralis major muscle may be useful, as this muscle may be spared or partially preserved given its multilevel (C5–C7) innervation. The clavicular part of the pectoralis muscle can help with active expiration.

Medications

People with cervical SCI have bronchial hyperresponsiveness due to loss of sympathetic input with unopposed vagal stimulation and altered mechanical lung properties with decreased deep breathing and "stretching" of airways.[83,84] Bronchodilators are a routinely recommended therapy in other conditions with airway hyperreactivity, such as chronic obstructive pulmonary disease and asthma, but their usage is less clear in the SCI population. The use of anticholinergic bronchodilators, such as ipratropium (Atrovent) and metaproterenol (Alupent; a beta 2 selective agonist), in acute SCI has not been well studied. A randomized control trial by Barratt demonstrated that salbutamol (Ventolin) had a beneficial effect on forced expiratory volume in FEV1, FVC, and peak expiratory flow rate in patients with acute motor complete tetraplegia.[85] The use of salbutamol, ipratropium, and metaproterenol appear to be effective in improving pulmonary function short term, whereas salmeterol (Serevent) appears effective in long-term use. Ipratropium's anticholinergic effects can potentially cause thickening of secretions and block surfactant, which could compromise its effects on respiratory function. For mechanically ventilated patients, bronchodilators are administered for dyspnea, shortness of breath, and reverse bronchoconstriction by metered dose inhaler or nebulizer.

Electrical Stimulation

For patients with SCI level above C3–C5 with intact phrenic nerves, phrenic and diaphragmatic pacing are alternative means for respiratory support. Laparoscopic implantation of electrodes in diaphragmatic pacing involves a simpler surgical procedure than pacemaker implantation on the phrenic nerves. Patients with diaphragmatic pacer systems have been shown to have improved quality of life, attributable to increased mobility and being non–ventilator dependent[86]; however, implantation is resource-intensive with considerable perioperative risk. Onders documented in a multicenter experience that laparoscopic diaphragm motor point mapping, electrode implantation, and pacing can be safely performed both in SCI and in amyotrophic lateral sclerosis (ALS). In SCI, 96% of the individuals were able to use diaphragmatic pacer systems to provide ventilation, replacing their mechanical ventilators. In ALS, individuals have been able to delay the need for mechanical ventilation up to 24 months, increasing survival.[87] Improvements in quality of life, defined as a success either by partial or complete independence from ventilatory support, have been reported.[86,88]

Respiratory Management in Chronic Spinal Cord Injury

The incidence of respiratory complications remains the leading cause of mortality in patients with chronic SCI. The decreased ability to take a deep breath and effectively cough to clear secretions puts patients with SCI at high risk for atelectasis and pneumonia.

Promoting Respiratory Health

People with SCI should follow preventive health measures such as immunization, counseling, and resources for smoking cessation and weight management, similar to the general population. Lung function and FEV1 in people with SCI naturally declines with age at a similar rate that in the general population. Decline in FVC and FEV1 is accelerated in SCI by an increase in body mass index and by persistent smoking. This decline is not predicted by level or severity of injury.[20,89] In 2016, individuals with SCI were classified by the Centers for Disease Control as being at high risk for influenza, so annual immunization should be encouraged.[90] Pneumococcal vaccination is also recommended, although SCI is not yet formally included in the high-risk group. Centers for Disease Control and Prevention recommends pneumococcal vaccination for Adults 19-65 years old with certain underlying medical conditions or other risk factors and Adults 65 years old and older.

For those who have never received a pneumococcal vaccine or with unknown vaccination history, a single dose of PCV15 (15-valent Pneumococcal Conjugate Vaccine – Vaxneuvance™) or PCV20 (20-valent Pneumococcal Conjugate vaccine – Prevnar20®) is recommended. If PCV20 is used, their pneumococcal vaccinations are complete. If PCV15 is used, this should be followed by one dose of PPSV23 (23-valent Pneumococcal Polysaccharide Vaccine – Pneumovax®). The recommended interval is at least 1 year. The minimum interval is 8 weeks and can be considered in adults with immunocompromising condition, cochlear implant or cerebrospinal fluid leak. For adults 65 years or older without an immunocompromising condition, cerebrospinal fluid leak or cochlear implant who previously received PCV13 (13-valent pneumococcal conjugate vaccine – Prevnar13®), 1 dose of PPSV23 should be administered at least a year after PCV13 was received. For adults 19 years old or older with cerebrospinal fluid leak or cochlear implant or with an immunocompromising condition, 1 dose of PPSV23 before age 65 years and 1 dose of PPSV23 at age 65 years or older recommended. Administer a single dose of PPSV23 at least 8 weeks after PCV13 was received.[91] Annual follow-up with an individual with SCI's medical provider should include measurement of FVC, seating posture in a wheelchair to address functional kyphosis or scoliosis, obesity, and neurologic change from posttraumatic cystic myelopathy.

Review Questions

1. TRUE OR FALSE: Respiratory complications are the most common cause of morbidity and mortality in patients with acute SCI.
2. In acute SCI, which is at highest risk for respiratory failure and likely require mechanical ventilation?
   a. C5 AIS D
   b. T12 AIS A
   c. C6 AIS D
   d. Above C5 AIS A
3. Unlike the general population, people with acute complete cervical and high thoracic complete SCI experience a "perfect storm" that increases their risk for respiratory impairment that will lead to respiratory muscle fatigue and failure.
   a. Decreased inspiration and loss of ability to cough (loss of expiratory muscles)
   b. Increased bronchial secretions, accumulation of secretions
   c. Autonomic dysfunction, loss of sympathetic tone, unopposed vagal activity
   d. Alterations in chest wall, lung, and abdominal compliance
   e. All of the above
4. Which muscle can predict ability to wean off the ventilator in a high cervical complete SCI?
   a. External intercostals
   b. Accessory muscles of inspiration (scalene/sternocleidomastoids)
   c. Abdominal muscles
   d. Diaphragm

REFERENCES

1. Brown R, DiMarco AF, Hoit JD, et al. Respiratory dysfunction and management in spinal cord injury. *Respir Care.* 2006;51:853–868; discussion 869-870.
2. Shavelle RM, DeVivo MJ, Strauss DJ, et al. Long-term survival of persons ventilator dependent after spinal cord injury. *The Journal of Spinal Cord Medicine.* 2006;29:511–519.
3. Jackson AB, Groomes TE. Incidence of respiratory complications following spinal cord injury. *Archives of Physical Medicine and Rehabilitation.* 1994;75:270–275.
4. Ragnarsson KT, Hall KM, Wilmot CB, et al. Management of pulmonary, cardiovascular, and metabolic conditions after spinal cord injury. In: Stover SL, Delisa JA, Whiteneck GG, eds. *Spinal Cord Injury: Clinical Outcomes From the Model Systems.* Gaithersburg, MD: Aspen Publishers Inc.; 1995:79–99.
5. DeVivo MJ, Kartus PL, Stover SL, et al. Cause of death for patients with spinal cord injuries. *Arch Intern Med.* 1989;149:1761–1766.
6. Wuermser LA, Chiodo A, Ho C. Spinal cord injury medicine. 2. Acute care management of traumatic and nontraumatic injury. *Arch Phys Med Rehabil.* 2007;88:S55–S61.
7. McMichan JC, Michel L, Westbrook PR. Pulmonary dysfunction following traumatic quadriplegia. *Recognition, prevention, and treatment. JAMA.* 1980;243:528–531.
8. Lanig IS, Peterson WP. The respiratory system in spinal cord injury. *Phys Med Rehabil Clin N Am.* 2000;11:29–43. vii.
9. Winslow C, Rozovsky J. Effect of spinal cord injury on the respiratory system. *American Journal of Physical Medicine & Rehabilitation.* 2003;82:803–814.
10. Ledsome JR, Sharp JM. Pulmonary function in acute cervical cord injury. *Am Rev Respir Dis.* 1981;124:41–44.
11. Derenne JP, Macklem PT, Roussos C. The respiratory muscles: mechanics, control, and pathophysiology. *Am Rev Respir Dis.* 1978;118:119–133.
12. Gross D, Ladd HW, Riley EJ, et al. The effect of training on strength and endurance of the diaphragm in quadriplegia. *American Journal of Medicine.* 1980;68:27–35.
13. Maarsingh EJ, van Eykern LA, Sprikkelman AB, et al. Respiratory muscle activity measured with a noninvasive EMG technique: technical aspects and reproducibility. *J Appl Physiol (1985).* 2000;88:1955–1961.
14. Han JN, Gayan-Ramirez G, Dekhuijzen R, et al. Respiratory function of the rib cage muscles. *Eur Respir J.* 1993;6:722–728.
15. Estenne M, De Troyer A. Cough in tetraplegic subjects: an active process. *Ann Intern Med.* 1990;112:22–28.
16. Terson de Paleville DGL, McKay WB, Folz RJ, et al. Respiratory motor control disrupted by spinal cord injury: mechanisms, evaluation, and restoration. *Transl Stroke Res.* 2011;2:463–473.
17. Danon J, Druz WS, Goldberg NB, et al. Function of the isolated paced diaphragm and the cervical accessory muscles in C1 quadriplegics. *Am Rev Respir Dis.* 1979;119:909–919.
18. Baydur A, Adkins RH, Milic-Emili J. Lung mechanics in individuals with spinal cord injury: effects of injury level and posture. *J Appl Physiol (1985).* 2001;90:405–411.
19. Kang SW, Shin JC, Park CI, et al. Relationship between inspiratory muscle strength and cough capacity in cervical spinal cord injured patients. *Spinal Cord.* 2006;44:242–248.
20. Schilero GJ, Bauman WA, Radulovic M. Traumatic spinal cord injury: pulmonary physiologic principles and management. *Clin Chest Med.* 2018;39:411–425.
21. Spungen AM, Dicpinigaitis PV, Almenoff PL, et al. Pulmonary obstruction in individuals with cervical spinal cord lesions unmasked by bronchodilator administration. *Paraplegia.* 1993;31:404–407.
22. De Troyer A, Kirkwood PA, Wilson TA. Respiratory action of the intercostal muscles. *Physiol Rev.* 2005;85:717–756.
23. De Troyer A, Legrand A, Gevenois PA, et al. Mechanical advantage of the human parasternal intercostal and triangularis sterni muscles. *J Physiol.* 1998;513(Pt 3):915–925.

24. Loring SH, Woodbridge JA. Intercostal muscle action inferred from finite-element analysis. *J Appl Physiol.* 1985;1991(70): 2712–2718.
25. De Troyer A, Estenne M, Heilporn A. Mechanism of active expiration in tetraplegic subjects. *N Engl J Med.* 1986;314: 740–744.
26. DeVivo MJ, Black KJ, Stover SL. Causes of death during the first 12 years after spinal cord injury. *Arch Phys Med Rehabil.* 1993;74:248–254.
27. Radulovic M, Schilero GJ, Wecht JM, et al. Airflow obstruction and reversibility in spinal cord injury: evidence for functional sympathetic innervation. *Arch Phys Med Rehabil.* 2008;89:2349–2353.
28. Mateus SRM, Beraldo PSS, Horan TA. Cholinergic bronchomotor tone and airway caliber in tetraplegic patients. *Spinal Cord.* 2006;44:269–274.
29. Bhaskar KR, Brown R, O'Sullivan DD, et al. Bronchial mucus hypersecretion in acute quadriplegia. Macromolecular yields and glycoconjugate composition. *Am Rev Respir Dis.* 1991;143:640–648.
30. Berlly M, Shem K. Respiratory management during the first five days after spinal cord injury. *The Journal of Spinal Cord Medicine.* 2007;30:309–318.
31. Slonimski M, Aguilera EJ. Atelectasis and mucus plugging in spinal cord injury: case report and therapeutic approaches. *J Spinal Cord Med.* 2001;24:284–288.
32. Wong SL, Shem K, Crew J. Specialized respiratory management for acute cervical spinal cord injury: a retrospective analysis. *Top Spinal Cord Inj Rehabil.* 2012;18:283–290.
33. Ditunno JF, Little JW, Tessler A, et al. Spinal shock revisited: a four-phase model. *Spinal Cord.* 2004;42:383–395.
34. Mortola JP, Sant'Ambrogio G. Motion of the rib cage and the abdomen in tetraplegic patients. *Clin SCI Mol Med.* 1978;54:25–32.
35. Ben-Dov I, Zlobinski R, Segel MJ, et al. Ventilatory response to hypercapnia in C(5-8) chronic tetraplegia: the effect of posture. *Arch Phys Med Rehabil.* 2009;90:1414–1417.
36. Wadsworth BM, Haines TP, Cornwell PL, et al. Abdominal binder improves lung volumes and voice in people with tetraplegic spinal cord injury. *Arch Phys Med Rehabil.* 2012;93:2189–2197.
37. Kulnik ST, MacBean V, Birring SS, et al. Accuracy of portable devices in measuring peak cough flow. *Physiol Meas.* 2015;36:243–257.
38. Cameron GS, Scott JW, Jousse AT, et al. Diaphragmatic respiration in the quadriplegic patient and the effect of position on his vital capacity. *Ann Surg.* 1955;141:451–456.
39. Hemingway A, Bors E, Hobby RP. An investigation of the pulmonary function of paraplegics. *J Clin Invest.* 1958;37: 773–782.
40. Kokkola K, Möller K, Lehtonen T. Pulmonary function in tetraplegic and paraplegic patients. *Ann Clin Res.* 1975;7:76–79.
41. Ohry A, Molho M, Rozin R. Alterations of pulmonary function in spinal cord injured patients. *Paraplegia.* 1975;13:101–108.
42. Braun NM, Arora NS, Rochester DF. Respiratory muscle and pulmonary function in polymyositis and other proximal myopathies. *Thorax.* 1983;38:616–623.
43. De Troyer A, Heilporn A. Respiratory mechanics in quadriplegia. The respiratory function of the intercostal muscles. *Am Rev Respir Dis.* 1980;122:591–600.
44. Morgan MD, Gourlay AR, Silver JR, et al. Contribution of the rib cage to breathing in tetraplegia. *Thorax.* 1985;40:613–617.
45. Polkey MI, Green M, Moxham J. Measurement of respiratory muscle strength. *Thorax.* 1995;50:1131–1135.
46. Carter RE. Respiratory aspects of spinal cord injury management. *Paraplegia.* 1987;25:262–266.
47. Slack RS, Shucart W. Respiratory dysfunction associated with traumatic injury to the central nervous system. *Clin Chest Med.* 1994;15:739–749.
48. Forner JV, Llombart RL, Valledor MC. The flow-volume loop in tetraplegics. *Paraplegia.* 1977;15:245–251.
49. Velmahos GC, Toutouzas K, Chan L, et al. Intubation after cervical spinal cord injury: to be done selectively or routinely? *Am Surg.* 2003;69:891–894.
50. Wing PC. Early acute management in adults with spinal cord injury: a clinical practice guideline for health-care providers. *Who should read it? J Spinal Cord Med.* 2008;31:360.
51. Claxton AR, Wong DT, Chung F, et al. Predictors of hospital mortality and mechanical ventilation in patients with cervical spinal cord injury. *Can J Anaesth.* 1998;45: 144–149.
52. Bach JR. Noninvasive respiratory management of high level spinal cord injury. *J Spinal Cord Med.* 2012;35:72–80.
53. Berney S, Stockton K, Berlowitz D, et al. Can early extubation and intensive physiotherapy decrease length of stay of acute quadriplegic patients in intensive care? A retrospective case control study. *Physiother Res Int.* 2002;7:14–22.
54. Como JJ, Sutton ERH, McCunn M, et al. Characterizing the need for mechanical ventilation following cervical spinal cord injury with neurologic deficit. *J Trauma.* 2005;59: 912–916; discussion 916.
55. Romero J, Vari A, Gambarrutta C, et al. Tracheostomy timing in traumatic spinal cord injury. *Eur Spine J.* 2009;18: 1452–1457.
56. Berney S, Opdam H, Bellomo R, et al. An assessment of early tracheostomy after anterior cervical stabilization in patients with acute cervical spine trauma. *J Trauma.* 2008;64: 749–753.
57. O'Keeffe T, Goldman RK, Mayberry JC, et al. Tracheostomy after anterior cervical spine fixation. *J Trauma.* 2004;57:855–860.
58. Ganuza JR, Garcia Forcada A, Gambarrutta C, et al. Effect of technique and timing of tracheostomy in patients with acute traumatic spinal cord injury undergoing mechanical ventilation. *J Spinal Cord Med.* 2011;34:76–84.
59. Ben Nun A, Orlovsky M, Best LA. Percutaneous tracheostomy in patients with cervical spine fractures--feasible and safe. *Interact Cardiovasc Thorac Surg.* 2006;5:427–429.
60. Sustić A, Krstulović B, Eskinja N, et al. Surgical tracheostomy versus percutaneous dilational tracheostomy in patients with anterior cervical spine fixation: preliminary report. *Spine (Phila Pa 1976).* 2002;27:1942–1945; discussion 1945.
61. Mallick A, Bodenham AR. Tracheostomy in critically ill patients. *Eur J Anaesthesiol.* 2010;27:676–682.
62. Babu R, Owens TR, Thomas S, et al. Timing of tracheostomy after anterior cervical spine fixation. *J Trauma Acute Care Surg.* 2013;74:961–966.
63. Ball PA. Critical care of spinal cord injury. *Spine (Phila Pa 1976).* 2001;26:S27–S30.
64. Royster RA, Barboi C, Peruzzi T. Critical care in the acute cervical spinal cord injury. *Topics in Spinal Cord Injury Rehabilitation.* 2004;9:11–32.
65. Wallbom A, Naran B, Thomas E. Acute ventilator management and weaning in individuals with high tetraplegia. *Topics in Spinal Cord Injury Rehabilitation.* 2005;10:1–7.

66. Consortium for Spinal Cord Medicine. Respiratory management following spinal cord injury: a clinical practice guideline for health-care professionals. *J Spinal Cord Med.* 2005; 28:259–293.
67. Peterson P, Brooks C, Mellick D, et al. Protocol for ventilator management in high tetraplegia. *Topics in Spinal Cord Injury Rehabilitation.* 1997;2:101–106.
68. Peterson WP, Barbalata L, Brooks CA, et al. The effect of tidal volumes on the time to wean persons with high tetraplegia from ventilators. *Spinal Cord.* 1999;37:284–288.
69. Fenton JJ, Warner ML, Lammertse D, et al. A comparison of high vs standard tidal volumes in ventilator weaning for individuals with sub-acute spinal cord injuries: a site-specific randomized clinical trial. *Spinal Cord.* 2016;54:234–238.
70. Watt JW, Devine A. Does dead space ventilation always alleviate hypocapnia? Long-term ventilation with plain tracheostomy tubes. *Anaesthesia.* 1995;50:688–691.
71. Gutierrez CJ, Harrow J, Haines F. Using an evidence-based protocol to guide rehabilitation and weaning of ventilator-dependent cervical spinal cord injury patients. *JRRD.* 2003;40:99.
72. Weinberger SE, Weiss JW. Weaning from ventilatory support. *N Engl J Med.* 1995;332:388–389.
73. Peterson W, Charlifue W, Gerhart A, et al. Two methods of weaning persons with quadriplegia from mechanical ventilators. *Paraplegia.* 1994;32:98–103.
74. Brochard L, Rauss A, Benito S, et al. Comparison of three methods of gradual withdrawal from ventilatory support during weaning from mechanical ventilation. *Am J Respir Crit Care Med.* 1994;150:896–903.
75. Esteban A, Frutos F, Tobin MJ, et al. A comparison of four methods of weaning patients from mechanical ventilation. Spanish Lung Failure Collaborative Group. *N Engl J Med.* 1995;332:345–350.
76. Petrof BJ, Jaber S, Matecki S. Ventilator-induced diaphragmatic dysfunction. *Curr Opin Crit Care.* 2010;16:19–25.
77. Pillastrini P, Bordini S, Bazzocchi G, et al. Study of the effectiveness of bronchial clearance in subjects with upper spinal cord injuries: examination of a rehabilitation programme involving mechanical insufflation and exsufflation. *Spinal Cord.* 2006;44:614–616.
78. Berlowitz DJ, Tamplin J. Respiratory muscle training for cervical spinal cord injury. *Cochrane Database Syst Rev.* 2013:CD008507.
79. Roth EJ, Stenson KW, Powley S, et al. Expiratory muscle training in spinal cord injury: a randomized controlled trial. *Arch Phys Med Rehabil.* 2010;91:857–861.
80. Postma K, Haisma JA, Hopman MTE, et al. Resistive inspiratory muscle training in people with spinal cord injury during inpatient rehabilitation: a randomized controlled trial. *Phys Ther.* 2014;94:1709–1719.
81. Mueller G, Hopman MTE, Perret C. Comparison of respiratory muscle training methods in individuals with motor and sensory complete tetraplegia: a randomized controlled trial. *J Rehabil Med.* 2013;45:248–253.
82. Sheel AW, Reid WD, Townson AF, et al. Effects of exercise training and inspiratory muscle training in spinal cord injury: a systematic review. *J Spinal Cord Med.* 2008;31:500–508.
83. Dicpinigaitis PV, Spungen AM, Bauman WA, et al. Bronchial hyperresponsiveness after cervical spinal cord injury. *Chest.* 1994;105:1073–1076.
84. Singas E, Grimm DR, Almenoff PL, et al. Inhibition of airway hyperreactivity by oxybutynin chloride in subjects with cervical spinal cord injury. *Spinal Cord.* 1999;37:279–283.
85. Barratt DJ, Harvey LA, Cistulli PA, et al. The use of bronchodilators in people with recently acquired tetraplegia: a randomised cross-over trial. *Spinal Cord.* 2012;50:836–839.
86. DiMarco AF, Onders RP, Ignagni A, et al. Inspiratory muscle pacing in spinal cord injury: case report and clinical commentary. *J Spinal Cord Med.* 2006;29:95–108.
87. Onders RP, Elmo M, Khansarinia S, et al. Complete worldwide operative experience in laparoscopic diaphragm pacing: results and differences in spinal cord injured patients and amyotrophic lateral sclerosis patients. *Surg Endosc.* 2009;23:1433–1440.
88. Le Pimpec-Barthes F, Legras A, Arame A, et al. Diaphragm pacing: the state of the art. *J Thorac Dis.* 2016;8:S376–S386.
89. Stolzmann KL, Gagnon DR, Brown R, et al. Longitudinal change in FEV1 and FVC in chronic spinal cord injury. *Am J Respir Crit Care Med.* 2008;177:781–786.
90. Goldstein B, Weaver FM, Hammond MC. New CDC recommendations: annual influenza vaccination recommended for individuals with spinal cord injuries. *J Spinal Cord Med.* 2005;28:383–384.
91. Pneumococcal Vaccine Timing for Adults. National Center for Immunization and Respiratory Diseases. Centers for Disease Control and Prevention.

Sleep Disorders in Individuals With Spinal Cord Injury

CHAPTER 15

Oksana Witt and Teodoro Castillo

OUTLINE

Anatomic and Physiologic Changes After Spinal Cord Injury Predisposing to Sleep Disorders

Spinal cord injury (SCI) can lead to alterations in lung, chest wall, and airway mechanics. The degree of respiratory dysfunction closely correlates with the neurological level of injury and degree of motor impairment. Individuals with cervical and thoracic SCI have:

- Decreased lung volumes
- Decreased thoracic wall compliance due to restriction caused by respiratory muscle weakness
- Airway hyperreactivity due to parasympathetic predominance
- Pulmonary function tests show a reduction of vital capacity, total lung capacity, expiratory reserve volume, and inspiratory capacity. Pulmonary function tests also show an increase in residual volume (increased in sitting position due to gravity) and little or no change in functional residual capacity.[1]

A bedside spirometer can be used to measure vital capacity to assess respiratory muscle strength instead of manual muscle test.

Primary muscles of inspiration include the diaphragm, innervated by the phrenic nerve (C3–C5). Accessory muscles of inspiration include the sternocleidomastoid (C2–C4), trapezius muscles (C1–C4), scalene muscles (C3–C8), and external intercostals (T1–T11). Primary muscles of expiration include the abdominal muscles made up of the rectus abdominis, transversus abdominis, internal/external obliques (T4–L2), and internal intercostals (T6–T12). The use of an abdominal binder in sitting position can help by allowing more efficient diaphragmatic resting position. Inspiratory resistive training and aerobic exercise training at a high level (70%–80% of maximum heart rate) in individuals with tetraplegia have been shown to improve the strength and endurance of a weak diaphragm and improve lung function.[2]

Sleep Disordered Breathing

Sleep disordered breathing (SDB) in SCI includes obstructive sleep apnea (OSA), hypoventilation at sleep onset, and central sleep apnea.[3–6]

Definitions

Obstructive sleep apnea is characterized by a repetitive collapse of the upper airway during sleep, usually associated with recurrent episodes of oxygen desaturation, sympathetic hyperactivity, large intrathoracic pressure swings, and can cause fragmentation of sleep and loss of the restorative function of sleep.[2,7]

- Compared to able-bodied individuals with OSA, individuals with American Spinal Injury Association (ASIA) impairment scale (AIS) A and B injuries at C4–C6 with OSA have reduced protective reflex to maintain upper airway patency (genioglossus reflex).[8]
- Loss of sympathetic modulation to the airways with resultant unopposed parasympathetic activation can lead to bronchoconstriction and increased nasal resistance, contributing to upper airway narrowing

by increasing negative pressure in the upper airway.[9,10]

- The apnea–hypopnea index (AHI) is used to classify the severity of OSA: mild OSA if 5–14 events/hour, moderate OSA if 15–29 events/hour, and severe OSA if more than 30 events/hour.
- Sleep-onset hypoventilation with impaired respiratory control and neuroplastic changes contribute to SDB given absence of upper airway resistance after spinal cord injury.

Hypoventilation at sleep onset is not associated with airway obstruction after SCI. Similar to healthy adults, individuals with SCI have decreased ventilation during sleep and increase in carbon dioxide. However, ventilation is decreased significantly more in individuals with C4–C7 injuries (complete and incomplete) than in those with T2–T6 injuries with greater drop in tidal volumes and rise in end-tidal carbon dioxide, indicating alveolar hypoventilation during sleep.[11]

Central sleep apnea is less common than OSA and represents recurrent episodes of diminished drive to the major inspiratory muscles resulting in apneic episodes. Central apnea could be a result of the weakened auxiliary respiratory muscles or a response to potentially respiratory-depressant medications.[12]

Etiology

Factors such as normal aging and comorbidities can disrupt the normal sleep pattern after SCI and in the general population.[13–15] Chronic spasticity and pain may also contribute to disrupted sleep. Cervical SCIs have been associated with greater difficulty falling asleep, more frequent awakenings, greater prescription of sleeping aids, and a higher incidence of snoring when compared with able-bodied controls.[16]

Epidemiology

The prevalence in the general population is estimated to be 24% in men and 9% in women, ages 30–60 years.[17] Prevalence of OSA, even mild, is approximately 40%–50% in chronic SCI and 65%–75% in acute SCI.[12,18–26] Individuals with tetraplegia, especially those with motor level C5 and above, are more likely to have sleep apnea compared with paraplegics.[23,27] Prevalence among adults with paraplegia is not significantly different from what is seen in the general population.[15,16,23,25,28–30] SDB in individuals with tetraplegia may be a biphasic disorder that is (1) acutely caused by the cervical SCI with partial resolution during injury recovery, and (2) increased with age, weight gain, ongoing chronic intermittent hypoxia, and the use of medications that compromise respiration.[20,29,31]

SDB was shown to develop early after onset of SCI with 62% of individuals having it by 4 weeks postinjury.[20]

Risk Factors

In chronic SCI, associations have been reported between OSA prevalence and increasing age, body mass index (BMI), and neck circumference, but these relationships are weaker in the acute postinjury period.[16,20,23,29,32]

- BMI is directly correlated with apnea severity, and is even stronger for people with tetraplegia screened by polysomnography[16,23,25,33,34]
- Neck circumference correlates with apnea severity in individuals with tetraplegia[16,25]
- Medications such as opiates, benzodiazepines, antispasticity, and antiarrhythmics can worsen both central and obstructive sleep apnea by depressing the central nervous system[35,36]
- Some individuals may be genetically predisposed to sleep apnea given a higher incidence in first-degree relatives[37]
- Supine sleeping position imposes greater gravitational narrowing of the upper airway and increases risk for OSA
- Greater adiposity for any given BMI compared with the general population, which leads to greater fat accumulation in the cervical region[38]

Other potential factors: Poor coordination between respiratory and pharyngeal dilator muscles, increased upper airway collapsibility (due to obesity), a reduced arousal threshold, and an unstable ventilatory control system.[10,12,29,39–42]

Assessment

OSA is characterized by loud snoring, witnessed pauses in breathing (apnea) during sleep, gasping arousals, excessive daytime sleepiness, fatigue, nocturia, and morning headaches.[6,43] Persons with SCI may also be taking medications that affect breathing, including sedatives, muscle relaxants, and narcotics.[26] In the Stockhammer study, most of the participants with apnea were not obese and few had daytime complaints.[16] The Epworth sleepiness scale can be used to assess the degree of daytime sleepiness. Due to the high prevalence of sleep apnea, especially with long-standing SCI, people with symptoms of SDB should be interviewed carefully and undergo polysomnography for definitive diagnosis of SDB.[21,24,44]

Complications

OSA results in excessive sleepiness, and increases risk for systemic and pulmonary hypertension, congestive heart failure, depression, increased mortality, decreased quality of life, functional impairment, and an increased risk for stroke or myocardial infarction.[2,43,45–50] Disruptions in gas exchange, intrathoracic pressure swings, and arousals during SDB can lead to autonomic nervous system fluctuations and cardiac arrhythmias.[51] Snoring is an independent predictor of ischemic heart disease and stroke in the general population and is more prevalent, more intense, and more persistent in people with SCI compared with the general population.[6,52] Sleep-related hypoxemia is correlated to cognitive changes, and severe OSA (AHI >30) in individuals with tetraplegia is associated with poorer attention, information processing, and recall compared with milder OSA.[53]

Management

Lifestyle interventions, such as exercise and weight loss, should be encouraged for people with SDB.[54,55] Positive airway pressure (PAP) is the main treatment of sleep apnea for people with and without SCI. There are three basic designs of facial masks: covering nose (nasal mask), fitting into the nostrils (nasal pillow mask), or covering both the nose and mouth (full-face mask). Nasal pillows may be better suited for tetraplegic individuals with limited upper extremity mobility.[56]

Types of PAP therapy include:

- *Fixed continuous positive airway pressure (CPAP)*: side effects of CPAP can include nasal congestion (60%), mask discomfort (40%), dryness (30%), frequent awakenings (30%), and complaints from bed partner (5%).[57]
- *Bilevel positive airway pressure:* is used for individuals with high pressure requirements. It has two pressure settings: one for inspiration and one for expiration.
- *Adaptive servo-ventilation:* provides support to the person's breathing pattern and is designed to treat central sleep apnea, complex sleep apnea, and Cheyne–Stokes respiration.
- *Automatic positive airway pressure:* pressure is delivered automatically, changing as needed to deliver the minimal pressure required to maintain airway patency.

Despite PAP being an effective treatment for OSA and showing improvement even with partial adherence, only 20%–50% of individuals with chronic SCI and SDB report adherence with CPAP due to an inability to fall asleep while wearing CPAP (63%), lack of improvement in symptoms (25%), or belief that treatment was unnecessary (8%).[15,16,23,57–60]

Other treatment options for mild or moderate OSA include oral appliances that move the mandible forward, or tongue retaining devices to open the posterior airspace.[61,62] Although they are less effective than PAP at improving AHI, the impact on symptoms and other health outcomes is the same. Dental conditions are relative contraindications to oral appliance therapy.[63] Other alternative treatments for SDB include upper airway surgery for adenotonsillar hypertrophy or retrognathia and hypoglossal nerve stimulation, although they have not been studied in the SCI population.[63–66]

Periodic Leg Movement and Restless Leg Syndrome

Etiology

Periodic leg movements (PLM) are characterized by periodic episodes of repetitive and highly stereotyped limb movements, involving great toe and ankle dorsiflexion, often accompanied by knee and hip flexion.[67,68] There are several conditions that fall under PLM, including periodic leg movement syndrome, periodic limb movement disorder, and restless leg syndrome.

Periodic limb movement disorder (PLMD) occurs when periodic leg movement syndrome (PLMS), an incidental finding on polysomnography of five or more PLM events per hour of sleep without clinical consequences, is accompanied by nonrestorative sleep or daytime sleepiness.[69] Using these criteria, PLMD should be diagnosed and treatments explored. PLMS can be present in up to 80% of individuals with restless leg syndrome.[70] PLMS predominate in nonrapid eye movement (NREM) sleep in the general population but occur in both NREM and rapid eye movement (REM) sleep in individuals with tetraplegia and paraplegia with complete and incomplete lesions, suggesting the existence of a spinal cord central pattern generator of PLMS.[67,68,70–72]

Restless leg syndrome (RLS) or Ekbom syndrome is characterized by uncomfortable leg sensations usually prior to sleep onset that causes an urge to move.[73] Possible etiologies of RLS include iron deficiency, neurotransmitter dysfunction, circadian rhythm disruption, and genetic factors. RLS may also be related to mesencephalic or other supraspinal neuroplastic changes, such as impaired dopaminergic regulation.[74]

Epidemiology

PLM indexes are higher in individuals with tetraplegia and paraplegia, especially with AIS C and D, compared with healthy controls based on polysomnography studies with prevalence 58% among those with complete and incomplete tetraplegia.[27,67] Severity and prevalence were not affected by SDB.[67] Patients with tetraplegia have greater tendency toward PLM arousals compared with paraplegic individuals and controls.[75] It has been reported that 28.6% of tetraplegic and paraplegic individuals had PLMS within the first year post-injury and it is more frequent in incomplete motor injuries compared with complete injuries.[27] PLMD prevalence has been reported to be 50%–100% among individuals with an injury above T10.[27,68,71,72,75–82] Of note, having SDB precludes the diagnosis of PLMD according to the International Classification of Sleep Disorders (ICSD-3).[20,29]

Complications

RLS can cause sleep-onset insomnia and interfere with sleep quality. Lower quality of life has been reported based on Short Form 36 Health Survey Questionnaire (SF-36).[83]

Assessment

RLS is a clinical diagnosis, characterized by an uncomfortable feeling in the lower extremities and occasionally in the upper extremities, with an irresistible urge to move, which usually provides partial or complete relief. Although people with SCI do not always have voluntary control of their lower extremities, they report similar complaints of leg discomfort that is relieved by massage or moving their legs. RLS can be confounded by neuropathic pain and muscle spasticity. Refractory "spasticity" despite maximal antispasticity therapy can be undiagnosed and/or untreated PLM.[69]

Considering RLS etiologies include iron deficiency, workup should include iron stores level with iron supplementation if iron is below 45 µg/dL.[84] MRI has demonstrated decreased iron in the substantia nigra of individuals with RLS, indicating that central nervous system iron deficiency may result in the inability of neurons in the substantia nigra pars compacta to transport dopamine.[85]

Management

Physical exercise is the first-line treatment of RLS, since it releases endorphins and dopamine, which leads to the activation of opiate and dopamine receptors.[80] Dopamine agonists, such as ropinirole (Requip) or pramipexole (Mirapex), should be trialed if symptoms persist despite exercise and iron supplementation. Individuals with confirmed PLM had substantial reduction in PLM index and arousals from sleep with low-dose pramipexole treatment.[86,87] If symptoms worsen on dopamine agonists, serum ferritin levels should be checked and a different agent should be tried, such as gabapentin (Neurontin).[88]

Circadian Rhythm Sleep–Wake Disorders

General Principles

In healthy individuals, light striking the retina stimulates the suprachiasmatic nuclei, which subsequently inhibits melatonin via the superior cervical ganglion before reaching the pineal gland that produces melatonin. Thus, melatonin production is inhibited during the daytime, but darkness removes this inhibition. Circadian rhythm disruption can lead to dysregulation of other hormones, such as cortisol, aldosterone, and growth hormone.[89]

Etiology

Since the superior cervical ganglion plays a role in melatonin inhibition, SCI's affecting this region can lead to significant disruption in circadian rhythm.[31] After a complete cervical SCI, the afferent input of and the efferent sympathetic innervation of the pineal gland via the superior cervical ganglion gets interrupted. Thus, circadian rhythmicity of melatonin is disrupted in tetraplegia.[90–95] Compared to healthy subjects, individuals with cervical SCI have significantly higher morning serum concentrations of melatonin, and lower evening and nighttime melatonin levels, along with statistically significant differences in the evening and midnight levels of cortisol levels.[89] This disturbance in the circadian pattern of melatonin and cortisol release in the SCI population could partially explain the disturbed sleep–wake cycle often observed in these individuals.

Phase advancement of temperature seen in tetraplegia, but not paraplegia, may contribute to poor sleep quality.[96] Antidiuretic hormone (ADH) increases at night in able-bodied individuals, resulting in lower urine output; however, people with SCI do not have a significant change in ADH during the day and at night, irrespective of whether the SCI was above or below T6.[97] Although there is paucity of studies on urinary problems and sleep, 17% of SCI individuals have reported voiding as their primary problem with sleep.[6]

Epidemiology

Tetraplegic individuals with complete and incomplete lesions at C4–T1 have fragmented sleep architecture and reduced slow wave and REM sleep based on electroencephalogram sleep, whereas paraplegic individuals have normal sleep stages.[9,98] Compared to control populations, individuals with tetraplegia were also shown to have an increase in percentage of stage 1 and decrease in the percentages of stage 2 and REM sleep.[32,39] Delayed REM onset has been reported in people with tetraplegia, especially in those with AIS A compared with other AIS classifications.[29] Environmental, social, and physiological effects may also contribute to sleep disturbances.

Management

Treatment of circadian rhythm disorders includes sleep hygiene, exogenous melatonin, and light therapy.[99,100] Melatonin in low doses (~1 mg) helps shift the circadian clock, whereas larger doses (greater than 3 mg) produce a hypnotic effect. Thus, chronic melatonin supplementation may help with sleep-onset insomnia and sleep phase entrainment.[101,102] Exogenous melatonin has been shown to be safe in tetraplegia, can normalize clock gene expression in peripheral blood, and is associated with significant subjective improvements in sleep quality, time to sleep initiation, and measures of psychological well-being; proportion of light sleep (stages 1 and 2) also increased significantly.[90–93] Melatonin is also a potent scavenger of reactive oxygen species and its neuroprotective or antioxidant properties have been shown in animal models of traumatic brain injury and SCI.[103]

Insomnia

General principles

Chronic insomnia is defined as difficulty initiating or maintaining sleep occurring at least 3 days per week for greater than 4 weeks with daytime consequences.[69]

Etiology

Insomnia has a higher prevalence in individuals with SCI compared to the general population, likely due to voiding problems, muscle spasms, and pain.[6] Individuals with SCI have greater difficulty with both sleep initiation and maintenance and have a higher rate of use of sleep aids. Compared with people without SCI, individuals with SCI have significantly greater incidence of sleep-related problems, with younger individuals having more sleep problems compared with older ones.[104]

Epidemiology

Insomnia is prevalent in the general population and is present in 15%–30% and women have higher risk than men, with contributing factors including pain, mood disorders, medications, circadian rhythm disruption, and other medical comorbidities.[18,105] Based on a survey, 57% of SCI individuals had insomnia symptoms, although it could have been confounded by SDB.[106] Another study has found that 49% of people with SCI complained of sleep dysfunction in the past year, with a higher percentage of cigarette smokers, asthma or chronic obstructive pulmonary disease, hypertension, and alcohol related issues in that group.[18]

Complications

Insomnia disorder can increase the risk for intolerance of PAP therapy for SDB and should be addressed prior to initiation of PAP therapy.[107]

Management

Initial treatment should start with proper sleep hygiene and other behavioral aspects.[69] Pharmacological therapy should be used only after cognitive-behavioral therapy for insomnia (CBT-I) has been attempted given concerns for fall risk and impaired cognition.[108] CBT-I includes behavioral techniques (stimulus control, sleep restriction therapy, sleep hygiene, and relaxation/arousal reduction strategies) in addition to cognitive therapy to address sleep-related thoughts and beliefs. Unfortunately, no formal studies of CBT-I have been conducted in SCI. Hypnotic medications should only be used on a short-term basis, since they have poor long-term efficacy in the general adult population.[43] Comorbid conditions should be addressed if present.[69]

Review Questions

1. Obstructive sleep apnea:
   a. Is more prevalent in tetraplegic and paraplegic individuals compared with the general population
   b. Is defined by greater than 90% loss of airflow with continued or increased thoracic and abdominal effort for at least 10 seconds
   c. Is defined as greater than 90% loss of airflow with absent thoracic and abdominal effort for at least 10 seconds
   d. Represents exaggerated response to hypoventilation or rise in partial pressure of carbon dioxide (pCO_2) that leads to a rapid increase in ventilation and subsequent rapid decline in pCO_2.
2. Sleep-disordered breathing can be treated with all of the following, EXCEPT:
   a. APAP
   b. Melatonin
   c. Adaptive servo-ventilation
   d. Oral appliances
3. Periodic leg movements are defined as:
   a. Periodic episodes of repetitive and highly stereotyped limb movements, involving great toe and ankle dorsiflexion, often accompanied by knee and hip flexion
   b. Five or more PLM events per hour of sleep, found on polysomnography and is an usually incidental finding without clinical consequences
   c. Five or more PLM events per hour of sleep, found on polysomnography, accompanied by nonrestorative sleep or daytime sleepiness
   d. Uncomfortable feeling in the lower extremities and occasionally in the upper extremities prior to sleep onset that causes an irresistible urge to move, which usually provides partial or complete relief.
4. Compared to the general population, individuals with SCI:
   a. Have the same variability in circadian rhythm of leg resistance and flow
   b. Have higher 24-hour heart rate values

c. Do not have nocturnal decrease in blood pressure or significant blood pressure variability over 24 hours
d. Have the same energy expenditure and sleeping metabolic rate

5. Initial treatment of insomnia should start with:
a. Dopamine agonists
b. Proper sleep hygiene
c. Hypnotic medications
d. Cognitive-behavioral therapy for insomnia

REFERENCES

1. Schilero G, Spungen A, Bauman W, Radulovic M, Lesser M. Pulmonary function and spinal cord injury. *Respir Physiol Neurobiol.* 2009;166(3):129–141.
2. Cifu D. *Braddom's Physical Medicine and Rehabilitation.* 6th ed. Philadelphia, PA: Elsevier; 2020.
3. Ancoli-Israel S, Kripke D, Mason W, Messin S. Sleep apnea and nocturnal myoclonus in a senior population. *Sleep.* 1981;4:349–358.
4. Carskadon M, Brown E, Dement W. Sleep fragmentation in the elderly: relationship to daytime sleep tendency. *Neurobiol Aging.* 1982;3:321–327.
5. Czeisler C, Moore-Ede M, Coleman R. Rotating shift work schedules that disrupt sleep are improved by applying circadian principles. *Science.* 1982;217(4558):460–463.
6. Biering-Sorensen F, Biering-Sorensen M. Sleep disturbances in the spinal cord injured: an epidemiological questionnaire investigation, including a normal population. *Spinal Cord.* 2001;39(10):505–513.
7. Bascom A, Sankari A, Goshgarian H, Badr M. Sleep onset hypoventilation in chronic spinal cord injury. *Physiol Rep.* 2015;3(8):e12490.
8. Castriotta R, Wilde M, Sahay S. Sleep disorders in spinal cord injury. *Sleep Med Clin.* 2012;7(4):643–653.
9. Giannoccaro M, Moghadam K, Pizza F, et al. Sleep disorders in patients with spinal cord injury. *Sleep Med Rev.* 2013;17(6):399–409.
10. Sankari A, Bascom A, Chowdhuri S, Badr M. Tetraplegia is a risk factor for central sleep apnea. *J Appl Physiol 1985.* 2014;116(3):345–353.
11. Kryger M, Roth T, Dement W. *Principles and Practice of Sleep Medicine.* 6th ed. New York: Elsevier; 2016.
12. Wijesuriya N, Gainche L, Jordan A, et al. Genioglossus reflex responses to negative upper airway pressure are altered in people with tetraplegia and obstructive sleep apnoea. *J Physiol.* 2018;596(14):2853–2864.
13. Krassioukov A. Autonomic function following cervical spinal cord injury. *Respir Physiol Neurobiol.* 2009;169(2):157–164.
14. Wijesuriya N, Lewis C, Butler J, et al. High nasal resistance is stable over time but poorly perceived in people with tetraplegia and obstructive sleep apnoea. *Respir Physiol Neurobiol.* 2017;235:27–33.
15. Sankari A, Bascom A, Oomman S, Badr M. Sleep disordered breathing in chronic spinal cord injury. *J Clin Sleep Med.* 2014;10(1):65–72.
16. Stockhammer E, Tobon A, Michel F, et al. Characteristics of sleep apnea syndrome in tetraplegic patients. *Spinal Cord.* 2002;40(6):286–294.
17. Young T, Palta M, Dempsey J, Skatrud J, Weber S, Badr S. The occurrence of sleep-disordered breathing among middle-aged adults. *N Engl J Med.* 1993;328(17):1230–1235.
18. Lavela S, Burns S, Goldstein B. Dysfunctional sleep in persons with spinal cord injuries and disorders. *Spinal Cord.* 2012;50(9):682–685.
19. Burns S, Rad M, Bryant S, Kapur V. Long-term treatment of sleep apnea in persons with spinal cord injury. *Am J Phys Med Rehabil.* 2005;84(8):620–626.
20. Berlowitz D, Brown D, Campbell D, Pierce R. A longitudinal evaluation of sleep and breathing in the first year after cervical spinal cord injury. *Arch Phys Med Rehabil.* 2005;86(6):1193–1199.
21. Chiodo A, Sitrin R, Bauman K. Sleep disordered breathing in spinal cord injury: a systematic review. *J Spinal Cord Med.* 2016;39(4):374–382.
22. Klefbeck B, Sternhag M, Weinberg J, Levi R, Hultling C, Borg J. Obstructive sleep apneas in relation to severity of cervical spinal cord injury. *Spinal Cord.* 1998;36(9):621–628.
23. Burns S, Kapur V, Yin K, Buhrer R. Factors associated with sleep apnea in men with spinal cord injury: a population-based case-control study. *Spinal Cord.* 2001;39(1):15–22.
24. Sankari A, Martin J, Bascom A, Mitchell M, Badr M. Identification and treatment of sleep-disordered breathing in chronic spinal cord injury. *Spinal Cord.* 2015;53(2):145–149.
25. Leduc B, Dagher J, Mayer P, Bellemare F, Lepage Y. Estimated prevalence of obstructive sleep apnea–hypopnea syndrome after cervical cord injury. *Arch Phys Med Rehabil.* 2007;88(3):333–337.
26. Bauman K, Kurili A, Schotland H, Rodriguez G, Chiodo A, Sitrin R. Simplified approach to diagnosing sleep-disordered breathing and nocturnal hypercapnia in individuals with spinal cord injury. *Arch Phys Med Rehabil.* 2016;97:363–371.
27. Proserpio P, Lanza A, Sambusida K, et al. Sleep apnea and periodic leg movements in the first year after spinal cord injury. *Sleep Med.* 2015;16(1):59–66.
28. Kim A, Keenan B, Jackson N, et al. Tongue fat and its relationship to obstructive sleep apnea. *Sleep.* 2014;37(10):1639–1648.
29. Berlowitz D, Spong J, Gordon I, Howard M, Brown D. Relationships between objective sleep indices and symptoms in a community sample of people with tetraplegia. *Arch Phys Med Rehabil.* 2012;93(7):1246–1252.
30. Tran K, Hukins C, Geraghty T, Eckert B, Fraser L. Sleep-disordered breathing in spinal cord-injured patients: a short-term longitudinal study. *Respirology.* 2010;15(2):272–276.
31. Sankari A, Badr M, Martin J, Ayas N, Berlowitz D. Impact of spinal cord injury on sleep: current perspectives. *Nat Sci Sleep.* 2019;11:219–229.
32. McEvoy R, Mykytyn I, Sajkov D, et al. Sleep apnoea in patients with quadriplegia. *Thorax.* 1995;50(6):613–619.
33. Flavell H, Marshall R, Thorton A, Clements P, Antic R, McEvoy R. Hypoxia episodes during sleep in high tetraplegia. *Arch Phys Med Rehabil.* 1992;73(7):623–627.
34. Young T, Peppard P, Gottlieb D. Epidemiology of obstructive sleep apnea: a population health perspective. *AM J Respir Crit Care Med.* 2002;165(9):1217–1239.
35. Dolly F, Block A. Effect of flurazepam on sleep-disordered breathing and nocturnal oxygen desaturation in asymptomatic subjects. *Am J Med.* 1982;73:239–243.
36. Ramsawh H, Bloom H, Ancoli-Israel S. Sleep, aging and late-life insomnia. In: Fillit HM, Rockwood K, Woodhouse K, eds. 7th ed. *Brocklehurst's Textbook of Geriatric Medicine and Gerontology.* Philadelphia: Saunders Elsevier; 2010: 943–948.

37. Redline S, Tishler P. The genetics of sleep apnea. *Sleep Med Rev*. 2000;4(6):583–602.
38. Spungen A, Adkins R, Stewart C, et al. Factors influencing body composition in persons with spinal cord injury: a cross sectional study. *J Appl Physiol*. 2003;95(6):2398–2407.
39. Cahan C, Gothe B, Decker M, Arnold J, Stohl K. Arterial oxygen saturation over time and sleep studies in quadriplegic patients. *Paraplegia*. 1993;31:172–179.
40. Rizwan A, Sankari A, Bascom A, Vaughan S, Badr M. Nocturnal swallowing and arousal threshold in individuals with chronic spinal cord injury. *J Appl Physiol*. 2018;125(2): 445–452.
41. Fuller D. How does spinal cord injury lead to obstructive sleep apnoea? *J Physiol*. 2018;596(14):2633.
42. Sankari A, Bascom A, Badr M. Upper airway mechanics in chronic spinal cord injury during sleep. *J Appl Physiol. 1985*. 2014;116(11):1390–1395.
43. Avidan A, Zee P. *Handbook of Sleep Medicine*. Philadelphia: Lippincott Williams and Wilkins; 2011.
44. Berry R, Brooks R, Gamaldo C, et al. The AASM Manual for the Scoring of Sleep and Associated Events: Rules, Terminology and Technical Specifications, Version 2.2. [Internet]. *American Academy of Sleep Medicine*. 2015 https://aasm.org/.
45. Scheer F, Zeitzer J, Ayas N, Brown R, Czeisler C, Shea S. Reduced sleep efficiency in cervical spinal cord injury; association with abolished night time melatonin secretion. *Spinal Cord*. 2006;44(2):78–81.
46. Bahammam A. Factors that may influence apnea–hypopnea index in patients with acute myocardial infarction. *Chest*. 2009;136(5):1444–1445.
47. Somers V, White D, Amin R, et al. Sleep apnea and cardiovascular disease: an American Heart Association/American College of Cardiology Foundation Scientific Statement from the American Heart Association Council for High Blood Pressure Research Professional Education Committee, Council on Clinical Cardiology, Stroke Council, and Council on Cardiovascular Nursing. In collaboration with the National Heart, Lung, and Blood Institute National Center on Sleep Disorders Research (National Institutes of Health). *Circulation*. 2008;118(10):1080–1111.
48. Garvey J, Pengo M, Drakatos P, Kent B. Epidemiological aspects of obstructive sleep apnea. *J Thorac Dis*. 2015;7(5):920–929.
49. Shahar E, Whitney C, Redline S, et al. Sleep disordered breathing and cardiovascular disease: cross-sectional results of the Sleep Heart Health Study. *AM J Respir Crit Care Med*. 2001;163(1):19–25.
50. Young T, Finn L, Peppard P, et al. Sleep disordered breathing and mortality: eighteen year follow-up of the Wisconsin Sleep Cohort. *Sleep*. 2008;31(8):1071–1078.
51. Fuller D, Lee K, Tester N. The impact of spinal cord injury on breathing during sleep. *Respir Physiol Neurobiol*. 2013;188(3):344–354.
52. Koskenvuo M, Kaprio J, Telakivi T. Snoring as a risk factor for ischaemic heart disease and stroke in men. *Br Med J*. 1987;294:16–19.
53. Schembri R, Spong J, Graco M, Berlowitz D, COSAQ study team Neuropsychological function in patients with acute tetraplegia and sleep disordered breathing. *Sleep*. 2017;40(2):zsw037.
54. Shojaei M, Alavinia S, Craven B. Management of obesity after spinal cord injury: a systematic review. *J Spinal Cord Med*. 2017;40(6):783–794.
55. Iftikhar I, Bittencourt L, Youngstedt S, et al. Comparative efficacy of CPAP, MADs, exercise-training, and dietary weight loss for sleep apnea: a network meta-analysis. *Sleep Med*. 2017;30:7–14.
56. Le Guen M, Cistulli P, Berlowitz D. Continuous positive airway pressure requirements in patients with tetraplegia and obstructive sleep apnoea. *Spinal Cord*. 2012;50(11):832–835.
57. Engleman H, Asgari-Jirhandeh N, McLeod A, Ramsay C, Deary I, Douglas N. Self-reported use of CPAP and benefits of CPAP therapy. *Chest*. 1996;109:1470–1476.
58. Berlowitz D, Schembri R, Graco M, et al. Positive airway pressure for sleep-disordered breathing in acute quadriplegia: a randomized controlled trial. *Thorax*. 2019;74(3):282–290.
59. Berlowitz D, Spong J, Pierce R, Ross J, Barnes M, Brown D. The feasibility of using auto-titrating continuous positive airway pressure to treat obstructive sleep apnea after acute tetraplegia. *Spinal Cord*. 2009;47(12):868–873.
60. Graco M, Green S, Tolson J, et al. Worth the effort? Weighing up the benefit and burden of continuous positive airway pressure therapy for the treatment of obstructive sleep apnea in chronic tetraplegia. *Spinal Cord*. 2019;57(3):247–254.
61. Gotsopoulos H, Chen C, Qian J, Cistulli P. Oral appliance therapy improves symptoms in obstructive sleep apnea: a randomized, controlled trial. *Am J Respir Crit Care Med*. 2002;166(5):743–748.
62. Ferguson K, Cartwright R, Rogers R, Schmidt-Nowara W. Oral appliances for snoring and obstructive sleep apnea: a review. *Sleep*. 2006;29(2):244–262.
63. Epstein L, Kristo D, Strollo PJ, et al. Clinical guideline for the evaluation, management and long- term care of obstructive sleep apnea in adults. *J Clin Sleep Med*. 2009;5(3): 263–276.
64. Strollo PJ, Soose R, Maurer J, et al. Upper airway stimulation in obstructive sleep apnea. *N Engl J Med*. 2014;370(2): 139–149.
65. Wong K, Marshall N, Grunstein R, Dodd M, Rogers N. Comparing the neurocognitive effects of 40 h sustained wakefulness in patients with untreated OSA and healthy controls. *J Sleep Res*. 2008;17(3):322–330.
66. Caples S, Rowley J, Prinsell J, et al. Surgical modifications of the upper airway for obstructive sleep apnea in adults: a systematic review and meta-analysis. *Sleep*. 2010;33 (10):1396–1407.
67. Peters A, van Silfhout L, Graco M, Schembri R, Thijssen D, Berlowitz D. Periodic limb movements in tetraplegia. *J Spinal Cord Med*. 2018;41(3):318–325.
68. Dickel M, Renfrow S, Moore P, Berry R. Rapid eye movement sleep periodic leg movements in patients with spinal cord injury. *Sleep*. 1994;17(8):733–738.
69. Kirshblum S, Lin V. *Spinal Cord Medicine*. 3rd ed. New York: Demos Medical Publishing; 2018.
70. Ferri R, Proserpio P, Rundo F, et al. Neurophysiological correlates of sleep leg movements in acute spinal cord injury. *Clin Neurophysiol*. 2015;126(2):333–338.
71. de Mello M, Lauro F, Silva A, Tufik S. Incidence of periodic leg movements and of the restless legs syndrome during sleep following acute physical activity in spinal cord injury subjects. *Spinal Cord*. 1996;34(5):294–296.

72. Mello M, Silva A, Rueda A, Poyares D, Tufik S. Correlation between K complex, periodic leg movements (PLM), and myoclonus during sleep in paraplegic adults before and after an acute physical activity. *Spinal Cord.* 1997;35(4):248–252.
73. Manconi M, Ferri R, Zucconi M, et al. Dissociation of periodic leg movements from arousals in restless legs syndrome. *Ann Neurol.* 2012;71(6):834–844.
74. Kang S, Lee H, Jung S, et al. Characteristics and clinical correlates of restless legs syndrome in schizophrenia. *Neuropsychopharmacol Biol Psychiatry.* 2007;31(5):1078–1083.
75. Telles S, Alves R, Chadi G. Periodic limb movements during sleep and restless legs syndrome in patients with ASIA A spinal cord injury. *J Neurol Sci.* 2011;303(1–2):119–123.
76. Salminen A, Manconi M, Rimpilä V, et al. Disconnection between periodic leg movements and cortical arousals in spinal cord injury. *J Clin Sleep Med.* 2013;9(11):1207–1209.
77. Esteves A, de Mello M, Lancellotti C, Natal C, Tufik S. Occurrence of limb movement during sleep in rats with spinal cord injury. *Brain Res.* 2004;1017(1–2):32–38.
78. Ondo W. Movements mimicking myoclonus associated with spinal cord pathology: is this a "pure motor restless legs syndrome.". *Tremor Hyperkinetic Mov N.* 2012:2.
79. Telles S, Alves R, Chadi G. Spinal cord injury as a trigger to develop periodic leg movements during sleep: an evolutionary perspective. *Arq Neuro-Psiquiatra.* 2012;70(11):1–6.
80. de Mello M, Esteves A, Tufik S. Comparison between dopaminergic agents and physical exercise as treatment for periodic limb movements in patients with spinal cord injury. *Spinal Cord.* 2004;42(4):218–221.
81. Yokota T, Hirose K, Tanabe H, Tsukagoshi H. Sleep-related periodic leg movements (nocturnal myoclonus) due to spinal cord lesion. *J Neurol Sci.* 1991;104(1):13–18.
82. Lee M, Choi Y, Lee S, Lee S. Sleep-related periodic leg movements associated with spinal cord lesions. *Mov Disord.* 1996;11(6):719–722.
83. Winkelman J, Redline S, Baldwin C, Resnick H, Newman A, Gottlieb D. Polysomnographic and health-related quality of life correlates of restless legs syndrome in the sleep Heart Health Study. *Sleep.* 2009;32(6):772–778.
84. Allen R, Earley C. The role of iron in restless legs syndrome. *Mov Disord.* 2007;22(Suppl):S440–S448.
85. Connor J, Want X, Allen R, et al. Altered dopaminergic profile in the putamen and substantia nigra in restless legs syndrome. *Brain.* 2009;132(Pt 9):2403–2412.
86. Nilsson S, Levi R, Nordstrom A. Treatment-resistant sensory motor symptoms in persons with SCI may be signs of restless legs syndrome. *Spinal Cord.* 2011;49:754–756.
87. Levy J, Hartley S, Mauruc-Soubirac E, et al. Spasticity or periodic limb movements? *Eur J Phys Rehabil Med.* 2018;54(5):698–704.
88. Happe S, Sauter C, Klosch G, Saletu B, Zeitlhofer J. Gabapentin versus ropinirole in the treatment of idiopathic restless legs syndrome. *Neuropsycholobiology.* 2003;48(2):82–86.
89. Fatima G, Sharma V, Verma N. Circadian variations in melatonin and cortisol in patients with cervical spinal cord injury. *Spinal Cord.* 2016;54:364–367.
90. Spong J, Kennedy G, Brown D, Armstrong S, Berlowitz D. Melatonin supplementation in patients with complete tetraplegia and poor sleep. *Sleep Disord.* 2013:128197.
91. Spong J, Kennedy G, Tseng J, Brown D, Armstrong S, Berlowitz D. Sleep disruption in tetraplegia: a randomized, double-blind, placebo-controlled crossover trial of 3 mg melatonin. *Spinal Cord.* 2014;52(8):629–634.
92. Kostovski E, Frigato E, Savikj M, et al. Normalization of disrupted clock gene expression in males with tetraplegia: a crossover randomized placebo-controlled trial of melatonin supplementation. *Spinal Cord.* 2018;56(11):1076–1083.
93. Zeitzer J, Ku B, Ota D, Kiratli B. Randomized controlled trial of pharmacological replacement of melatonin for sleep disruption in individuals with tetraplegia. *J Spinal Cord Med.* 2014;37(1):46–53.
94. Verhegen R, Jones H, Nyakayiru J, et al. Complete absence of evening melatonin increase in tetraplegics. *Faseb J.* 2012;26(7):3059–3064.
95. Kostovski E, Dahm A, Mowinckel M, et al. Circadian rhythms of hemostatic factors in tetraplegia: a double-blind, randomized, placebo-controlled cross-over study of melatonin. *Spinal Cord.* 2015;53(4):285–290.
96. Thijssen D, Eijsvogels T, Hesse M, Ballak D, Atkinson G, Hopman M. The effects of thoracic and cervical spinal cord lesions on the circadian rhythm of core body temperature. *Chronobiol Int.* 2011;28(2):146–154.
97. Kilinc S, Akman M, Levendoglu F, Ozker R. Diurnal variation of antidiuretic hormone and urinary output in spinal cord injury. *Spinal Cord.* 1999;37(5):332–335.
98. Adey W, Bors E, Porter R. EEG sleep patterns after high cervical lesions in man. *Arch Neurol.* 1968;19:377–383.
99. Mundey K, Benloucif S, Harsanyi K. Phase-dependent treatment of delayed sleep phase syndrome with melatonin. *Sleep.* 2005;28(10):1271–1278.
100. Rosenthal N, Joseph-Vanderpool J, Levendosky A, et al. Phase-shifting effects of bright morning light as treatment for delayed sleep phase syndrome. *Sleep.* 1990;13(4):354–361.
101. Fischer S, Smolnik R, Herms M, Born J, Fehm H. Melatonin acutely improves the neuroendocrine architecture of sleep in blind individuals. *J Clin Endocrinol Metab.* 2003; 88(11):5315–5320.
102. Skene D, Arendt J. Circadian rhythm sleep disorders in the blind and their treatment with melatonin. *Sleep Med.* 2007;8(6):651–655.
103. Naseem M, Parvez S. Role of melatonin in traumatic brain injury and spinal cord injury. *Scientific World Journal.* 2014;2014:1–13.
104. Jensen M, Hirsh A, Molton I, Bamer A. Sleep problems in individuals with spinal cord injury: frequency and age effects. *Rehabil Psychol.* 2009;54(3):323–351.
105. Davenport P, Chan P, Zhang W, Chou Y. Detection threshold for inspiratory resistive loads and respiratory-related evoked potentials. *J Appl Physiol.* 2007;102(1):s276–S285.
106. Shafazand S, Anderson K, Nash M. Sleep complaints and sleep quality in spinal cord injury: a web-based survey. *J Clin Sleep Med.* 2019;15(5):719–724.
107. Wallace D, Sawyer A, Shafazand S. Comorbid insomnia symptoms predict lower 6-month adherence to CPAP in US veterans with obstructive sleep apnea. *Sleep Breath.* 2018;22(1):5–15.
108. Qaseem A, Kansagara D, Forciea M, Cooke M, Denberg T. Management of chronic insomnia disorder in adults: a clinical practice guideline from the American college of physicians. *Ann Intern Med.* 2016;165(2):125–133.

Thromboembolism/Deep Vein Thrombosis

CHAPTER 16

Audrey Leung and Hetal Patel

OUTLINE

Epidemiology

Venous thromboembolism (VTE), which includes deep venous thrombosis (DVT) and pulmonary embolism (PE), is a major complication affecting individuals with acute spinal cord injuries (SCI).[1] The incidence of DVT in acute SCI varies greatly, ranging anywhere between 9% and 90%.[2–12] In patients with SCI who do not receive prophylaxis, over 80% of DVTs occur within the first 2 weeks of injury.[6] VTE can lead to significant mortality and morbidity, with death secondary to PE being about 3.5% in the first 3 months following injury.[2] Thus, prevention and management of VTE remain important considerations when caring for patients with SCIs.

Risk factors for VTE in spinal cord injury[13]

- Paraplegia vs. tetraplegia
- Increasing age
- Complete injuries (AIS A)
- Concomitant lower extremity or pelvic fractures
- Previous VTE
- History of thrombophilia

The high risk of VTE in acute SCI patients is thought to be due to the presence of the three risk factors that are part of the classic Virchow triad: hypercoagulable state, venous stasis, and endothelial injury. Fibrinogen metabolism has been shown to be abnormal in acute SCI compared with able body individuals.[14] Venous stasis after SCI is a result of decreased venous distensibility and increased venous flow resistance in addition to relaxation of muscles, which results in decreased venous blood flow.[1] Lastly, endothelial injury is very common due to trauma and resulting concomitant injuries.[15]

Evaluation and Diagnosis

Deep Vein Thrombosis

Clinical diagnosis of DVT is often unreliable, especially in individuals with SCI, as they frequently have sensory loss and almost always have lower extremity swelling.[13] Therefore diagnostic testing is necessary to confirm the diagnosis.

Classic signs and symptoms of DVT

- Pain
- Swelling and/or edema
- Skin discoloration
- Increased warmth
- Low-grade fever

Contrast venography is considered the gold standard test for evaluation of DVTs, but due to the invasive nature and cost of this study, it is not commonly used.[16] Instead venous duplex ultrasound is the primary diagnostic test for DVTs. Venous ultrasound has a sensitivity of 63.5% for distal clots but 96.5% for proximal clots.[17] A negative duplex ultrasound does not completely exclude DVTs, particularly distal DVTs, and therefore, if there is high clinical suspicion or if the patient has persistent or worsening symptoms, repeat duplex ultrasound scan 5–7 days later should be considered.[18]

D-dimer assay, which is a marker for fibrin turnover, is a rapid test that has high sensitivity (95.2%) but low specificity (55.3%) for DVT as it may be elevated in other disease states,[17] which can limit its use in diagnosing DVT or PE particularly in acute SCI as tissue injury can result in elevated D-dimer levels.[19,20] However, D-dimer assay does have a high negative predictive value (96.2%), so a negative D-dimer test can be used to help rule out thromboembolism even in the acute setting.[17,19]

Despite a higher risk of VTE in individuals with acute SCI, routine screening for DVT is not recommended in individuals who are asymptomatic due to the low sensitivity of duplex ultrasound[21] and the fact that no clinical trials have assessed the benefit of routine screening of SCI patients for DVT.[13]

Pulmonary Embolism

Clinical diagnosis of PE is also unreliable, and patients may present with nonspecific clinical symptoms that can mimic other cardiopulmonary illnesses.[22]

Classic signs and symptoms of PE

- Chest pain
- Dyspnea
- Tachypnea
- Tachycardia
- Hemoptysis
- Hypoxemia

Pulmonary angiography is the reference standard for diagnosis of PE. However, like venography, due to the invasive and expensive nature of the test as well as the risk of complications, it is now only used when a concomitant endovascular treatment is planned. Instead, computed tomography pulmonary angiogram (CTPA) is the modality of choice for workup of suspected PE. CTPA has been shown to have high sensitivity (83%) and specificity (96%).[23] It has advantages over other imaging modalities in that it is minimally invasive, fast, and can evaluate for other potential etiologies of chest pain (i.e., pneumonia, musculoskeletal injuries, pericardial abnormalities).[24]

Ventilation and perfusion (VQ) scan was previously the diagnostic study of choice prior to the advent of CTPA. However, in patients with renal failure, contrast material allergies, patients who cannot fit in the scanner, and young women who are pregnant where radiation exposure should be minimized, VQ scan can be used.[24] Magnetic resonance (MR) pulmonary angiogram is not used routinely because of the large portion of technically inadequate studies, long examination times, contraindications to MR imaging in patients with implanted devices, and claustrophobia.[24]

Prophylaxis

Mechanical Methods for Thromboprophylaxis

Current SCI Consortium guidelines recommend initiation of intermittent pneumatic compression devices with or without graduated compression stockings as soon as possible after acute spinal cord injury, except if contraindicated due to a concomitant lower extremity injury.[13] However, there are few high-quality studies looking at the use of pneumatic compression devices for thromboprophylaxis in spinal cord injury, and graduated compression stockings have demonstrated relatively poor protection against DVT in comparison to low molecular weight heparin (LMWH).[25]

Anticoagulant Methods for Thromboprophylaxis

Current SCI Consortium guidelines recommend the use of LMWH for thromboprophylaxis in acute SCI once there is no evidence of active bleeding, and it should be combined with mechanical thromboprophylaxis unless contraindicated.[13] Moreover, LMWH is favored over the use of low-dose unfractionated heparin (LDUH) for prophylaxis. Several studies have shown that LMWH is associated with a significant decrease in PE compared to LDUH following acute SCI.[21,26] In addition to this, LDUH is associated with a 40 times greater risk of heparin-induced thrombocytopenia compared with LMWH.[27] Current standard of practice is to continue anticoagulant prophylaxis for at least 8 weeks after injury in spinal cord injury patients with limited mobility, with consideration for longer duration based on risk factors including motor complete injuries, lower extremity fractures, older age, previous VTE, cancer, and obesity.

Oral anticoagulants are less well studied in SCI. Neither warfarin or direct oral anticoagulants (DOACs) are recommended in the early acute-care stage after SCI due to the risk of postinjury bleeding. However, in the postacute, rehabilitation phase either warfarin or DOACs can be considered.[13] DOACs offer the benefit of not needing routine laboratory monitoring and fewer drug interactions compared to warfarin.

Inferior Vena Cava Filter Use in Spinal Cord Injury

Inferior vena cava (IVC) filters are not recommended as first-line thromboprophylaxis in SCI and are generally indicated for use only in those who have a contraindication to anticoagulation.[13] Current evidence for the use of prophylactic IVC filters in trauma patients so far has not been shown to reduce PE-related mortality or overall mortality[28–32] and systematic review of prospective studies has found no evidence of decreased rate of PE in patients with and without prophylactic IVC filters.[33] In addition to this, complications of IVC filters include migration, perforation, cough-assist restrictions, and insertion site DVT.[13] If used, IVC filters should be removed when they are no longer required.

Venous Thromboembolism Prophylaxis in Chronic Spinal Cord Injury

Use of VTE prophylaxis in individuals with chronic SCI hospitalized for medical complications has not been well studied. It is thought that individuals with chronic SCI are at similar or greater risk of VTE compared with individuals without SCI. Current guidelines recommend routine use of thromboprophylaxis as one would for individuals without SCI in the same clinical setting during the period of increased risk.[13]

Venous Thromboembolism in Pediatric Spinal Cord Injury

Because DVT is rare in children 12 years of age and under, routine use of anticoagulants for VTE prophylaxis is not recommended. This risk increases to 8% in those injured between 13 and 15 years of age and 9% to those injured between 16 and 21 years of age,[34,35] so for adolescents with acute SCI, the current SCI Consortium guidelines recommend anticoagulant for thromboprophylaxis for at least 8 weeks.[13]

Treatment of Acute Venous Thromboembolism

There is currently a paucity of data evaluating treatment of VTE after SCI, as most research is focused on prevention in the acute stage. Standard treatment is anticoagulation, generally with intravenous unfractionated heparin or LMWH with transition to oral anticoagulation, which is generally maintained for 3–6 months.[36,37] There was a single study by Tomaio and colleagues that studied six SCI patients with acute DVT, which found that subcutaneous enoxaparin is a safe, cost-effective treatment for DVT while being less labor-intensive in comparison to intravenous heparin.[38] There are currently no studies available comparing the effectiveness of warfarin and DOACs for treatment of acute VTE in individuals with SCI.

Review Questions

1. Which of the following is not a risk factor for VTE in patients with SCI?[39,40,41]
   a. Complete SCI
   b. History of prior VTE
   c. Tetraplegia
   d. Age
2. Based on 2016 Consortium for Spinal Cord Medicine guidelines, a patient with an uncomplicated SCI and limited mobility should undergo anticoagulant thromboprophylaxis for at least what duration?
   a. 6 weeks
   b. 8 weeks
   c. 12 weeks
   d. 16 weeks
3. Mr. Johnson is a 56-year-old male admitted following a new C7 AIS A SCI injury secondary to motor vehicle collision. He has completed a 2-week acute-care stay and is planning to transfer to inpatient rehabilitation tomorrow. He has been receiving LMWH since admission and has no clinical signs of VTE. What is the appropriate management upon admission to rehabilitation?
   a. Doppler ultrasonography; if negative, discontinue LMWH
   b. Doppler ultrasonography; continue LMWH regardless of results
   c. No doppler ultrasonography; discontinue LMWH
   d. No doppler ultrasonography; continue LMWH
4. Ms. Smith is a 32-year-old female who sustained a T1 AIS B SCI 8 years ago after a fall from a ladder. She was recently admitted for sepsis secondary to urinary tract infection. What VTE prophylaxis, if any, should she receive?
   a. LMWH
   b. Initiate warfarin dosing
   c. Sequential Compression Device (SCD) only
   d. No prophylaxis necessary
5. Which of the following is not a main factor within Virchow triad?
   a. Venostasis
   b. Hypercoagulability
   c. Edema
   d. Endothelial injury
6. Of the following level of injuries, assuming all are complete, which would be at highest risk for VTE?[40]
   a. C1
   b. C3
   c. C4
   d. T1
7. According to 2016 Consortium Clinical Practice Guidelines, which of the following is not an appropriate thromboprophylaxis option during the postacute rehabilitation of a patient's new SCI admission?
   a. Warfarin
   b. LMWH
   c. Aspirin
   d. Apixaban

REFERENCES

1. Miranda RA, Hassouna HI. Mechanisms of thrombosis in spinal cord injury. *Hematol Oncol Clin North Am.* 2000 Apr;14(2):401–416.
2. Casas ER, Sanchez MP, Arias CR, Masip JP. Prophylaxis of venous thrombosis and pulmonary embolism in patients with acute traumatic spinal cord lesions. *Paraplegia.* 1977;14(3):178–183.
3. Frisbie JH, Sasahara AA. Low dose heparin prophylaxis for deep venous thrombosis in acute spinal cord injury patients: a controlled study. *Paraplegia.* 1981;19:343–346.
4. Brach BB, Moser KM, Cedar L, Minteer M, Convery R. Venous thrombosis in acute spinal cord paralysis. *J Trauma.* 1977;17(4):289–292.
5. Powell M, Kirshblum S, O'Connor KC. Duplex ultrasound screening for deep vein thrombosis in spinal cord injured

patients at rehabilitation admission. *Arch Phys Med Rehabil.* 1999 Sep;80(9):1044–1046.
6. Merli GJ, Crabbe S, Paluzzi RG, Fritz D. Etiology, incidence, and prevention of deep vein thrombosis in acute spinal cord injury. *Arch Phys Med Rehabil.* 1993;74(11):1199–1205.
7. Rossi E, Green D, Rosen JS, Spies SM, Jao JS. Sequential changes in factor VIII and platelets preceding deep vein thrombosis in patients with spinal cord injury. *Br J Haematol.* 1980;45(1):143–151.
8. Myllynen P, Kammonen M, Rokkanen P. Böstman O, Lalla M, Laasonen E. Deep vein thrombosis and pulmonary embolism in patients with acute spinal cord injury: a comparison with non-paralysed patients immobilised due to spinal fractures. *J Trauma.* 1985;25:541–543.
9. Gündüz S, Oğur E, Möhür H, Somuncu I, Açjksöz E, Ustünsöz B. Deep vein thrombosis in spinal cord injured patients. *Paraplegia.* 1993;31(9):606–610.
10. Perkash A. Experience with the management of deep vein thrombosis in patients with spinal cord injury. Part II: a critical evaluation of the anticoagulant therapy. *Paraplegia.* 1980;18(1):2–14.
11. Merli GJ, Herbison GJ, Dittuno JF, et al. Deep vein thrombosis: prophylaxis in acute spinal cord injured patients. *Arch Phys Med Rehabil.* 1988;69:661–664.
12. Waring WP, Karunas RS. Acute spinal cord injuries and the incidence of clinically occurring thromboembolic disease. *Paraplegia.* 1991;29(1):8–16.
13. Prevention of Venous Thromboembolism in Individuals with Spinal Cord Injury Clinical Practice Guideline for Health Care Providers Third Edition. Paralyzed Veterans of America Clinical Practice Guidelines. 2016.
14. Frisbie J. Fibrinogen metabolism in patients with spinal cord injury. *J Spinal Cord Med.* 2006;29(5):507–510.
15. Kearon C, Julian JA, Newman TE, Ginsberg JS. Noninvasive diagnosis of deep venous thrombosis. *Ann Intern Med.* 1998;128(8):663–677.
16. Goodacre S, Sampson F, Thomas S. vanBeek E, Sutton A. Systematic review and meta-analysis of the diagnostic accuracy of ultrasonography for deep vein thrombosis. *BMC Med Imaging.* 2005;5:6.
17. Akman MN, Cetin N, Bayramoglu M, Isiklar I, Kilinc S. Value of the D-dimer test in diagnosing deep vein thrombosis in rehabilitation inpatients. *Arch Phys Med Rehabil.* 2004;85:1091–1094.
18. Needleman L, Cronan JJ, Lilly MP, et al. Ultrasound for lower extremity deep venous thrombosis: multidisciplinary recommendations from the society of radiologists in ultrasound consensus conference. *Circulation.* 2018;137(14): 1505–1515.
19. Owings JT, Gosselin RC, Anderson JT, Battistella FD, Bagley M, Larkin EC. Practical utility of the D-dimer assay for excluding thromboembolism in severely injured trauma patients. *J Trauma.* 2001 Sep;51(3):425–429.
20. Johna S, Cemaj S, O'Callaghan T, Catalano R. Effect of tissue injury on D-Dimer levels: a prospective study in trauma patients. *Med Sci Monit.* 2002 Jan;8(1). CR5-8.
21. Spinal Cord Injury Thromboprophylaxis Investigators Prevention of venous thromboembolism in the rehabilitation phase after spinal cord injury: prophylaxis with low-dose heparin or enoxaparin. *J Trauma.* 2003;54(6):1111–1115.
22. Goldhaber SZ. Pulmonary embolism. *N Eng J Med.* 1998;339:93–104.
23. Stein PD, Fowler SE, Goodman LR, et al. Multidetector computed tomography for acute pulmonary embolism. *N Engl J Med.* 2006 Jun 1;354(22):2317–2327.
24. Moore AJE, Wachsmann J, Chamarthy MR, Panjikaran L, Tanabe Y, Rajiah P. Imaging of acute pulmonary embolism: an update. *Cardiovasc Diagn Ther.* 2018 Jun;8(3):225–243.
25. Halim TA, Chhabra HS, Arora M, Kumar S. Pharmacological prophylaxis for deep vein thrombosis in acute spinal cord injury: an Indian perspective. *Spinal Cord.* 2014;52(7):547–550.
26. Paciaroni M, Ageno W, Agnelli G. Prevention of venous thromboembolism after acute spinal cord injury with low-dose heparin or low-molecular-weight heparin. *Thromb Haemost.* 2008;99(5):978–980.
27. Martel N, Lee J, Wells PS. Risk of heparin-induced thrombocytopenia with unfractionated and low-molecular-weight heparin thromboprophylaxis: a meta-analysis. *Blood.* 2005;106(8):2710–2715.
28. Wojcik R, Cipolle MD, Fearen I, Newcomb J, Pasquale MD. Long-term follow-up of trauma patients with a vena caval filter. *J Trauma.* 2000;49(5):839–843.
29. Antevil JL, Sise MJ, Sack DI, et al. Retrievable vena cava filters for preventing pulmonary embolism in trauma patients: a cautionary tale. *J Trauma.* 2006;60(1):35–40.
30. Cherry RA, Nichols PA, Snavely TM, David MT, Lynch FC. Prophylactic inferior vena cava filters: do they make a difference in trauma patients? *J Trauma.* 2008;65(3): 544–548.
31. Singh S, Haut ER, Brotman DJ, et al. *Pharmacologic and Mechanical Prophylaxis of Venous Thromboembolism Among Special Populations [Internet].* Rockville (MD): Agency for Healthcare Research and Quality (US); 2013 May. Report No.: 13-EHC082-1.
32. Haut ER, Garcia LJ, Shihab HM, et al. The effectiveness of prophylactic inferior vena cava filters in trauma patients: a systematic review and meta-analysis. *JAMA Surg.* 2014 Feb;149(2):194–202.
33. Velmahos GC, Kern J, Chan LS, Oder D, Murray JA, Shekelle P. Prevention of venous thromboembolism after injury: an evidence-based report–part II: analysis of risk factors and evaluation of the role of vena caval filters. *J Trauma.* 2000 Jul;49(1):140–144.
34. Vogel L, Betz R, Mulcahey M. Pediatric spinal cord disorders. In: Kirshblum S, Campagnolo DI, eds. *Spinal Cord Medicine.* 2nd ed. Philadelphia: Lippincott Williams & Wilkins; 2011:533–564.
35. Schottler J, Vogel LC, Sturm P. Spinal cord injuries in young children: a review of children injured at 5 years of age and younger. *Dev Med Child Neurol.* 2012 Dec;54(12): 1138–1143.
36. Teasell RW, Hsieh JT, Aubut JA, Eng JJ, Krassioukov A, Tu L. Spinal Cord Injury Rehabilitation Evidence Review Research Team. Venous thromboembolism after spinal cord injury. *Arch Phys Med Rehabil.* 2009 Feb;90(2): 232–245.
37. Green D. Diagnosis, prevalence, and management of thromboembolism in patients with spinal cord injury. *J Spinal Cord Med.* 2003;26:329–334.

38. Tomaio A, Kirshblum SC, O'Connor KC, Johnston M. Treatment of acute deep vein thrombosis in spinal cord injured patients with enoxaparin: a cost analysis. *J Spinal Cord Med.* 1998 Jul;21(3):205–210.
39. Jones T, Ugalde V, Franks P, Zhou H, White RH. Venous thromboembolism after spinal cord injury: incidence, time course, and associated risk factors in 16,240 adults and children. *Arch Phys Med Rehabil.* 2005 Dec;86(12):2240–2247.
40. Maung AA, Schuster KM, Kaplan LJ, Maerz LL, Davis KA. Risk of venous thromboembolism after spinal cord injury: not all levels are the same. *J Trauma.* 2011 Nov;71(5): 1241–1245.
41. Giorgi Pierfranceschi M, Donadini MP, Dentali F, et al. The short- and long-term risk of venous thromboembolism in patients with acute spinal cord injury: a prospective cohort study. *Thromb Haemost.* 2013 Jan;109(1):34–38.

Neurogenic Bowel

CHAPTER 17

Lance L. Goetz

OUTLINE

Introduction

While the effects of spinal cord injury (SCI) on mobility and self-care are often obvious, the impact on other body systems, including bowel and bladder function, are less apparent. Persons living with SCI, however, often rate these problems as having severe impacts on their quality of life.[1,2] Things that nondisabled persons take for granted, such as access to restrooms and being able to defer a bowel movement until the appropriate time, can present severe problems for persons with SCI. This chapter outlines issues related to loss of normal bowel function, termed *neurogenic bowel dysfunction* (NBD). NBD has been identified as an area of "least competence" among persons with SCI.[1]

Anatomy and Physiology

The gut is composed of layered smooth muscle, both circularly and longitudinally oriented. These muscle layers cause both forward (propulsion) and backward (mixing) actions.

Neuroanatomy

Enteric Nervous System

The colon has its own "enteric" nervous system that can function even when removed from the body. This consists of Auerbach myenteric (within muscle layers) plexus and Meissner submucosal (under the mucosa) plexus.

- The myenteric plexus coordinates muscle contractions, whereas the submucosal plexus is involved with gut signaling and secretion.
- Early physiologists Bayless and Starling coined the term "the law of the intestine" to describe the gut's polarity: the sum of gut contractions is cephalad movement of gut contents.

Autonomic Nervous System (Fig. 17.1)

Parasympathetic

- Cranial nerve X, the vagus (vagabond, wanderer) travels from the oral cavity to the splenic flexure and innervates the gut to that point.
- The last one-third of colon, from the splenic flexure distally, is the only part of the gut innervated by the spinal cord. The pelvic splanchnic nerves, also called the nervi erigentes (nerve root levels S2–S4), supplies parasympathetic innervation to this area. Parasympathetic stimulation increases colonic motility.

Sympathetic Innervation

- Arises from approximately T11–L3 nerve root levels and projects to sympathetic chain ganglia (inferior mesenteric, celiac).
- Sympathetic stimulation inhibits gut motility.
- The colon is innervated by the hypogastric nerve (L1–L3).
- The internal anal sphincter relaxes in response to sympathetic stimuli, which facilitates storage of stool.

Somatic

- Oral cavity muscles that are under voluntary control are innervated by multiple cranial nerves.
- The external anal sphincter is composed of striated muscle, innervated by the pudendal nerve (somatic nervous system nerve root levels S2–S4) and is normally under voluntary control.[3]

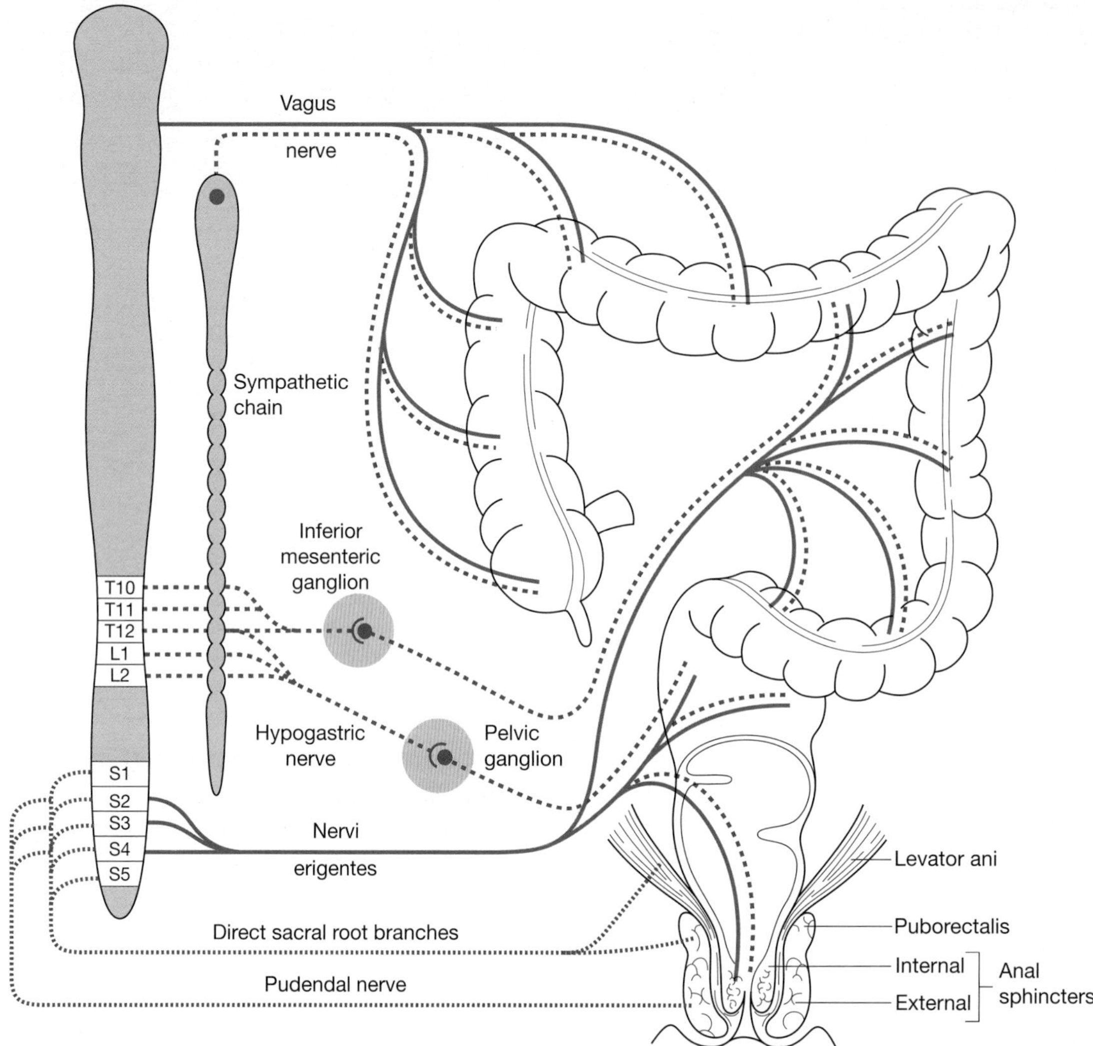

Fig. 17.1 The bowel has three nervous systems. Neurologic levels and pathways for the sympathetic, parasympathetic, and somatic nervous system innervation of the colon and anorectum. Not shown is the enteric nervous system, which travels along the bowel wall from esophagus to internal anal sphincter and forms the final common pathway to control the bowel wall smooth muscle. (Courtesy John C. King, MD.)

Normal Defecation/Events[4]

- Reflex activity giant migratory contractions start at the cecum and propel stool through the colon.
- Stool fills and distends the rectum. The internal anal sphincter relaxes. This is known as the rectal inhibitory reflex or sampling reflex.
- Contraction of the external anal sphincter (striated muscle) and pelvic floor muscles, especially the puborectalis muscle occurs to hold stool ("holding reflex").

Voluntary Activity

- When the person is ready, they relax the external sphincter and pelvic floor.
- Valsalva and abdominal muscles assist with stool expulsion as needed.

History and Physical Examination

The International Standards for Neurologic Classification of Spinal Cord Injury examination should be performed on all persons with new myelopathy. In 2015, International Standards to Document Remaining Autonomic Function after Spinal Cord Injury were published. These incorporate important components of the anorectal examination. The anorectal examination is critical to predicting the neurologic status of the individual's bowel function, initially and on an ongoing basis. Key components include anal sensation, voluntary anal contraction, anal tone, reflexes, bulbocavernosus reflex (BCR), and anal wink (S2–S4). In upper motor neuron (UMN) SCI, sacral reflexes return as spinal shock resolves.

Pathophysiology of Neurogenic Bowel Dysfunction

SCI exerts a direct neurologic effect on the distal one-third (descending) colon. UMN, reflexic, "spastic" NBD results from a lesion above the conus medullaris and presents with colonic distension, overactive segmental but underactive propulsive peristalsis, a hyperactive holding reflex,[4] increased/spastic external anal sphincter (EAS) tone, BCR, and anal wink (after spinal shock resolves). Lower motor neuron, areflexic or flaccid NBD results from a lesion affecting the parasympathetic and somatic cell bodies in the conus, cauda equina, or inferior splanchnic nerve and pudendal nerve. It presents with decreased descending colon tone, fecal distension, decreased EAS and pelvic floor tone, and absent BCR and anal wink.

Treatment for Neurogenic Bowel Dysfunction

To utilize gravity, upright position for bowel care is desired, but not always feasible, due to balance or other issues.

Bowel Program Versus Bowel Care

The term *bowel program* refers to the total package, an individualized comprehensive management plan including medications, diet, fluid intake, exercise, and bowel care interventions used in bowel management. *Bowel care* refers to a specific procedure used to eliminate stool. Bowel care is ideally performed about 20 minutes after a meal.

Bristol Stool Scale

The Bristol stool scale (BSS) is being increasingly used, especially in inpatient settings, as it offers a convenient way to report and follow stool consistency and can be taught to clients and caregivers. A BSS of 3–4 is the recommend goal in NBD (Fig. 17.2).[5]

Medications

Multiple types of oral medications are used empirically in patients with SCI, as in other medical populations, despite a lack of rigorous research defining their comparative efficacy.

Bulking Agents

- Not all persons need fiber supplements in addition to dietary fiber.
- This generally refers to various types of fiber, such as psyllium, calcium polycarbophil, methylcellulose, wheat dextrin, and others that absorb water and increase stool bulk.

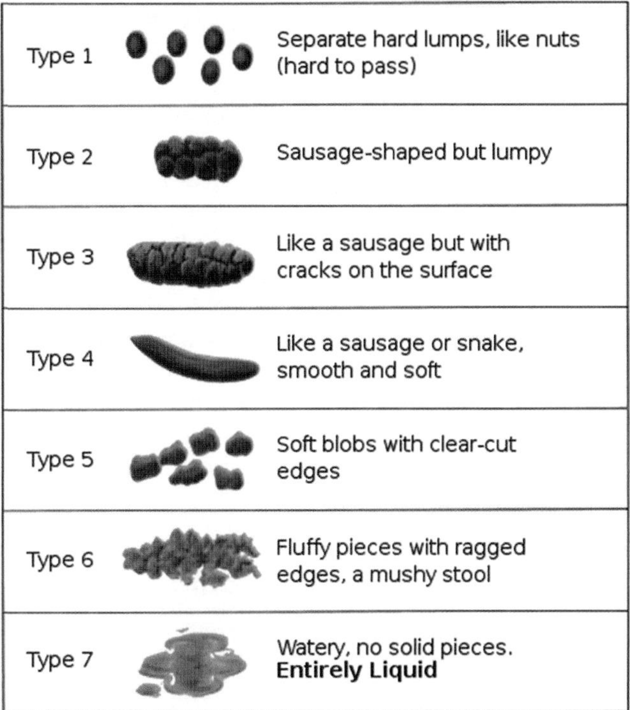

Fig. 17.2 The Bristol Stool Scale (BSS). (Marcus K.H. Auth, Rakesh Vora and George Kokai. Investigation of chronic diarrhoea. Paediatrics and Child Health, 2016-10-01, Volume 26, Issue 10, Pages 423–432.)

- Some but not all persons can benefit from fiber supplements apart from dietary fiber. Many different fiber types exist, with different effects on stool bulk and motility.
- Persons may need to trial different agents.

Stool Softeners

Stool softeners, such as docusate, should only be used in persons with excessively hard stool.

Electrolyte and Osmotic Agents

- These pull fluid into the gut, resulting in increased motility.
- When using oral agents such as milk of magnesia and magnesium citrate, there is a need to watch for electrolyte imbalance or excessively soft stool.
- Polyethylene glycol powder, when mixed with 8 ounces (225 mL) of water, has the advantage of being nonabsorbed, and does not cause electrolyte imbalance. It is used in small doses that can be titrated. In much larger doses (e.g., 4–8 L or more) it is used for bowel preparation.

Stimulants

- Oral bisacodyl is sometimes used but can cause cramping and urgent bowel movements. The preferred method of administration is rectally timed with bowel care.
- Anthraquinone based stimulants (rhubarb, senna, cascara, aloe) have been suspected of being associated with damage to gut mucosa and melanosis coli, a brown staining of the colon. There is no proven association for colorectal cancer (CRC), but concern exists.[6]

Suppositories

- These are rectal contact irritants that cause a chemical reflex peristalsis. Bisacodyl is the most common agent.
- Glycerin suppositories are less potent and can be used in incomplete injuries or persons transitioning to digital stimulation alone.
- Polyethylene glycol–based bisacodyl suppositories have been demonstrated to provide faster bowel movement results when compared to hydrogenated vegetable-based suppositories in persons with SCI.[7–9]
- Mini-enemas (5 mL volume) usually contain docusate and glycerin and can be used for reflex bowel care. They may contain benzocaine, an anesthetic that can reduce autonomic dysreflexia (AD) symptoms during bowel care.

Enemas

- Routine enema use is generally discouraged after SCI, as enemas can have unpredictable onset and duration. They are generally reserved for intermittent use or when no other agents are effective.

Table 17.1 Overview of Basic Bowel Management According to NBD Classification

Reflexic Neurogenic Bowel Dysfunction	Areflexic Neurogenic Bowel Dysfunction
Lifestyle modifications: adequate fluid and fiber intake, physical exercise, and an individualized bowel care plan	
Daily but can be a minimum of three times per week	One or more times each day
Lifestyle +/− medication regimen to achieve a Bristol stool form scale score of 3 (firm) or 4 (smooth soft)	Lifestyle +/− medication regimen to achieve a Bristol stool form scale score of 3 (firm) or 4 (smooth soft)
Rectal stimulants (suppository or mini enema)	
Digital rectal stimulation and manual evacuation of stool	Manual removal of stool
Medication options: oral laxatives (stimulants, bulk-forming agents, and stool softeners) and prokinetics	

Adapted and modified from the Multidisciplinary Association of Spinal Cord Injury Professionals (MASCIP) Guidelines for Management of Neurogenic Bowel Dysfunction in Individuals with Central Neurological Conditions. https://www.mascip.co.uk/wp-content/uploads/2015/02/CV653N-Neurogenic-Guidelines-Sept-2012.pdf.

- The use of phosphate enemas, when necessary, should be limited to once in 24 hours due to risk of absorption and hyperphosphatemia.

Upper Motor Neuron/Reflexic Specific Care

Digital Rectal Stimulation

- Digital or manual rectal stimulation is recommended as part of bowel care in persons with UMN or reflexic NBD.
- Stimulus causes reflex peristalsis of the colon.
- Typically performed for 10–20 seconds and repeated every 5–10 minutes until the bowel is empty.
- The end of bowel care has been defined in the past as no results after two successive digital stimulations.[4]
- Closure of the internal rectal sphincter can also be a signal for the end of bowel care. Caregivers can sometimes manually sense, and persons with SCI can also sometimes sense this closure.
- Some persons with SCI can manage with digital stimulation alone and do not require any rectal medications.

Lower Motor Neuron/Areflexic Specific Care

- There is not good evidence that abdominal massage or the Valsalva maneuver are effective for bowel emptying after SCI (see Table 17.1).[5]
- Manual evacuation of stool is recommended for bowel care for persons with areflexic or lower motor

neuron type NBD.[5] Due to low exterior anal sphincter tone and lack of reflex peristalsis, persons with lower motor neuron NBD cannot retain or eliminate stool and must manually remove stool one or more times daily.
- Due to lack of spinal cord-mediated reflex peristalsis, rectal stimulants such as bisacodyl are often of limited effectiveness.

Neurogenic Bowel and Gastrointestinal Complications

(See GI chapter 18 for a more detailed discussion.)

Volvulus

- From Latin *volvere* meaning "to twist"
- In chronic SCI, colonic constipation and increased weight of a loop of bowel elongates mesentery, predisposing to twisting
- Cecum and sigmoid colon most common sites
- Increased risk in multiple sclerosis and SCI[10]
- Presents with abdominal distension, nausea, and vomiting; abdominal pain can be absent in SCI
- Surgical emergency can lead to abdominal perforation, ischemia, and gangrene

Autonomic Dysreflexia

- Any source of intraabdominal irritation or acute abdomen, or less serious problems such as impaction can cause AD.
- Common with digital stimulation during bowel care.
- Persons at risk for AD with bowel care and their caregivers should be educated about signs and symptoms.
- May need to monitor blood pressure; use generous amount of lidocaine jelly 5 minutes before digital stimulation.
- If severe, use nitropaste and AD protocol.
- If severe, may need to use suppository only or consider ostomy.

Hemorrhoids

- Common in SCI, may be related to straining, inadequate pelvic floor tone, muscle atrophy
- Conservative treatment is preferred with suppositories or ointments to shrink and reduce inflammation
- Banding or surgical removal can be performed but can cause AD

Impaction

Occurs due to inadequate or too infrequent bowel care.

Obstruction

- Most commonly due to scar tissue/adhesions
- History of bowel exploration or prior surgery puts persons with SCI at risk

Cancer Risk

- Persons with SCI should be offered colorectal cancer screening at least at the same intervals as persons without SCI.
- May require more time to obtain adequate bowel preparation for colonoscopy.

Other Management Strategies

Transanal Irrigation

- Based on a recent randomized, multicenter trial, the use of transanal irrigation for NBD is recommended for persons with SCI who have "insufficient results" with basic bowel management.[5,11]
- Transanal irrigation was associated with improved satisfaction vs. usual care.

Surgical Options

Antegrade Continence Enema/Malone Procedure

- The appendix is used to create a small continent internal stoma/channel
- Tubing is inserted and enema fluid is used to flush from ascending colon usually one to two times weekly
- Performed mostly in children with myelomeningocele, less experience in adult SCI

Sacral Anterior Root Stimulation

- Bowel and bladder emptying can be electrically stimulated on demand in selected persons
- Requires spine surgery including laminectomy and dorsal rhizotomy
- Limited availability

Ostomy

- Some persons get an ostomy soon after injury, electively, or in persons with pressure ulcers, to help prevent bacterial contamination of the wound bed and improve healing.[12]
- For others, ostomy is a last resort due to aesthetic perceptions and the need for surgery.
- AD with bowel care, bleeding hemorrhoids, prolonged bowel care, lack of caregivers, difficulty with transfers, and incontinence can all be indications for ostomy.
- Studies of persons who undergo ostomy demonstrate that they do not frequently have the procedure reversed, and often wish that they had undergone the procedure sooner. Large reductions in caregiver

burden, the need for transfers to the commode, and reductions in incontinence are all reported benefits of the procedure.[12]

- Persons with SCI may benefit from high stoma placement for ease of access.
- Fear of incontinence following a meal, fear of intolerance of certain foods, and the need to stay near a restroom, can be a great relief after ostomy for some persons with SCI.
- There is little written about pouch management after SCI ostomy. Persons who are ambulatory can sit on a commode and empty a one-piece pouch easily. Persons with SCI may benefit from a two-piece pouching system to allow easier disposal of pouch contents. While emptying their pouch, clothing and lap should be protected with tissue.
- There is little information about use of digital stimulation or suppositories with stomas.
- A few persons use irrigation sleeves to facilitate timed emptying.

Conclusions

Persons with SCI are at risk for gastrointestinal tract complications during the acute period and throughout their lifetime. Due to sensorimotor deficits, diagnosis may be delayed, and a high index of suspicion is indicated. Neurogenic bowel dysfunction has important medical and psychosocial implications for persons with SCI.

Review Questions

1. Causes of diarrhea in persons with SCI include:
   a. Overtreatment with laxatives
   b. Flow of stool around an impaction
   c. *Clostridium difficile* colitis
   d. Food intolerance
   e. All of the above
2. Bowel care for persons with SCI and "flaccid" or areflexic NBD would typically involve:
   a. Repeated digital rectal stimulations and/or suppositories
   b. Three times per week frequency
   c. Manual removal of stool
   d. Large volume enemas
3. You are consulted on a 22-year-old woman who incurred C5 complete (AIS A) spinal cord injury from a diving accident 4 days ago. She had no other major injuries. On examination, you find extensor plantar responses, absent patellar and Achilles reflexes, no anal sensation, or voluntary anal sphincter contraction, low anal sphincter tone, and absent positive bulbocavernosus reflex or anal wink. Which of the following is true?
   a. She is likely to recover anal sensation within 4–6 weeks.
   b. An areflexic bowel care program with daily manual stool removal is indicated.
   c. Anal sphincter tone is likely to remain low.
   d. Daily enemas should be utilized as a first-line treatment strategy.
4. The emergency department pages you regarding a 58-year-old man who has had C6 complete (AIS A) tetraplegia for 33 years. He has no bowel movement for 4 days, so he started taking polyethylene glycol at home. However, he has developed nausea and vomiting since yesterday. He denies any fevers, chills, malodorous or cloudy urine. His spasms are subjectively increased over baseline. On examination, his abdomen is nontender but palpation elicits leg spasms, sweating, and headache. What should you recommend?
   a. Continue oral hydration and laxatives, as bowel obstruction is unlikely.
   b. Urgent abdominal imaging, including plain X-rays followed by CT scan, are not warranted.
   c. A broad list of potential causes for the person's presentation should be considered.
   d. Index of suspicion for acute abdomen is low in this scenario.
5. A 58-year-old man with C5 tetraplegia for 25 years has caregivers who come in every other day to assist him with bowel care. He notes that about 3 hours is required for complete emptying. A workup reveals colonic distension with stool but no obstruction. In considering whether ostomy is a good choice for him, which of the following is true?
   a. Transanal irrigation is not an option for this person.
   b. Ostomy management generally reduces caregiver burden compared to bowel care.
   c. Ostomy reversal is not possible following stoma placement after SCI.
   d. Autonomic dysreflexia is often worsened after ostomy placement.

REFERENCES

1. Stiens SA, Bergman SB, Goetz LL. Neurogenic bowel dysfunction after spinal cord injury: clinical evaluation and rehabilitative management. *Arch Phys Med Rehabil.* 1997;78 (3 Suppl):S86–S102.
2. Levi R, Hultling C, Nash MS, Seiger A. The Stockholm spinal cord injury study: 1. Medical problems in a regional SCI population. *Paraplegia.* 1995;33(6):308–315.
3. Rodriguez G, Stiens SA. Neurogenic bowel: dysfunction and rehabilitation. In: Cifu DX, Kaelin DL, Kowalske KJ, eds. *Braddom's Physical medicine and rehabilitation.* 5th ed. New York: Elsevier; 2016.
4. Stiens SA, Goetz LL, Strayer J. Neurogenic bowel dysfunction: evaluation and adaptive management. In: O'Young B, Young M, Stiens SA, eds. *Physical Medicine and Rehabilitation Secrets.* 3rd ed. Philadelphia: Mosby Elsevier; 2008: 531–538.

5. Management of neurogenic bowel dysfunction in adults after spinal cord injury. Clinical practice guideline for health care providers. Consortium for Spinal Cord Medicine. Paralyzed Veterans of America: Washington, DC; 2020.
6. Lombardi N, Bettiol A, Crescioli G, et al. Association between anthraquinone laxatives and colorectal cancer: protocol for a systematic review and meta-analysis. *Syst Rev*. 2020; 9(1):19.
7. Stiens SA, Luttrel W, Binard JE. Polyethylene glycol versus vegetable oil based bisacodyl suppositories to initiate side-lying bowel care: a clinical trial in persons with spinal cord injury. *Spinal Cord*. 1998;36(11):777–781.
8. Stiens SA, Singal AK, Korsten MA. The gastrointestinal system after spinal cord injury: assessment and intervention. In: Lin VW, ed. *Spinal Cord Medicine: Principles and Practice*. 2nd ed. New York: Demos Medical; 2010:382–408.
9. Stiefel DJ, Truelove EL, Persson RS, Chin MM, Mandel LS. A comparison of oral health in spinal cord injury and other disability groups. *Spec Care Dent Off Publ Am Assoc Hosp Dent Acad Dent Handicap Am Soc Geriatr Dent*. 1993;13(6):229–235.
10. Thornton S, Pal J, Geibel J. Sigmoid and cecal volvulus [Internet]. Medscape; 2020. https://emedicine.medscape.com/article/2048554-overview.
11. Christensen P, Bazzocchi G, Coggrave M, et al. A randomized, controlled trial of transanal irrigation versus conservative bowel management in spinal cord-injured patients. *Gastroenterology*. 2006;131(3):738–747.
12. Stone JM, Wolfe VA, Nino-Murcia M, Perkash I. Colostomy as treatment for complications of spinal cord injury. *Arch Phys Med Rehabil*. 1990;71(7):514–518.

CHAPTER 18

Dysphagia and Common GI Issues After SCI

Stacy Gross, Katelyn Barley, and Keith Burau

OUTLINE

Introduction

Swallowing is a complex process by which saliva, food, or liquids are transported from the oral cavity and through the esophagus while maintaining airway protection. Dysphagia is an impairment in the anatomic or physiologic components of typical swallow function. Dysphagia can occur in any or all three phases of the swallow: oral, pharyngeal, and esophageal. Dysphagia after spinal cord injury (SCI) is relatively common, secondary to a result of impaired neurological control of swallowing, structural disorders, or iatrogenic complications.[1] The incidence and prevalence of dysphagia in the SCI population is difficult to determine due to varying definitions of dysphagia, different settings across the continuum of care, and a variety of measurement tools. Early identification of patients who are at high risk of dysphagia is critical to preventing life-threatening complications, such as aspiration pneumonia. Of note, diseases of the respiratory system are the leading cause of death in patients with spinal cord injuries. Of these, greater than 65% are cases of pneumonia.[2]

Predictors of Risk of Dysphagia in Spinal Cord Injury Population

- Age[3,4]
- Cervical spine surgery, especially the anterior approach[3,4]
- Presence of a tracheostomy[3,4]

Cuff deflation does not eliminate nor reduce the risk of aspiration[5]

- Level and severity of injury[3]
- Cervical bracing[6]
- Intubation[3]
- Pneumonia and other infectious processes
- Altered mental status
- Medications

Evaluation of Swallowing[7]

- Aspiration and aspiration pneumonia
- Malnutrition and dehydration
- Reduced quality of life

Dysphagia is often diagnosed based on the presence of aspiration before, during, or after the swallow. However, aspiration is not the only characteristic of dysphagia. Impairments can occur across the phases of the swallow (Table 18.1).[8,9]

Clinical Swallow Examination[10]

Patients may be referred for a clinical swallow examination (CSE) due to increased risk of dysphagia or failure of a screening. A CSE is an assessment of dysphagia that relies on symptoms reported and signs observed without direct visualization. The CSE helps the speech-language pathologist to determine immediate safety and efficiency for oral intake, if an instrumental assessment is warranted, and if further referrals are needed. Information gathered during a CSE helps a clinician build hypotheses regarding swallowing impairment that can then be verified through instrumental evaluation. Unlike an instrumental evaluation, the CSE cannot

Table 18.1 Components of the Swallow and Clinical Features of Dysphagia[9]

	Oral Phase	Pharyngeal Phase	Esophageal Phase
Components	Lip closure Tongue control Bolus preparation Bolus mastication Bolus transport	Initiation of the swallow Soft palate elevation Laryngeal elevation Hyoid excursion Epiglottic inversion Laryngeal vestibule closure Pharyngeal stripping Pharyngeal contraction Tongue base retraction	Esophageal clearance
Clinical Features of Dysphagia	Anterior spillage from lips Oral residue Pocketing Poor bolus control Impaired mastication Premature spillage to pharynx Extra effort or time needed to chew or swallow Inability to eat certain foods	Aspiration Penetration Pharyngeal residue Wet, altered, and/or absent vocal quality Multiple swallows Throat clearing Coughing Unexplained weight loss Difficulty initiating swallow	Sensation of food sticking in the throat or chest Regurgitation Expectoration Unexplained weight loss Difficulty with solid food Coughing Effortful swallow

rule-in or rule-out aspiration. Compared with an instrumental evaluation, the CSE is more readily available, relatively inexpensive, and easily repeatable.

Instrumental Assessment

An instrumental evaluation is not a pass/fail assessment of the swallow. The purpose of imaging is to identify physiologic impairments across the phases of the swallow to target treatment.

Videofluoroscopic Swallow Study or Modified Barium Swallow[7]

A videofluoroscopic swallow study (VFSS) is an objective evaluation of swallowing completed under fluoroscopy in the radiology suite. It provides a comprehensive view of the swallow from the lips through the esophagus. The study is noninvasive and consists of providing trials of contrast material in varying amounts and textures to the patient while imaging.

Clinical indications:

- Need to assess for specific oral concerns
- Need to assess for specific esophageal concerns
- Need to assess for oral, pharyngeal, or esophageal anatomical changes

Fiberoptic Endoscopic Evaluation of Swallowing[7]

A fiberoptic endoscopic evaluation of swallowing (FEES) is an objective evaluation of swallowing completed with flexible endoscopy, which offers a superior evaluation of anatomy and secretion management. Accessibility is a strength of FEES, as the equipment is portable and does not carry the risk of radiation exposure that VFSS does, allowing for increased duration and repeatability. Unlike the VFSS, the oral cavity and esophagus are not included in imaging. The view is from the nasopharynx to the hypopharynx only. Additionally, the image is lost at the peak of the swallow or when the endoscope is covered.

Clinical indications:

- Patient positioning or equipment (i.e., halo bracing, head-of-bed elevation restrictions), which limits the ability to complete VFSS
- Need to assess laryngeal functioning for voice
- Need to assess for fatigue (increased duration allows assessment of fatigue without radiation)
- Need to assess specific textures
- Need to assess secretion management
- Need to assess for laryngeal or pharyngeal sensory deficits

Treatment of Dysphagia

Following an instrumental evaluation of the patient's oropharyngeal swallowing skills, a speech-language pathologist makes recommendations for compensatory and/or rehabilitative strategies to aid in the safety and efficiency of the patient's swallow. Treatment options seek to balance protecting the patient's airway, maintaining nutrition and hydration, and upholding quality of life.

Compensatory[7]

These strategies compensate for impaired function without changing underlying physiology and may be recommended for short-term or long-term use. Adjustments can be made to posture, food and liquid, or swallowing patterns. Compensatory strategies should not be employed unless trialed during instrumental evaluation. The effectiveness of strategies may be overestimated in the CSE, as it facilitates no benefit or results in poor outcomes.

- Diet and liquid modifications
- Sensory adjustments
- Volume modification
- Method of bolus delivery
- Body positioning (e.g., chin tuck, head turn)
- Head or facial position
- Swallowing maneuvers (e.g., supraglottic swallow, super-supraglottic swallow, effortful swallow)

Rehabilitative[7]

Rehabilitative strategies focus on exercise principles to create long-term physiologic improvements in components of the oropharyngeal swallow. Biofeedback, such as surface electromyography, may be used.

- Exercises to improve oral motor control
- Stimulation of swallow reflex
- Exercises to improve airway closure
- Exercises to improve cough effectiveness (e.g., expiratory muscle strength training)

Nonoral

Following evaluation, it may be determined that alternate means of nutrition need to be considered if the patient's oropharyngeal swallow is unsafe for nutrition or hydration by mouth (PO). In these instances, the speech-language pathologist will continue to address dysphagia through treatment, with the goal of returning to PO. Although inappropriate for PO, certain patients may meet requirements for the Frazier Free Water Protocol, allowing them small sips of water for pleasure.[11,12]

Complications of Dysphagia

Dysphagia can have both medical and psychosocial consequences.

Aspiration and Aspiration Pneumonia

While dysphagia is a risk factor for aspiration, not all patients with dysphagia will aspirate. Additionally, aspiration alone is insufficient for the development of aspiration pneumonia. Aspiration pneumonia develops in the presence of aspiration plus additional risk factors, such as poor oral hygiene and reduced mobility.[13]

Reduced Quality of Life

Being unable to eat one's favorite food or ingest meals normally has an understandable impact on quality of life. A speech-language pathologist must consider not only the safety and efficiency of the patient's swallow but also the patient's quality of life when making recommendations. Questionnaires such as the Swallowing Quality of Life[14] and Dysphagia Handicap Index[15] were developed to measure the effect of dysphagia on quality of life and have great benefit as outcome measures.

Malnutrition or Dehydration

Maintaining adequate nutrition and hydration is more difficult for those with dysphagia.[16,17] Patients may have an overall lower rate of intake, due to fear and discomfort surrounding eating or drinking or discontentment with a modified diet. Patients requiring thickened liquids are at greater risk of dehydration not because of the thickener agent itself, but its impact on palatability.

Gastrointestinal Complications After Spinal Cord Injury

Gastrointestinal (GI) dysfunction occurs in 27% to 62% of persons with SCI with common complaints including constipation, distention, abdominal pain, rectal bleeding, incontinence, diarrhea, and hemorrhoids.[18,19] Furthermore, gastroenterological complications are one of the most common complications following SCI, accounting for 1.9% to 11%, including paralytic ileus, gastroparesis, peptic ulcer disease, acute pancreatitis, etc.[20] Risk factors include older age, male sex, head injury, multisystem trauma, and cervical spine injury. These are severe complications that substantially increase the morbidity rate of spinal cord injury; therefore, it is important to distinguish and diagnose these conditions early to avoid the high mortality rate associated with them.[21]

Spinal shock, resulting in loss of all autonomic and reflex behaviors below the level of cord lesion, occurs shortly after injury and may last several days to weeks. During the first 4 weeks from injury, 4.7% of patients reported acute abdominal symptoms, whereas 4.2% reported acute gastroduodenal ulceration and hemorrhage.[18,19] During spinal shock, the abdomen is distended and flaccid and there are absent or hypoactive bowel sounds, with loss of sensation below the level of the lesion often associated with paralytic ileus. When shock resolves, there is a return and then exaggeration of reflex activity below the level of the lesion in the case of upper motor neuron involvement.

The alteration in sensory, motor, autonomic, and reflex functions lead to impaired pain sensation, making the diagnosis of abdominal pathology particularly difficult in the SCI population. These patients will not present with the typical acute abdominal symptoms seen in the able-bodied population (i.e., sharp pain, rigidity, and guarding).[21] Persons with a spinal cord lesion will likely present with a predominance of vague and poorly localized abdominal pain and distention, which may lead to a delay in diagnosis.

Review of Gastrointestinal Neuroregulatory Control

Intrinsic (Enteric) Nervous System[22]

Submucosal Plexus (Meissner Plexus)

- Relays information from the mucosa to the intrinsic and extrinsic nervous systems of the GI tract
- Controls local secretion and absorption

Myenteric Plexus (Auerbach Plexus)

- Sits between the two layers of smooth muscle of the muscularis propria
- Provides intrinsic regulation to the GI tract that results in peristalsis

Extrinsic Nervous System[23,24]

Parasympathetic Communication Via the Vagus and Pelvic Splanchnic Nerves

- Increases peristalsis, secretions, relaxation of sphincters, and assists with pancreatic and hepatic functions

Sympathetic Communication Via T5–L2

- Decreases peristalsis, secretions, absorption, and the release of insulin and digestive enzymes
- Contracts sphincters
- Increases hepatic glycogenolysis and gluconeogenesis
- T5–T9 → greater splanchnic nerve → celiac ganglion → esophagus, stomach, liver, gallbladder, pancreas
- T10–T12 → lesser splanchnic nerve → superior mesenteric ganglion → small intestines, ascending colon, and two-thirds of the transverse colon
- L1–L2 → hypogastric plexus → inferior mesenteric ganglion → one-third of the transverse colon, descending colon, anorectal region, internal anal sphincter

Somatic innervation via pudendal nerve (S2–S4) to the external anal sphincter and pelvic floor muscles (Fig. 18.1)

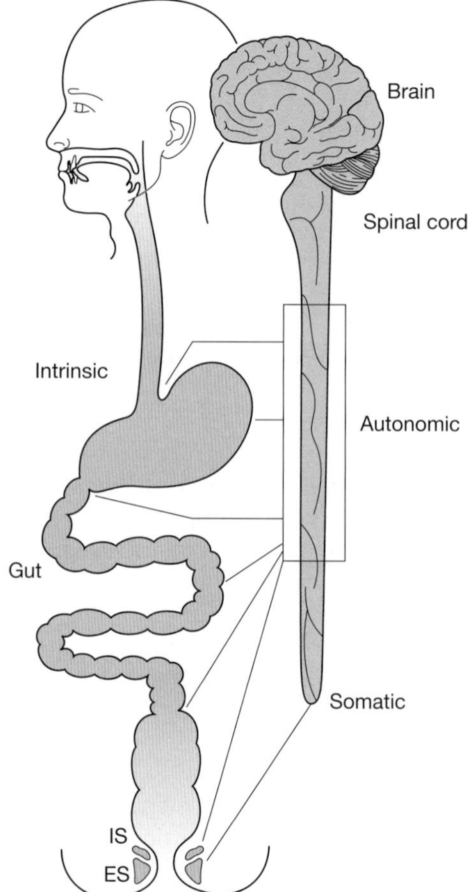

Fig. 18.1 Gastrointestinal function is coordinated by three nervous systems: somatic, autonomic, and the enteric nervous system intrinsic to the gut wall. *ES*, External sphincter; *IS*, internal sphincter. (Courtesy John C. King, MD.)

Early Symptoms of Abdominal Pathology After Spinal Cord Injury

- Fever
- Nausea/vomiting and anorexia
- Increased spasticity
- Referred shoulder tip pain
- Alteration in bowel or bladder function
- Autonomic dysreflexia
- Feeling there is 'something wrong'

Complications of Gastrointestinal Dysfunction After Spinal Cord Injury

Paralytic Ileus

- Obstruction of the gastrointestinal tract due to paralysis of intestinal muscles without evidence of mechanical obstruction[25,26]
  - Often associated with spinal shock after an acute spinal cord injury
  - More often seen in cervical and upper thoracic level cord lesions
- Clinical Presentation
  - Nausea and vomiting
  - Lack of output of gas and stool
  - Abdominal distention and tenderness

- Abdominal distention may increase the work of breathing and vomiting, which may increase the risk of respiratory complications and aspiration pneumonia
- Evaluation
  - Abdominal radiographs
- Treatment
  - Nil by mouth (NPO)
  - Nasogastric suction and intravenous fluids

Pancreatitis

- Inflammation of the pancreas with intraparenchymal corrosion caused by the pancreatic juice[27]
  - Most common the first 4 weeks postinjury
  - Three times greater risk in SCI
- Predisposing factors
  - Direct trauma to pancreas and/or to the structures connected to it[27,28]
  - Abnormal gallbladder motility in lesions above T10
  - Abnormal biliary secretion
- Clinical presentation: often subtle
  - Abdominal pain (may be absent in quadriplegic patients)
  - Nausea and vomiting
  - Poor appetite
- Evaluation
  - Labs: elevated amylase, lipase
  - Abdominal ultrasonography and, preferably, computed tomography (CT)
- Treatment
  - Medical observation; antibiotics

Superior Mesenteric Artery Syndrome

- Condition in which the third part of the duodenum is compressed between the superior mesenteric artery (SMA) and aorta, resulting in GI obstruction[29,30]
  - The duodenum lies anterior to the spine and aorta but posterior to the SMA
  - Anything that results in less space between these structures can result in compression and obstruction of the duodenum
  - In normal circumstances, retroperitoneal fat and lymphatic tissues cushion the SMA off the spine and protect the duodenum from compression
- Predisposing factors
  - Rapid weight loss (with loss of retroperitoneal fat)
  - Prolonged supine positioning
  - Decreased abdominal tone
  - Use of spinal orthosis
- Clinical presentation
  - Postprandial nausea and bilious vomiting[29]
  - Epigastric pain
  - Abdominal distention
- Evaluation
  - Abdominal radiographs
  - Barium study shows dilation of the first and second part of the duodenum with abrupt cutoff at the third part
- Treatment
  - Eat small, frequent meals in upright body position[30]
  - Lie in left lateral decubitus position after meals[29]
  - Remove spinal orthosis if able
  - Metoclopramide may improve upper GI motility
  - In severe forms, a nasogastric tube is inserted beyond the obstruction to enable continued nutritional support, while parenteral nutrition is initiated[31]
  - If conservative management fails, surgical duodenojejunostomy is indicated

Appendicitis

- Inflammation of the appendix
- Clinical presentation: often subtle[32]
  - Anorexia
  - A change in bladder pattern
  - Unexplained fatigue
  - Vague abdominal discomfort
  - Fever may be present
  - Abdominal tenderness is uncommon
  - Autonomic dysreflexia may be seen in T6 SCI and above
- Evaluation
  - May have leukocytosis
  - Abdominal imaging including CT and ultrasound
- Treatment
  - Delay in diagnosis results in appendix perforation in 92% to 100% of patients
  - Surgical removal

Cholecystitis

- Occurs when a stone in the cystic duct causes gallbladder inflammation
  - Cholelithiasis is two times as prevalent in those with SCI[33,34]
  - Altered innervation to the gallbladder can cause dysmotility and reduced ejection fraction, which can lead to cholestasis and subsequent sludge and stone formation[21,35]

- Predisposing factors
  - Rapid weight loss is a risk factor for stone formation acutely following SCI[36]
  - Acute acalculous cholecystitis can occur in those with critical illness or polytrauma[37]
- Clinical presentation
  - The presenting symptom may only be referred pain in the right shoulder, but even with high cervical injuries some patients were able to report right upper quadrant pain.[38]
- Evaluation
  - Ultrasound is the preferred method as it has a high sensitivity (>95%), is fast, noninvasive and does not involve radiation.[39]
  - A hepatobiliary iminodiacetic acid scan is used if ultrasound is negative or inconclusive.
  - CT has a low specificity and can miss ~20% of stones, so it is not routinely used to diagnose acute cholecystitis.
- Treatment
  - Surgery is indicated for symptomatic cholelithiasis, cholecystitis, choledocholithiasis, and pancreatitis.[40]
  - Prophylactic cholecystectomy for asymptomatic stones in SCI patients is debated but serial ultrasounds to assess for the development of gallbladder disease may be indicated.

Gastroparesis

- Impaired gastric emptying
  - Common, especially in the first few weeks for those with cervical and thoracic injuries[35]
  - GI motility time in SCI vs. able-bodied participants showed delayed gastric emptying (10.6 vs. 3.5 hours), colonic transit time (52.3 vs. 14.2 hours), and whole gut transit time (3.3 vs. 1.0 days)[41]
- Clinical Presentation
  - Postprandial fullness, epigastric pain, nausea, vomiting, bloating, and/or early satiety
  - In those who have cervical and thoracic injuries, symptoms may not be as prominent or may be limited to constipation, distension, or signs of aspiration[24]
- Evaluation[42,43]
  - Esophagogastroduodenoscopy and CT/magnetic resonance (MR) enterography to rule out mechanical obstruction
  - Gastric emptying scintigraphy
  - ^{13}C breath test
- Treatment[44]
  - Behavioral modifications: diet low in fat and nondigestible fiber, control of acute hyperglycemia
  - Prokinetic agents 15 minutes before meals
    - Metoclopramide: use should be limited to <3 months unless benefits outweigh risks – black box warning for extrapyramidal side effects[45]
    - Erythromycin: use limited to <4 weeks due to tachyphylaxis[46]

Gastroduodenal Ulceration

- Peptic ulcers in the stomach and/or duodenum
  - Highest occurrence of peptic ulcer formation and perforation is within the first 10 to 30 days after SCI[47]
- Predisposing factors[48,49]
  - Higher level of injury
  - Complete injury
  - Respiratory failure
- Clinical presentation
  - About 70% of peptic ulcers are asymptomatic in the general population[50]
  - When symptoms occur, gastric ulcers tend to cause pain upon eating and duodenal ulcers cause pain 2–4 hours after a meal, but this can be obscured following SCI[51]
  - Symptoms may be limited to heartburn, bloating, nausea, early satiety that is worsened by eating
- Evaluation
  - Rule-out perforation with KUB
  - Esophagogastroduodenoscopy w/ biopsy to test for *H. pylori*
- Prophylaxis
  - H2 blockers or proton pump inhibitors for at least 4 weeks is recommended for all patients after SCI[52]
    - PPIs have a quicker, more sustained increase in gastric pH compared to H2 blockers
    - Tolerance can occur with H2 blockers requiring dosage adjustment
    - H2 blockers must be renally dosed[53]
  - May be required beyond 4 weeks for those with other risk factors such as[48,54]:
    - Premorbid peptic ulcers
    - Prolonged mechanical ventilation
    - Coagulopathy
    - Live failure
    - Burns
    - Ongoing use of corticosteroids
  - Maintaining adequate nutrition that meets the increased energy requirements during the acute

phase of SCI has shown to decrease the risk of PUD[55]
  - Enteral nutrition has lower infectious complications and lower incidence of hyperglycemia compared to parenteral nutrition[56]
- Treatment
  - Eradicate *H. pylori* with triple therapy if present and confirm eradication with fecal antigen or urea breath testing
  - Antisecretory therapy with a PPI, durations depends on ulcer size and other comorbidities

Review Questions

1. A patient complains of odynophagia, globus sensation, and coughing following meals. Based on these symptoms alone, who should receive the initial consult?
   a. Otolaryngologist
   b. Speech-language pathologist
   c. Dietician
   d. Gastroenterologist
2. In which of the following may aspiration occur?
   a. Cuffed tracheostomy tube with cuff deflated
   b. Cuffless tracheostomy
   c. Cuffed tracheostomy tube with cuff inflated
   d. All of the above.
3. Which of the following is NOT a significant risk factor for dysphagia in those with cervical spinal cord injury?
   a. Age
   b. Medication induced xerostomia
   c. Cervical spine surgery
   d. Presence of tracheostomy tube
4. A 48-year-old man was involved in a bicycle accident in which he sustained a T6–T7 vertebral fracture with ASIA A T5 paraplegia. He underwent surgical intervention consisting of laminectomy and posterior fusion of T6–T7 with body plaster cast placed for immobilization. Three weeks later, the patient began to experience nausea and vomiting with epigastric abdominal pain, worse after eating meals. He has lost 25 pounds since the accident. What is the best treatment at this time?
   a. Medical observation
   b. Antibiotics
   c. Small, frequent meals in upright body position
   d. Surgical correction
5. A 54-year-old man with a T6 ASIA A injury sustained 12 years ago presents with fever. Review of systems notes intermittent vague right shoulder pain. Vital signs are stable. Initial labs show an increased white blood cell count, normal comprehensive metabolic panel, and normal urinalysis. Right upper quadrant ultrasound is inconclusive. What is the best next step to evaluate the patient's underlying diagnosis?
   a. Magnetic resonance cholangiopancreatography
   b. Endoscopic retrograde cholangiopancreatography
   c. CT abdomen
   d. Hepatobiliary iminodiacetic acid scan

REFERENCES

1. Wolf C, Meiners TH. Dysphagia in patients with acute cervical spinal cord injury. *Spinal Cord.* 2003;41(6):347–353.
2. National Spinal Cord Injury Statistical Center (US). 2020 Annual Report – Complete Public Version. Birmingham, AL: National Spinal Cord Injury Statistical Center; 2020:47.
3. Iruthayarajah J, McIntyre A, Mirkowski M, Welch-West P, Loh E, Teasell R. Risk factors for dysphagia after a spinal cord injury: a systematic review and meta-analysis. *Spinal Cord.* 2018 Dec;56(12):1116–1123.
4. Kirschblum S, Johnston MV, Brown J, O'Connor KC, Jarosz P. Predictors of dysphagia after spinal cord injury. *Arch Phys Med Rehabil.* 1999 Sep;80(9):1101–1105.
5. Ding R, Logemann J. Swallow physiology in patients with trach cuff inflated or deflated: a retrospective study. *Head Neck.* 2005 Sep;27(9):809–813.
6. Stambolis V, Brady S, Klos D, Wesling M, Fatianov T, Hildner C. The effects of cervical bracing upon swallowing in young, normal, healthy volunteers. *Dysphagia.* 2003;18(1):39–45.
7. Groher ME, Cary MA. *Dysphagia: Clinical Management in Adults and Children.* 3rd ed. St. Louis: Elsevier; 2020.
8. Valenzano TJ, Waito AA, Steele CM. A review of dysphagia presentation and intervention following traumatic spinal injury: an understudied population. *Dysphagia.* 2016 Oct;31(5):598–609.
9. Martin-Harris BM, Brodsky MB, Michel Y, Castell DO, Schleicher M, Sandidge J. MBS measurement tool for swallow impairment–MBSImp: establishing a standard. *Dysphagia.* 2008 Dec;23(4):392–405.
10. Garand KLF, McCullough G, Crary M, Arvedson JC, Dodrill P. Assessment across the life span: the clinical swallow evaluation. *Am J Speech Lang Pathol.* 2020;29(2):919–933.
11. Panther K. The Frazier free water protocol. *Perspectives on Swallowing and Swallowing Disorders.* 2005;14(1):4–9.
12. Gillman A, Winkler R, Taylor NF. Implementing the free water protocol does not result in aspiration pneumonia in carefully selected patients with dysphagia: a systematic review. *Dysphagia.* 2017 Jun;32(3):345–361.
13. Langmore SE, Terpenning MS, Schork A, et al. Predictors of aspiration pneumonia: how important is dysphagia? *Dysphagia.* 1998;13(2):69–81.
14. McHorney CA, Bricker DE, Kramer AE, et al. The SWAL-QOL outcomes tool for oropharyngeal dysphagia in adults: I. conceptual foundation and item development. *Dysphagia.* 2000;15(3):115–121.
15. Silbergleit AK, Schultz L, Jacobson BH, Beardsley T, Johnson AF. The dysphagia handicap index: development and validation. *Dysphagia.* 2012 Mar;27(1):46–52.
16. Crary MA, Humphrey JL, Carnaby-Mann G, Sambandam R, Miller L. Silliman S. Dysphagia, nutrition, and hydration in ischemic stroke patients at admission and discharge from acute care. *Dysphagia.* 2013 Mar;28(1):69–76.

17. Crary MA, Carnaby GD, Shabbir Y, Miler L, Silliman S. Clinical variables associated with hydration status in acute ischemic stroke patients with dysphagia. *Dysphagia.* 2016 Feb;31(1):60–65.
18. Ebert E. Gastrointestinal involvement in spinal cord injury: a clinical perspective. *J Gastrointestin Liver Dis.* 2012;21(1): 75–82.
19. Hagen EM. Acute complications of spinal cord injuries. *World J Orthop.* 2015 J18;6(1):17.
20. Sarıfakıoğlu B, Afşar SI, Yalbuzdağ ŞA, et al. Acute abdominal emergencies and spinal cord injury; our experiences: a retrospective clinical study. *Spinal Cord.* 2014;52:697–700.
21. Miller BJ, Geraghty TJ, Wong CH, Hall DF, Cohen JR. Outcome of the acute abdomen in patients with previous spinal cord injury. *ANZ J Surg.* 2001;71:407–411.
22. Barrett KE. Functional anatomy of the GI tract and organs draining into it. In: Barrett KE, ed. *Gastrointestinal Physiology.* 2nd ed. New York: McGraw-Hill Education LLC; 2014.
23. Chen D, Anschel AS. Gastrointestinal disorders. In: Kirshblum S, Campagnolo DI, eds. *Spinal Cord Medicine.* 2nd ed. Philadelphia: Wolters Kluwer Health Aids; 2011.
24. Waxman SG. The autonomic nervous system. In: Waxman SG, ed. *Clinical Neuroanatomy.* 27th ed. New York: McGraw-Hill Education; 2013.
25. Harvey L. *Management of Spinal Cord Injuries: A Guide for Physiotherapists.* Elsevier Health Sciences; 2008 Jan 10.
26. Watson N. Late ileus in paraplegia. *Paraplegia.* 1981;19:13–16.
27. Pirolla EH, de Barros Filho TE, Godoy-Santos AL, Fregni F. Association of acute pancreatitis or high level of serum pancreatic enzymes in patients with acute spinal cord injury: a prospective study. *Spinal Cord.* 2014 Nov;52(11):817–820.
28. Nobel D, Baumberger M, Eser P, Michel D, Knecht H, Stocker R. Nontraumatic pancreatitis in spinal cord injury. *Spine (Phila Pa 1976).* 2002 May 1;27(9):E228–E232.
29. Shapiro G, Green DW, Fatica NS, Boachie-Adjei O. Medical complications in scoliosis surgery. *Curr Opin Pediatr.* 2001;13:36–41.
30. Van Brussel JP, Dijkema WP, Adhin SK, Jonkers GJPM. Wilkie's syndrome, a rare cause of vomiting and weight loss: diagnosis and therapy. *Neth J Med.* 1997;51:179–181.
31. Laffont I, Bensmail D, Rech C, Prigent G, Loubert G, Dizien O. Late superior mesenteric artery syndrome in paraplegia: case report and review. *Spinal Cord.* 2002;40(2):88–91.
32. Strauther GR, Longo WE, Virgo KS, Johnson FE. Appendicitis in patients with previous spinal cord injury. *Am J Surg.* 1999;178:403–405.
33. Rotter KP, Larrain CG. Gallstones in spinal cord injury (SCI): a late medical complication? *Spinal Cord.* 2003;41(2):105–108.
34. Apstein MD, George B, Tchakarova B. Spinal cord injury is a risk factor for cholesterol gallstone disease: a prospective study. *J Am Paraplegia Soc.* 1991;14:197–198.
35. Stiens SA, Singal AK, Korsten MA. The gastrointestinal system after spinal cord injury: assessment and intervention. In: Lin VW, ed. *Spinal Cord Medicine.* 2nd ed. Principles and Practice. New York: Demons Medical Publishing, Inc; 2010:382–408.
36. Everhart JE. Contributions of obesity and weight loss to gallstone disease. *Ann Intern Med.* 1993;119(10):1029–1035.
37. Romero Ganuza FJ, La Banda G, Montalvo R, et al. Acute acalculous cholecystitis in patients with acute traumatic spinal cord injury. *Spinal Cord.* 1997;35(2):124–128.
38. Tola VB, Chamberlain S, Kostyk SK, et al. Symptomatic gallstones in patients with spinal cord injury. *J Gastrointest Surg.* 2000;4(16):642–647.
39. Heuman DM, Mihas AA, Allen J. Gallstones (cholelithiasis) workup. In: Anand BS, ed. *Medscape Online*; 2016;2017. https://emedicine.medscape.com/article/175667-workup#-showall.
40. Moonka R, Stiens SA, Eubank WB, et al. The presentation of gallstones and results of biliary surgery in a spinal cord injured population. *Am J Surg.* 1999;178(3):246–250.
41. Williams III RE, Bauman WA, Spungen AM, et al. SmartPill technology provides safe and effective assessment of gastrointestinal function in persons with spinal cord injury. *Spinal Cord.* 2012;50:81–84.
42. Sarnelli G, Caenepeel P, Geypens B, et al. Symptoms associated with impaired gastric emptying of solids and liquids in functional dyspepsia. *Am J Gastroenterol.* 2003;93(4): 783–788.
43. Mukand JA, Kaplan MS, Blackinton DD, et al. The gastric emptying scan as a tool for surgical management of severe bowel dysfunction in spinal cord injury: 2 case reports. *Arc Phys Med Rehabil.* 2000;81(11):1531–1534.
44. Camilleri M, Parkman HP, Shafi MA, et al. Clinical guideline: management of gastroparesis. *Am J Gastroenterol.* 2013;108:18.
45. Rao AS, Camilleri M. Review article: metoclopramide and tardive dyskinesia. *Ailment Pharmacol Ther.* 2010;31:11.
46. Richards RD, Davenport K, McCallum RW. The treatment of idiopathic and diabetic gastroparesis with acute intravenous and chronic oral erythromycin. *Am J Gastroenterol.* 1993;88:203–207.
47. Bar-On Z, Ohry A. The acute abdomen in spinal cord injury individuals. *Paraplegia.* 1995;33(12):704–706.
48. Albert TJ, Levine MJ, Balderston RA, Cotler JM. Gastrointestinal complications in spinal cord injury. *Spine.* 1991; 16(10 Suppl):S522–S525.
49. Cook D, Heyland D, Griffith L, et al. Risk factors for clinically important upper gastrointestinal bleeding in patients requiring mechanical ventilation. Canadian Critical Care Trials Group. *Critical Care Medicine.* 1999;27(12):2812–2817.
50. Lu CL, Chang SS, Wang SS, et al. Silent peptic ulcer disease: frequency, factors leading to "silence," and implications regarding the pathogenesis of visceral symptoms. *Gastrointest Endosc.* 2004;60:34.
51. Gururatsakul M, Holloway RH, Talley NJ, Holtmann GJ. Association between clinical manifestations of complicated and uncomplicated peptic ulcer and visceral sensory dysfunction. *J Gastroenterol Hepatol.* 2010;25:1162.
52. Consortium for Spinal Cord Medicine Early acute management in adults with spinal cord injury: clinical practice guidelines for healthcare professionals. *J Spinal Cord Med.* 2008;31(4):403–479.
53. Welage LS. Overview of pharmacologic agents for acid suppression in critically ill patients. *Am J Health Syst Pharm.* 2005;62(10 Suppl 2):S4–S10.
54. Kiwerski J. Bleeding from the alimentary canal during the management of spinal cord injury patients. *Paraplegia.* 1986;24(2):92–96.
55. Kuric J, Lucas CE, Ledgerwood AM, et al. Nutritional support: a prophylaxis against stress bleeding after spinal cord injury. *Paraplegia.* 1989;27(2):140–145.
56. Gramlich L, Kichian K, Pinilla J, et al. Does enteral nutrition compared to parenteral nutrition result in better outcomes in critically ill adult patients? A systematic review of the literature. *Nutrition.* 2004;20(10):843–848.

Neurogenic Bladder

CHAPTER 19

Rajbir Chaggar and Lance L. Goetz

OUTLINE

Introduction

Neurogenic bladder, also known as neurogenic lower urinary tract dysfunction, is one of the most common complications in spinal cord injury (SCI) patients. Neurogenic bladder is defined as disruption of normal central and/or peripheral nervous system regulation to the bladder, resulting in dysfunction. Approaches to the management of neurogenic bladder vary based on patient presentation and associated complications.

Anatomy and Physiology

Upper Tract: Kidneys and Ureters

- Renal parenchyma produces urine, emptying into renal calyces, and eventually renal pelvis (forming the beginning of the collecting system).
- Renal pelvis ultimately becomes ureter after ureteropelvic junction, a relatively narrow region where obstruction can frequently occur.
- Ureters enter the bladder wall obliquely, permitting increasing bladder pressures to force ureters shut between layers of the bladder wall; this one-way valve reduces the risk of vesicoureteral reflux (VUR) of urine into the upper tract.[1]

Lower Tract: Bladder and Urethra

- From the bladder, urine passes through the bladder outlet and internal urinary sphincter into urethra.
- In males, urethra is further subclassified in relation to the prostate and penis.
- Distally, the external urinary sphincter normally provides the last site of restriction.
- Pelvic floor is thought to promote ideal conditions for the urinary system.[2]

Regulation

- Coordinated effort of several portions of the nervous system (Fig. 19.1).[3]
- The autonomic system coordinates involuntary aspects of emptying and storage through parasympathetic and sympathetic fibers involved in the sacral micturition center.
- Somatic fibers provide voluntary input to the external sphincter.
- The central nervous system (CNS) allows for high-level regulation of micturition activity via communication between pontine and sacral micturition centers, through the micturition reflex. This reflex is in part mediated by afferent A-delta fibers traveling in the pelvic nerve, utilizing a spinobulbospinal reflex arc with a pathway to the pontine micturition center with regulatory input from more rostral structures, which subsequently utilize spinal efferent pathways and ultimately peripheral nerves to affect the detrusor and related structures for micturition.[4]

Innervation

Pelvic Nerve

- Formed by S2–S4 roots
- Parasympathetic innervation
- Muscarinic receptors (M2 predominantly with some M3), which utilize acetylcholine as neurotransmitter. Receptors are located throughout bladder but concentrated in bladder dome
- Receptor activation leads to detrusor contraction
- A-delta afferent fibers also travel with the pelvic nerve, and provide sensory information regarding bladder filling when threshold met as part of micturition reflex to more rostral structures[4]

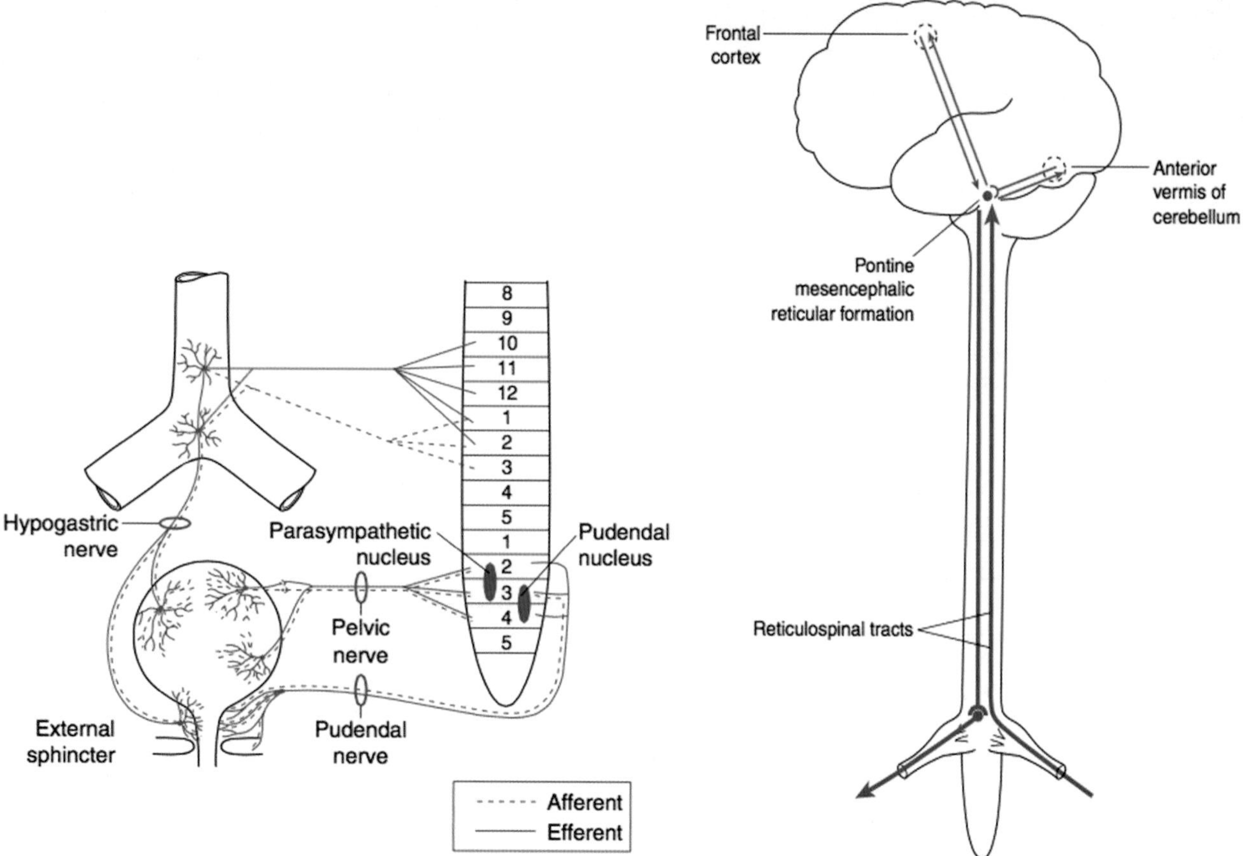

Fig. 19.1 Primary Neural Pathways Involved in Micturition. (From Cifu DX. *Braddom's Physical Medicine and Rehabilitation*. 6th ed. Elsevier; 2021.)

Hypogastric Nerve

- Formed by T11–L2 roots
- Sympathetic innervation
- Primary receptor types are alpha and beta, utilizing norepinephrine as primary neurotransmitter
  - Alpha 1 receptors: around the bladder outlet and internal sphincter, prostatic urethra; activation promotes smooth muscle contraction.
  - Beta 2 receptors: throughout bladder, though more concentration in body than outlet; activation promotes smooth muscle relaxation.
  - Beta 3 receptors: concentrated within body, dome of bladder; activation promotes smooth muscle relaxation.[5]

Pudendal Nerve

- Formed by S2–S4 roots
- Somatic innervation
- Utilizes acetylcholine as a neurotransmitter
- Allows for voluntary control of external urinary sphincter (striated muscle)[6]

Bladder Function

Bladder Storage

- Stimulated sympathetic alpha-receptors close off bladder outlet, whereas stimulated beta-receptors promote relaxation of the detrusor muscle to promote filling.
- Simultaneous inhibition of parasympathetic activity with internal, external sphincter remaining closed, known as the guarding reflex, mediated by bladder afferents.[7]

Bladder Voiding

- Loss of inhibition to sacral micturition center.
- Relaxation of pelvic floor and bladder outlet, stimulation of parasympathetic muscarinic receptors in bladder preferentially in more cranial aspects (dome) promotes contraction in a caudal direction.[6]
- Voluntary relaxation of external sphincter allows for passage of urine.

Pathophysiology and Presentation

Interruption in the innervation and regulation of the bladder leads to neurogenic bladder; however, the site of the lesion, the completeness of the lesion, the presence of multiple lesions, and preexisting urogenital conditions may all affect the clinical presentation. Pathophysiologic changes are mediated by contributions of these factors. Additionally, changes to adrenergic and cholinergic receptor density and responsiveness to neurotransmitters,[8] the development of a suprasacral spinal micturition reflex with upper motor neuron injury to bladder,[4] and aberrant activation of C-afferent fibers[4] may all also be part of pathophysiologic changes in neurogenic bladder.

Types of Lesions

Suprapontine Lesion

- Rostral CNS lesion with preservation of pontine micturition center
- Would not be seen in SCI, unless concomitant brain injury or other CNS disorder[9]
- May cause issues with void initiation and inappropriate timing, and neurogenic detrusor overactivity (NDO)
- May have preservation of detrusor sphincter synergy, depending on etiology of CNS lesion[10]

Suprasacral Spinal Cord/Infrapontine Lesion

- Suprasacral dysfunction can be caused by a variety of traumatic and nontraumatic events.
- Infrapontine/suprasacral lesions, pontine regulation for detrusor and sphincter synergy is interrupted, promoting detrusor sphincter dyssynergia (DSD).[10]
- May, but not always, have DSD, NDO, depending on extent and etiology of lesion, which may be associated autonomic dysreflexia (AD) if the lesion is at or cranial to T6.[9]

Sacral Spinal Cord Lesion

- Similar potential etiologies as suprasacral lesions
- Loss of bladder contractions (areflexic)
- Impaired bladder compliance may be present and may have dysfunctional sphincter[10]

Infrasacral (Cauda Equina and Peripheral Nerves) Lesion

- Traumatic and nontraumatic etiologies
- May be caused by peripheral neuropathy; notably, diabetes mellitus can cause autonomic neuropathy
- Depending on etiology, can have sensory, sensory and motor, or autonomic dysfunction[11]
- Areflexic bladder and sphincter dysfunction may be present; diabetes may additionally cause NDO[10]

Mixed Lesion

- Lesions at several levels simultaneously
- Neurogenic bladder where multiple lesions of similar completeness are present would foreseeably present, based on the lowest level of injury; however, will likely require urodynamics for more definitive analysis[9,10]

Evaluation

History

A detailed history and examination is critical in the evaluation of neurogenic bladder. Conversations with the patient may reveal information regarding incontinence, dysuria, intake and output volumes, bladder spasms, history of urinary tract infections, and other medical conditions that may affect their urologic or renal function. Similarly, determining baseline renal and urologic function is often critical in workup and later management; for example, does a patient suffer from end-stage renal disease and is on dialysis? Do they make any urine, and if so, how much? Does a patient have a history of stress incontinence or overactive bladder? Is there a history of renal, urologic, or gynecologic conditions, injuries, or malignancies? Is the patient taking medication that may affect these systems? Neurogenic bowel, bowel habits, and stool burden may also affect urinary sphincter activity and thus affect urologic symptoms.[9]

In the presence of a neurologic disorder such as SCI, certain key lower urinary tract symptoms can be considered neurogenic (Table 19.1).[10]

Table 19.1 Key Lower Urinary Tract Symptoms

Storage Symptoms	Voiding Symptoms	Post Micturition Symptoms
Frequency	Stream strength, continuity, splitting, and/or hesitancy	Feeling of incomplete emptying
Nocturia		Post micturition leakage
Urgency	Straining	
Incontinence (multiple types)	Terminal dribble	

Physical Examination

A detailed neurologic examination according to the International Standards for Neurological Classification of Spinal Cord Injury, formerly known as the American Spinal Cord Injury Association (ASIA) examination, should be performed. The bulbocavernosus reflex, anocutaneous reflex, and anal tone provide useful information regarding the state of spinal shock and a prediction of reflexic versus areflexic bladder.[3] Additional components to consider are a gastrointestinal, penile, scrotal, prostate, rectal, or pelvic exam if warranted based on history.

Laboratory Tests

Baseline urinalysis and urine culture may be useful in anticipation of future bladder colonization. Urinalysis and urine culture may also be helpful prior to urologic procedures, during workup of new urinary symptoms, or change in routine elimination management strategies. Baseline renal function (glomerular filtration rate, or GFR) is classically estimated by creatinine clearance,

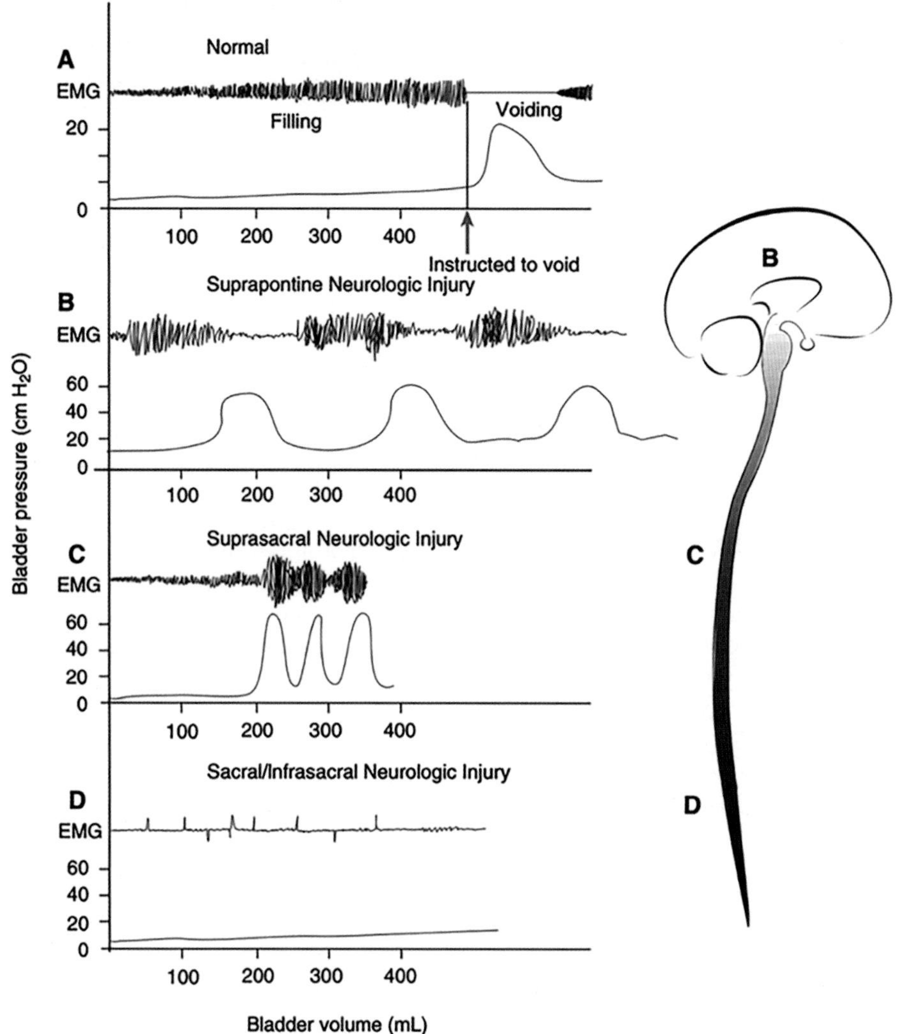

Fig. 19.2 Bladder Pressures During Filling and Voiding, With Expected Electromyographic Activity. (A) Normal pattern; acontractile during filling phase, with voiding phase that occurs by intentional sphincter relaxation with subsequent bladder contraction. (B) Suprapontine lesion; inappropriate contractions during filling with coordinated sphincter relaxation, causing incontinence. (C) Infrapontine/suprasacral lesion; inappropriate contractions during filling with inappropriate concomitant sphincter contraction (i.e., DSD). (D) Sacral/infrasacral lesion; near or total acontractile bladder or sphincter. (From Cifu D. *Braddom's Physical Medicine and Rehabilitation* 6th ed. Elsevier; 2021.)

which can be calculated with a 24-hour urine collection in tandem with a serum value. However, creatinine clearance is an imperfect predictor of GFR, and may overestimate GFR due to intrinsic secretion of creatinine by proximal renal tubular cells. Serum creatinine may also be less reliable over time as muscle mass breaks down.[3] Other measures of GFR, such as cystatin C, which is not affected by muscle mass, may be superior in estimating GFR in these cases.[12]

Imaging and Special Tests (discussed further in Chapter 20)

- Renal, bladder ultrasound
- Computed tomography urogram, renal colic
- X-ray imaging (kidney, ureter, and bladder)
- Post-void residual
- Cystoscopy, cystography
- Urodynamic studies with or without fluoroscopy (Fig. 19.2)
- Sphincter electromyography (Fig. 19.2)
- Isotope studies (dimercapto succinic acid, MAG-3 scans)[3]

Management

Management of neurogenic bladder is determined by acuity of injury, site of injury, functional status, and associated comorbidities. Typically, in the acute setting, patients experience spinal shock, during which time reflexes below the site of injury are absent. During this time, the bladder may be areflexic. An indwelling catheter is frequently used during the acute management of neurogenic bladder, particularly in the critical care setting where patients may be receiving large volumes of fluid, require intensive input and output monitoring, and may not be able to communicate voiding needs. After a period lasting typically between 72 hours and a few weeks, reflexes below the level of injury return, signaling the end of spinal shock, though some consider the presence of involuntary bladder contractions to indicate the end of spinal shock, a process that can last weeks to even years.[13] Patients may develop a spastic bladder with possible DSD, with upper motor neuron injury, or continue to demonstrate a flaccid, areflexic bladder with variable sphincter activity in the setting of a lower motor neuron injury, such as cauda equina syndrome. Once out of spinal shock, bladder management is determined based on the type of neurogenic bladder and the patient's functional status.

Upper Motor Neuron Injuries

Bladder Incontinence

- Neurogenic lower urinary tract dysfunction from a suprasacral spinal cord/infrapontine lesion is typically managed with clean intermittent catheterization (CIC) with daily 2-L volumes and a goal of less than 400 mL per catheterization. This has the benefit of reducing infection rates associated with chronic indwelling urinary catheter use, decreasing potential traumatic traction injuries, liberalizing the genital system for sexual intercourse, reducing the risk of decreased bladder compliance, and potentially lowering the incidence of bladder cancers when compared with indwelling catheter use.[14] Potential disadvantages of CIC include nonsterile environment with potential for urinary tract infections, potential for false tract formation and trauma with repeated use, and potential to trigger AD in some individuals.[9]
- Nursing initially performs aseptic intermittent catheterization (IC), and depending on the patient's functional status and comfort, the patient may participate in performing CIC, or family members may be taught how to perform this. IC should be avoided if the patient and caretaker are unable to perform the procedure, aberrant urogenital anatomy is present, there is a need for high-volume fluid intake, there is a low bladder capacity (<200 mL), the patient is unable or unwilling to follow the regimen, or complications (including AD) exist.[14]
- When IC is not appropriate, or for temporary purposes, indwelling urethral catheters may be used. Suprapubic catheters or urinary diversion procedures may be required, particularly in the chronic setting. This is discussed more in Chapter 20.
- Other potential options include reflex bladder voiding or allowing bladder pressures to fill to a volume that induces bladder contractions and subsequent voiding reflexively; typically, medical and/or surgical treatment of the sphincter is required to allow for voiding with this method (see Chapter 20 for surgical options). VUR, stones, and infections are also risks with indwelling urethral catheters.[9] Close monitoring is indicated in this situation.
- Medications: For NDO, anticholinergics can be used; ongoing research suggests beta-3 agonists may also be beneficial.[15,16] If the bladder is refractory to medications, botulinum toxin A injected into the bladder wall may be useful.[3]

Sphincter Incontinence

- For those with sphincter incompetence/under activity (which is unusual with suprasacral spinal cord/infrapontine lesion), timed voiding before full capacity (when pressures exceed resistance of sphincter) is useful. External collection devices and garments may be worn in between scheduled voids, or if incontinence is significant, an indwelling catheter may be required. Pelvic floor exercises do not have strong evidence to suggest large-scale benefit in this population.[17,18] Urethral bulking agents and surgical procedures may also be utilized.
- Medications: For underactive sphincter, alpha agonists for cases of sphincter incompetence have weak evidence for use; however, these agents may cause systemic side effects, and may cause VUR and/or AD in patients with excessive bladder contractions with increased outflow resistance.[9]

Bladder Retention

- For retention due to weak bladder contractions (sphincter contraction greater than bladder contraction), suprapubic bladder tapping can be used, though this may trigger DSD and subsequent AD. Catheterization, supportive garments, and external collection devices may be used.
- Medications: Bethanechol (Urecholine) is a cholinergic that might help augment weak contractions (it is not useful if the bladder is completely areflexic), but the medication may also increase external sphincter pressures, so it should not be used if DSD or high levels of outlet resistance are present.[19]
- Potential surgical options are discussed in the Chapter 20.

Sphincter Retention

- For retention due to outlet/sphincter, specific bladder reflex triggering methods can potentially be used, such as anal stretching or suprapubic tapping. Anal stretch with a gloved finger can relax the pelvic floor, then a subsequent Valsalva maneuver can utilize the underlying spastic bladder to void. This may also promote reflex bowel activity. Given the need/ability to perform Valsalva maneuver and anal stretching, which may be uncomfortable in some patients with incomplete lesions, this technique may be limited to

certain patient groups.[19] IC or indwelling catheterization may otherwise be required.
- For overactive sphincter, alpha-blockers or botulinum toxins injected into the sphincter can be helpful in decreasing DSD and promoting voiding.
- Potential surgical options are discussed in Chapter 20.

Lower Motor Neuron Injuries

Bladder Incontinence

- Bladder incontinence may be due to bladder overdistension. A timed voiding schedule with IC to prevent overdistension and overflow is critical. If incontinence between timed voids with IC is medically, psychologically, or functionally harmful, indwelling catheters may be more appropriate.[9]
- Medication: If there is a completely areflexic bladder without contractions, bethanechol is not thought to be helpful.[20]

Sphincter Incontinence

- Sphincter under activity is more common in lower motor neuron injuries. Timed voiding is utilized. External collection devices and garments may be worn in between scheduled voids, or if incontinence is significant, an indwelling catheter may be required. Pelvic floor exercises for associated pelvic floor weakness do not have strong evidence to suggest large-scale benefit in this population.[17,18]
- Medications: Alpha agonists for cases of sphincter incompetence have weak evidence for use but may cause other systemic side effects, and may cause VUR and/or AD in patients with excessive bladder contractions with increased outflow resistance.[9]
- Urethral bulking agents and surgical procedures may also be utilized and are discussed in subsequent chapters.

Bladder Retention

- Urinary retention due to lack of bladder contractions can use timed voids with IC, or voids with Credé or Valsalva maneuvers, particularly with cauda equina and peripheral nerve lesions that cause pelvic floor weakness (however, IC is preferred due to risk of complications with bladder expression).[3,14] Indwelling catheterization, external devices, or garments may instead need to be utilized.
- Medications: Bethanechol is not generally found to be effective with a completely areflexic bladder, and may also increase outlet resistance, which can be potentially harmful in these patients.[19]
- Potential surgical options are discussed in Chapter 20.

Sphincter Retention

- For urinary retention due to sphincter tone, therapeutic behaviors typically cannot utilize any bladder contraction to overcome outlet resistance. IC or indwelling catheterization may be required.
- Medications: With sphincter overactivity, alpha-blockers and botulinum injections into the sphincter may be employed.

Medication Management

(See Table 19.2.)

Complications

Various acute and chronic sequelae exist from neurogenic bladder and its management. These are primarily discussed in other chapters, but include:

- Aberrant anatomy (trabeculations, sacculations, diverticula, etc.)
- VUR, upper tract dilation, renal failure
- Hypercalciuria and bladder/kidney stones
- Bacteriuria, urinary tract infection, and perioperative prophylaxis
- Management of AD
- Sexual dysfunction
- Bladder cancer
- Hematuria
- Renal amyloidosis

Review Questions

1. A patient with a history of end-stage renal disease on hemodialysis and lumbar spinal stenosis is admitted to the acute care hospital for a lumbar laminectomy after developing progressive lower extremity weakness. The SCI team is consulted for further management recommendations. Which of the following topics is critical to address during the interview process?
   a. History of urinary tract infections
   b. Baseline urine production
   c. Assessment of bladder spasms
   d. Presence of dysuria
2. Which of the following would be a contraindication to suprapubic tube placement?
   a. Urethral diverticula
   b. Spastic bladder
   c. Bladder cancer
   d. Anti-muscarinic use
3. A patient with overactive sphincter activity is to be started on tamsulosin (Flomax). When asked about some of the side effects this medication has over others in the same class of agents, you note:
   a. Tamsulosin has a higher rate of retrograde ejaculation then less selective agents
   b. Tamsulosin has a higher rate of hypotension than less selective agents
   c. Tamsulosin does not differ in side effect profile compared with less selective agents
   d. Tamsulosin may cause hypertension, and is contraindicated in patients with AD

Table 19.2 Typical Agents Used in Management of Neurogenic Lower Urinary Tract Dysfunction

Agent	Use	Side Effects	Examples
Muscarinic antagonists	Treatment of NDO	Dry mouth, constipation, blurry vision, tachycardia	Propantheline, trospium, hyoscyamine, oxybutynin, tolterodine/fesoterodine, darifenacin/solifenacin, imipramine, propiverine[3,9]
Muscarinic agonists	Enhance weak bladder contractions	Salivation, vomiting, diarrhea, dizziness, flushing, bradycardia, cardiac arrhythmia[21]	Bethanechol, though limited in use[20]
Adrenergic antagonists	Decrease sphincter, bladder outlet activation; may provide antihypertensive effects	Dizziness/hypotension. Less selective: more hypotensive effects; more selective: higher risk of retrograde ejaculation[3]	Phenoxybenzamine (alpha, less selective, less favored); prazosin/terazosin/doxazosin (alpha 1, more selective); tamsulosin/ alfuzosin/ silodosin (alpha 1a, most selective)[3]
Adrenergic agonists	Increase outlet resistance (alpha 1) typically in stress incontinence; detrusor relaxation (beta 3)	Alpha 1: may increase stroke risk, worsen DSD if untreated contractions; arrhythmia, nausea, vomiting (not typically used).[22] Beta 3: usually well tolerated, may have hypertension, dry mouth, constipation, tachycardia, headache, dizziness[23]	Ephedrine (alpha 1, beta 1, beta 2 agonist): not typically used; mirabegron (beta 3 agonist)[15,16]
Estrogens	Denervation with resultant/concomitant stress incontinence in women (hormonally sensitive urethral submucosa)[3]	Uncommonly, vaginal discharge or pruritus, breast tenderness. Risk of stimulation of hormonally sensitive cancers	Estrogen creams, rings, patches, or tablets[24]
Onabotulinum-toxinA	Interrupt presynaptic transmission; intravesical administration into bladder for NDO, sphincter overactivity	Spread to other nontarget areas, risk of infection, may trigger AD	Botox

AD, Autonomic dysreflexia; DSD, detrusor sphincter dyssynergia; NDO, neurogenic detrusor overactivity.

4. Which of the following are considered bladder storage symptoms?
   a. Hematuria, urethral discharge, bladder spasms
   b. Frequency, nocturia, urgency, incontinence (multiple types)
   c. Stream strength/continuity/splitting/hesitancy; straining, terminal dribble
   d. Feeling of incomplete emptying, post-micturition leakage
5. A patient with dual traumatic brain injury and SCI is admitted to your service. His acute course was complicated by behavioral changes from frontal lobe dysfunction, neurostorming, and later autonomic dysreflexia. Which of the below are likely sites of neurologic injury (mixed lesions) that may impair micturition in this patient?
   a. Suprasacral spinal cord/infrapontine lesion, cauda equina and peripheral nerve lesion
   b. Suprapontine lesion, sacral spinal cord lesion
   c. Suprasacral spinal cord/infrapontine lesion, sacral spinal cord lesion
   d. Suprapontine lesion, suprasacral spinal cord/ infrapontine lesion

REFERENCES

1. Stephens FD, Lenaghan D. The anatomical basis and dynamics of vesicoureteral reflux. *J Urol.* 1962;87(5):669–680.
2. Grimes WR, Stratton M. *Pelvic floor dysfunction. StatPearls [Internet]*. Treasure Island (FL): StatPearls Publishing; 2020. https://www.ncbi.nlm.nih.gov/books/NBK559246/.
3. Cifu DX. *Braddom's Physical Medicine and Rehabilitation.* 6th ed. : Elsevier; 2021.
4. de Groat WC, Yoshimura N. Changes in afferent activity after spinal cord injury. *Neurourol Urodyn.* 2010;29(1):63–76.
5. Wang P, Luthin GR, Ruggieri MR. Muscarinic acetylcholine receptor subtypes mediating urinary bladder contractility and coupling to GTP binding proteins. *J Pharmacol Exp Ther.* 1995;273(2):959–966.
6. Fletcher TF, Bradley WE. Neuroanatomy of the bladder-urethra. *J Urol.* 1978;119(2):153–160.
7. Fowler CJ, Griffiths D, de Groat WC. The neural control of micturition. *Nat Rev Neurosci.* 2008;9(6):453–466.
8. Norlén L, Dahlström A, Sundin T, Svedmyr N. The adrenergic innervation and adrenergic receptor activity of the feline urinary bladder and urethra in the normal state and after hypogastric and/or parasympathetic denervation. *Scand J Urol Nephrol.* 1976;10(3):177–184.
9. Kirshblum S, Lin VW, eds. *Spinal Cord Medicine.* 3rd ed. New York: Demos Medical Publishing; 2019.

10. Gajewski JB, Schurch B, Hamid R, et al. An International Continence Society (ICS) report on the terminology for adult neurogenic lower urinary tract dysfunction (ANLUTD). *Neurourol Urodyn.* 2018;37(3):1152–1161.
11. Freeman R. Diabetic autonomic neuropathy. In: Zochodne DW, Malik RA, eds. *Handbook of Clinical Neurology [Internet].* Elsevier; 2014:63–79. https://linkinghub.elsevier.com/retrieve/pii/B9780444534804000060.
12. Dharnidharka VR, Kwon C, Stevens G. Serum cystatin C is superior to serum creatinine as a marker of kidney function: a meta-analysis. *Am J Kidney Dis.* 2002;40(2):221–226.
13. Ditunno JF, Little JW, Tessler A, Burns AS. Spinal shock revisited: a four-phase model. *Spinal Cord.* 2004;42(7):383–395.
14. Consortium for Spinal Cord Medicine Bladder management for adults with spinal cord injury: a clinical practice guideline for health-care providers. *J Spinal Cord Med.* 2006;29(5):527–573.
15. Chapple C, Khullar V, Nitti VW, et al. Efficacy of the β3-adrenoceptor agonist mirabegron for the treatment of overactive bladder by severity of incontinence at baseline: a post hoc analysis of pooled data from three randomised phase 3 trials. *Eur Urol.* 2015;67(1):11–14.
16. El Helou E, Labaki C, Chebel R, et al. The use of mirabegron in neurogenic bladder: a systematic review. *World J Urol.* 2020;38(10):2435–2442.
17. Vásquez N, Knight SL, Susser J, Gall A, Ellaway PH, Craggs MD. Pelvic floor muscle training in spinal cord injury and its impact on neurogenic detrusor over-activity and incontinence. *Spinal Cord.* 2015;53(12):887–889.
18. Zhou X, Williams AMM, Lam T. Effects of exercise-based interventions on urogenital outcomes in persons with spinal cord injury: a systematic review and meta-analysis. *J Neurotrauma.* 2021;38(9):1225–1241.
19. Sporer A, Leyson JFJ, Martin BF. Effects of bethanechol chloride on the external urethral sphincter in spinal cord injury patients. *J Urol.* 1978 Jul;120(1):62–66.
20. Finkbeiner AE. Is bethanechol chloride clinically effective in promoting bladder emptying? A literature review. *J Urol.* 1985;134(3):443–449.
21. Padda IS, Derian A. *Bethanechol. [Updated 2021]. StatPearls [Internet].* Treasure Island (FL): StatPearls Publishing; 2020. https://www.ncbi.nlm.nih.gov/books/NBK560587/.
22. Statler AK, Maani CV, Kohli A. *Ephedrine. [Updated 2021]. StatPearls [Internet].* Treasure Island (FL): StatPearls Publishing; 2020. https://www.ncbi.nlm.nih.gov/books/NBK547661/.
23. Dawood O, El-Zawahry A. *Mirabegron. [Updated 2021]. StatPearls [Internet].* Treasure Island (FL): StatPearls Publishing; 2020. https://www.ncbi.nlm.nih.gov/books/NBK538513/.
24. Flores SA, Hall CA. *Atrophic vaginitis. [Updated 2021]. StatPearls [Internet].* Treasure Island (FL): StatPearls Publishing; 2020. https://www.ncbi.nlm.nih.gov/books/NBK564341/.

CHAPTER 20

Urological Conditions in Persons With Spinal Cord Injury

William R. Visser, Shira Lanyi, Adam P. Klausner, and Sarah C. Krzastek

OUTLINE

Introduction

Urological conditions afflict 10% of the general population and up to 69.3% of the geriatric population.[1,2] Persons with spinal cord injuries (SCI) face these same conditions and are also at increased risk for unique urological pathology due to urinary stasis and neurological voiding dysfunction. This chapter provides an overview of urological conditions specific to the SCI population and offers guidance on evaluation and management of these conditions.

Urological Pathology in Persons With Spinal Cord Injury

Neurogenic Bladder

Optimal bladder management is a key component of improving health and limiting long-term complications in the person with SCI. Neurogenic bladder (NGB) management varies widely depending on type of neurologic injury. As the type of neurological injury greatly affects the voiding pathology, each person with SCI should have an individualized plan given their urologic needs, functional ability, and additional medical conditions.

Diagnostic Evaluation: Urodynamics

While the level of the neurologic injury may allow the person's medical team to estimate the type of resultant bladder pathophysiology, evaluation with urodynamic testing should be performed. Urodynamics to assess bladder pressures and volume, combined with a voiding diary to assess voiding or catheterization frequency, volume of urine output, intake quantity, and/or incontinence episodes over a 3-day period, can improve diagnostic accuracy. Video urodynamics is considered the gold standard to assess bladder pathophysiology. This study involves placing a small catheter in the bladder and an additional catheter in either the vagina, rectum, or intestinal stoma to measure bladder and abdominal pressures. The person is placed on a fluoroscopy-enabled bed to allow for a concordant voiding cystourethrogram. Additional electromyography leads are placed on either side of the perineum to allow for measurement of pelvic floor activity during storage and voiding phases of the study. Multiple fill/void cycles can be performed for improved accuracy. Incorporating additional techniques such as provocative maneuvers (coughing, laughing, abdominal compression) and pressure flow studies may aid in diagnosis.

Voiding patterns can be broadly classified based on level of neurologic insult (Table 20.1).[3] It cannot be assumed that a certain type or level of injury will result in a specific storage or voiding pattern for any given patient. Urodynamics should be performed on all persons with SCI after the acute phase of the injury has resolved.[4,5] Some persons may appear to have full neurologic recovery, especially in partial SCI with recovery of ambulatory status; however, these individuals should still undergo a urodynamic study due to clinically significant underlying silent bladder dysfunction.[4] Repeat urodynamics should be considered in all persons with SCI with changes in clinical status such as increased incontinence episodes, worrisome imaging findings

Table 20.1 Location of Neurologic Injury and Corresponding Voiding Pathophysiology

Level of Injury	Voiding Pathophysiology
Suprapontine	Physiological reflex voiding
Pons–Sacrum	NDO, hyperreflexic voiding +/− DSD
Sacral	Hypocontractility, areflexic voiding

DSD, Detrusor sphincter dyssynergia; *NDO*, neurogenic detrusor overactivity.

(hydronephrosis), or recurrent urinary tract infections (UTIs). It should be noted that persons with SCI are at increased risk of autonomic dysreflexia (AD) with injuries or lesions above T6 and must be monitored appropriately throughout the study. Although this type of study is valuable, results may be variable.[6–8] Clinical presentation and diagnostic imaging should be paired with urodynamics to form a well-rounded understanding of each patient's bladder physiology.

Medical Management

Management options for NGB, including medical and surgical modalities, are summarized in Table 20.2. Medications are aimed at improving symptoms of urinary urgency, frequency, and incontinence, and decreasing intravesical pressure, as well as improving bladder capacity and reducing detrusor leak point pressures.[9–13] Alpha-blockers, such as tamsulosin (Flomax), can decrease bladder outlet resistance for improved voiding and has been shown to help decrease symptoms of AD in 44% of persons with SCIs.[14,15] These medications are generally well tolerated and may be used as first line options in persons with SCIs.

Surgical Management

Endoscopic intradetrusor injection of botulinum neurotoxin is a safe and effective strategy for improved bladder management in persons with SCI and can decrease neurogenic detrusor overactivity, decrease incontinence episodes, and increase bladder capacity.[16] Typically, 200 units are injected in divided doses around the bladder with effects lasting 6–12 months, at which point the procedure must be repeated. Alternatively, botulinum neurotoxin can be injected into the external urethral sphincter to temporarily decrease bladder outlet resistance and improve voiding in persons with SCI who have detrusor sphincter dyssynergia or who can spontaneously void.[16]

Utilization of sacral neuromodulation has also been shown to improve bladder capacity, decrease the number of catheterizations required per day, and decrease overall detrusor activity on urodynamics studies. This form of therapy is accomplished via electrical stimulation of the S3 nerve root by inserting an electrode through the sacral foramen connected to a permanently implanted sacral nerve stimulator underneath this skin of the buttocks. Rhythmic impulses help to alter the reflex pathways in the central nervous system and improve symptoms of NGB.[17]

Table 20.2 Management Options for the Neurogenic Bladder

Therapy	Mechanism of Action
Medications	
Antimuscarinics	Inhibit the action of acetylcholine on detrusor smooth muscle, antispasmodic
Oxybutynin	
Trospium	
Tolterodine	
β-3 Agonists	Result in detrusor smooth muscle relaxation
Mirabegron	
α Antagonists	Decrease bladder outlet resistance
Tamsulosin	
Surgeries	
Intradetrusor botulinum toxin	Inhibits acetylcholine release from the parasympathetic nerves in the detrusor muscle
Sacral neuromodulation	Stimulates S3 nerve root to alter the reflex voiding pathway

Urinary Diversion

The goal of bladder management in persons with SCI is to optimize bladder emptying to reduce UTIs and elevated bladder pressures, which may result in long-term renal damage (Table 20.3).

Catheterization

Historically, persons with SCI were started on "sterile" intermittent catheterization (IC) in an effort to reduce bacterial inoculation of the urinary tract.[18] Subsequent research showed that "clean" IC decreased cost, simplified the procedure, and posed no significant increased risk of UTI.[19,20] Since its emergence in the 1970s, IC has been the preferred method of bladder drainage.[21] Inability or unwillingness to perform IC, body habitus, urethral damage or strictures, and incontinence are some reasons that may prevent successful implementation of an IC program. These individuals may proceed to management with an indwelling urethral catheter or placement of a suprapubic catheter. Chronically indwelling catheters have up to a six fold increase in the rate of UTI compared with individuals performing IC.[22,23] Additionally, indwelling urethral catheters have been associated with high rates of urethral erosion, fistula formation, epididymitis, and periurethral abscess, and should not be used as long-term bladder management solutions if possible.[16] Condom catheters should only be used in individuals demonstrated to have complete

Table 20.3 Methods of Urinary Diversion

Catheterization
External
Clean intermittent
Indwelling (urethral vs. suprapubic)
Surgical Diversion
Ileal conduit
Ileovesicostomy
Appendicovesicostomy
Augment cystoplasty

emptying with low bladder pressures, as persons with incomplete emptying or high bladder pressures are at risk of upper tract deterioration. If an external urethral sphincterotomy has been performed, external catheters may be the preferred long-term method to divert urine away from the skin of the scrotum and perineum.[16] Reflex voiding via external stimulation, such as suprapubic tapping, touching the external genitalia, or pulling pubic hair, as well as bladder expression via the Valsalva or Credé maneuver may be feasible for some individuals with SCI.[24–26]

Surgical Urinary Diversion

If noninvasive strategies are unsuccessful or only partially successful, operative strategies may be implemented for improved bladder management. Endoscopic injection of periurethral bulking agents, bladder neck reconstruction, and bladder neck closure with diversion are theoretical strategies for treatment of incontinence in the individual with an SCI. They are frequently utilized in children with NGB; however, more research is needed to convey effectiveness in the adult SCI population.[27–30] Mid-urethral autologous and synthetic slings can be a crucial part of managing urinary incontinence. They have an overall low complication rate with >80% continence reported in some articles.[31,32] Artificial urinary sphincters are used for urinary incontinence in males with intrinsic sphincter deficiency and have been used with some success in persons with SCI, although complication rates remain high and individuals with elevated bladder pressures are at increased risk for upper tract damage.[33–35]

When conservative therapy fails to control urodynamic findings such as detrusor leak point pressure, bladder compliance, and detrusor overactivity, providers should consider invasive surgical management. Surgical urinary diversion has long been a mainstay in urology. During these procedures, the operative team harvests the appendix or a portion of small intestine and, by means of direct anastomosis or retubularization, can create an alternate route of urinary drainage such as an ileal conduit, ileovesicostomy, or appendicovesicostomy.[36] Additionally, in cases of severely limited bladder capacity or significantly elevated bladder pressures, the surgeons may elect to pursue an augmentation cystoplasty. During this procedure, a portion of the small intestine is harvested and anastomosed to a clam-shelled bladder to increase storage capacity.[36] Creation of a continent-catheterizable channel using the appendix can be employed if catheterization of the urethra is difficult or impossible.[36]

Urinary Tract Infections

UTIs are the number-one cause of emergency department visits and admission diagnoses for persons with SCIs.[37] Persons with NGB have multiple risk factors for UTI (Table 20.4). Underlying neurologic abnormalities often allow for atypical presenting signs and symptoms, which can delay appropriate medical treatment. Alterations in physiologic micturition can lead to stasis of urine.[37] This in turn places individuals at risk of both acute cystitis as well as chronic colonization of the bladder. Chronic indwelling catheters (urethral or suprapubic), condom catheters, and IC are all associated with increased UTI risk. Primary neurologic injuries and underlying bladder ischemia from elevated intravesical pressures may further impair the ability of persons with SCI to clear bacteria from the urinary tract secondary to an altered immunologic response in both antiinflammatory and proinflammatory states.[38] Studying and treating UTIs in persons with NGB is difficult, as there is no consensus among providers about the true definition of a UTI in this population. The National Institute on Disability and Rehabilitation Research provides a recommendation on defining UTI in persons with SCIs, which may be used as a guide.

Table 20.4 Risk Factors for Urinary Tract Infections in Persons With Neurogenic Bladder

- Altered micturition
  - Detrusor sphincter dyssynergia
  - High-pressure voiding
  - Bladder ischemia
    - Vesicoureteral reflux
    - Large postvoid residuals
- Nonphysiologic bladder emptying
  - Clean intermittent catheterization
  - Chronic indwelling urethral or suprapubic catheter
  - Surgical urinary diversion
- Altered immune response

Definition of UTI in persons with SCIs[39]: Pyuria, signs or symptoms of UTI, and one of the following:

1. $>10^2$ colony-forming units (CFU)/mL from a straight-catheterized specimen
2. $>10^4$ CFU/mL from a condom catheter
3. Any value from indwelling or suprapubic catheters

Typical signs and symptoms of a UTI, including dysuria, frequency, urgency, and suprapubic or perineal pain, are generally not present in persons with SCIs, but rather individuals present with:

- AD
- Increased spasticity
- New or worsening urinary incontinence
- Vague back or abdominal pain
- Foul-smelling urine

Upon presentation, a broad differential diagnosis must be maintained until a definitive diagnosis can be reached.[40] Asymptomatic bacteriuria is a frequent confounding laboratory finding in a patient with SCI. Antibiotic treatment may be warranted for this group of individuals only if colonized with urea-splitting species *(Proteus, Pseudomonas, Klebsiella, Staphylococcus)* due to the increased risk of urolithiasis formation.[41] Mild and moderate presentations of acute bacterial cystitis can be appropriately managed with oral antibiotics in the outpatient setting. Longer antibiotic regimens of 10–14 days as opposed to the standard 3–7 days for uncomplicated UTIs are more effective in persons with SCI. The specific antibiotic of choice is dependent upon the local antibiogram, but may consist of cephalexin (Keflex), trimethoprim-sulfamethoxazole (Bactrim), or nitrofurantoin (Macrobid).[42] Individuals presenting with signs of sepsis or systemic infection should be treated with broad-spectrum antibiotics and supportive care until the offending bacterial species can be isolated along with susceptibilities. If left untreated, bacteria can ascend into the upper urinary tract and lead to pyelonephritis or spread via reflux into the prostatic ducts or vas deferens in men to cause prostatitis and epididymoorchitis. If there is associated ureteral obstruction, this should be managed appropriately with either an indwelling ureteral stent or a percutaneous nephrostomy tube.

As many persons with SCIs will present with atypical symptoms and may suffer significant complications from an untreated UTI, minimization of recurrent UTIs is imperative. Providers should create an individualized bladder management plan for each person, aimed at improving bladder capacity and emptying and reducing intravesical pressures.[43] Additional measures to reduce recurrent symptomatic infections have shown mixed success. Bladder irrigation, cranberry supplements, D-mannose, and methenamine are all strategies that have been shown to reduce recurrent UTIs in persons without SCI,[40] but equivalent success rates have yet to be demonstrated in the SCI population. Regardless, these strategies may be attempted for refractory cases. Antibiotic prophylaxis is discouraged in the SCI population due to incomplete eradication of bacteria, development of antibiotic resistance, and frequent rapid recolonization of the bladder once treatment has stopped. However, persons with NGB undergoing urologic procedures should have preoperative urine cultures obtained with enough time to obtain sensitivity information. It is both safe and effective to treat persons with asymptomatic bacteriuria with one dose of preprocedural antibiotics, assuming the bacteria is appropriately covered by the antibiotic of choice. Symptomatic individuals should be treated with a standard treatment course.[44]

Stone Disease

Kidney stones are a common and pervasive medical condition in the general population. Similarly, the lifetime risk of urolithiasis in the SCI population is 12% for males and 6% for females, with recurrence rates of 35%–64%.[45]

The primary composition of 80% of stones worldwide is calcium-oxalate, but stones may also contain calcium phosphate, struvite (resulting from infection with urea-splitting organisms), uric acid, and cystine.[46–48] The pathophysiology of stone formation is complex and diverse. Recurrent stone formers are at risk of progression to hypertension, chronic kidney disease, and end-stage renal disease without appropriate diagnosis, work up, and treatment.

Although persons with SCI are susceptible to the common causes of stones, including dietary habits, obesity, diabetes, hypertension, genetic, metabolic and anatomic factors, certain medications, and hot, arid climates,[46–50] several specific risk factors apply uniquely to persons with SCIs[51]:

- Increased urinary calcium
- Reduced urinary citrate
- Increased urinary specific gravity
- High urinary pH

Hypercalciuria is a direct result of immobilization with subsequent bone resorption. Hypocitraturia appears to be a consequence of a decreased filtered load of citrate.[52,53] Other risk factors that may play a role in kidney stone formation include bladder catheterization, bladder debris, vesicoureteral reflux, and environmental factors.[45] Persons with SCIs are also at high risk for bladder stones due to urinary stasis associated with incomplete bladder emptying and urinary colonization from catheterization.

The typical clinical presentation of a kidney stone is renal colic with flank pain radiating to the groin. Additional symptoms may include nausea, vomiting, fever, and chills due to underlying obstruction or infection. The initial diagnosis of a kidney stone in persons with SCI may be made via screening imaging (recommended annually) or with atypical signs and symptoms upon presentation, including frequent UTIs, sepsis, and AD.[45–47,54]

For those individuals who present with nephrolithiasis without the indication for immediate intervention, initial steps should include a urinalysis and urine culture to rule out infection. Renal ultrasound and abdominal X-ray may be performed as initial diagnostic imaging modality due to cost-effectiveness and decreased radiation exposure; however, noncontrast computed tomography (CT) should be obtained prior to surgical intervention due to higher sensitivity and specificity.[46,47,54]

Symptomatic ureteral stones <10 mm may be followed with conservative management, or medical expulsive therapy, in the absence of urosepsis, acute kidney injury, and/or unrelenting pain. Approximately 86% of stones pass spontaneously within 4–6 weeks.[49] Increased fluid intake up to 2 L per day is recommended, as well as straining the urine for collection of a specimen for biochemical analysis. Additional medical therapy with alpha-1 antagonists may be used, as they may assist with stone passage. Biochemical analysis of the stone, whether collected from a urine sample or retrieved during surgery, is helpful in directing further investigation of the underlying cause of stone formation.[48–50]

Indications for urgent treatment include uncontrolled pain, intractable nausea and vomiting, significant renal dysfunction, anuria, or signs of systemic infection. Typically, individuals that need urgent treatment undergo a retrograde or percutaneously placed antegrade ureteral stent to bypass the stone and allow for appropriate drainage of urine, with or without concurrent treatment of the stone. In the setting of infection, definitive intervention for the stone is deferred until adequate treatment of the infection. Definitive management of kidney stones can be achieved through three main pathways. Extracorporeal shock wave lithotripsy has the lowest risk profile; unfortunately, stone passage rates are the lowest for this modality.[45] During this procedure, external shockwaves are directed at radiopaque kidney stones using fluoroscopy. As stone fragments rely on gravity and ureteral peristalsis for passage after fragmentation by extracorporeal shock wave lithotripsy, this treatment modality is not recommended for bedbound individuals. It is also contraindicated in persons with solitary kidneys or persons on anticoagulation. Ureteroscopy with laser lithotripsy and/or stone basket extraction is another important tool for kidney stone removal.[55] This modality allows the surgical team to insert an endoscopic instrument through the urethra and into the ureter in a retrograde fashion, which allows access to the upper tracts. In cases of very large kidney stone burden, percutaneous nephrolithotomy (PCNL) may provide the best stone-free outcome for the patient.[47,50] In this surgery, a percutaneous access sheath is inserted directly through the back or flank and into the renal collecting system. Persons with SCI who undergo ureteroscopy and PCNL are at significant risk of developing sepsis secondary to translocation of bacteria into the circulatory system.[45] Furthermore, persons with SCI who undergo PCNL have risk of pneumothorax or hydrothorax, acute blood loss anemia requiring transfusion, intensive care unit admission due to sepsis, fistula formation, and death.[45] Providers that perform these procedures should have an in-depth understanding of this and plan for close postoperative monitoring. Bladder stones, if small enough, can be irrigated out of the bladder, or crushed or lasered and extracted. Occasionally, for large bladder stones, a small incision is made directly through the suprapubic region into the bladder and stones are extracted manually.

Men's Health

Persons with SCI are at increased risk of developing men's health related issues. Disruption of the physiologic neural network and hormonal imbalances are the key factors that cause the associated issues. Several of these topics are covered in greater detail in other sections but mentioned here for completeness.

Erectile Dysfunction

Several complex feedback mechanisms work simultaneously to help men achieve and maintain an erection. In persons with SCIs, the neurologic input to this equation may be damaged or nonexistent. Preganglionic sympathetic neurons arise from thoracolumbar segments T11–L2 and provide stimulus for psychogenic erections.[56] Preganglionic parasympathetic neurons arising from S2–S4 and the somatic nerve fibers that originate in the Onuf nucleus of the lumbosacral region provide the mechanism for reflexogenic erections.[57] Treating erectile dysfunction in the SCI population may be achieved by use of pharmaceutical therapy including PDE-5 inhibitors, intracavernosal injections (prostaglandin E1, papaverine, phentolamine and/or atropine), and urethral suppositories (prostaglandin E1).[58] Implantable penile prosthetic devices should be considered for individuals that fail medical management. Inflatable two-piece and three-piece prosthetics are effective and safe alternatives for persons with SCI but require good hand dexterity to inflate and deflate by way of an intrascrotal pump. The malleable penile prosthesis is another option. In addition to improved sexual health, individuals may have improved ability to perform IC and to secure condom catheters.[58] Both of these options require preoperative and postoperative counseling regarding the risk of device infection and erosion, as bladder dysfunction, catheterization, and decreased penile sensation increase these risks in the SCI population.

Hypogonadism

Hypogonadism is another prevalent issue in the SCI population. Low testosterone is observed in 39% to 46% of men with SCI and is directly related to increased fat mass and time elapsed since injury.[59,60] Dysfunction of the hypothalamic–pituitary–gonadal axis in the first year after injury can lead to hypogonadism. Furthermore, persons with SCI are at higher risk of comorbidities that cause hypogonadism, such as head injury, obesity, diabetes, metabolic syndrome, and hyperlipidemia.[59] Treatment of hypogonadism may be achieved with testosterone replacement therapy or with gonadotropin stimulation.

Fertility

Erectile dysfunction, ejaculatory dysfunction, and hypogonadism predispose persons with SCI to infertility issues. Initiation of pharmacologic treatment with clomiphene citrate (Clomid) can promote sperm production in individuals with oligospermia and low testosterone. Penile vibratory stimulation, electroejaculation, or surgical sperm retrieval (sperm aspiration or extraction) can be utilized to obtain sperm for use with assisted reproductive technologies.

Conclusion

Persons with SCI are at increased risk for urological pathology including incontinence, incomplete bladder emptying, high bladder pressures, urinary tract infection, and stones, which may lead to progressive renal deterioration. Sexual function may also be impaired, as individuals have high rates of erectile dysfunction, hypogonadism, and infertility. Pathophysiology is highly dependent on the neurologic injury, and treatments should be targeted to improve quality of life and prevent long-term kidney dysfunction and infectious complications.

Review Questions

1. The urodynamic finding of detrusor sphincter dyssynergia is most frequently observed in persons with:
   a. Stroke
   b. T11 injury
   c. Pudendal nerve injury
   d. Atherosclerosis
   e. Normal pressure hydrocephalus
2. A 33-year-old male is involved in a motor vehicle collision and has a partial injury to C4–C6. Initially, he requires intermittent catheterization of his bladder due to urinary retention, but slowly regains the ability to void spontaneously. His postvoid residual is 30 cc and renal ultrasound does not show any abnormalities at 6 months follow-up. What is the next best step?
   a. Schedule follow-up in 3 months
   b. Prescribe tamsulosin (Flomax)
   c. Prescribe oxybutynin (Ditropan)
   d. Schedule for urodynamics
3. A 45-year-old SCI male with C3–C6 injury currently manages his bladder with reflex voiding into a diaper. His provider notices a sacral wound during his annual review and believes urine may be preventing the healing process. Unfortunately, a condom catheter is not currently feasible due to body habitus. Urodynamics showed adequate bladder capacity and a detrusor leak point pressure within the normal range. He has poor hand dexterity. What is the best long-term management option for this patient?
   a. Malleable penile prosthesis
   b. Augmentation cystoplasty
   c. Appendicovesicostomy
   d. Artificial urinary sphincter
   e. Botulinum neurotoxin injection
4. During a recent follow-up visit to her primary care provider, a 60-year-old female with SCI was diagnosed with a urinary tract infection and started on a 5-day course of cephalexin (Keflex) for treatment. When she follows up in SCI clinic, she tells her provider this is the seventh UTI she has had this year. She currently performs IC without issues and had a recent renal bladder ultrasound that showed no hydronephrosis and a normal-appearing bladder. Which of the following is the next best step in management?
   a. Prophylactic antibiotics
   b. Repeat urine culture to ensure eradication of bacteria
   c. Suprapubic catheter placement
   d. Cystoscopy
   e. Counsel the patient on asymptomatic bacteriuria
5. A patient presents to the emergency department with elevated blood pressure and headache. He appears flush and states he has felt unwell since this morning. His autonomic dysreflexia is medically managed, and a subsequent CT scan reveals a 1.5 cm kidney stone at the ureteropelvic junction. He undergoes emergent retrograde ureteral stent placement, and his clinical signs improve. He has a history of atrial fibrillation and is prescribed apixaban (Eliquis). What procedure should this patient be scheduled for?
   a. Urodynamics
   b. Extracorporeal shock wave lithotripsy
   c. Percutaneous nephrolithotomy
   d. Ureteroscopy and laser lithotripsy
   e. No treatment. The stone is passed on its own

REFERENCES

1. Suh J, Kim KH, Lee SH, et al. Prevalence and management status of urologic disease in geriatric hospitals in South Korea: a population-based analysis. *Investig Clin Urol.* 2017;58(4):281–288.
2. Jewett MA, Fernie GR, Holliday PJ, Pim ME. Urinary dysfunction in a geriatric long-term care population: prevalence and patterns. *J Am Geriatr Soc.* 1981;29(5):211–214.
3. Schurch B, Iacovelli V, Averbeck MA, Carda S, Altaweel W, Agrò EF. Urodynamics in patients with spinal cord injury: a clinical review and best practice paper by a working group of the international continence society urodynamics committee. *Neurourol Urodyn.*. 2018;37(2):581–591.
4. Patki P, Woodhouse J, Hamid R, Shah J, Craggs M. Lower urinary tract dysfunction in ambulatory patients with incomplete spinal cord injury. *J Urol.* 2006;175(5):1784–1787. discussion 1787.
5. Vince RA, Klausner AP. Surveillance strategies for neurogenic lower urinary tract dysfunction. *Urol Clin North Am.* 2017;44(3):367–375.
6. Bellucci CHS, Wöllner J, Gregorini F, et al. Neurogenic lower urinary tract dysfunction–do we need same session repeat urodynamic investigations? *J Urol.* 2012 Apr;187(4):1318–1323.
7. Abrams P, Agarwal M, Drake M, et al. A proposed guideline for the urological management of patients with spinal cord injury. *BJU Int.* 2008;101(8):989–994.

8. Lien WC, Kuan TS, Lin YC, Liang FW, Hsieh PC, Li CY. Patients with neurogenic lower urinary tract dysfunction following spinal cord injury are at increased risk of developing type 2 diabetes mellitus: a population-based cohort study. *Medicine (Baltimore)*. 2016;95(2):e2518.
9. Stöhrer M, Madersbacher H, Richter R, Wehnert J, Dreikorn K. Efficacy and safety of propiverine in SCI-patients suffering from detrusor hyperreflexia–a double-blind, placebo-controlled clinical trial. *Spinal Cord*. 1999;37(3):196–200.
10. Bakheit AM, Thilmann AF, Ward AB, et al. A randomized, double-blind, placebo-controlled, dose-ranging study to compare the efficacy and safety of three doses of botulinum toxin type A (Dysport) with placebo in upper limb spasticity after stroke. *Stroke.*. 2000;31(10):2402–2406.
11. Madhuvrata P, Singh M, Hasafa Z, Abdel-Fattah M. Anticholinergic drugs for adult neurogenic detrusor overactivity: a systematic review and meta-analysis. *Eur Urol*. 2012;62(5):816–830.
12. Han S-H, Cho IK, Jung JH, Jang SH, Lee B-S. Long-term efficacy of mirabegron add-on therapy to antimuscarinic agents in patients with spinal cord injury. *Ann Rehabil Med.*. 2019 Feb;43(1):54–61.
13. Vasudeva P, Prasad V, Yadav S, et al. Efficacy and safety of mirabegron for the treatment of neurogenic detrusor overactivity resulting from traumatic spinal cord injury: a prospective study. *Neurourol Urodyn.*. 2021;40(2):666–671.
14. Chancellor MB, Erhard MJ, Hirsch IH, Stass WE. Prospective evaluation of terazosin for the treatment of autonomic dysreflexia. *J Urol*. 1994;151(1):111–113.
15. Kakizaki H, Ameda K, Kobayashi S, Tanaka H, Shibata T, Koyanagi T. Urodynamic effects of alpha1-blocker tamsulosin on voiding dysfunction in patients with neurogenic bladder. *Int J Urol Off J Jpn Urol Assoc*. 2003;10(11):576–581.
16. Romo PGB, Smith CP, Cox A, et al. Non-surgical urologic management of neurogenic bladder after spinal cord injury. *World J Urol*. 2018;36(10):1555–1568.
17. Leng WW, Chancellor MB. How sacral nerve stimulation neuromodulation works. *Urol Clin North Am*. 2005;32(1): 11–18.
18. Guttmann L, Frankel H. The value of intermittent catheterisation in the early management of traumatic paraplegia and tetraplegia. *Paraplegia.*. 1966;4(2):63–84.
19. Wyndaele JJ. Intermittent catheterization: which is the optimal technique? *Spinal Cord*. 2002;40(9):432–437.
20. Lapides J, Diokno AC, Silber SJ, Lowe BS. Clean, intermittent self-catheterization in the treatment of urinary tract disease. *J Urol*. 1972;107(3):458–461.
21. Consortium for Spinal Cord Medicine Bladder management for adults with spinal cord injury: a clinical practice guideline for health-care providers. *J Spinal Cord Med*. 2006; 29(5):527–573.
22. Esclarín De Ruz A, García Leoni E, Herruzo Cabrera R. Epidemiology and risk factors for urinary tract infection in patients with spinal cord injury. *J Urol*. 2000;164(4): 1285–1289.
23. Weld KJ, Dmochowski RR. Effect of bladder management on urological complications in spinal cord injured patients. *J Urol*. 2000;163(3):768–772.
24. Cardenas DD, Kelly E, Mayo ME. Manual stimulation of reflex voiding after spinal cord injury. *Arch Phys Med Rehabil*. 1985 Jul;66(7):459–462.
25. Wyndaele JJ, Madersbacher H, Kovindha A. Conservative treatment of the neuropathic bladder in spinal cord injured patients. *Spinal Cord*. 2001;39(6):294–300.
26. Groen J, Pannek J, Castro Diaz D, et al. Summary of European Association of Urology (EAU) Guidelines on Neuro-Urology. *Eur Urol*. 2016;69(2):324–333.
27. Bennett JK, Green BG, Foote JE, Gray M. Collagen injections for intrinsic sphincter deficiency in the neuropathic urethra. *Paraplegia*. 1995;33(12):697–700.
28. Pérez LM, Smith EA, Parrott TS, Broecker BH, Massad CA, Woodard JR. Submucosal bladder neck injection of bovine dermal collagen for stress urinary incontinence in the pediatric population. *J Urol*. 1996;156(2 Pt 2):633–636.
29. Nakamura S, Hyuga T, Kawai S, Nakai H. Long-term outcome of the Pippi Salle Procedure for intractable urinary incontinence in patients with severe intrinsic urethral sphincter deficiency. *J Urol*. 2015;194(5):1402–1406.
30. Nguyen HT, Baskin LS. The outcome of bladder neck closure in children with severe urinary incontinence. *J Urol*. 2003;169(3):1114–1116. discussion 1116.
31. Lombardi G, Musco S, Celso M, et al. A retrospective study on female urological surgeries over the 10 years following spinal cord lesion. *Spinal Cord*. 2013;51(9):688–693.
32. Losco GS, Burki JR, Omar YAI, Shah PJR, Hamid R. Long-term outcome of transobturator tape (TOT) for treatment of stress urinary incontinence in females with neuropathic bladders. *Spinal Cord*. 2015;53(7):544–546.
33. Farag F, Koens M, Sievert KD, De Ridder D, Feitz W, Heesakkers J. Surgical treatment of neurogenic stress urinary incontinence: a systematic review of quality assessment and surgical outcomes. *Neurourol Urodyn*. 2016;35(1):21–25.
34. Murphy S, Rea D, O'Mahony J, et al. A comparison of the functional durability of the AMS 800 artificial urinary sphincter between cases with and without an underlying neurogenic aetiology. *Ir J Med Sci*. 2003;172(3):136–138.
35. Chartier Kastler E, Genevois S, Gamé X, et al. Treatment of neurogenic male urinary incontinence related to intrinsic sphincter insufficiency with an artificial urinary sphincter: a French retrospective multicentre study. *BJU Int*. 2011;107(3):426–432.
36. Wyndaele J-J, Birch B, Borau A, et al. Surgical management of the neurogenic bladder after spinal cord injury. *World J Urol*. 2018;36(10):1569–1576.
37. García Leoni ME, Esclarín De Ruz A. Management of urinary tract infection in patients with spinal cord injuries. *Clin Microbiol Infect*. 2003;9(8):780–785.
38. McKibben MJ, Seed P, Ross SS, Borawski KM. Urinary tract infection and neurogenic bladder. *Urol Clin North Am*. 2015;42(4):527–536.
39. Disability NI. on, Rehabilitation Research Consensus Statement January 27–29 1992. The prevention and management of urinary tract infections among people with spinal cord injuries. *J Am Paraplegia Soc*. 1992;15(3):194–207.
40. Goetz LL, Klausner AP. Strategies for prevention of urinary tract infections in neurogenic bladder dysfunction. *Phys Med Rehabil Clin N Am*. 2014;25(3):605–618. viii.
41. Schaeffer AJ, Matulewicz RS, Klumpp DJ. Infections of the urinary tract. In: Wein AJ, Kavoussi LR, Partin AW, Peters CA, eds. *Campbell-Walsh Urology.*. 11th ed. : Elsevier; 2016:301.

42. Hooton TM, Bradley SF, Cardenas DD, et al. Diagnosis, prevention, and treatment of catheter-associated urinary tract infection in adults: 2009 International Clinical Practice Guidelines from the Infectious Diseases Society of America. *Clin Infect Dis.* 2010;50(5):625–663.
43. Gamé X, Castel-Lacanal E, Bentaleb Y, et al. Botulinum toxin A detrusor injections in patients with neurogenic detrusor overactivity significantly decrease the incidence of symptomatic urinary tract infections. *Eur Urol.* 2008;53(3):613–618.
44. Chong JT, Klausner AP, Petrossian A, et al. Pre-procedural antibiotics for endoscopic urological procedures: initial experience in individuals with spinal cord injury and asymptomatic bacteriuria. *J Spinal Cord Med.* 2015;38(2):187–192.
45. Welk B, Fuller A, Razvi H, Denstedt J. Renal stone disease in spinal-cord-injured patients. *J Endourol.* 2012;26(8):954–959.
46. Dawson CH, Tomson CRV. Kidney stone disease: pathophysiology, investigation and medical treatment. *Clin Med Lond Engl.* 2012;12(5):467–471.
47. Khan SR, Pearle MS, Robertson WG, et al. Kidney stones. *Nat Rev Dis Primer.* 2016;2:16008.
48. Sakhaee K, Maalouf NM, Sinnott B. Kidney stones 2012: pathogenesis, diagnosis, and management. *J Clin Endocrinol Metab.* 2012;97(6):1847–1860.
49. Fontenelle LF, Sarti TD. Kidney stones: treatment and prevention. *Am Fam Physician.* 2019;99(8):490–496.
50. Worcester EM, Coe FL. Clinical practice. Calcium kidney stones. *N Engl J Med.* 2010;363(10):954–963.
51. Burr RG, Nuseibeh IM. Urinary catheter blockage depends on urine pH, calcium and rate of flow. *Spinal Cord.* 1997;35(8):521–525.
52. Naftchi NE, Viau AT, Sell GH, Lowman EW. Mineral metabolism in spinal cord injury. *Arch Phys Med Rehabil.* 1980;61(3):139–142.
53. Burr RG, Chem C, Nuseibeh I. Creatinine, calcium, citrate and acid-base in spinal cord injured patients. *Paraplegia.*. 1993;31(11):742–750.
54. Vitale C, Croppi E, Marangella M. Biochemical evaluation in renal stone disease. *Clin Cases Miner Bone Metab.* 2008;5(2):127–130.
55. Wolfe T, Klausner AP, Goetz LL, King AB, Hudson T, Gater DR. Ureteroscopy with laser lithotripsy for urolithiasis in the spinal cord injury population. *Spinal Cord.* 2013;51(2):156–160.
56. Giuliano F. Neurophysiology of erection and ejaculation. *J Sex Med.* 2011 Oct;8(Suppl 4):310–315.
57. Giuliano F, Clement P. Neuroanatomy and physiology of ejaculation. *Annu Rev Sex Res.* 2005;16:190–216.
58. Ibrahim E, Lynne CM, Brackett NL. Male fertility following spinal cord injury: an update. *Andrology.* 2016;4(1):13–26.
59. Bauman WA, La Fountaine MF, Cirnigliaro CM, Kirshblum SC, Spungen AM. Lean tissue mass and energy expenditure are retained in hypogonadal men with spinal cord injury after discontinuation of testosterone replacement therapy. *J Spinal Cord Med.* 2015;38(1):38–47.
60. Durga A, Sepahpanah F, Regozzi M, Hastings J, Crane DA. Prevalence of testosterone deficiency after spinal cord injury. *PM R.*. 2011;3(10):929–932.

CHAPTER 21

Sexuality and Reproduction After Spinal Cord Injury

Jennifer Weekes

OUTLINE

Introduction

Most traumatic spinal cord injuries (SCIs) occur during an individual's reproductive years. SCIs can impact fertility and sexuality in both men and women.[1] Evidence has shown that the top priorities of individuals with SCIs include motor function, bowel, bladder, and sexual function.[2] SCIs can affect physical and psychological aspects of sexual function. Importantly, sex can still be enjoyed and experienced after an injury. The degree of impact depends on the level and severity of injury.[2]

Sexual Activity and Satisfaction After Spinal Cord Injury

Components of the Sexual Response

- Excitement/arousal phase
- Plateau phase
- Orgasm phase
- Resolution phase
- Refractory phase (men only)[3]

In able-bodied individuals, excitement/arousal involves all three nervous systems[4]

- Sacral parasympathetic via pelvic nerve(S2–S4)
- Thoracic sympathetic via hypogastric nerve and the lumbar sympathetic chain (T11–T12)
- Somatic (pudendal nerve)

Neurophysiology of Arousal: Psychogenic and Reflexogenic

- In able-bodied individuals, arousal occurs via two pathways labeled psychogenic and reflexogenic stimulation. These typically occur simultaneously; however, in rapid-eye-movement sleep the psychogenic pathway predominates.[4]
- Psychogenic
  - Afferent: Stimuli generated in the brain (by thoughts) or consciously received by the brain (such as with erotica), with inputs get integrated in the hypothalamus.
  - Efferent: Via thoracolumbar sympathetic outflow with the preservation of the T11–T12 pinprick (spinothalamic tract) serving as a marker of preserved outflow function.
- Reflexogenic
  - Requires an intact sacral reflex arc (S2–S4)[4]
  - Afferent limb inputs:
    - Primarily via pudendal nerve, which provides cutaneous sensation from the clitoris or penis.
    - Also receives some input from pelvic (parasympathetic) and hypogastric (sympathetic) nerves via deep pressure and visceral receptors.
  - Efferent limb:
    - Pudendal nerve enters the pelvic plexus; the cavernous nerves then exit that plexus and innervate the erectile structures of the penis and clitoris (Fig. 21.1).

Sexual Function in Women With Spinal Cord Injury

Pelvic Innervation in Women

The female pelvic structures receive innervation from both the sympathetic and parasympathetic pathways. The sympathetic pathways (via the hypogastric nerve)

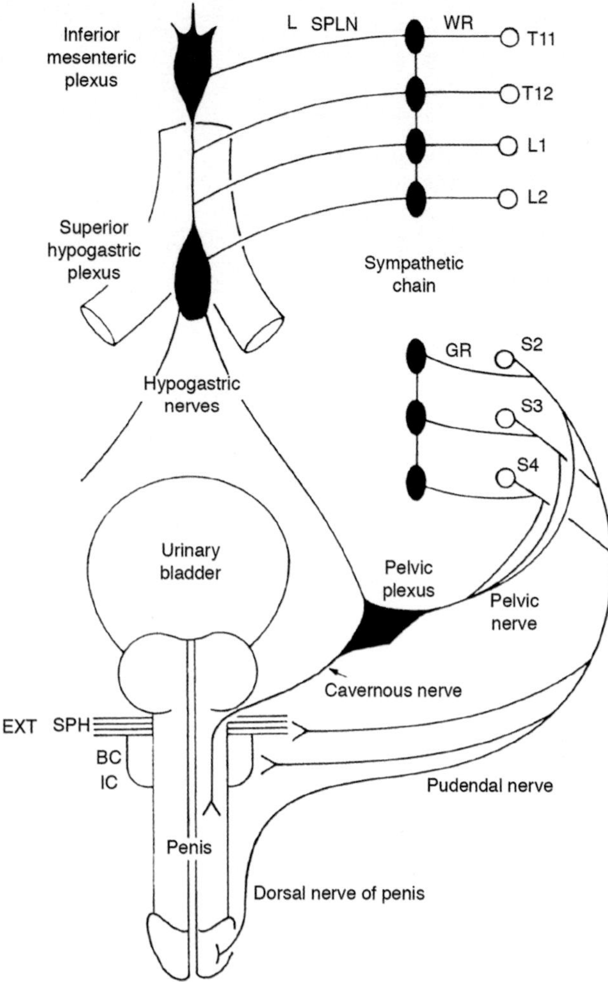

Fig. 21.1 Neuroanatomy innervation of the Penis. *BC*, Bulbocavernosis; *EXT SPH*, Sphincter; *GR*, Grey Ramus; *IC*, Ischiocavernosus; *SPLN*, Splannic nerve; *WR*, White Ramus. (Adapted from De Groat WC, Steers WD. Neuroanatomy and neurophysiology of penile erection. In: Tanagho EA, Lue TF, McClure RD, eds. *Contemporary Management of Impotence and Infertility*. Baltimore, MD: Williams & Wilkins; 1988:3-27.)

enable muscular contraction and vasoconstriction. The parasympathetic pathway is via the pelvic nerve and it causes genital muscular relaxation and vasodilation. It also causes vaginal lubrication.

Arousal

In women with SCI, it has been shown that injury level and completeness are key predictors to sexual function following SCI.

In complete injuries,[5]

- Women with complete upper motor neuron (UMN) injuries have an intact sacral reflex arc and so are able to have reflexogenic but not psychogenic arousal.
- Women with complete lower motor neuron (LMN) injuries do not have an intact sacral reflex arc and are only able to have psychogenic arousal.

In incomplete injuries,[6]

- Women with incomplete injuries have the ability to achieve both reflexogenic and psychogenic arousal. However, ability to achieve psychogenic arousal was found to correlate with the degree of preservation of pinprick sensation for T11–T12 dermatomes.
- This is thought to be due to the fact that the spinothalamic outflow (which is part of the psychogenic efferent pathway) that transmits pinprick sensation for T11–L2 is very close to the sympathetic cell bodies.

Orgasm

Orgasm is the peak of sexual excitement and/or the release of vasocongestion that was generated during the arousal period.[1] Women are able to achieve orgasm regardless of level and completeness of injury.[7,8] However, it has been shown that women with complete LMN lesions affecting the sacral region (S2–S4) have a harder time achieving orgasm. It is thought that orgasm requires an intact sacral reflex, but this is not always the case. Key differences in achieving orgasm for women after SCI include:

- Longer time to reach orgasm than able-bodied individuals
- Different experiences such as flushing, mild to severe autonomic dysreflexia (AD) (in women with injuries higher than T6).

Although to a lesser extent, some individuals with complete LMN injuries (S2–S5) are found to be able to have orgasms.[7,8] There have been some suggestions that there are alternate afferent pathways via the vagus nerve that can bypass the spinal cord and help generate orgasm.[9,10]

Treating Sexual Dysfunction in Women

Counseling and rehabilitation programs play a key role in addressing both the physical and psychological aspects of sexual dysfunction following SCI.[9]

Arousal and Orgasm

- There are some nonpharmacologic methods to increase arousal, such as self-exploration with stimulation of the clitoris and nipples.[11] Stimulation may need to be for a longer time than in able-bodied individuals.
- Pharmacologic options include phosphodiesterase type 5 (PDE-5) inhibitors. There was a small study that demonstrated increased pelvic vasocongestion and vaginal lubrication, but these results were not supported on a large scale, and other studies have had inconclusive data.[12]
- It is also important to manage sexual drive and other medical factors such as low estrogen (leading to vaginal dryness and atrophy, postinjury bowel and bladder management, and issues with incontinence and depression).[13]

Fertility in Women With Spinal Cord Injury

Following SCI, women can experience amenorrhea for 3–12 months (50% have return of normal menses by 6 months and 90% have return to normal menses by 1 year) followed by the return of normal menses. When normal menses returns after SCI, individuals will normally return to their previous fertility status.[14] Ovulation may still occur despite absence of menses, so women will need to consider contraception options if they are sexually active and do not wish to conceive during that time. Women with SCIs resulting in limited mobility are recommended to use birth control pills with lower doses of estrogen due to deep vein thrombosis risks.[14,15]

Sexual Function in Men With Spinal Cord Injury

Pelvic Innervation

As with women, an intact sacral reflex arc is important for control of erection in men. The penis is controlled by both autonomic (parasympathetic and sympathetic) and somatic nervous systems

- **Parasympathetic:** Preganglionic parasympathetic fibers enter the pelvic plexus via the pelvic nerve.
- **Sympathetic**: Postganglionic sympathetic fibers also enter the pelvic plexus via the hypogastric nerve.
- **Somatic:** Tactile stimulation is transmitted via the dorsal nerve of the penis to the pudendal nerve.

Erection is mediated by parasympathetic stimulation, and ejaculation is mediated by sympathetic stimulation. Somatic stimulation is important for stimulation and contraction of the genital skeletal muscles during erection and ejaculation.[15]

Erectile Dysfunction (Fig. 21.2)

There is a period of spinal shock following the initial injury that lasts from a few hours to a few weeks. Most men regain erectile function within a year.[15] Similar to women, level and completeness of injury determine preservation of erection.

In UMN lesions:

- Individuals with both complete and incomplete UMN are able to achieve reflexogenic erections and obtain rigidity.
- Men with lesions above T6 may experience AD during the period of arousal/erection.

In LMN lesions:

- Complete injuries are less likely to be able to achieve reflexogenic erection leading to rigidity.
- There are inconclusive data around incomplete LMN.[16]

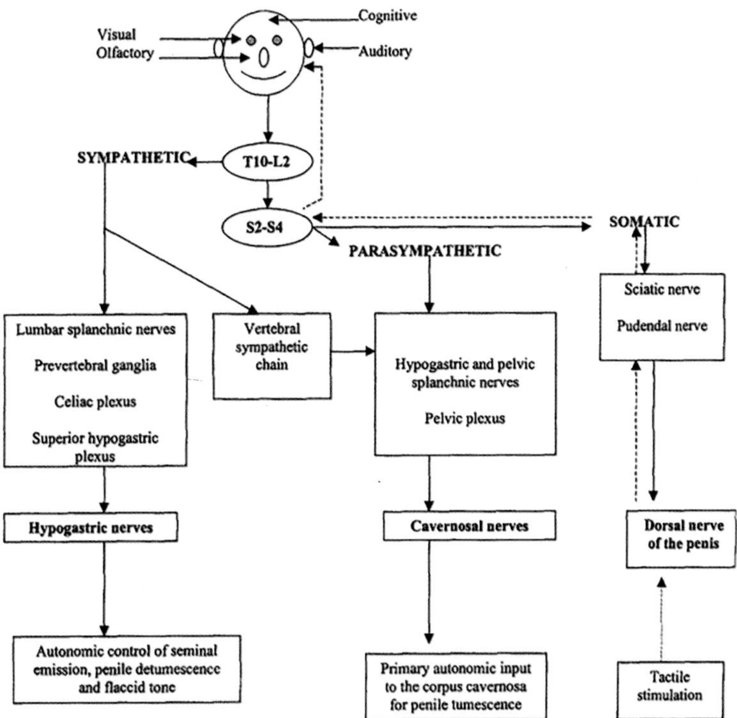

Fig. 21.2 Innervention of the Penis. (From Monga M, Bernie J, Rajasekaran M. Male infertility and erectile dysfunction in spinal cord injury: a review. *Archives of Physical Medicine and Rehabilitation*. 1999;80(10):1331-1339.)

Ejaculation in Men With Spinal Cord Injury

The two parts to ejaculation are seminal emission and expulsion. One or both phases may be disrupted. Seminal emission is controlled by sympathetic outflow and expulsion is controlled by parasympathetic outflow.[17] Additional complications with ejaculations following SCI include premature ejaculation, retrograde ejaculation, and delayed appearance of ejaculate (requires gravity).[17] A significant number of individuals are unable to ejaculate and often require methods to assist. Penile vibratory stimulation is used to assist with increasing sexual pleasure, whereas retrieval techniques will be required if ejaculation is needed for sexual reproduction.[18]

Treatment of Erectile Dysfunction in Men

Treatment options include:

- Oral agents
- Noninvasive therapies such as vacuum erection devices
- Minimally invasive therapies such as intraurethral suppositories, intracavernosal injections, topical agents (PDE-1)
- Surgical options: penile prosthesis

Pharmacological Agents

The most common oral agents used are phosphodiesterase inhibitors (PDE-5). For erection to occur, the smooth muscle of the corpus cavernosum must relax to allow increase in blood flow. The most commonly used is sildenafil (Viagra), which works to selectively inhibit PDE-5 and, with the assistance of nitrous oxide, reduces inactivation of cyclic guanosine monophosphate, thus promoting smooth muscle relaxation.[19] The most common side effects in individuals with SCI are headache, flushing, and mild hypotension.[15,19]

Vacuum Erection Devices

A rigid vacuum device is placed over the penis and creates a seal, which works to draw blood into the penis and create tumescence. A rigid ring is placed at the base of the penis to sustain the erection. This must be used with caution in individuals with no sensation. Individuals with poor hand function will require adaptive approaches for usage.[15]

Minimally Invasive Therapies

Intracavernosal injections including vasoactive agents such as papaverine, phentolamine (Regitine), and alprostadil (PDE-1) have also been used. They bypass the nitrous oxide-pathway that maintains high levels of cyclic guanosine monophosphate and work more rapidly than the PDE-5 inhibitors. The downside of this process is that it can lead to priapism and prolonged erections if not dosed appropriately.[19]

Penile Prosthesis

Penile prosthesis is one of the first significant treatments for erectile dysfunction. However, there have been a significant number of complications, including mechanical failure and infection, that have been demonstrated.[15]

Infertility in Men With Spinal Cord Injury

Infertility is more common in men than women following SCIs. This is multifactorial and due to the decrease in quality and quantity of male sperm, erectile dysfunction, and issues with ejaculation.[15] Erectile and ejaculatory dysfunction have been discussed previously.

Semen Quality

Individuals with SCIs typically will have normal sperm count but low motility and thus viability. This decrease in viability has been shown to occur within the first few weeks postinjury. Studies have shown that years postinjury there is no difference in semen quality. Lifestyle factors such as scrotum hyperthermia, prolonged time in a wheelchair, and issues with bladder are also thought to contribute to poor semen quality.

Semen Retrieval

Despite the initial change in semen quality, there are ways to assist with sperm retrieval for individuals with ejaculatory dysfunction. Methods include penile vibratory stimulation (PVS), electroejaculation, prostate massage, and surgical sperm retrieval.

- PVS[20]
  - First line of treatment.
  - Vibrator is placed over the frenulum of the glans penis. Stimulation leads to ejaculation. This is shown to work better in individuals with intact ejaculatory reflex arcs, such as those with complete UMNs at level T10 or above.[20] Vibrators with higher amplitudes have proven to be more effective. Can elicit AD (Fig. 21.3).
- Electroejaculation
  - Rectal probe is placed in the rectum. The electric current directly stimulates the prostate and leads to seminal emission. As with PVS, can elicit AD.[20]
- Prostate massage
  - Physicians insert a finger into rectum with the attempt to manually move semen through the ejaculation duct system. This has a lower success rate.[20]
- Surgical sperm retrieval
  - Sperm is directly removed from the vas deferens via various techniques such as open testis biopsy, testicular aspiration, microsurgical epididymal sperm aspiration, percutaneous epididymal sperm aspiration, etc.[20]

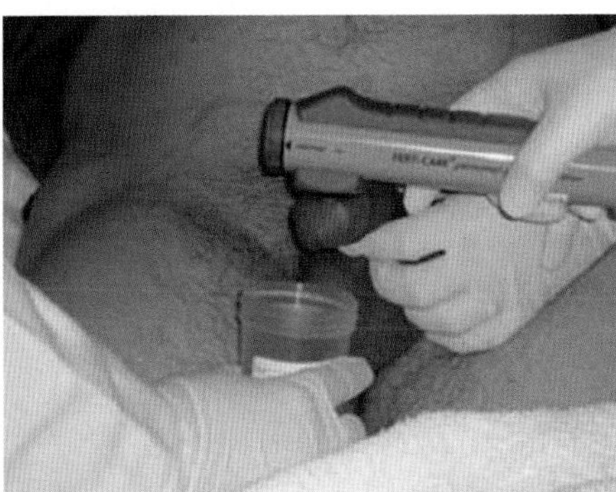

Fig. 21.3 Penile Vibratory Stimulation. (Adapted from Elliott SL. Sexual dysfunction and infertility in individuals with spinal cord disorders. In: Kirshblum S, Lin VW, eds. *Spinal Cord Medicine*. 3rd ed. New York: Springer Publishing; 2019:411-435.)

Upon retrieval, individuals can then work with their practitioner on various insemination techniques.

Conclusion

A comprehensive plan is needed to address sexual dysfunction and infertility in patients with SCIs. Rehabilitation should address the full range of sexuality and sexual function that include unique challenges, both medical and nonmedical, based on level of injury.

Review Questions

1. In women with SCIs, level and completeness are key indicators of sexual function following injury. Women with complete UMN injuries are able to have which type of orgasm?
   a. Psychogenic but not reflexogenic
   b. Reflexogenic but not psychogenic
   c. Psychogenic and reflexogenic
   d. Not able to have orgasms at all
2. Women with incomplete injuries have the ability to achieve both reflexogenic and psychogenic arousal. The ability to achieve psychogenic arousal best correlates with:
   a. Level of injury
   b. Preservation of light touch sensation for T11–T12 dermatomes
   c. Preservation of pinprick sensation for T11–T12 dermatomes
   d. All of the above
3. Orgasms are thought to require an intact sacral reflex; however, women with complete LMN injuries were found to be able to have orgasms. How is this so?
   a. It is an unknown phenomenon
   b. An alternate vagus nerve pathway
   c. Both
   d. None of the above
4. Complications with ejaculation for men following SCI include:
   a. Premature ejaculation
   b. Retrograde ejaculation
   c. Delayed appearance of ejaculate
   d. All of the above
5. What is the most common side effect in individuals who utilize phosphodiesterase inhibitors (PDE-5) to assist with erection post-SCI?
   a. Headaches
   b. Flushing
   c. Hypotension
   d. All of the above

REFERENCES

1. Stoffel JT, Van der Aa F, Wittmann D, Yande S, Elliott S. Fertility and sexuality in the spinal cord injury patient. *World J Urol.* 2018;36(10):1577–1585.
2. Anderson KD. Targeting recovery: priorities of the spinal cord-injured population. *J Neurotrauma.* 2004;21(10):1371–1383.
3. Parr D. Human sexual response By William H. Masters and Virginia E. Johnson, London: J. & A. Churchill. 1966. Pp. 366. Price 70s. *Br J Psychiatry.* 1968;114(507):259–260.
4. Kirshblum S, Lin V, eds. *Spinal Cord Injury Medicine.* 3rd ed. New York: Springer Publishing; 2019.
5. Sipski ML, Alexander CJ, Rosen RC. Physiological parameters associated with psychogenic sexual arousal in women with complete spinal cord injuries. *Arch Phys Med Rehabil.* 1995;76(9):811–818.
6. Sipski ML, Alexander CJ, Rosen RC. Physiologic parameters associated with sexual arousal in women with incomplete spinal cord injuries. *Arch Phys Med Rehabil.* 1997;78(3):305–313.
7. Sipski ML, Alexander CJ, Rosen RC. Orgasm in women with spinal cord injuries: a laboratory-based assessment. *Arch Phys Med Rehabil.* 1995;76(12):1097–1102.
8. Sipski ML, Alexander CJ, Rosen R. Sexual arousal and orgasm in women: effects of spinal cord injury. *Ann Neurol.* 2001;49(1):35–44.
9. Brackett NL, Lynne CM, Sønksen J, Ohl DA. Sexual function and fertility after spinal cord injury. In: Kirshblum S, Campagnolo DI, Gorman P, eds. *Spinal Cord Medicine.* 2nd ed. Philadelphia: Wolters Kluwer Health/Lippincott Williams & Wilkins; 2011:410–426.
10. Courtois F, Charvier K. Sexual dysfunction in patients with spinal cord lesions. *Handb Clin Neurol.*. 2015;130:225–245.
11. Lombardi G, Musco S, Kessler TM, Marzi VL, Lanciotti M, Del Popolo G. Management of sexual dysfunction due to central nervous system disorders: a systematic review. *BJU International.* 2015;115:47–56.
12. Rutberg L, Fridén B, Karlsson A-K. Amenorrhoea in newly spinal cord injured women: an effect of hyperprolactinaemia? *Spinal Cord.* 2007;46(3):189–191.
13. Courtois F, Alexander M, McLain AB. Women's sexual health and reproductive function after SCI. *Top Spinal Cord Inj Rehabil.* 2017;23(1):20–30.
14. Monga M, Bernie J, Rajasekaran M. Male infertility and erectile dysfunction in spinal cord injury: a review. *Arch Phys Med Rehabil.* 1999;80(10):1331–1339.

15. Comarr AE. Sexual function among patients with spinal cord injury. *Urol Int.* 1970;25(2):134–168.
16. Ohl DA, Quallich SA, Sønksen J, Brackett NL, Lynne CM. Anejaculation and retrograde ejaculation. *Urol Clin North Am.* 2008;35(2):211–220.
17. Brown DJ, Hill ST, Baker HWG. Male fertility and sexual function after spinal cord injury. *Prog Brain Res.* 2006;152:427–439.
18. Biering-Sørensen F, Sønksen J. Sexual function in spinal cord lesioned men. *Spinal Cord.* 2001;39(9):455–470.
19. Lamid S. Nocturnal penile tumescence studies in spinal cord injured males. *Spinal Cord.* 1986;24(1):26–31.
20. Löchner-Ernst D, Mandalka B, Kramer G, Stöhrer M. Conservative and surgical semen retrieval in patients with spinal cord injury. *Spinal Cord.* 1997;35(7):463–468.

CHAPTER 22

Women's Health After Spinal Cord Injury

Jennifer Weekes

OUTLINE

Introduction

Spinal cord injuries (SCIs) can affect all aspects of women's health, including gynecologic, obstetric, and psychosocial. Evaluation and management are best accomplished by a holistic and planned approach with a knowledgeable provider and team.

Gynecological Health

The female reproductive system is controlled by both sympathetic and parasympathetic nervous systems. Research evaluating gynecologic health pre- and post-SCI has identified similar issues to able bodied individuals with the exception of urinary tract infections (UTIs) and vaginal yeast infections that have been documented to occur with increased frequency following SCI[1] (Fig. 22.1).

After a traumatic SCI, individuals will often experience amenorrhea, but up to 50% will regain normal menses within 6 months and approximately >90% within 1 year.[1] A number of gynecologic issues have been shown to follow preinjury risks; however, there are complications following SCI. Women with injuries above T6 are at risk for autonomic dysreflexia that can be triggered by menstruation, sexual intercourse, labor and delivery, and gynecological examinations.[1] Additionally, spasticity can be increased during an individual's menstrual cycle. Endocrine-associated conditions associated with SCI include prolactinemia and galactorrhea.

Fertility

It has been well proven that fertility is often not affected in women with SCIs. Women with SCIs are no different than able-bodied women in their desire to reproduce. For those who do not wish to conceive, birth control is an option that needs to be explored.[2]

Obstetric Care

Pregnancy

Once the decision is made to pursue pregnancy following an SCI, all individuals are encouraged to seek preconception care, with a planned pregnancy being most likely to limit complications. Many of the medications SCI patients use for pain control, spasticity, blood pressure regulation, and bladder infection

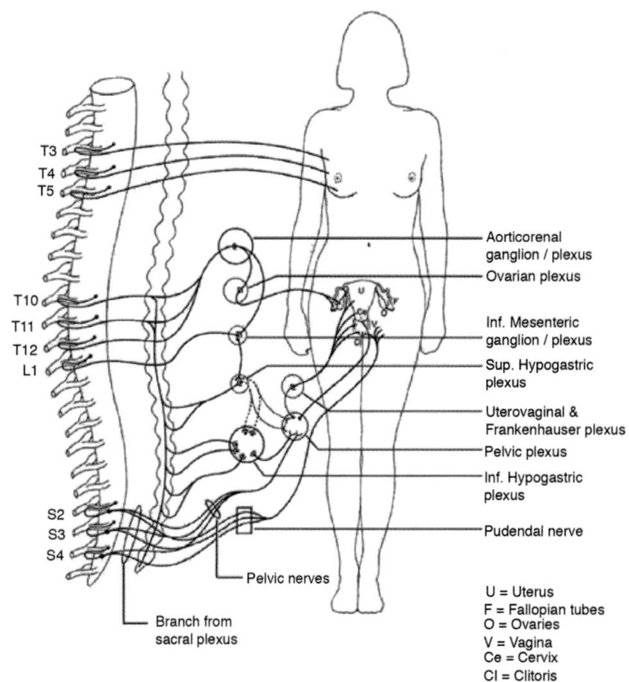

Fig. 22.1 Neurology of the Female Reproductive System. Adopted from McLain AJ, Alexander MCS. Women's health challenges after spinal cord injuries and disorders. In: Kirshblum S, Lin V, eds. *Spinal Cord Medicine*. 3rd ed. New York: Springer Publishing; 2019:955–986.

prophylaxis, such as tizanidine (Zanaflex), clonidine (Catapres), diazepam (Valium), and opioids, are contraindicated during pregnancy and should be changed prior to conception. Pregnancy can be high risk in individuals with SCI due to increased risk of autonomic dysreflexia, contractures, pressure injuries, spasticity, and other complications depending on level of injury (Fig. 22.2).[3]

Antenatal Care

The T10 spinal level is key, as it relates to fetal movement and position. Individuals with injuries above T10 have difficulty perceiving fetal movement as well as uterine contractions.[3] Antenatal complications in individuals with SCIs can affect all systems and lead to pregnancy complications.

Common Complications

Autonomic Dysreflexia

Autonomic dysreflexia (AD) is typically experienced by individuals with injuries T6 or above. It can be seen in 50% of pregnant women with SCI. If severe, it can lead to maternal intracranial bleeding, death, heart rate issues, or fetal bradycardia.

- Maternal signs: Headache, blood pressure rise (greater than 20 mmHg), nausea, anxiety, sweating, blushing, irregularities in heart rate. Fetal signs: Fetal bradycardia[1]

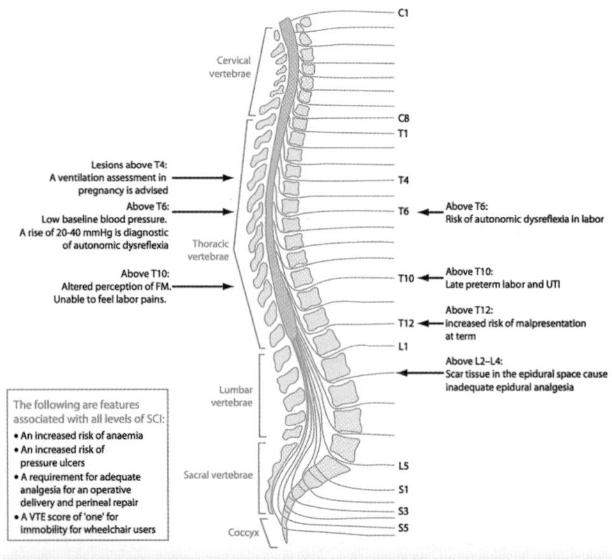

Fig. 22.2 Diagram Showing Features of Spinal Cord Injury at Various Vertebrae in Relation to Pregnancy. *FM*, Fetal movements; *SCI*, spinal cord injury; *UTI*, urinary tract infection; *VTE*, venous thromboembolism. (Adapted from Dawood R, Altanis E, Ribes-Pastor P, Ashworth F. Pregnancy and spinal cord injury. *The Obstetrician & Gynaecologist*. 2014;16(2):99–107.)

AD needs to be distinguished from preeclampsia.

- Differentiation between preeclampsia: can be hard to distinguish. However, in AD, blood pressure will continue to rise until noxious stimuli are eliminated. Both can coexist and be difficult to manage.[1]
- If there is a history of AD, oftentimes a prophylactic epidural is recommended early in labor.[3]

Urinary Tract Infections

Women with SCIs are at higher risk for UTIs during pregnancy. This is the most frequent pregnancy complication.[4] Indwelling catheters should typically be avoided due to increased risk of infection; however, they may be needed in the first and third trimesters to help with AD.[3]

Deep Vein Thrombosis

Women with SCIs have a higher risk for deep vein thrombosis (DVT). The reason for increased risk is due to hormonal changes supporting venous dilation (progesterone) and clotting (estrogen) and increased immobility. Six months after SCI, the DVT risk is nearly the same as the general population.[3] Passive range-of-motion exercises, elevations of legs, and compression stockings can all lessen the risk.

Spasticity

Spasticity can worsen while pregnant. If treatment is needed, oral baclofen (Lioresal) is the drug of choice. However, it can be associated with withdrawals in the neonate.[3] Tizanidine (Zanaflex) and clonidine (Catapres) are contraindicated.

Skin and Seating

During pregnancy, there is an increased risk of pressure injuries due to the increased immobility, weight gain, and improper seating. There is a need to ensure regular skin assessments and proper offloading.[3]

Labor and Delivery

Labor symptoms are dependent upon the level of injury. Typically, persons with injuries T10 and below are able to perceive labor and feel contractions.[3] Uterine contractions travel into the spinal cord at T10 via the Frankenhauser plexus.[3] Women with injuries below this level will feel labor pain contractions. Labor contraction pain in individuals above this level will vary but can be perceived as referred pain to the upper extremities, increased spasticity, AD, and/or nonspecific pain.[5] Unless clinically indicated, vaginal deliveries are recommended.[3] AD is the most serious and critical complication of labor and delivery in women with injuries at the T6 level and above,[6] and delayed management can lead to intracranial bleeding of the mother, fetal death, and fetal bradyarrhythmias.[3,7] It is of course important to differentiate AD from preeclampsia. The optimal treatment is to remove the stimuli and deliver. For patients who have a history of AD, early epidurals have been recommended.[3,7]

Postpartum

Following delivery, the desire to breastfeed is normal for women with SCIs. For individuals with complete lesions above T4, it may be delayed and require additional tactics and stimulation.[3] For women who have spasticity, baclofen has been proven to be safe in breastfeeding mothers, as little is excreted via breast milk. Individuals with SCIs may also experience postpartum depression (which is often under diagnosed), fatigue, and difficulty with caring for the newborn depending on injury level.[8]

Review Questions

1. A major pregnancy complication for women with injuries T6 or higher is autonomic dysreflexia. How can this be distinguished from preeclampsia?
   a. Monitoring both maternal and fetal heartrate
   b. Autonomic dysreflexia only occurs during the first trimester
   c. With autonomic dysreflexia the patient's blood pressure will continue to rise until the noxious stimuli have been removed
   d. None of the above
2. Following SCI, women are at increased risk for UTIs during pregnancy. What are recommendations regarding Foley placement as a way to prevent this?
   a. Foley catheter placement early in pregnancy (i.e., first trimester)
   b. Can consider changing to an indwelling catheter in the third trimester
   c. Transition to a suprapubic catheter if possible
   d. Both a and b
3. Which pharmacologic agents for spasticity are contraindicated during pregnancy?
   a. Baclofen
   b. Tizanidine
   c. Clonidine
   d. Both b and c
4. Spinal cord lesions at what level can lead to altered/limited sensation during pregnancy?
   a. T10
   b. T6
   c. T4
   d. T12
5. Above what level do individuals experience breastfeeding challenges following SCI?
   a. T6
   b. T10
   c. T4
   d. C6

REFERENCES

1. Jackson AB, Wadley V. A multicenter study of women's self-reported reproductive health after spinal cord injury. *Arch Phys Med Rehabil.* 1999;80(11):1420–1428.
2. DeForge D, Blackmer J, Garritty C, et al. Fertility following spinal cord injury: a systematic review. *Spinal Cord.* 2005;43(12):693–703.
3. Dawood R, Altanis E, Ribes-Pastor P, Ashworth F. Pregnancy and spinal cord injury. *The Obstetrician & Gynaecologist.* 2014;16(2):99–107.
4. Pannek J, Bertschy S. Mission impossible? Urological management of patients with spinal cord injury during pregnancy: a systematic review. *Spinal Cord.* 2011;49(10):1028–1032.
5. Greenspoon JS, Paul RH. Paraplegia and quadriplegia: special considerations during pregnancy and labor and delivery. *Am J Obstet Gynecol.* 1986;155(4):738–741.
6. Wanner MB, Rageth CJ, Zäch GA. Pregnancy and autonomic hyperreflexia in patients with spinal cord lesions. *Spinal Cord.* 1987;25(6):482–490.
7. McGregor JA, Meeuwsen J. Autonomic hyperreflexia: a mortal danger for spinal cord-damaged women in labor. *Am J Obstet Gynecol.* 1985;151(3):330–333.
8. Lee AH, Wen B, Walter M, et al. Prevalence of postpartum depression and anxiety among women with spinal cord injury. *J Spinal Cord Med.* 2019;44(2):1–6.

Musculoskeletal Disorders

CHAPTER 23

Deborah Caruso

OUTLINE

Introduction

The increased reliance on the upper extremities for mobility and activities of daily living (ADLs) is a major contributor to individuals with spinal cord injury (SCI) having a higher incidence of reported musculoskeletal (MSK) pain. The overall incidence ranges from 50%–81% and correlates with lower quality-of-life scores.[1]

Shoulder Pain

Overview

Shoulder pain is the most and second-most common MSK complaint in tetraplegia and paraplegia, respectively.[2] The higher prevalence of shoulder pain has been attributed to overuse injuries in a joint that is primarily structured for flexibility and motion but not weight bearing. The dynamics of heavy reliance on the shoulder for mobility tasks (e.g., propelling a wheelchair, transferring) can overload the shoulder's soft tissues due to muscular imbalance and poor biomechanics.

Impingement Syndrome

The most common diagnosis, encompassing two-thirds of shoulder pain complaints, is subacromial impingement syndrome.[3] Subacromial impingement syndrome consists of a spectrum of clinical findings and not an injury to a specific structure. Symptoms include anterolateral shoulder pain that is typically worse with overhead movements. On physical exam, a positive Neer sign, Hawkins sign, or Jobe Empty Can sign may be elucidated. A positive drop arm test suggests a rotator cuff tear, namely in the supraspinatus. The diagnosis for these conditions is made clinically, with imaging reserved for cases that do not respond to conservative interventions.

Bicipital Tendonitis

Bicipital tendonitis presents with anterior shoulder pain with occasional radiation to the arm, deltoid, or base of neck. Physical exam reveals pain to palpation of the bicipital tendon in the bicipital groove, positive Yergason sign, and/or positive Speed test. The diagnosis is made clinically, with ultrasound/MRI being utilized if diagnosis is not clear.

Diagnostics

Although the diagnosis of shoulder pain in individuals with SCI relies on clinical history and examination, given the heavy dependence of individuals with SCI on their upper extremities for mobility and ADLs, MRI should be considered early if rotator cuff tear is suspected, as surgical repair is most effective in the first 3 weeks following injury.[4]

Treatments

Treatment of shoulder pain is predominantly rehabilitation-based, with physical therapy and modifications to equipment. Corticosteroid injections may provide short-term reduction in pain. Emerging therapies include platelet rich plasma injections for tendonosis.[5] Surgical debridement can be considered after 3 months of conservative care.

Elbow Pain

Overview

Elbow pain (prevalence 6%–15%)[1] is primarily related to overuse injuries of the muscle and tendons, with secondary nerve impingement in some cases.

Lateral Epicondylitis

Lateral epicondylitis is an overuse injury involving the origin of the wrist extensors, with the extensor carpi radialis brevis being the most common tendon affected. Wheelchair users are at elevated risk due to repetitive forceful elbow extension, maximal pronation, and wrist flexion needed for propulsion. Clinically, individuals present with pain and tenderness over the forearm extensor tendon origin on the lateral epicondyle, with pain being worse with resisted wrist extension. Treatment is conservative and includes forearm cuff, counterforce bracing, and occasionally a cock-up wrist splint to decrease motion of the wrist extensors. Other considerations include local corticosteroid injections, ultrasound, extracorporeal shock wave, and iontophoresis. Emerging treatments include platelet rich plasma injections. Surgical debridement can be considered after 6 months of conservative care. For prevention, the final push phase in wheelchair propulsion should be done with forearm and wrist in neutral, not hyperpronation and ulnar deviation. [4]

Cubital Tunnel Syndrome

The ulnar nerve is susceptible to chronic traction and tension due to its vulnerable location in the ulnar groove and the cubital tunnel. Overall prevalence of cubital tunnel syndrome in SCI is 22%–45%.[6] Etiologies include prolonged pressure from resting arms on the wheelchair arm rests and repetitive flexion and extension at the elbow. Symptoms include pain and paresthesias down the medial aspect of the forearm and hand. On physical exam, Tinel sign might be positive at the medial epicondyle. There may be wasting of intrinsic hand muscles and decreased sensation in the fifth digit and medial aspect of the fourth digit. Diagnosis is made via nerve conduction studies. Treatment is rehabilitation-based and includes protection with an elbow pad and avoidance of prolonged elbow flexion using extension splinting at night. Exercises should target elbow flexibility and forearm strength. If there are prolonged sensory or motor deficits, surgical referral should be placed for decompression and possible transposition.[4]

Wrist and Hand Pain

de Quervain Tenosynovitis

de Quervain tenosynovitis is an overuse injury to the abductor pollicis longus and extensor digitorum brevis tendons over the first compartment in the wrist. Wheelchair users are at risk due to the finishing push stroke with wrists in ulnar deviation.[4] Pain is located on the radial aspect of the wrist and is increased with passive stretching of the tendons as done with the Finkelstein maneuver. Thumb axial grind test should be done to evaluate for carpometacarpal pain as a contributor. Evidence suggests that corticosteroids injected along the tendon sheaths are more effective as a supplement to rehabilitation treatments consisting of opponens splinting and/or nonsteroidal antiinflammatory drugs (NSAIDs).[7] Surgical decompression can be considered after 6 weeks of conservative care.

Carpal Tunnel Syndrome

Carpal tunnel syndrome involves compression of the median nerve as it traverses the carpal tunnel. Prevalence ranges between 40%–66%, with higher rates seen in individuals with paraplegia compared with tetraplegia.[6] Severity is associated with duration of wheelchair use and age. Etiology is thought to be secondary to repetitive strain and overuse of the wrist flexor tendons. Symptoms include pain and paresthesias on the dorsum of the hand and the 3.5 radial digits. Physical exam signs include a positive Phalen maneuver or Tinel sign and weakness and/or atrophy of the thenar eminence. Diagnosis of choice is nerve conduction and electromyography studies. Treatment is usually rehabilitation based, initially with resting wrist splints and corticosteroid injections. If there is poor response to conservative measures or in individuals with severe symptoms, surgical decompression carpal tunnel is therapeutic.[4]

Prevention

Ergonomics

Individuals with SCI should avoid:[1]

- Extreme positions of the wrist, particularly maximal extension during transfers to help protect the median nerve in the carpal tunnel (i.e., transfers with closed fist technique).
- Positioning of the hand above the shoulder, as the association between overhead activity and shoulder pain is strong.
- Extreme positions at the shoulder, particularly extreme internal rotation and abduction, which can predispose to impingement.
- Unlevel transfers, if possible.

Equipment Selection

Manual wheelchair users should have a customized manual wheelchair constructed with the lightest possible material to decrease rolling resistance.

The rear axle should be as far forward as possible, increased incrementally, without compromising stability. This decreases stroke frequency, rate of rise of force, and the push angle.

Seat height should allow for the elbow to be flexed between 100 and 120 degrees when the hand rests on the top center of the push-rim (Fig. 23.1).[6]

Individuals should use long, smooth strokes. The hand should drift down to below the push-rim after contact using a semicircular pattern (Fig. 23.2).[6] Seating should provide adequate trunk support so that upper extremities have a stable base to decrease risk of injury.

Positioning

For individuals with tetraplegia, the upper limb should have support across all potential pressure points when lying supine. The upper limb should be in abduction and external rotation regularly. Caregivers should grasp individuals with SCI at the back of the scapula and avoid pulling on the arm when positioning patients.

Extremity Fractures and Contractures in Spinal Cord Injury

Individuals with SCI often have significant acute and chronic MSK sequela. Long term, immobility and alterations in bone metabolism result in increased fracture risk, posing unique treatment challenges. In addition, neurologic injury compromises muscle balance and mobility, predisposing individuals with SCI to potentially disabling contractures.

Fractures in Acute Spinal Cord Injury

Fractures in acute SCI typically coincide with the initial traumatic events with an incidence of 28%.[1] The most common acute long bone fractures occur in the femur, followed by the tibia, humerus, radius, and ulna. While postacute long bone fracture rates the first year after SCI are no different than age-matched controls,[8] medical complications related to these fractures are more frequent. Surgical management of femoral and tibial fractures in individuals with SCI is associated with fewer medical complications and more rapid union than nonoperative management.

The most common acute upper extremity fracture after acute SCI is the humerus. Unlike lower extremity fractures, upper extremity fractures do not differ significantly in time to union, range of motion, and rehabilitation time when comparing operative and nonoperative management. Importantly, early orthopedic fixation facilitates rehabilitation care and thus should be recommended in individuals with SCI given their high reliance on the upper extremity.[1]

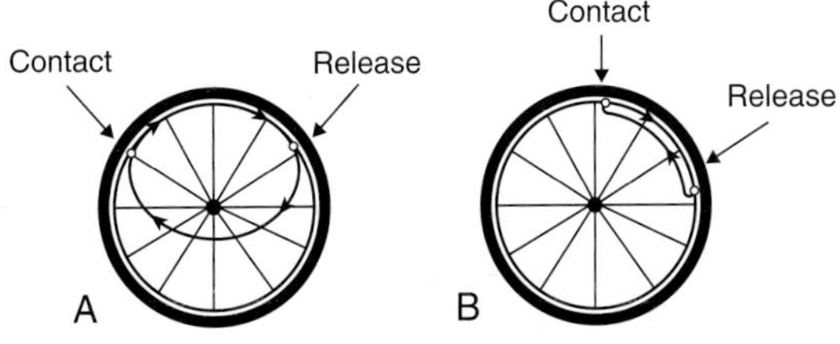

Fig. 23.2 (A) Indicates the recommended propulsion technique; (B) is an example of a poor propulsion pattern.[6]

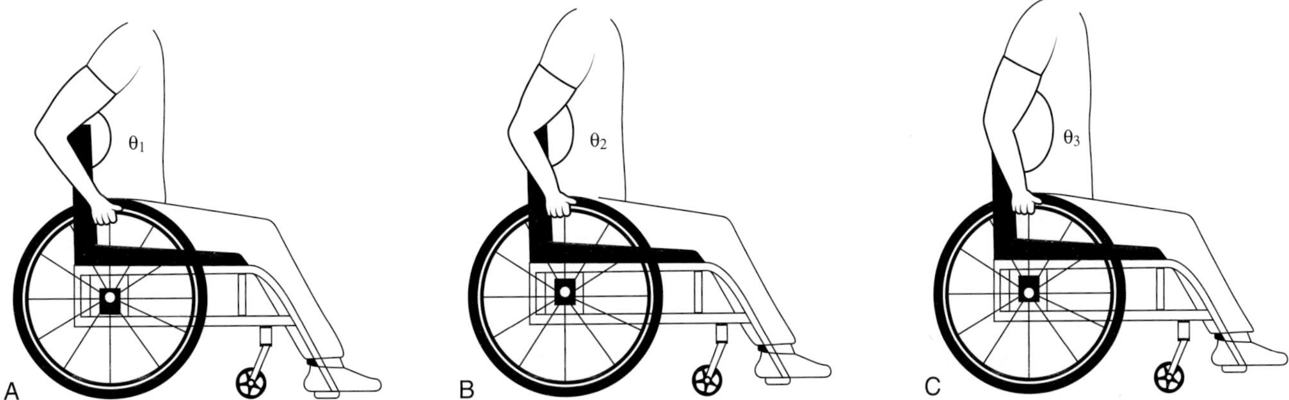

Fig. 23.1 Shows the difference in elbow angles with change of seat height; with (B) showing the recommended elbow angle of 100–120 degrees.[6]

Fractures in Chronic Spinal Cord Injury

Incidence of pathologic fractures, most commonly extraarticular, in individuals with chronic SCI is estimated to be as high as 40%. The fractures typically result from mild trauma, with higher rates seen in paraplegics, presumably due to their increased mobility.[1] The most common injury mechanism is fall from the wheelchair, followed by accidents during transfer and unnoticed traumas.[9]

Risk factors for fractures include time from injury and motor complete SCI, presumably due to impaired bone metabolism and remodeling below the level of injury. The cause is multifactorial and can include decreased mechanical loading and hormonal and autonomic dysregulation. Bone mineral density decreases to about 50% at 3–4 years after SCI.

Fracture location correlates with bone mineral density level, with supracondylar factures of the femur being the most common, followed by proximal tibia and proximal femur fractures.[9]

Symptoms include soft tissue edema, increase in limb girth, warmth, spasticity, deformity, and/or autonomic dysreflexia. There may be no pain depending on the level and completeness of injury.

Secondary complications of long bone fractures include, in decreasing order of frequency, implant failure or dislocation, pressure injuries, venous thrombosis, malalignment, nonunion, infections, and compartment syndrome.[9]

Treatments are personalized to the individual's functional status, location of fracture, and comorbidities. Risk factors for nonunion include open reduction, open fracture, severity of fracture, smoking, and osteoporosis.[9] Studies investigating the use of modalities to best manage nonunions, such as low-intensity pulse ultrasound or electromagnetic coils, are lacking.

Femoral Neck Fractures

Femoral neck fractures are challenging to treat due to poor fixation in osteoporotic bone, high risk of nonunion, and increased risk for angulation and malformation in nonoperative patients. Endoscopic replacement is the standard of care.

Distal Femur and Proximal Tibia Fractures

The distal femur and proximal tibia are the most common locations of pathologic fractures in chronic SCI, related to torsion across the knee with transfers. Although these fractures have historically been managed nonoperatively with well-padded splints, knee immobilizers and frequent skin inspections, operative fixation is becoming more common. There is some literature to suggest that the time to union is shorter and there is a decreased frequency of complications with operative interventions.[10]

Ankle Fractures

Ankle fractures typically unite with well-padded splints. Alignment is essential to help prevent malleolar pressure injuries from varus and/or valgus deformities.

Upper Extremity Fractures

Nondisplaced upper extremity fractures are typically treated with splinting. Displaced fractures should be considered for operative fixation to help preserve upper extremity function.[1]

Prevention

There is no compelling evidence for routine dual-energy X-ray absorptiometry (DEXA) scans, the use of bisphosphonates, and/or calcium and vitamin D in fracture prevention.[11] The use of functional electrical stimulation via surface electrodes to produce functional movement, tilt table standing, standing frame, or robotic treadmill walking have not been shown to attenuate bone loss.[12]

Contractures in Spinal Cord Injury

Contractures are an abnormal shortening of muscle leading to a high resistance to stretching. They are caused by the loss of extensibility of skin, ligaments, muscles, and joint capsules that restrict joint mobility in the setting of prolonged immobilization and chronic use of the soft tissues in a shortened range, usually due to muscle imbalance seen in SCI.

Contractures in SCI can lead to deformity, limitations in motor task performance, pain, sleep disturbance, increased caregiver needs, difficulty with bladder/bowel management, difficulty with seating/positioning, increased fall risk, and pressure injuries. They may limit the patient's candidacy for tendon transfer surgeries aimed at improving upper extremity function.

Contractures in Acute Spinal Cord Injury

Risk factors for contractures in acute SCI include pressure injuries, spasticity requiring medication, and traumatic brain injury.[13]

Contractures in Chronic Spinal Cord Injury

The incidence of contractures in major joints 1 year after spinal cord injuries range from 11%–43%, with ankle, wrist, and shoulder contractures being the most commonly encountered.[14] Risk factors for shoulder contractures include tetraplegia, shoulder pain, spasticity, time to admission to rehabilitation, and increased age. Denervation/weakness of the triceps is associated with elbow flexion contractures.[15]

The most common interventions for contractures are stretch and passive movements. It is typically recommended that muscles should have 20–30 minutes of sustained stretch daily to prevent contractures; however, there is no clinical evidence to support this.[16] A Cochrane systematic review indicated that stretch has no clinically important short-term or long-term effects on joint mobility in patients with neurologic conditions.[17] To apply a stretch for more than 30 minutes, it is typically recommended to use orthotics to assist.

Surgical interventions include peripheral neurectomies, myotomies, tenotomies, or tendon lengthening procedures.[1] Surgical interventions for common SCI contractures include[18]:

- Elbow flexion contracture—biceps brachii tenotomy or lengthening or brachialis myotomy
- Hip flexion—iliopsoas myotomy or tenotomy
- Hip adduction—obturator neurectomy with adductor tenotomy
- Knee flexion—careful MSK examination is needed to differentiate genuine hamstring contracture versus flexion deformity of the hip or equinus deformity of the ankle. Hamstring tenotomy results may not be satisfactory without correction of hip flexion and/or ankle deformities
- Ankle equinus—Achilles tenotomy, Achilles tendon lengthening, tibialis posterior rerouted anteriorly to medial malleolus (severe inversion contracture)
- Ankle valgus deformity—peroneal tendons rerouted to lateral malleolus
- Ankle varus deformity—anterior versus posterior tibial tendon transfer

Summary

There is a high incidence of MSK pain and overuse injuries in the SCI population, which is largely due to reliance on the upper extremities for mobility and ADLs.

Fractures and contractures are debilitating MSK sequela of SCI that pose challenges to both the individual with SCI and the treating clinical team.

Review Questions

1. A 35-year-old male with T6 motor/sensory complete paraplegia reports an abrupt onset of right shoulder pain after a fall out of his chair onto his outstretched arm 2 days ago. On physical exam, patient has tenderness to palpation over the subacromial bursa, positive Hawkins and Jobe Empty Can sign. Drop arm test is positive. What is the next step in your treatment plan?
   a. Rest, ice, elevation, NSAIDs
   b. Urgent MRI with possible need for orthopedic referral
   c. Physical therapy referral
   d. Corticosteroid injection for pain management
2. A 70-year-old patient with long-standing paraplegia reports more pains in his upper extremities. He is interested in making conservative modifications that may improve his pain. Which of the following should NOT be advised?
   a. Patient should avoid maximal extension of the wrist
   b. Rear axle should be placed as far backward as possible
   c. Use a semicircular pattern with long smooth strokes during manual wheelchair propulsion
   d. Avoid unlevel transfers if possible
3. A 45-year-old female patient with T10 motor complete paraplegia presents to your clinic with complaints of bilateral wrist pain over her thumbs. The pain started insidiously and become worse with manual wheelchair propulsion. On physical exam, she has pain over the first compartment of her wrists and a positive Finkelstein test. The initial treatment of choice is:
   a. NSAIDs
   b. Long opponens splint + NSAIDs
   c. Corticosteroid injections to the first compartment tendon sheath
   d. Surgical release
4. A 55 year old female with motor complete paraplegia presents to your office with complaints of numbness in the first 3 digits of her dominant right hand that started 3 months ago. She has no thenar atrophy on exam and no sensory deficits. When you tap over the palmar surface of her wrist crease, paresthesias radiate to her first three digits. Your initial plan of care should not include:
   a. Corticosteroid injection into the wrist
   b. Neutral wrist splint
   c. Education to avoid extreme positions of the wrist
   d. NSAIDs
5. What is not true regarding MSK complaints in SCI?
   a. Shoulder pain is the most common MSK complaint in tetraplegia
   b. Carpal tunnel syndrome is the most common cause of upper extremity pain in patients with paraplegia
   c. Patients with SCI should avoid positioning their hands above the shoulder, as there is a strong association between overhead activity and shoulder pain

d. For manual wheelchair propulsion, the seat height should be set so that elbow flexion ranges between 90 and 110 degrees.

6. What is the most common location of a fracture in SCI?
   a. Proximal tibia
   b. Proximal humerus
   c. Supracondylar femur
   d. Proximal femur
7. Which of the following is NOT true regarding fractures in chronic SCI?
   a. There is a higher rate of fractures in patients with paraplegia versus tetraplegia
   b. Fractures are most commonly caused by nonsignificant force/trauma
   c. Fractures are more common in complete versus incomplete SCI
   d. Fractures are most commonly intraarticular
8. You are evaluating a 55-year-old female with chronic motor complete paraplegia who has now entered menopause. She would like to know more about fracture prevention. You inform her that:
   a. There is no compelling evidence for the use of Vitamin D and calcium supplementation in the prevention of lower extremity fractures in SCI
   b. She should be monitored yearly with DEXA scans
   c. She should be using a standing frame daily for 30 minutes
   d. She should be started on a bisphosphonate for fracture prophylaxis
9. Which of the following is not a risk for shoulder contractures in SCI?
   a. Tetraplegia
   b. Spasticity
   c. Shoulder pain
   d. Time to admission to rehabilitation
   e. Autonomic dysreflexia
10. Your patient with C7 motor complete tetraplegia has a significant flexion deformity of his right knee, which causes difficult positioning in his wheelchair. Why might a hamstring tenotomy perhaps not be effective?
    a. The knee flexion deformity may be secondary to a hip flexion deformity, not increased hamstring tone
    b. The knee flexion deformity may be secondary to a talipes equinus deformity at the ankle, not increased hamstring tone
    c. The knee flexion deformity may be secondary to a talipes calcaneus deformity at the ankle, not increased hamstring tone
    d. a + b
    e. a + c

REFERENCES

1. Lin VW, Bono CM. *Spinal Cord Medicine: Principles and Practice*. New York: Demos Medical; 2010.
2. Sie IH, Waters RL, Adkins RH, et al. Upper extremity pain in the postrehabilitation spinal cord injured patient. *Arch Phys Med Rehabil*. 1992;73:44–48.
3. Ferrero G, Mijno E, Actis MV, et al. Risk factors for shoulder pain in patients with spinal cord injury: a multicenter study. *Musculoskelet Surg*. 2015;99(Suppl 1):S53–S56.
4. Dyson-Hudson TA, Hogaboom NS, Nakamura R, et al. Ultrasound-guided platelet-rich plasma injection for the treatment of recalcitrant rotator cuff disease in wheelchair users with spinal cord injury: a pilot study. *J Spinal Cord Med*. 2022;45(1):42–48.
5. Apple Jr. DF. *Physical Fitness: A Guide for Individuals with Spinal Cord Injury*. Diane Pub Co; 2004.
6. Paralyzed Veterans of America Consortium for Spinal Cord Medicine. Preservation of upper limb function following spinal cord injury: a clinical practice guideline for health-care professionals. *J Spinal Cord Med*. 2005;28(5):434–470.
7. Rowland P, Phelan N, Gardiner S, et al. The effectiveness of corticosteroid injection for de Quervain's stenosing tenosynovitis (DQST): a systematic review and meta-analysis. *Open Orthop J*. 2015;9:437–444.
8. Vestergaard P, Krogh K, Rejnmark L, et al. Fracture rates and risk factors for fractures in patients with spinal cord injury. *Spinal Cord*. 1998;36:790–796.
9. Grassner L, Klein B, Maier D, et al. Lower extremity fractures in patients with spinal cord injury characteristics, outcome and risk factors for non-unions. *J Spinal Cord Med*. 2018;41:676–683.
10. Koong DP, Symes MJ, Sefton AK, et al. Management of lower limb fractures in patients with spinal cord injuries. *ANZ J Surg*. 2020;90:1743–1749.
11. Carbone LD, Gonzalez B, Miskevics S, et al. Association of bisphosphonate therapy with incident of lower extremity fractures in persons with spinal cord injuries or disorders. *Archives of Physical Medicine and Rehabilitation*. 2020; 101:633–641.
12. Soleyman-Jahi S, Yousefian A, Maheronnaghsh R, et al. Evidence-based prevention and treatment of osteoporosis after spinal cord injury: a systematic review. *Eur Spine J*. 2018;27:1798–1814.
13. Dalyan M, Sherman A, Cardenas DD. Factors associated with contractures in acute spinal cord injury. *Spinal Cord*. 1998;36:405–408.
14. Diong J, Harvey LA, Kwah LK, et al. Incidence and predictors of contracture after spinal cord injury–a prospective cohort study. *Spinal Cord*. 2012;50:579–584.
15. Hardwick D, Bryden A, Kubec G, et al. Factors associated with upper extremity contractures after cervical spinal cord injury: a pilot study. *J Spinal Cord Med*. 2018;41:337–346.
16. Harvey LA, Glinsky JA, Katalinic OM, et al. Contracture management for people with spinal cord injuries. *NeuroRehabilitation.*. 2011;28:17–20.
17. Harvey LA, Katalinic OM, Herbert RD, et al. Stretch for the treatment and prevention of contracture: an abridged republication of a Cochrane Systematic Review. *J Physiother*. 2017;63:67–75.
18. Eltorai I, Montroy R. Muscle release in the management of spasticity in spinal cord injury. *Paraplegia.*. 1990;28:433–440.

CHAPTER 24

Heterotopic Ossification

Audrey Chun

OUTLINE

Epidemiology

Heterotopic ossification (HO) is the pathologic formation of lamellar bone in soft tissues including around muscles surrounding peripheral joints. Following spinal cord injury (SCI):

- HO most commonly develops around the hip, followed by the knee, elbow, shoulder, and, rarely, in smaller joints of the hands and feet.[1–3]
- HO most commonly develops 3–12 weeks after injury with peak incidence at 8 weeks.
- The incidence of HO has been reported to vary greatly, from 10%–78%.[2]
- Clinically significant HO causes a loss of range of motion (ROM) and function and has been shown to occur in 10%–20% of persons with SCI[1,3–8]

Risk factors associated with HO include[1–3,8–10]:

- Motor complete injury
- Male gender
- Presence of a deep vein thrombosis (DVT)
- Spasticity
- Pressure injury
- Nicotine use
- Tracheostomy placement
- Urinary tract infections

Genetic predisposition to HO has not yet been established and there is variable evidence regarding an association with human leukocyte antigen (HLA) serotypes, such as HLA-B27.[11,12]

HO may present with:

- Fever
- Joint swelling
- Decreased ROM
- Pain

The differential diagnosis for this presentation should include[1–3]:

- HO
- Fracture
- DVT
- Septic arthritis
- Cellulitis
- Impending pressure injury

Complications of HO can include[1,3,13–17]:

- Impaired ROM that can cause difficulty with self-care, progressing in therapies and/or fitting into equipment like wheelchairs
- Worsened spasticity
- Worsened pressure injuries
- More symptomatic DVTs
- Nerve entrapment (for example, sciatic nerve entrapment when the hip is involved)

Pathogenesis

The pathogenesis of HO after SCI is poorly understood, but it has been suggested that damage to the blood–spinal cord barrier may allow for the passage of inflammatory mediators and growth factors that are normally concentrated in the central nervous system into the peripheral circulation, driving HO formation.[1–3,18–23] Inflammatory mediators and growth factors released after injury are thought to stimulate fibroblastic proliferation and collagen deposition at peripheral soft tissue sites. The involved area becomes hypoxic and releases factors like bone morphogenic proteins that trigger the formation of mesenchymal and osteoprogenitor cell clusters.

These clusters then differentiate into chondrocytes that hypertrophy and rapidly divide, eventually secreting a cartilaginous matrix. Remodeling of this matrix then occurs following the release of angiogenic factors and microvascularization, allowing for osteoblastic differentiation and mineralization. Eventually, this woven bone is further remodeled into mature lamellar bone with Haversian canals, a marrow cavity, and blood vessels.[1–3,24–27]

Diagnosis

In early HO, triple phase bone scan is more sensitive than plain X-rays.[1–3]

- Bone scans evaluate for the increased uptake of osteotropic radionucleotides and have been shown to reveal HO as early as 2.5 weeks after injury.[28]
- Calcification requires 2–6 weeks to become apparent on X-ray and usually occurs after diagnosis can be made by bone scan.[29,30]
- Bone scans can also be helpful for determining the maturity of HO, where a decreasing or steady-state uptake ratio of radionucleotides indicates maturity.[1,3]

Computed tomography (CT) or magnetic resonance imaging (MRI), which allows for better visualization of formed heterotopic bone, may be useful for planning surgical HO excision.[2,31] CT is rarely indicated for establishing an early diagnosis of HO but increased T2 signal, representative of edema in muscle, fascia, and/or subcutaneous tissue, can make MRI helpful in early HO.[1,32] Ultrasound has been suggested as a reliable and sensitive method for HO screening after SCI.[33–36] Ultrasound offers various advantages over the other modalities, including relative ease of performance and decreased radiation exposure. It has also been suggested to have a diagnostic accuracy comparable to CT and MRI, including the ability to identify about 90% of HO cases at 62 days postinjury.[33,37,38]

The Brooker classification scheme classifies the progression of HO at the hip based on X-rays of the pelvis.[1,2,39]

- Class 0: absence of ossification.
- Class 1: islands of bone within soft tissue of any size.
- Class 2: bone spurs from pelvis/femur with ≥1 cm between opposing bone surfaces.
- Class 3: bone spurs from pelvis and femur with <1 cm between opposing bone surfaces.
- Class 4: complete ankylosis of the hip.

Other classification systems include those that allow for grading of HO at locations other than the hip and those that more closely evaluate the site of HO including surrounding neurovascular structures to better assess prognosis or plan subsequent surgical excisions.[1,2,40–42]

Serum markers for HO are neither sensitive nor specific enough to diagnose HO.[43,44] Serum alkaline phosphatase (ALP) is historically the most commonly ordered lab when HO is suspected; however, ALP is nonspecific. ALP can be elevated in HO, reflecting osteoblastic activity in ectopic bone formation, but it is not always elevated. Serum ALP can also be elevated with nonspecific trauma, surgery, or abdominal conditions.[1,2] Elevated serum creatine phosphokinase may be a more reliable predictor of HO.[45,46]

Treatment

Treatment options for HO include ROM with stretching, nonsteroidal antiinflammatory drugs (NSAIDs), bisphosphonates, radiotherapy, and surgical excision. When HO is diagnosed, aggressive ROM is usually avoided as forceful joint manipulation is thought to induce additional tissue microtrauma, contributing to increased HO formation.[1,3,47,48] Functional electrical stimulation is relatively contraindicated acutely after HO.[1,49] One systematic review suggested that etidronate and indomethacin may reduce HO risk post-operatively. Another review suggested that early treatment with rofecoxib and indomethacin may prevent HO after SCI but only limited evidence supported warfarin, pulse low intensity electromagnetic field (PLIMF) therapy, or radiotherapy.[51] Bisphosphonates were supported by strong evidence for early HO therapy, but once HO was already formed, only surgical resection was deemed effective.[51] Pharmacological prophylaxis of HO after SCI with indomethacin, rofecoxib, warfarin, or etidronate are not recommended given the relatively low morbidity of HO, potential adverse drug effects, and limited availability of the medications.[1–3,6,51,52]

NSAIDs have been thought to reduce the development of HO when given early after SCI.[2]

- Two randomized control trials (RCTs) examined the early use of NSAIDs to reduce the development of HO after SCI. One showed a lower incidence of early HO diagnosed on bone scan and fewer patients who received indomethacin vs. placebo developing X-ray evidence of HO,[6] and the second showed a lower incidence of HO and a lower relative risk of developing HO in patients who received rofecoxib vs. placebo.[53]
- Indomethacin, a nonselective COX-1 and COX-2 inhibitor, has been the historical gold standard.[54]
- NSAIDs have a limited therapeutic window just prior to bone formation and can have various adverse effects on patients with polytrauma beyond just bleeding risk.[1–3,18]
- Rofecoxib was once often prescribed for HO prophylaxis but was withdrawn from the market after an RCT found that chronic use elevated the risk of myocardial infarction and stroke.[55]
- Indomethacin has also been shown to interfere with fracture healing.[48,56,57]

One study has suggested that warfarin may inhibit the development of HO after SCI.[2]

- The observational retrospective study noted an association between warfarin use and HO after SCI. In this study, warfarin administration and HO development were found to be significantly related; none of the patients treated with warfarin developed HO and none of the patients with HO were treated with warfarin.[58]

Etidronate is a first-generation nonnitrogen bisphosphonate that has been shown to halt the progression of HO, but its use in current practice is largely limited by lack of availability.[1–3]

- One study compared patients treated with 3 days of intravenous (IV) etidronate followed by 6 months of oral (PO) etidronate vs. patients treated with 6 months of PO etidronate only. The effect on HO did not differ significantly between IV- and PO-treated groups.[1,59]

- One study of patients diagnosed early with positive bone scans who were treated with 3 days of IV followed by 6 months of PO etidronate, and found that 27% of patients developed subsequent X-ray evidence of HO 1.5–6 years after therapy initiation.[60] Etidronate may halt the progression of HO, but its use is most effective if it is used early when X-rays are still negative.[61]
- In addition to the lack of availability, other barriers to etidronate treatment include gastrointestinal side effects, renal toxicity, increased risk of skeletal fragility, and high cost.[62]
- Clodronate is another first-generation bisphosphonate that could be an alternative to etidronate, but its use for treating HO after SCI has not yet been adequately studied and it is not currently available for use in the United States.[1,3]

There are limited reports on second- and third-generation bisphosphonates that are more potent aminobisphosphonates with higher affinity for bone.

- Pamidronate has been suggested to halt the secondary progression of HO after surgical excision. A study of seven patients treated with pamidronate before and after surgical HO excision showed that none of the patients treated with pamidronate showed clinical, X-ray, or laboratory signs of HO recurrence at 5–54 months follow-up.[63]
- Alendronate (Fosamax) has not been found to directly prevent the development of HO and has been suggested to cause contractures.[1–3] A study of patients treated with weekly alendronate vs. no treatment showed no direct correlation between HO prevention and alendronate use but suggested an indirect link between the two. Abnormal serum ALP levels were significantly correlated with HO, whereas normal ALP levels were significantly correlated with alendronate use (i.e., the drug may help reduce a risk factor for HO instead of providing a direct prophylactic effect). This study, however, also suggested that patients who received alendronate treatment were more likely to develop contractures vs. the control group.[64]

PLIMF therapy, which uses magnetic fields to increase oxygen levels and blood flow to reduce toxic by-products at areas of inflammation, may help prevent HO after SCI but is not commonly used.[1,2]

Radiotherapy has been shown to reduce the progression of HO, but its long-term risks have not been adequately studied, so it is generally not used as a first-line option.[1–3]

- One RCT of 29 patients found significant differences in the incidence of HO between PLIMF treatment and control groups.[65]
- Radiotherapy is thought to prevent HO formation and/or progression by inhibiting the differentiation of osteoprogenitor cells.[66]
- Radiotherapy has been shown to inhibit bone morphogenic protein-2 signaling, reduce osteoblast proliferation and differentiation, and promote apoptosis.[67,68]
- Two case series studies have suggested that radiotherapy after surgical excision of HO helps to reduce the progression of HO.[69,70]
- Although radiotherapy may decrease HO recurrence postoperatively, potential complications may also include delayed wound healing, osteonecrosis, and, rarely, sarcoma.[71,72]

Surgical excision can improve ROM after hip HO but recurrence can be common post-operatively.[1–3]

- Surgical excision of HO generally occurs when ectopic bone is completely mature on a bone scan (can take 12–18 months to occur); however, earlier excision has been reported.[1–3,73]
- One review on recurrence rates after surgical excision was unable to clarify ideal timing for excision due to a lack of consensus on HO classification and recurrence rates.[74]
- Studies suggest surgical excision should be followed by prophylaxis with NSAIDs, bisphosphonates, or radiotherapy due to high recurrence rates with surgery alone.[1–3,75–77]

Review Questions

1. Where is the most common site of HO after SCI?
   a. Knee
   b. Hip
   c. Elbow
   d. Shoulder
2. How long after SCI does HO most commonly develop?
   a. 1–4 days
   b. 1–4 weeks
   c. 1–4 months
   d. 1–4 years
3. What is the most sensitive imaging method for detecting early HO?
   a. Triple phase bone scan
   b. X-ray
   c. CT
   d. MRI
4. Serum ALP is the most specific test for diagnosing HO, true or false?
   a. True
   b. False
5. How long do providers typically wait for surgical excision of HO?
   a. 12–18 months
   b. 1–4 months
   c. 6–10 months
   d. 24 months

REFERENCES

1. Bauman WA, Nash MS. Endocrinology and metabolism of persons with spinal cord injury. In: Kirshblum S, Lin VW, eds. *Spinal Cord Medicine*. 3rd ed. Springer Publishing Company; 2019:278–317.
2. Alibrahim F, McIntyre A, Serrato J, Mehta S, Loh E, Teasell RW. Heterotopic ossification following spinal cord injury. In: Eng JJ, Teasell RW, Miller WC, et al., eds. *Spinal Cord Injury Rehabilitation Evidence*. Version 6.0; 2016:1-20.
3. Bryce TN, Huang V, Escalon MX. Spinal cord injury. In: Cifu DX, ed. *Braddom's Physical Medicine and Rehabilitation*. 6th ed. Elsevier; 2021:1096–1098.
4. Subbarao JV, Garrison SJ. Heterotopic ossification: diagnosis and management, current concepts and controversies. *J Spinal Cord Med*. 1999;22(4):273–283.
5. Van Kuijk AA, Geurts AC, van Kuppevelt HJ. Neurogenic heterotopic ossification in spinal cord injury. *Spinal Cord*. 2002;40(7):313–326.
6. Banovac K, Williams JM, Patrick LD, Haniff YM. Prevention of heterotopic ossification after spinal cord injury with indomethacin. *Spinal Cord*. 2001;39(7):370–374.
7. Kirshblum S, Donovan J. Medical complications of SCI: bone, metabolic, pressure ulcers and sexuality and fertility. In: Weidner N, Rupp R, Tansey K, eds. *Neurological Aspects of Spinal Cord Injury*. Germany: Springer Publishing; 2017: 463–499.
8. Ranganathan K, Loder S, Agarwal S, et al. Heterotopic ossification: basic-science principles and clinical correlates. *J Bone Joint Surg Am*. 2015;97(13):1101–1111.
9. Razavi SZE, Aryan A, Kazemi S, et al. Prevalence of hip ossification and related clinical factors in cases with spinal cord injury. *Arch Neurosci*. 2015;2(4):e25395.
10. Citak M, Suero EM, Backhaus M, et al. Risk factors for heterotopic ossification in patients with spinal cord injury: a case-control study of 264 patients. *Spine*. 2012;37(23):1953–1957.
11. Larson JM, Michalski JP, Collacott EA, et al. Increased prevalence of HLA-B27 in patients with ectopic ossification following traumatic spinal cord injury. *Rheumatol Rehabil*. 1981;20(4):193–197.
12. Hunter T, Dubo HI, Hildahl CR, Smith NJ, Schroeder ML. Histocompatibility antigens in patients with spinal cord injury or cerebral damage complicated by heterotopic ossification. *Rheumatol Rehabil*. 1980;19(2):97–99.
13. Cipriano CA, Pill SG, Keenan MA. Heterotopic ossification following traumatic brain injury and spinal cord injury. *J Am Acad Orthop Surg*. 2009;17(11):689–697.
14. Nauth A, Giles E, Potter BK, et al. Heterotopic ossification in orthopaedic trauma. *J Orthop Trauma*. 2012;26(12):684–688.
15. Genêt F, Kulina I, Vaquette C, et al. Neurological heterotopic ossification following spinal cord injury is triggered by macrophage-mediated inflammation in muscle. *J Pathol*. 2015;236(2):229–240.
16. Jodoin M, Rouleau DM, Therrien E, et al. Investigating the incidence and magnitude of heterotopic ossification with and without joints involvement in patients with a limb fracture and mild traumatic brain injury. *Bone Rep*. 2019;11:100222.
17. Salga M, Jourdan C, Durand MC, et al. Sciatic nerve compression by neurogenic heterotopic ossification: use of CT to determine surgical indications. *Skelet Radiol*. 2015;44(2):233–240.
18. Wong KR, Mychasiuk R, O'Brien TJ, et al. Neurological heterotopic ossification: novel mechanisms, prognostic biomarkers and prophylactic therapies. *Bone Res*. 2020;8:42.
19. Alves JL. Blood–brain barrier and traumatic brain injury. *J Neurosci Res*. 2014;92(2):141–147.
20. Stamatovic SM, Keep RF, Andjelkovic AV. Brain endothelial cell-cell junctions: how to "open" the blood brain barrier. *Curr Neuropharmacol*. 2008;6(3):179–192.
21. Wilson EH, Weninger W, Hunter CA. Trafficking of immune cells in the central nervous system. *J Clin Invest*. 2010;120(5):1368–1379.
22. Wolburg H, Wolburg-Buchholz K, Engelhardt B. Involvement of tight junctions during transendothelial migration of mononuclear cells in experimental autoimmune encephalomyelitis. *Ernst Schering Res Found Workshop*. 2004;47:17–38.
23. Shlosberg D, Benifla M, Kaufer D, Friedman A. Blood–brain barrier breakdown as a therapeutic target in traumatic brain injury. *Nat Rev Neurol*. 2010;6(7):393–403.
24. Pape HC, Marsh S, Morley JR, Krettek C, Giannoudis PV. Current concepts in the development of heterotopic ossification. *J Bone Joint Surg Br*. 2004;86(6):783–787.
25. Tannous O, Stall AC, Griffith C, Donaldson CT, Castellani Jr RJ, Pellegrini Jr VD. Heterotopic bone formation about the hip undergoes endochondral ossification: a rabbit model. *Clin Orthop Relat Res*. 2013;471(5):1584–1592.
26. Davies OG, Grover LM, Eisenstein N, Lewis MP, Liu Y. Identifying the cellular mechanisms leading to heterotopic ossification. *Calcif Tissue Int*. 2015;97(5):432–444.
27. Winkler S, Niedermair T, Fuchtmeier B, et al. The impact of hypoxia on mesenchymal progenitor cells of human skeletal tissue in the pathogenesis of heterotopic ossification. *Int Orthop*. 2015;39(12):2495–2501.
28. Shehab D, Elgazzar AH, Collier BD. Heterotopic ossification. *J Nucl Med*. 2002;43(3):346–353.
29. Orzel JA, Rudd TG. Heterotopic bone formation: clinical, laboratory, and imaging correlation. *J Nucl Med*. 1985;26(2):125–132.
30. Freed JH, Hahn H, Menter R, Dillon T. The use of the three-phase bone scan in the early diagnosis of heterotopic ossification (HO) and in the evaluation of didronel therapy. *Paraplegia*. 1982;20(4):208–216.
31. Amendola MA, Shirazi K, Amendola BE, Kuhns LR, Tisnado J, Yaghmai I. Computed tomography of malignant tumors of the osseous pelvis. *Comput Radiol*. 1983;7(2): 107–117.
32. Wick L, Berger M, Knecht H, Glucker T, Ledermann HP. Magnetic resonance signal alterations in the acute onset of heterotopic ossification in patients with spinal cord injury. *Eur Radiol*. 2005;15(9):1867–1875.
33. Rosteius T, Suero EM, Grasmucke D, et al. The sensitivity of ultrasound screening examination in detecting heterotopic ossification following spinal cord injury. *Spinal Cord*. 2017;55(1):71–73.
34. Wang Q, Zhang P, Li P, et al. Ultrasonography monitoring of trauma-induced heterotopic ossification: guidance for rehabilitation procedures. *Front Neurol*. 2018;9:771.
35. Stefanidis K, Brindley P, Ramnarine R, et al. Bedside ultrasound to facilitate early diagnosis and ease of follow-up in neurogenic heterotopic ossification: a pilot study from the intensive care unit. *J Head Trauma Rehabil*. 2017;32(6): E54–E58.

36. Ohlmeier M, Suero EM, Aach M, Meindl R, Schildhauer TA, Citak M. Muscle localization of heterotopic ossification following spinal cord injury. *Spine J.* 2017;17(10):1519–1522.
37. Cassar-Pullicino VN, McClelland M, Badwan DAH, McCall IW, Pringle RG, El Masry W. Sonographic diagnosis of heterotopic bone formation in spinal injury patients. *Paraplegia.* 1993;31(1):40–50.
38. Argyropoulou MI, Kostandi E, Kosta P, et al. Heterotopic ossification of the knee joint in intensive care unit patients: early diagnosis with magnetic resonance imaging. *Crit Care.* 2006;10(5):R152.
39. Brooker AF, Bowerman JW, Robinson RA, Riley Jr LH. Ectopic ossification following total hip replacement. Incidence and a method of classification. *J Bone Joint Surg Am.* 1973;55(8):1629–1632.
40. Garland DE, Orwin JF. Resection of heterotopic ossification in patients with spinal cord injuries. *Clin Orthop Relat Res.* 1989;242:169–176.
41. Mavrogenis AF, Guerra G, Staals EL, Bianchi G, Ruggieri P. A classification method for neurogenic heterotopic ossification of the hip. *J Orthop Traumatol.* 2012;13(2):69–78.
42. Arduini M, Mancini F, Farsetti P, Piperno A, Ippolito E. A new classification of peri-articular heterotopic ossification of the hip associated with neurological injury: 3D CT scan assessment and intra-operative findings. *Bone Joint J.* 2015;97-B(7):899–904.
43. Estrores IM, Harrington A, Banovac K. C-reactive protein and erythrocyte sedimentation rate in patients with heterotopic ossification after spinal cord injury. *J Spinal Cord Med.* 2004;27(5):434–437.
44. Citak M, Grasmucke D, Suero EM, et al. The roles of serum alkaline and bone alkaline phosphatase levels in predicting heterotopic ossification following spinal cord injury. *Spinal Cord.* 2016;54(5):368–370.
45. Singh RS, Craig MC, Katholi CR, Jackson AB, Mountz JM. The predictive value of creatine phosphokinase and alkaline phosphatase in identification of heterotopic ossification in patients after spinal cord injury. *Arch Phys Med Rehabil.* 2003;84(11):1584–1588.
46. Sherman AL, Williams J, Patrick L, Banovac K. The value of serum creatine kinase in early diagnosis of heterotopic ossification. *J Spinal Cord Med.* 2003;26(3):227–230.
47. Crawford CM, Varghese G, Mani MM, Neff JR. Heterotopic ossification: are range of motion exercises contraindicated? *J Burn Care Rehabil.* 1986;7(4):323–327.
48. Sullivan MP, Torres SJ, Mehta S, Ahn J. Heterotopic ossification after central nervous system trauma: a current review. *Bone Jt Res.* 2013;2(3):51–57.
49. Zotz TGG, de Paula JB. Influence of transcutaneous electrical stimulation on heterotopic ossification: an experimental study in Wistar rats. *Braz J Med Biol Res.* 2015;48(11): 1055–1062.
50. Aubut JL, Mehta S, Cullen N, Teasell RW. ERABI Group, the SCIRE research team. A comparison of heterotopic ossification treatment within the traumatic brain and spinal cord injured population: an evidence based systematic review. *Neuro Rehabil.* 2011;28(2):151–160.
51. Teasell RW, Mehta S, Aubut JL, et al. A systematic review of the therapeutic interventions for heterotopic ossification after spinal cord injury. *Spinal Cord.* 2010;48(7):512–521.
52. Stover SL, Hahn HR, Miller JM. Disodium etidronate in the prevention of heterotopic ossification following spinal cord injury (preliminary report). *Paraplegia.* 1976;14(2):146–156.
53. Banovac K, Williams JM, Patrick LD, Levi A. Prevention of heterotopic ossification after spinal cord injury with COX-2 selective inhibitor (rofecoxib). *Spinal Cord.* 2004;42(12): 707–710.
54. Ritter MA, Sieber JM. Prophylactic indomethacin for the prevention of heterotopic bone formation following total hip arthroplasty. *Clin Orthop Relat Res.* 1985;196:217–225.
55. Sibbald B. Rofecoxib (Vioxx) voluntarily withdrawn from market. *Can Med Assoc J.* 2004;171(9):1027–1028.
56. Rø J, Sudmann E, Marton PF. Effect of indomethacin on fracture healing in rats. *Acta Orthop Scand.* 1976;47(6): 588–599.
57. Baird EO, Kang QK. Prophylaxis of heterotopic ossification – an updated review. *J Orthop Surg Res.* 2009;4:12.
58. Buschbacher R, McKinley W, Buschbacher L, Devaney CW, Coplin B. Warfarin in prevention of heterotopic ossification. *Am J Phys Med Rehabil.* 1992;71(2):86–91.
59. Banovac K, Gonzalez F, Wade N, Bowker JJ. Intravenous disodium etidronate therapy in spinal cord injury patients with heterotopic ossification. *Paraplegia.* 1993;31(10): 660–666.
60. Banovac K. The effect of etidronate on late development of heterotopic ossification after spinal cord injury. *J Spinal Cord Med.* 2000;23(1);23:40–44.
61. Banovac K, Gonzalez F, Renfree KJ. Treatment of heterotopic ossification after spinal cord injury. *J Spinal Cord Med.* 1997;20(1):60–65.
62. Vasileiadis GI, Sakellariou VI, Kelekis A, et al. Prevention of heterotopic ossification in cases of hypertrophic osteoarthritis submitted to total hip arthroplasty. Etidronate or Indomethacin? *J Musculoskelet. Neuronal Interact.* 2010;10(2): 159–165.
63. Schuetz P, Mueller B, Christ-Crain M, Dick W, Haas H. Aminobisphosphonates in heterotopic ossification: first experience in five consecutive cases. *Spinal Cord.* 2005;43(10): 604–610.
64. Ploumis A, Donovan JM, Olurinde MO, et al. Association between alendronate, serum alkaline phosphatase level, and heterotopic ossification in individuals with spinal cord injury. *J Spin Cord Med.* 2015;38(2):193–198.
65. Durovic A, Miljkovic D, Brdareski Z, Plavsic A, Jevtic M. Pulse low-intensity electromagnetic field as prophylaxis of heterotopic ossification in patients with traumatic spinal cord injury. *Vojnosanit Pregl.* 2009;66(1):22–28.
66. Chao ST, Joyce MJ, Suh JH. Treatment of heterotopic ossification. *Orthopedics.* 2007;30(6):457–464.
67. Pohl F, Hassel S, Nohe A, et al. Radiation-induced suppression of the Bmp2 signal transduction pathway in the pluripotent mesenchymal cell line C2C12: an in vitro model for prevention of heterotopic ossification by radiotherapy. *Radiat Res.* 2003;159(3):345–350.
68. Szymczyk KH, Shapiro IM, Adams CS. Ionizing radiation sensitizes bone cells to apoptosis. *Bone.* 2004;34(1): 148–156.
69. Sautter-Bihl ML, Liebermeister E, Nanassy A. Radiotherapy as a local treatment option for heterotopic ossification in patients with spinal cord injury. *Spinal Cord.* 2000;38:33–36.

70. Sautter-Bihl ML, Hultenschmidt B, Liebermeister E, Nanassy A. Fractionated and single-dose radiotherapy for heterotopic bone formation in patients with spinal cord injury. A phase-I/II study. *Strahlenther Onkol.* 2001;177:200–205.
71. Haubner F, Ohmann E, Pohl F, Strutz J, Gassner HG. Wound healing after radiation therapy: review of the literature. *Radiat Oncol.* 2012;7:162.
72. Farris MK, Chowdhry VK, Lemke S, Kilpatrick M, Lacombe M. Osteosarcoma following single fraction radiation prophylaxis for heterotopic ossification. *Radiat Oncol.* 2012;7:140.
73. McAuliffe JA, Wolfson AH. Early excision of heterotopic ossification about the elbow followed by radiation therapy. *J Bone Joint Surg Am.* 1997;79(5):749–755.
74. Genêt F, Ruet A, Almangour W, Gatin L, Denormandie P, Schnitzler A. Beliefs relating to recurrence of heterotopic ossification following excision in patients with spinal cord injury: a review. *Spinal Cord.* 2015;53(5):340–344.
75. Van Kuijk AA, van Kuppevelt HJM, van der Schaaf DB. Osteonecrosis after treatment for heterotopic ossification in spinal cord injury with the combination of surgery, irradiation, and an NSAID. *Spinal Cord.* 2000;38(5):319–324.
76. Freebourn TM, Barber DB, Able AC. The treatment of immature heterotopic ossification in spinal cord injury with combination surgery, radiation therapy and NSAID. *Spinal Cord.* 1999;37(1):50–53.
77. Banovac K, Sherman AL, Estrores IM, Banovac F. Prevention and treatment of heterotopic ossification after spinal cord injury. *J Spinal Cord Med.* 2004;7(4):376–382.

CHAPTER 25

Spine Fractures, Dislocations, and Instability

Ricky Placide and Alden Newcomb

OUTLINE

Introduction

Traumatic injury to the spinal column includes vertebral fractures, dislocations, and ligamentous injuries. Approximately 2%–6% of blunt trauma patients sustain an injury to the spinal column with an annual health-care cost of over one billion dollars.[1,2] The majority of spinal trauma is caused by motor vehicle collisions, with high rates of speed, improper/lack of seat belt use, and intoxication as risk factors.[3] Spine trauma is not limited to high-energy mechanisms of injury; vertebral fractures are one of the most common geriatric fragility fractures. Both high- and low-energy spine trauma is associated with a high level of morbidity, such as spinal cord injury (SCI) and chronic pain.[4]

Injury patterns within the spine vary by spinal level. The cervical spine is commonly injured, as it has the highest inherent flexibility and rotational moment arm given its connection between the torso and head. There are more than 200,000 hospitalizations annually for cervical spine injuries.[5] The distribution of age and mechanism of cervical injury is bimodal, with motor vehicle collisions causing injury in young patients (15–24 years old) and low-energy mechanisms, such as ground-level falls, seen in patients older than 55 years. Other high-energy mechanisms of cervical injury include shallow water diving and gunshot wounds.[6]

Thoracolumbar injuries range from fragility compression fractures to high-energy fracture-dislocations. Ninety percent of all spine fractures involve the thoracic and lumbar regions, and 52% of those occur at the thoracolumbar junction. The thoracic spine has the least intrinsic flexibility of the entire spinal column due to its association with the rib cage and sternum; therefore, thoracic injuries generally require significantly more energy. The lumbar spine is significantly more mobile, which creates a transition zone of higher biomechanical stress between the thoracic and lumbar vertebrae between T11 and L1. Approximately half (52%) of all thoracolumbar fractures occur between these levels.[7] There are approximately 15,000 severe thoracolumbar injuries annually in the United States with an associated 33% incidence of severe neurologic sequelae from these injuries. Additionally, high-energy thoracolumbar trauma is associated with major visceral and axial injuries such as rib fractures, pneumothorax, hemothorax, and cardiac/pulmonary contusions.

Spinal Instability

There are numerous medical publications describing ways to categorize spinal instability (Table 25.1). Some classification schemes are mostly historic and not typically used in today's clinical practice. The focus of this chapter will be on traumatic spinal instability; however, other etiologies deserve consideration, such as the spine instability neoplastic score (SINs) in neoplastic disease (Table 25.2). There is significant variability among the published spinal instability classification schemes. For example, some are general and are to be applied anywhere in the spine, whereas some are specific to a particular region of the spine. Some are based on the mechanism of injury (compression, distraction, flexion, extension, rotation), whereas others use fracture patterns on spine imaging to guide their classification.

In the clinical setting it is important to be able to determine if a traumatic spine injury is stable (transverse process fracture) and only needs supportive care; intermediately unstable (L1 burst fracture without neurologic symptoms and/or signs); or a fracture-dislocation of the cervical spine with progressive tetraparesis requiring emergent operative intervention. In addition to the spine injury itself, other factors come into the decision-making process, including associated injuries and comorbidities; decisions are best made in consultation with the critical care/trauma team and appropriate medical services. In the case of traumatic spinal instability, the most recognized classification systems to aid in decision-making used today are the subaxial cervical spine injury classification system (SLIC)[8] and the thoracolumbar injury classification system (TLICS).[9] These classification systems assign points in each of three categories: fracture or dislocation morphology (burst fracture, translational dislocation, etc.), integrity of the soft tissues (disc, interspinous ligaments, facet joints, etc.), and the neurological status of the patient (nerve root injury, cord injury). Adding the numbers assigned from each category can aid in determining whether to proceed with nonoperative or operative intervention for that particular injury.

Table 25.1 Selected Descriptions and Classification Schemes Related to Spinal Instability

Allen and Ferguson[25]
AO spine classification[14]
Benzel[26]
Berg[27]
Chance[15]
Denis[28]
Kelly and Whiteside[29]
Magerl[30]
Watson-Jones[31]
White and Panjabi[32]
SLIC, TLICS[8,9]
SINs[33]

SINs, Spinal instability neoplastic score; *SLIC*, subaxial cervical spine injury classification; *TLICS*, thoracolumbar injury classification system.

Table 25.2 Selected Etiologies of Spinal Instability and Examples

Congenital	Upper cervical spine instability in many inherited syndromes (e.g., Down syndrome)
Degenerative	Degenerative L4–L5 spondylolisthesis
Iatrogenic	Resection of stabilizing structures in the setting of decompressive surgery (e.g., post laminectomy kyphosis in the cervical spine)
Infectious	Destructive spondylodiscitis often with progressive kyphosis and instability
Neoplastic	Tumor invasion and destruction of the bony and soft tissue stabilizers of the spine (SINs)
Traumatic	Traumatic thoracic fracture – dislocation
Posttraumatic	Charcot spine
Other	Destructive spondyloarthropathy in the setting of renal disease and amyloid deposition

SINs, Spinal instability neoplastic score.

Fractures/Dislocations

Traumatic spine injuries are typically categorized and discussed regionally. This is due to the particular spinal anatomy and surrounding structures, and unique biomechanics in the various regions of the spine. In the setting of trauma, the spine is usually divided into the craniocervical junction (occiput to C2), the subaxial cervical spine (C3–C7), the thoracolumbar spine (T1–L5), and the lumbosacral/lumbopelvic spine (L5–sacrum–pelvis). While injuries to the cervicothoracic and thoracolumbar transition zones deserve special attention, this chapter will review traumatic spine injuries as mentioned above. Fractures of the spinous process and transverse process tend to be stable injuries except in rare circumstances and will not be discussed further in this chapter.

Craniocervical Junction (Occiput–C2)

Occipital Condyle Fractures

Occipital condyle fractures (OCF) are relatively rare injuries with motor vehicle accidents being the most common mechanism of injury. There are several published classification systems to describe OCF. When they occur in isolation without any other regional associated injuries, OCFs tend to be relatively stable injuries and can be treated in a cervical orthosis. However, due to the mechanism of injury and location, OCF can be associated with traumatic brain injury (TBI) and/or occipitocervical dissociation (OCD).

OCD (also referred to as atlantooccipital dissociation and craniocervical dislocation) is a traumatic injury that causes dissociation of the occipital condyles from the C1 lateral masses. Most commonly, this injury is the result of a motor vehicle accident. OCD can be solely a soft tissue disruption or can be associated with fractures about the craniocervical junction. Historically, OCD was almost always a fatal injury. Associated TBI and SCI are not uncommon. However, significant advances in prehospital care, improvements in trauma centers, rapid imaging capabilities (computed tomography [CT]) leading to earlier diagnosis, and evolution of occipital

Table 25.3 Selected Imaging Methods for Diagnosing Occipital Cervical Dissociation

Condyle-C1 interval[34]
Powers ratio[35]
Harris basion-axis ratio[36]
Wholey basion-dens interval[37]

cervical stabilization techniques have led to improved survivorship and outcomes in patients with OCD.

There are several described methods to identify OCD (Table 25.3). With significantly better reliability than plain radiographs and rapid availability, CT scan is the initial imaging modality of choice (Fig. 25.1). However, in the case of spontaneous occiput–C1 reduction, magnetic resonance imaging (MRI) is warranted if there is any suspicion of OCD. In addition to pain from soft tissue disruption and fractures, TBI, and SCI, there may be involvement of lower cranial nerves. The hypoglossal and jugular foramen (glossopharyngeal, vagal, and accessory nerves) are adjacent to the occipital condyles and therefore can be injured in the setting of OCD as well as OCF.

Atlas–C1 Burst Fracture

Fractures of the atlas include the Jefferson burst fracture and fractures of the lateral masses/facet joints and are typically associated with an axial load. Atlas fractures are the second most common fracture of the upper cervical spine after odontoid fractures. Many fractures of the atlas are stable and may be treated in a cervical orthosis. Others that are associated with other injuries, either bony or soft tissue, may require operative intervention. One such injury includes disruption or avulsion of the transverse atlantal ligament. Although recently called into question, the "rule of Spence" can help determine if a C1 burst fracture is stable or unstable.[10] If there is concern for instability, CT and MRI are warranted (Fig. 25.2).

As with many injuries to the craniocervical junction, patients can have a variety of signs and symptoms. Neurological deficit due to SCI in the setting of a C1 fracture is rare; however, neck pain and headache are common. Patients may also have lower cranial nerve (IX–XII) dysfunction, and signs/symptoms associated with disruption of the vertebral artery; basilar circulation (nausea/vomiting, visual changes, tinnitus).

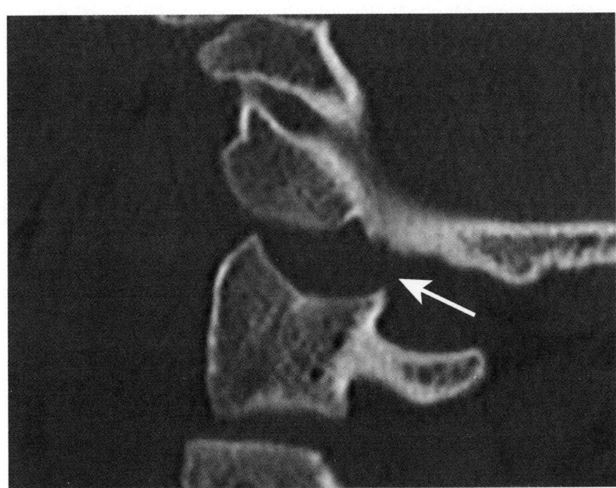

Fig. 25.1 Computed Tomography Scan Demonstrating Dissociation of the Occiput from C1.

Axis (C2) Fractures

Fractures of the axis include fractures of the odontoid process, pars interarticularis, C2 body, lateral masses, and facet joints. This section will discuss odontoid and pars fractures. Fractures of the odontoid process are the most common cervical spine fracture in the elderly. The mechanism is a flexion and/or extension force, often from a ground-level fall. The classification by Anderson and D'Alonzo is the one that is most commonly used.[11] It divides odontoid fractures into types I, II, or III based on fracture location, with some subcategorization. Type II is the most common and most likely to be problematic. Many can be managed in a rigid cervical orthosis; however, some warrant operative stabilization. There is controversy surrounding the ideal management of type II odontoid fractures in the elderly, as nonoperative as well as operative treatments are associated with morbidity and mortality. The younger patient with a type II odontoid fracture is typically the victim of a high-energy injury and is more likely to have other associated injuries. As with the elderly population, operative treatment for type II odontoid fractures in the young trauma patient is more likely if there is fracture comminution, fracture displacement, and angulation (Fig. 25.3). SCI is not common in the setting of a type II odontoid fracture; however, fracture instability allowing C1–C2 translation may affect the C2 nerve root, causing radiculopathy.

Fracture of the C2 pars interarticularis (hangmans fracture) is typically a traumatic spondylolysis/spondylolisthesis of C2. The Levine Edward classification is the most commonly used classification system to describe this injury.[12] The mechanism of injury is typically high-energy hyperextension in combination with compression, distraction, or additional flexion/extension. This injury can be associated with significant soft tissue disruption including a traumatic disc herniation at

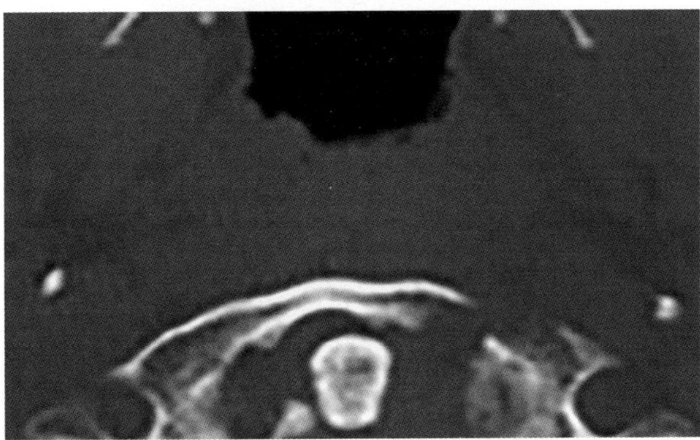

Fig.25.2 Axial Computed Tomography View of C1. Example of a C1 ring fracture (Jefferson burst fracture) and bony avulsion of the atlantodental ligament.

C2–C3. Depending on the severity of the injury, C2 pars fractures can be treated nonoperatively or operatively (Fig. 25.4).

Subaxial Cervical Spine (C3–C7)

Injuries to the subaxial cervical spine can range from insignificant, nondisplaced fractures to high-energy fracture-dislocation with bony and soft tissue disruption with complete SCI. Approximately 150,000 cervical spine injuries occur annually in North America, and 7%–8% are associated with SCI.[13] Subaxial spinal cord injuries account for about 75% of all spinal cord injuries. The mechanisms of traumatic injury include flexion, extension, compression, distraction, rotation, or a combination of any of these forces (Fig. 25.5).

A detailed review of all subaxial cervical spine injuries is beyond the scope of this chapter. A more comprehensive list of subaxial cervical spine injury types can be found in Table 25.4.

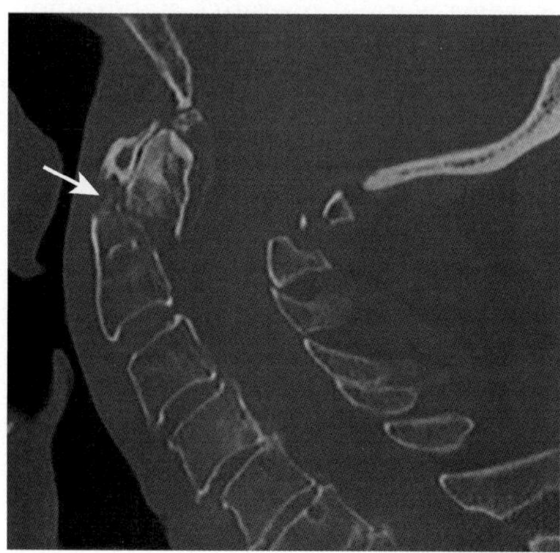

Fig. 25.3 Type II Odontoid Fracture.

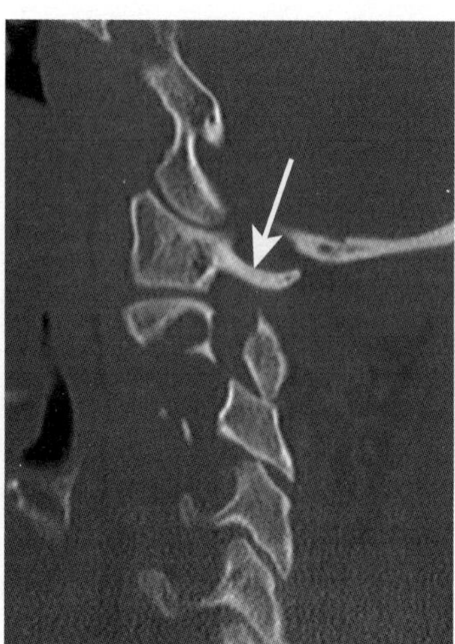

Fig. 25.4 C2 Pars Interarticularis Fracture (hangmans fracture/traumatic C2 spondylolisthesis).

Thoracolumbar (T1–L5)

Traumatic injury to the spinal column is a relatively common occurrence, and the majority of these injuries happen in the thoracic and lumbar spine, with the thoracolumbar region being the most commonly injured. As in other regions, the two main demographic groups suffering thoracolumbar trauma are young patients with a high-energy injury and the older population with low-energy injuries. The primary injury classification schemes are the TLICS and the AOSpine classification

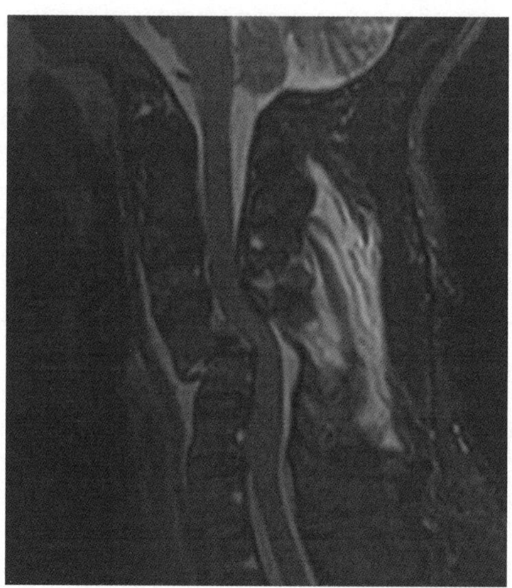

Fig. 25.5 Sagittal Magnetic Resonance Image (short tau inversion recovery) of the Cervical Spine Demonstrating a C4–C5 Fracture-Dislocation, Cord Compromise, and Significant Soft Tissue Disruption.

Table 25.4 Examples of Cervical Spine Structures Potentially Injured in Trauma

Vertebral body fractures	Compression, burst, teardrop
Posterior element fractures	Spinous process, transverse process, lateral mass/facet, lamina, pedicle
Soft tissue injury	Traumatic disc herniation, anterior longitudinal ligament, posterior longitudinal ligament, ligamentum flavum, facet capsule, interspinous/supraspinous ligaments, paraspinal muscle

and include not only injury classification but treatment recommendations as well (nonoperative, operative).[9,14]

As with the cervical spine, the thoracic and lumbar spinal column, spinal cord/nerve root, and surrounding soft tissues are subject to injury (Table 25.4). An important distinction between the cervical/thoracic spine and the lumbar spine is neuroanatomy. In most adults, the spinal cord ends at approximately L1, thereby typically transitioning from upper motor neuron to lower motor neuron physiology. In certain circumstances, this becomes important with regard to treatment and prognosis. Not only is pathophysiology different, the biomechanics of the neural structures themselves can affect treatment decisions.

One of the more common fractures of the thoracic and lumbar spine is a burst fracture, with the thoracolumbar junction accounting for most of these fractures (Figs. 25.6 and 25.7). By definition, a burst fracture is a fracture of the vertebral endplate and the posterior wall of the vertebral body, thereby involving the spinal canal. Even with modern classification systems, management of thoracolumbar burst fractures can be controversial, and there remains room for clinical decision-making. Bracing and surgery are both appropriate treatment options based on the overall clinical situation.

In addition to the fractures mentioned in Table 25.4, a traumatic injury to the spine that typically involves the thoracolumbar spine is the Chance fracture.[15] This is usually a flexion distraction injury and involves all three columns of the spine. The injury can be purely bony, purely soft, or a combination of bony and soft tissue disruption.

Lumbosacralpelvic (L5–Sacrum–Pelvis)

Sacral fractures

The sacrum provides an important junction to connect the spinal column to the pelvis, therefore sacral fractures can affect the lumbosacral junction, sacropelvic junction (including the sacroiliac joint), or both. As the sacrum forms part of the posterior pelvic ring, fractures of the sacrum can disrupt the integrity of the pelvic ring. Severe sacral fractures lead to dissociation of the spine from the pelvis and lower extremities, referred to as spinopelvic or lumbopelvic dissociation. Sacral fractures with comminution and/or displacement may cause injury to the surrounding neural structures, including nerve roots L5, and S1–S4. In severe sacral fractures and sacroiliac disruption, neurological injury can occur in greater than 50% of patients, and sacral nerve root involvement can result in a traumatic cauda equina syndrome.[16,17]

There are two main groups of patients that suffer sacral fractures: first is young adults involved in high-energy trauma such as a motor vehicle crash or fall from a height, and the second is the elderly population involved in low-energy trauma such as a ground-level fall. Insufficiency fractures of the pelvis may occur spontaneously in the patient with risk factors such as osteoporosis, chronic steroid use, or previous pelvic radiation.

Plain radiography for the initial evaluation of a patient with a sacral fracture has limited utility, as there are many overlying bony structures depending on the views obtained. CT scan is ideal to evaluate bony detail, evaluate the neural foramen, classify the fracture pattern, and help with treatment planning (Fig. 25.8).

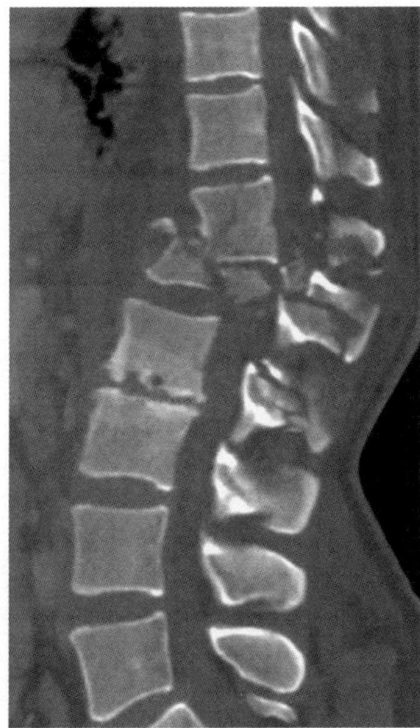

Fig. 25.6 Sagittal Computed Tomography Scan of an L1 Fracture-Dislocation.

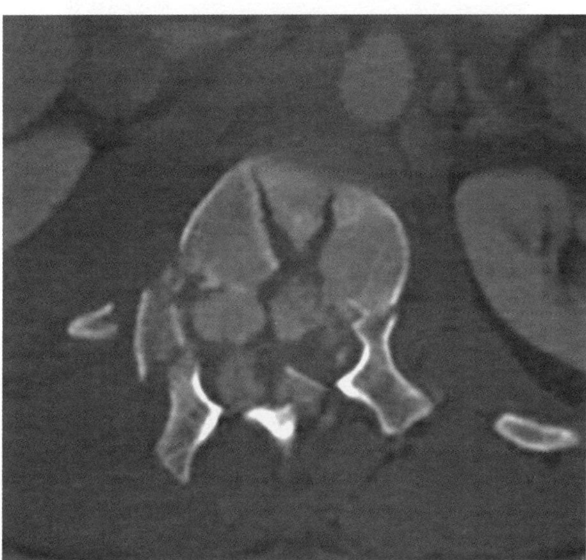

Fig. 25.7 Axial Computed Tomography Scan of an L1 Burst Fracture.

MRI is useful to assess the neural structures, surrounding soft tissues, and in the case of an insufficiency fracture that may not be obvious on CT (Fig. 25.9). There are several classification systems used to describe sacral fractures. One of the more common is the Denis classification where the sacrum is divided vertically into zones I, II, and III, with zone III having the highest rate of neurological injury.[16,17] The Denis classification of sacral fractures describes zone I as fracture lateral to the neural foramen, zone II as fracture within the neural foramen, and zone III as fracture medial to the neural foramen, within the spinal canal. Others include Roy-Camille[18] and the Orthopaedic Trauma Association pelvic fracture classification.[19] Sacral fractures are also described by the appearance of their fracture lines, for example U-shaped and H-shaped.

Management of sacral fractures ranges from symptomatic care with activity as tolerated to operative lumbopelvic stabilization procedures and decompression of the lumbosacral nerve roots. There are a variety of operative options including less invasive percutaneous procedures to more extensive open surgeries; however, this will depend on the fracture pattern, level of instability, and neurological involvement.

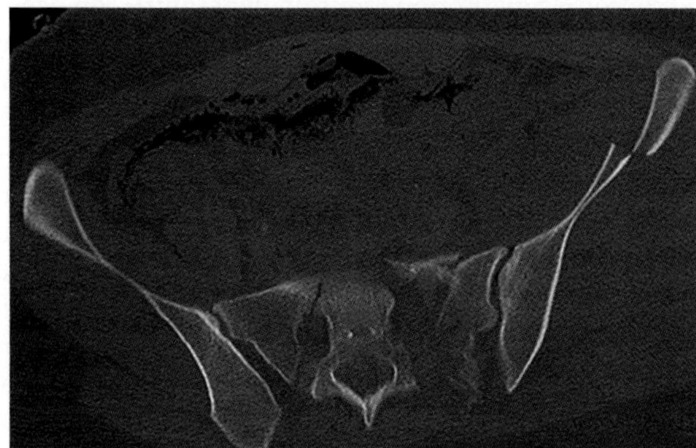

Fig. 25.8 Axial Computed Tomography Demonstrating an Unstable Sacral Fracture.

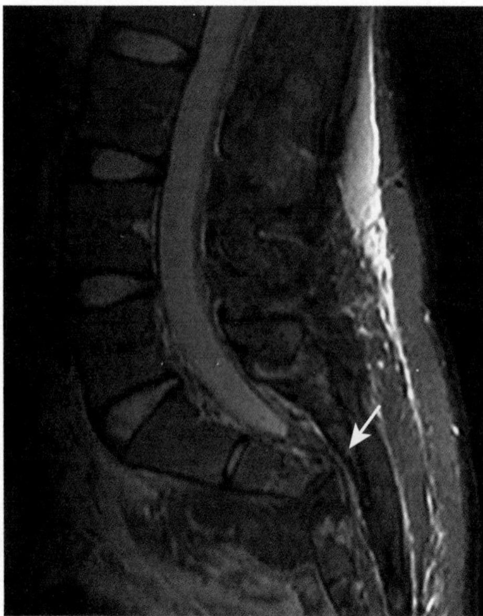

Fig. 25.9 Sagittal Magnetic Resonance Image Demonstrating a Sacral Fracture With Kyphotic Angulation and Involvement of the S2 and S3 Nerve Roots.

Pediatric Spine Trauma

Pediatric and adult spine injuries have many similarities with respect to mechanism of injury, patterns of injury, and treatment. However, there are important differences that are noteworthy and help with evaluation and management of the pediatric patient with a spinal injury. Pediatric spine trauma is relatively rare, accounting for only 2%–5% of all spinal injuries.[20] In recent decades, there has been a decrease in incidence of pediatric spinal cord and spinal column injuries in the United States.[21]

For this discussion, we will refer to children aged 0–14 years and adolescents aged 15–17 years. Motor vehicle accidents are the most common cause of spinal column injuries in adolescents and children.[21] Other causes include falls, pedestrian injuries, and nonaccidental trauma, particularly in children. The most common cause of SCI in adolescents and children is penetrating trauma, followed by sports injuries[21] (Fig. 25.10). Pediatric spine injuries are much less common than adult spine injuries, primarily due to regional differences in anatomy and biomechanics.

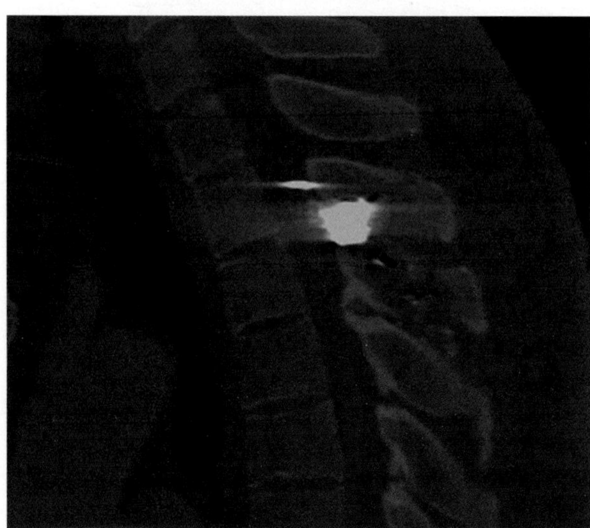

Fig. 25.10 Sagittal Computed Tomography Demonstrating a Penetrating Injury to the Upper Thoracic Spine.

Cervical Spine

Approximately 65% of pediatric spine injuries involve the cervical spine, and younger children are more likely to have craniocervical and upper cervical injuries.[22] In the pediatric population, the cervical spine has more range of motion and flexibility and less well-developed ligaments and paraspinal muscles compared with the adult. In the pediatric subaxial cervical spine, the articular processes (facet joints) are oriented more transversely than in adults and therefore have less resistance to translational forces. Also, the vertebral bodies are more wedge shaped anteriorly, allowing for physiologic translation (pseudosubluxation), especially at C2–C3 and C3–C4.

OCD is a traumatic separation of the occiput from C1 and is usually a purely ligamentous injury in the pediatric population. This injury is relatively more common in the pediatric population than in adults and is typically the result of a high-energy injury. It is often fatal and is not uncommonly associated with other injuries, including intracranial trauma. C1 (atlas) ring fractures (Jefferson burst fractures) are rare in children and can be confused with open synchondroses of C1. Typically, C1 vertebral synchondroses are not all fused until about 7 years of age. Atlantoaxial rotatory subluxation can be trauma-related in about one-third of cases but is more commonly associated with inflammatory conditions of the head and neck.[23] It is thought that C1–C2 joint hypermobility and/or redundant joint synovium that gets "trapped" in the C1–C2 joints leads to pain, muscle spasm, and torticollis. Hangman fracture is rare in children, otherwise it has a similar presentation as in adults. Subaxial (C3–C7) cervical spine injuries in the pediatric population are similar to the injuries seen in adults, including compression fractures, burst fractures, traumatic disc herniation, laminar fractures, facet fractures/dislocations, and pedicle fractures.

Thoracolumbar Spine

Thoracolumbar pediatric injuries are similar to the injuries seen in adults. Less than 1% of all spine trauma is pediatric thoracic and lumbar spine injuries.[19] However, a major difference is the more elasticity, flexibility, and compressibility of the pediatric spine compared with adults. Therefore, pediatric patients are less likely to fracture their vertebra. This is related to the condition unique to children, typically less than 8 years of age, referred to as SCI without radiographic abnormality.[24] In this situation, the spinal cord cannot stretch as much as the spinal column without injury. Compression fractures, burst fractures, Chance injuries, and traumatic spondylolisthesis have similar mechanisms, imaging findings, and treatment options as in adults. Although not studied as in adults, the TLICS has been applied to pediatric thoracolumbar injuries in clinical practice.

Summary

Spinal fractures, dislocations, and instability have many etiologies. This chapter is an overview focused on traumatic spinal injuries. Spinal injuries have the potential for significant morbidity and mortality. In the case of a severe spine injury, rapid assessment of history, physical examination, and imaging are critical, as treatment in a timely fashion yields improved outcomes. Ideally, this is accomplished through an interdisciplinary effort including trauma surgeons, critical care specialists, spine surgeons, and physical medicine and rehabilitation specialists.

Review Questions

1. The majority of spine fractures occur:
   a. At the craniocervical junction
   b. At the cervicothoracic junction
   c. At the thoracolumbar junction
   d. At the lumbopelvic junction
2. Examples of spinal instability include:
   a. Congenital and degenerative
   b. Iatrogenic and infectious
   c. Traumatic and neoplastic
   d. All of the above
3. The most commonly used classification system for traumatic thoracolumbar spine injuries and can also help with management decision-making is:
   a. White and Panjabi spinal instability scheme
   b. SINs (spinal instability neoplastic score)
   c. Thoracolumbar injury classification system (TLICS)
   d. Levine Edward
4. In the Denis classification of sacral fractures, which has the highest incidence of neurological injury?
   a. Denis zone I fractures
   b. Denis zone II fractures
   c. Denis zone III fractures
   d. They all have a high incidence of neurological injury
5. The majority of pediatric spine injuries occur:
   a. In the cervical spine
   b. In the thoracic spine
   c. In the lumbar spine
   d. In the sacrum/pelvis
6. The most common causes of spinal cord injuries in children and adolescents is:
   a. Motor vehicle accidents
   b. Penetrating trauma
   c. Sports injuries
   d. Pedestrian accidents

REFERENCES

1. Greenbaum J, Walters N, Levy PD. An evidenced-based approach to radiographic assessment of cervical spine injuries in the emergency department. *J Emerg Med.* 2009;36:64–71.
2. Kendler DL, Bauer DC, Davison KS, et al. Vertebral fractures: clinical importance and management. *Am J Med.* 2016;129(221):e1–e10.
3. van Den Hauwe L, Sundgren PC, Flanders AE. Spinal trauma and spinal cord injury (SCI). In: Hodler J, Kubik-Huch RA, von Schulthess GK, eds. *Diseases of the Brain, Head and Neck, Spine 2020–2023: Diagnostic Imaging.* Springer; 2020.
4. Bono CM, Schoenfield, AJ. *Orthopaedic Surgery Essentials: Spine.* Wolters Kluwer; 2017.
5. Baaj AA, Uribe JS, Nichols TA, et al. Health care burden of cervical spine fractures in the United States: analysis of a nationwide database over a 10-year period: presented at the 2009 Joint AANS/CNS Spine Section Meeting. *Journal of Neurosurgery: Spine.* 2010;13:61–66.
6. Marcon RM, Cristante AF, Teixeira WJ, Narasaki DK, Oliveira RP, de Barros Filho TE. Fractures of the cervical spine. *Clinics (Sao Paulo).* 2013;68(11):1455–1461.
7. Wood KB, Li W, Lebl DS, Ploumis A. Management of thoracolumbar spine fractures. *The Spine Journal.* 2014;14:145–164.
8. Vaccaro AR, Hulbert RJ, Patel AA, et al. The subaxial cervical spine injury classification system. *Spine.* 2007;32:2365–2374.
9. Vaccaro AR, Lehman Jr RA, Hurlbert RJ. A new classification of thoracolumbar injuries: the importance of injury morphology, the integrity of the posterior ligamentous complex, and neurologic status. *Spine.* 2005;30:2325–2333.
10. Woods RO, Inceoglu S, Akpolat YT, et al. C1 lateral mass displacement and transverse atlantal ligament failure in Jefferson's fracture: a biomechanical study of the "Rule of Spence". *Neurosurgery.* 2018;82(2):226–231.
11. Anderson LD, D'Alonzo RT. Fractures of the odontoid process of the axis. *J Bone Joint Surg Am.* 1974;56:1663–1674.
12. Levine AM, Edwards CC. The management of traumatic spondylolisthesis of the axis. *J Bone Joint Surg Am.* 1985;67:217–226.
13. Joaquim AF, Patrell AA. Subaxial cervical spine trauma: evaluation and surgical decision making. *Global Spine J.* 2014;4:63–70.
14. Bevevino AJ, Vaccaro AR, Rubenstein R.Vialle LR, ed. The AOSpine thoracolumbar injury classification, Chapter 1. In: *AOSpine Masters Series; Thoracolumbar Spine Trauma.* Vol. 6. Thieme Medical Publishers, Inc; 2016.
15. Chance GQ. Note on a type of flexion fracture of the spine. *Br J Radiol.* 1948;21:452.
16. Denis F, Davis S, Comfort T. Sacral fracture: an important problem. Retrospective analysis of 236 cases. *Clin Orthop Relat Res.* 1988;227:67–81.
17. Gibbons KJ, Soloniuk DS, Razack N. Neurological injury and patterns of sacral fractures. *J Neurosurg.* 1990;72:889–893.
18. Roy-Camille R, Saillant G, Gagna G, et al. Transverse fracture of the upper sacrum. Suicide jumper's fracture. *Spine.* 1985;10:838–845.
19. Marsh JL, Slongo TF, Agel J, et al. Fracture and dislocation classification compendium—2007: Orthopaedic Trauma Association classification, database, and outcome committee. *J Orthop Trauma.* 2007;21 S1-S33.
20. Srinivasan V, Jea A. Pediatric thoracolumbar spine trauma. *Neurosurg Clin N Am.* 2017;28:103–114.
21. Saunders LL, Selassie A, Cao Y, et al. Epidemiology of pediatric traumatic spinal cord injury in a population-based cohort, 1998–2012. *Top Spinal Cord Inj Rehabil.* 2015;21(4): 325–332.
22. Alanay A, Yilgor C. Pediatric cervical spine. In: Vialle LR, ed. *AOSpine Masters Series: Cervical Spine Trauma.* 5. Thieme Medical Publishers, Inc; 2015.
23. Goldstein HE, Anderson RCE. Classification and management of pediatric craniocervical injuries. *Neurosurg Clin N Am.* 2017;28:73–90.
24. Pang D, Wilberger JE. Spinal cord injury without radiographic abnormalities in children. *J Neurosurg.* 1982; 57(1):114–129.
25. Allen Jr BL, Ferguson RL, Lehmann T. A mechanistic classification of closed, indirect fractures and dislocation of the lower cervical spine. *Spine.* 1982;7:1–27.
26. Benzel EC, ed. *Biomechanics of Spine Stabilization.* Rolling Meadows: American Association of Neurological Surgeons; 2001.
27. Berg EE. The sternal-rib complex: a possible fourth column thoracic spine fractures. *Spine.* 1993;18:1916–1919.
28. Denis F. The three-column spine and its significance in the classification of acute thoracolumbar spine injuries. *Spine.* 1983;8:817–831.
29. Kelly RP, Whitesides Jr. TE. Treatment of lumbodorsal fracture-dislocations. *Ann Surg.* 1968;167:705–717.
30. Magerl F, Aebi M, Gertzbein SD, et al. A comprehensive classification of thoracic and lumbar injuries. *Eur Spine J.* 1994;3:184–201.
31. Watson-Jones R. The results of postural reduction of fractures of the spine. *J Bone Joint Surg Am.* 1938;20:567–586.
32. White AA, Panjabi MM. Physical properties and functional biomechanics of the spine. In: White AA, Panjabi MM, eds. *Clinical Biomechanics of the Spine.* 2nd ed. Philadelphia: Lippincott Williams & Wilkins; 1990.
33. Fisher CG, DiPaola CP, Ryken TC, et al. A novel classification system for spinal instability in neoplastic disease: an evidence-based approach and expert consensus from the Spine Oncology Study Group. *Spine.* 2010;35:E1221–E1229.
34. Gire JD, Roberto RF, Bobinski M, et al. The utility and accuracy of computed tomography in the diagnosis of occipitocervical dissociation. *Spine J.* 2013;13:510–519.
35. Powers B, Miller MD, Kramer RS, et al. Traumatic anterior atlanto-occipital dislocation. *Neurosurgery.* 1979;4:12–17.
36. Harris Jr JHJ, Carson GC, Wagner LK, et al. Radiologic diagnosis of traumatic occipitovertebral dissociation: 2. Comparison of three methods of detecting occipitovertebral relationships on lateral radiographs of supine patients. *AJR Am J Roentgenol.* 1994;162:887–892.
37. Wholey MH, Bruwer AJ, Baker Jr. HL. The lateral roentgenogram of the neck; with comments on the atlanto-odontoid-basion relationship. *Radiology.* 1958;71:350–356.

Spine Complications

CHAPTER 26

Kevin Forster and Lance L. Goetz

OUTLINE

Intradural Complications

Posttraumatic Syringomyelia

Overview

Posttraumatic syringomyelia (PTS) is defined by the formation of a cyst, or syrinx, within the spinal cord, which may expand and cause neurologic change and myelopathy.[1–3] PTS is most commonly located at vascular watershed areas in the central and dorsolateral gray matter.[1,3] Most syrinxes spread superiorly from the site of injury.[1]

Pathophysiology

PTS is thought to be related to spinal cord tethering that causes alterations in cerebrospinal fluid (CSF) flow in the region of the original traumatic lesion. (See also Chapter 28.) It can be related to[1,2,4]:

- Hemorrhagic necrosis of the spinal cord
- Ischemia
- Arachnoiditis
- Liquefaction of a hematoma

Clinical Presentation

PTS is most commonly asymptomatic,[1] and it can present 2 months to 30 years after spinal cord injury (SCI).[3] When symptomatic, PTS is often unilateral early in the disease course.[3] Patients often report[1,2]:

- Pain, which can worsen with a Valsalva maneuver, sneeze, or cough
- Dysesthesia
- Hyperesthesia
- Loss of pain and temperature
- Relative preservation of light touch and proprioception[2]
- Motor weakness

Imaging

Magnetic resonance imaging (MRI) is the gold standard for diagnosis.[1,2]

Management

Patients with symptomatic syrinx managed conservatively may have progression and worsening myelopathy.[1] Surgery is indicated in cases of progressive neurological change in the setting of progressive syrinx and cord compression. Shunting of CSF is often an initial treatment, although it has been reported that shunting has a low long-term success rate in PTS.[5] Postoperative complications include[1]:

- Shunt failure
- Infection
- Pseudomeningocele
- Peritoneal pseudocyst

Adhesive Arachnoiditis

Overview

Scarring of the pial and arachnoid membranes within the thecal sac is secondary to chronic inflammation.[6] Focal adhesions may progress to scarring that eradicates the subarachnoid space and impairs the flow of CSF.[1,4] This can be related to[1]:

- Trauma
- Infection
- Complication of myelography
- Intrathecal steroid injection
- Subarachnoid hemorrhage
- Lumbar degenerative disc
- Prior spine surgery

Pathophysiology

Adhesive arachnoiditis is an inflammation that causes proliferation of soft tissue and adhesions, which eventually progress to fibrosis. It may develop acutely after the initial insult or, most commonly, several years later.[1]

Signs and Symptoms

- Lumbar arachnoiditis
  - Radiculopathy
  - Sensory deficits
  - Back pain

- Cervicothoracic arachnoiditis
  - Myelopathy

Diagnosis

MRI is the preferred imaging method.[6] It may reveal:

- Clumped nerve roots in the thecal sac.
- Peripherally adherent nerve roots with an empty thecal sac appearance.
- Soft tissue mass in the spinal canal and obliteration of the subarachnoid space.[1,7]

Treatment

Conservative management includes oral steroids that may result in temporary improvement in symptoms only.[1] Intrathecal steroid injection is not recommended due to reports of arachnoiditis secondary to injection. Surgical management goals are to repair the CSF pathways and to dissect any adhering or scarring of the arachnoid membrane.[5,8]

Progressive Posttraumatic Myelopathy

Overview

Myelopathy in patients with chronic SCI may manifest with chronic, debilitating symptoms. Presentation may be variable depending on the level of injury and any late complications such as syringomyelia. Symptoms can include[1]:

- Focal neck or back pain
- Extremity pain
- Paresthesias
- Weakness
- Autonomic dysregulation
- Bowel changes
- Bladder changes
- Spasticity
- Hyperreflexia
- Clonus

Imaging

MRI is the gold standard; degeneration of the cord at the site of injury may be seen.

Treatment

The treatment goal is symptomatic pain control and prevention of worsening neurologic status. Surgical intervention is indicated in the setting of clinical decline, to attempt to prevent worsening myelopathy.[1]

Axial Complications

Structural changes to the spine can occur after an SCI. These changes can include abnormal curvatures of the spine, such as kyphosis, or scoliosis. Acutely, they are often a direct result of the inciting trauma, as the impact forces cause compression and instability in the spine. In the chronic setting, deformity may be related to surgical or nonsurgical complications.[1]

- Surgical complications[1,9]:
  - Implant failure
  - Excessive force at implant bone junction
  - Technical error
  - Osteoporotic bone
- Nonsurgical complications[1,9]:
  - Osteonecrosis of the spine
  - Charcot spine

Pseudoarthrosis

Overview

Pseudarthrosis is abnormal spinal motion at a site of fusion. It is often related to a failed surgical spinal fusion. The continuous low-grade motion present at a fusion site interferes with an osseous union at the bone-hardware interface.[10]

Symptoms

- Axial or radicular pain[10]
- Exacerbation of neurologic symptoms[11]

Imaging[10,11]

- Lucency through the bone graft
- Endplate erosion and sclerosis
- Loss of fixation

Charcot Spine

Overview

Charcot spinal arthropathy, also known as neuropathic spinal arthropathy, is uncommon. It is characterized by a progressive bony and ligamentous injury of the spine.[10] Charcot joints can develop in a variety of joints in the body as a result of a loss of deep sensation and proprioception in a joint that has preserved movement. They can be seen with diseases that cause a loss of peripheral sensation including[12,13]:

- SCI
- Syringomyelia
- Diabetic neuropathy
- Tertiary syphilis

In SCI, Charcot changes occur below the neurologic level of injury. Charcot spine is more common in neurologically complete SCI.[1] On average, it occurs 17.3 years after the initial trauma.[12]

Pathophysiology

Charcot spine is thought to be related to neurotraumatic and neurovascular injury. The loss of sensation interferes with the normal protective neuromuscular reflexes of the paraspinal musculature that would typically occur if significant stress were placed on a joint. The loss of joint protective mechanisms results in increased stress on the spinal ligaments. Repetitive stress results in injury and progressive instability.[10,14] This increased instability leads to repetitive trauma to the spine, causing[10,14]:

- Inflammation
- Callus formation
- Microfractures

Signs and Symptoms

Delayed diagnosis is common. The sensory deficits that lead to the Charcot joint can cause delayed symptom manifestation. When present, symptoms can include[10]:

- Low back pain
- Kyphosis
- Scoliosis
- Spinal crepitus
- Neurologic changes
  - Loss of sensation
  - Worsening weakness
  - Spasticity
  - Autonomic dysreflexia

Diagnosis

Charcot joint is most common at the thoracolumbar and lumbosacral junctions. Diagnosis can be difficult, as common imaging findings overlap with many diseases on the differential.[10]

Imaging[1,10]

- Early disease:
  - Hypertrophic bone around the vertebrae below the neurologic level of injury
- Late disease:
  - Destruction of joint surfaces
  - Fractures of the subchondral bone
  - Vertebral collapse
  - Pseudoarthrosis (Figs. 26.1 and 26.2)

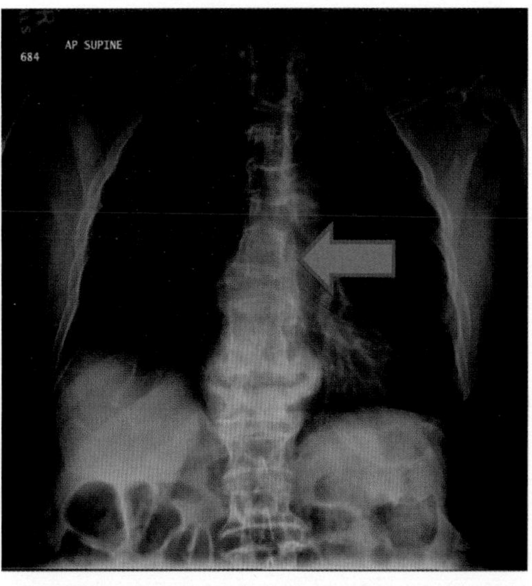

Fig. 26.1 Midthoracic Charcot deformity of the spine.

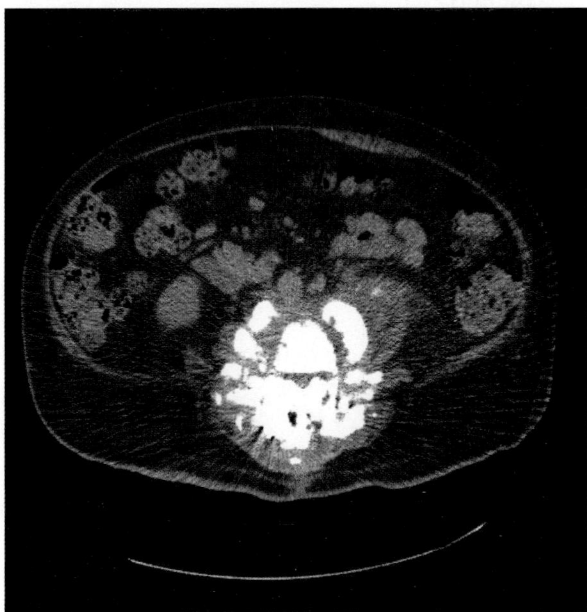

Fig. 26.2 Charcot deformity of the spine.

Differential[10]

- Pyogenic spinal infection
- Discitis osteomyelitis
- Atypical infection
  - Osseous tuberculosis
- Degenerative joint disease
- Hemodialysis-related spondyloarthropathy
- Pseudoarthrosis

Complications[1]

- Neurologic deficits secondary to degenerative changes in spine and ligaments causing disruption of neural structures
- Kyphosis
- Stenosis
- Scoliosis
- Arachnoiditis
- Cord tethering

Treatment

Treatment is often surgical. The goal of surgical treatment is to reconstruct the supporting structures of the injured spine.[10,13,14]

Kyphosis

Posttraumatic kyphosis can be seen after a traumatic injury. Its underlying cause is dependent upon the time from initial injury[1]:

- In the acute setting, kyphosis may be a result of compression and instability from the initial impact
- In the chronic setting, kyphosis can be related to surgical complications or nonsurgical causes (osteonecrosis of the vertebral spine, Charcot spine)

Signs and Symptoms[1]

- Spinal deformity
- Low back pain
- Change in neurologic status
- Autonomic dysreflexia
- Crepitus

Imaging

Measurement compares the angle between the superior and inferior endplates of the adjacent vertebra.

Treatment[1,9]

- Surgery is considered if:
  - The kyphotic curve is progressive
  - There are worsening neurologic deficits
- Goal of surgery:
  - Decompression of the neural structures
  - Provide support across the anterior and posterior columns[1]

Scoliosis

Scoliosis is less common than kyphotic deformity. It can be seen with lateral compression or burst injury.[1,9]

Treatment

Surgery is indicated with[9]:

- Progressive scoliotic curve that causes spinal imbalance
- Worsening neurologic deficits that are refractory to conservative management

Review Questions

1. The most common symptom of posttraumatic syringomyelia is:
   a. Pain
   b. Weakness
   c. Asymptomatic
   d. Loss of sensation to light touch
2. The underlying cause of Charcot spine is:
   a. Instability of the spine related to initial trauma
   b. Failure of surgical fusion
   c. Motor weakness of paraspinal musculature
   d. Loss of sensation in a joint with preserved motion
3. During an annual follow-up visit, a patient with a 5-year history of T3 sensory incomplete (AIS B) SCI notes that she has noted an increasingly stooped posture. You obtain plain film imaging of the cervical, thoracic, and lumbar spine and note that there is increased thoracic kyphosis with an angle of 15 degrees. Neurologic and functional history and examination are unchanged from previous years. You recommend:
   a. Referral for surgical fixation
   b. Obtain MRI of thoracic spine
   c. Order thoracolumbosacral orthosis bracing
   d. Obtain repeat imaging in 6 months
4. The gold standard imaging for posttraumatic syringomyelia is:
   a. Plain film
   b. Computed tomography
   c. MRI
   d. Computed tomography myelogram
5. Pseudarthrosis is caused by:
   a. Spinal motion at a site of spine fusion
   b. Traumatic injury to spinal joints
   c. Loss of protective reflexes of the paraspinal musculature
   d. Osteonecrosis of the spine

REFERENCES

1. Nehaw S, Lee BS, Benzel EC. Spine complications in patients with chronic spinal cord injury. In: Kirshblum S, Lin VW, eds. *Spinal Cord Medicine*. 3rd ed. New York: Demos Medical Publishing; 2019:559–566.
2. Karam Y, Hitchon PW, Mhanna NE, He W, Noeller J. Post-traumatic syringomyelia: outcome predictors. *Clinical Neurology and Neurosurgery*. 2014;124:44–50.
3. Little JW. Syringomyelia. In: Lin VW, Cardenas DD, eds. *Spinal Cord Medicine: Principles and Practice*. New York: Demos; 2003:501–507.
4. Holly LT, Johnson JP, Masciopinto JE, Batzdorf U. Treatment of posttraumatic syringomyelia with extradural decompressive surgery. *FOC*. 2000;8(3):1–6.
5. Aghakhani N, Baussart B, David P, et al. Surgical treatment of posttraumatic syringomyelia. *Neurosurgery*. 2010;66(6): 1120–1127, discussion 1127.
6. Waldman SD. Arachnoiditis. In: Waldman SD, ed. *Atlas of Common Pain Syndromes*. 4th ed. Philadelphia: Elsevier; 2019:328–331.
7. Delamarter RB, Ross JS, Masaryk TJ, Modic MT, Bohlman HH. Diagnosis of lumbar arachnoiditis by magnetic resonance imaging. *Spine (Phila Pa 1976)*. 1990;15(4):304–310.
8. Klekamp J, Batzdorf U, Samii M, Bothe HW. Treatment of syringomyelia associated with arachnoid scarring caused by arachnoiditis or trauma. *J Neurosurg*. 1997;86(2):233–240.
9. Vaccaro AR, Silber JS. Post-traumatic spinal deformity. *Spine*. 2001 Dec;26(Supplement):S111–S118.
10. Ledbetter LN, Salzman KL, Sanders RK, Shah LM. Spinal neuroarthropathy: pathophysiology, clinical and imaging features, and differential diagnosis. *RadioGraphics*. 2016;36(3):783–799.
11. Chun DS, Baker KC, Hsu WK. Lumbar pseudarthrosis: a review of current diagnosis and treatment. *FOC*. 2015;39(4):E10.
12. Grassner L, Geuther M, Mach O, Bühren V, Vastmans J, Maier D. Charcot spinal arthropathy: an increasing long-term sequel after spinal cord injury with no straightforward management. *Spinal Cord Ser Cases*. 20158;1(1):15022.
13. Suda Y, Shioda M, Kohno H, Machida M, Yamagishi M. Surgical treatment of Charcot spine. *J Spinal Disord Tech*. 2007;20(1):85–88.
14. Schwartz HS. Traumatic Charcot spine. *J Spinal Disord*. 1990;3(3):269–275.

CHAPTER

27 Spinal Orthoses

Jeffrey Tubbs

OUTLINE

Introduction

Spinal orthoses can be categorized by materials used, soft, rigid, or semirigid, and/or by spinal regions incorporated. General indications for spinal orthoses include:

- Pain control
- Spine stabilization and immobilization
  Preventing and correcting deformities[1]

Orthotics Biomechanics

The functional spinal unit is a three-joint complex with the vertebral body articulating with the intervertebral disc (anteriorly) and two facet joints (posteriorly).[2]

This joint complex allows movement in three planes:

- Sagittal (flexion/extension)
- Lateral bending
- Axial rotation

Movement of the trunk alters loading, strain, and shear forces on the spine.

- Loading forces: axial compression through the three-joint complex
- Strain forces: on disks and ligaments placed under stretch
- Shear forces: between disks and vertebral endplates horizontally[3] (Fig. 27.1)

Additional considerations for orthotic needs are taken into account after trauma and operative care, including spinal stability, fracture type, comorbidities, and goals of care.[4] Primary goals for orthoses treatment of spinal injuries include protecting the spinal column from stress that causes progression of deformity and inhibits healing.[5,6]

The Denis three column theory describes spinal instability in terms of the anatomical structures involved. The spine is considered unstable if two contiguous columns are affected:

- Anterior: anterior longitudinal ligament, anterior two-thirds vertebral body, anterior annulus fibrosis
- Middle: posterior one-third vertebral body, posterior annulus fibrosis, posterior longitudinal ligament
- Posterior: pedicles, facets, ligamentum flavum, spinous process, supraspinous and intraspinous ligaments

The Denis classification also describes four types of fractures: compression, burst, seatbelt, fracture/dislocation[7,8] (Table 27.1).

Cervical Orthoses

Cervical orthoses are commonly used to treat various causes of neck pain, trauma, and postoperative care.

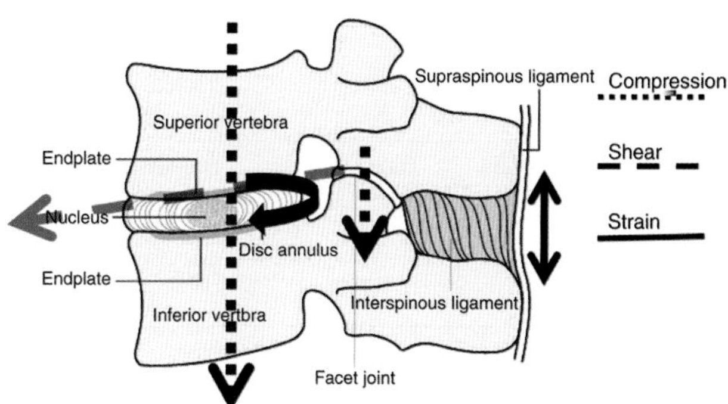

Fig. 27.1 Anteriorly, vertebral bodies articulate with a fibrocartilaginous intervertebral disc and posteriorly, with two facets. Trunk movements produce compressive loading forces *(dotted black arrows)* directed axially through the three-joint complex, strain forces *(solid black arrows)* stretch the elastic fibers within connective tissue, and shear forces *(dotted gray arrow)* are directed horizontally at the interface of articulating surfaces. (Courtesy Stellman JM. *Encyclopedia of Occupational Health and Safety*. 4th ed. Geneva Switzerland: International Labor Office; 1998. Adapted from Rolin OY, Carter III WE. Biomechanics of the spine. In: Webster JB, Murphy DP, eds. *Atlas of Orthoses and Assistive Devices*. 5th ed. Philadelphia: Elsevier; 2019:65.)

Table 27.1 Summary of Main Fracture Types

Level		Type		Mechanism of Injury	Remarks	Orthoses
Upper cervical	C1	Jefferson		Axial load	Triplanar instability	Halo vest
	C2	Hangman		Hyperextension plus distraction	Traumatic spondylolisthesis, triplanar instability	Halo vest
		Odontoid		Shear plus compression	Type I: stable; types II and III: unstable	Halo vest
Lower cervical	C3–C7	Anterior compression		Hyperflexion	C5 most common level, possible brachial plexus involvement	Rigid collar
		Whiplash		Hyperextension	Soft tissue injury to anterior longitudinal ligament likely, long-term risk for chronic forward head posture	Soft collar
CERVICOTHORACIC JUNCTION INJURIES SPANNING THIS LEVEL REQUIRE A CTO OR CTLSO						
Upper thoracic	T1–T8	Denis classification applies to all thoracic and lumbar levels	Denis I: anterior compression	Flexion plus compression	3/4 of thoracolumbar fractures are of this type, 2/3 of those occur at T12–L1–L2 Anterior column damage only in most cases Posterior ligamentous injury may indicate instability	Hyperextension is the mechanism of action Common choices: corsets, Jewett (milder injuries), and TLSOs (custom or prefabricated)
			Denis II: burst	Compression plus flexion	Anterior and middle columns are damaged Fracture of superior endplate is more commonThere may be retropulsion of one or more fragments from the posterior wall	
Lower thoracic	T9–T12		Denis III: chance and slice	Flexion plus distraction ("seat belt injury")	Chance: posterior and middle column damage to vertebral body Slice: posterior and middle column damage to intervertebral disc Surgery is indicated	
THORACOLUMBAR JUNCTION (T12–L1–2) ARE VERY COMMON FRACTURE SITES AND REQUIRE A TLSO						
Upper lumbar	L1–L2		Denis IV: fracture dislocation	Translation, flexion, rotation, shear	Complete disruption of anterior, middle, and posterior columns Surgery is indicated	N/A
Lower lumbar	L3–L5	Other	Spondylolysis and spondylolisthesis	May be a sports-related injury from gymnastic-sIn adults, may cause chronic LBP	Common in the lower lumbar spine, especially L4–L5 and L5–S1 Spondylolisthesis usually requires posterior pelvic tilt in the orthosis	Custom LSO or TLSO

CTLSO, Cervicothoracolumbosacral orthosis; *CTO*, cervicothoracic orthosis; *LBP*, lower back pain; *LSO*, lumbosacral orthosis; *TLSO*, thoracolumbosacral orthosis.

Courtesy Malas BS, Meade KP, Patwardhan AG, et al. Orthoses for spinal trauma and postoperative care. In Hsu JD, Michael JW, Fisk JR, eds. *AAOS Atlas of Orthoses and Assistive Devices.* 4th ed. Philadelphia: Mosby; 2008.

Adapted from Romanoski N, Schultz S, Gater Jr DR. Orthoses for spinal trauma and postoperative care. In: Webster JB, Murphy DP, eds. *Atlas of Orthoses and Assistive Devices.* 5th ed. Philadelphia: Elsevier; 2019:107.

Cervical Soft Collar

This collar provides minimal motion restriction of the cervical spine but can serve a role as a kinesthetic reminder and provide some warmth and comfort for muscle pain.[9,10] Indications include minor muscles spasm, muscle strain.

Rigid Cervical Collar

The rigid collar provides greater motion restriction than a soft collar but is less well tolerated due to discomfort. Examples of this collar include Miami J, Aspen, and Philadelphia (Fig. 27.2).

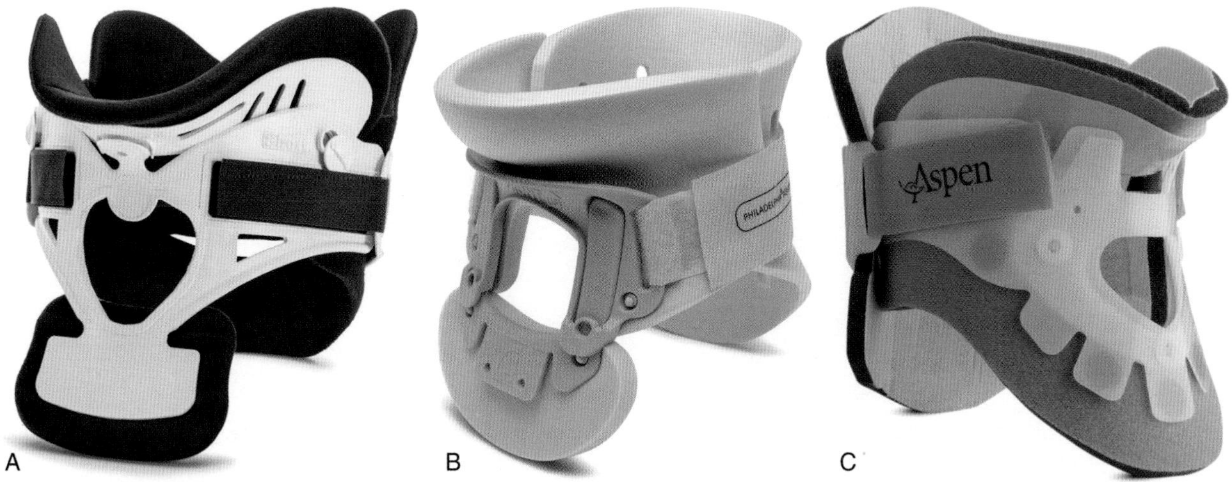

Fig. 27.2 Semirigid Collar: (A) Miami J collar. (B) Philadelphia collar. (C) Aspen collar. (A and B, Courtesy Össur, Inc.; C, Courtesy of Aspen Medical Products, copyright 2016.)

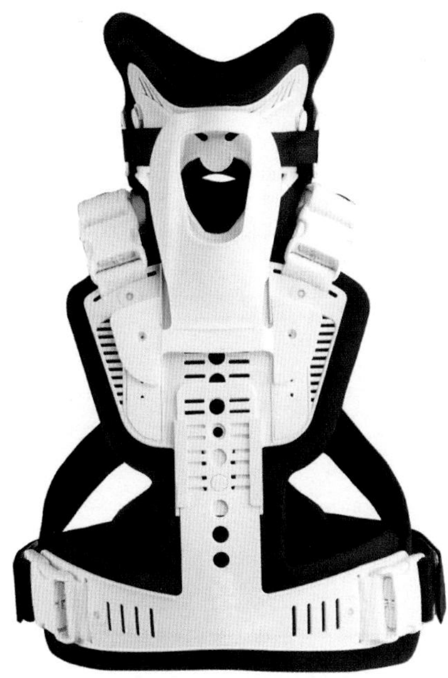

Fig. 27.3 Cervicothoracic Orthosis. Miami JTO. (Courtesy of: Össur, Inc.)

Cervical Thoracic Orthoses

Miami JTO

Offers a thoracic extension on the traditional Miami J. Indications include cervical and high thoracic injuries (Fig. 27.3).[11]

Sternal Occipital Mandibular Immobilizer

Provides good flexion control but allows some extension/rotation/lateral motion.[9] Indications include cervical strain/sprain, stable fractures with intact ligaments, postoperative support (Fig. 27.4).[10]

Halo Vest

Offers triplanar cervical spine motion control. Indications include unstable cervical fractures, high cervical injuries (occiput–C2), C1 fractures with transverse ligament rupture, dens fractures, C2 neural arch fractures, atlantoaxial instability (Fig. 27.5; Tables 27.2 and 27.3).[1,11]

Thoracolumbosacral Orthoses

Thoracolumbosacral orthoses (TLSOs) are largely designed with a three-point pressure application (sternum, spine, pelvis, ribs, etc.) for treatment of thoracolumbar pathology and postoperative care.

Molded Thoracolumbosacral Orthoses, Body Jacket, Clam Shell

This is a common TLSO that provides the most effective triplanar stabilization. It is a total contact orthotic that is the most restrictive in limiting thoracolumbar flexion/extension/rotation/lateral bending. Indications include middle to lower thoracic or lumbar fractures, postoperative immobilization after spinal decompression/fusion/stabilization (Fig. 27.6).[1]

Cruciform Anterior Spinal Hyperextension

The cruciform anterior spinal hyperextension (CASH) brace limits flexion. Indications include kyphosis/compression fracture (Fig. 27.7).

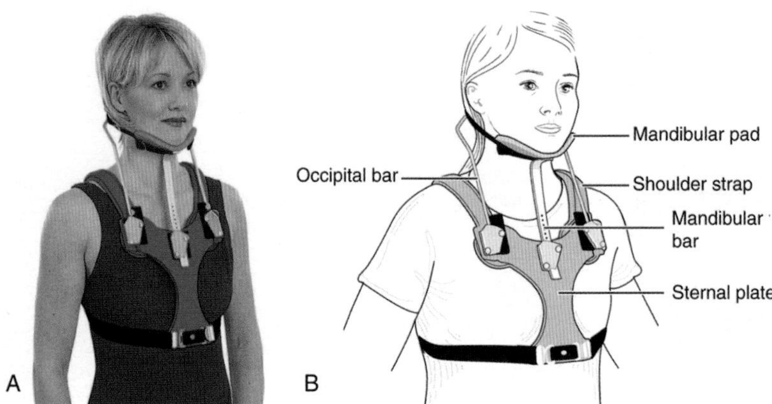

Fig. 27.4 Cervicothoracic Orthosis. (A) Sternal occipital mandibular immobilizer style. (B) Components of the sternal occipital mandibular immobilizer. (A, Courtesy of Trulife.)

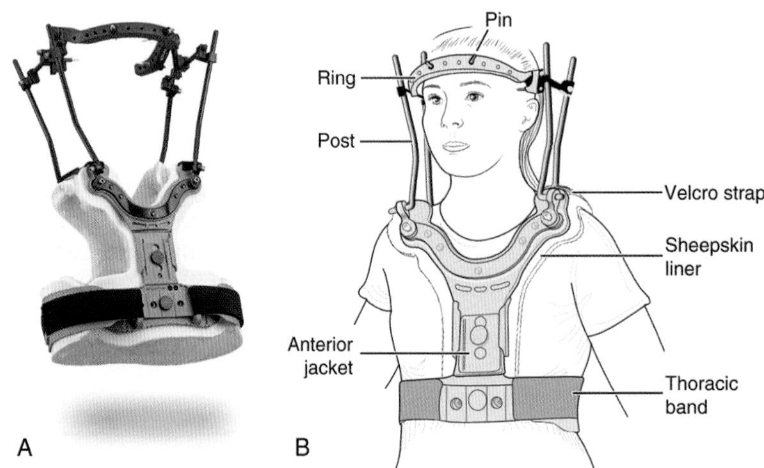

Fig. 27.5 (A) Ambulatory halo orthosis. (B) Components of the ambulatory halo orthosis. (A, Courtesy of Össur, Inc.)

Hyperextension (Jewett)

This brace limits flexions but has more lateral support compared with the CASH.[10,12] Indications include compression fractures (Fig. 27.8).

Taylor

This brace limits flexion/extension and allows minimal axial rotation. Indications include kyphosis, stable thoracolumbar fractures, and postoperative immobilization.

Knight-Taylor

This brace limits flexion/extension/lateral flexion and allows minimal axial rotation. Indications include stable thoracolumbar fractures and postoperative immobilization (Fig. 27.9).

Orthoses Thoracolumbar Fractures and Trauma

The lower thoracic spinal segments are more mobile as they do not have as many direct rib attachments to the sternum as the upper thoracic levels do. The T12–L1 level is at increased risk for traumatic injuries and degenerative disease over time as it is a junction between the thoracic spine and fixed sacrum.[1]

Compression Fractures

Compression fractures commonly occur due to poor bone density and are caused by minimal, if any, trauma. These fractures lead to anterior vertebral height loss and wedging of the anterior column on imaging.[13] Some single-level injuries may be managed with activity/ambulation and extension exercise alone. Typical

Table 27.2 Normal Cervical Motion From Occiput to First Thoracic Vertebra and the Effects of Cervical Orthoses

	Mean of Normal Motion (%)		
Orthosis	**Flexion or Extension**	**Lateral Bending**	**Rotation**
Normal[a]	100.0	100.0	100.0
Soft collar[a]	74.2	92.3	82.6
Philadelphia collar	28.9	66.4	43.7
Sternal occipital mandibular immobilizer orthosis	27.7	65.6	33.6
Four-poster brace	20.6	45.9	27.1
Yale cervicothoracic brace	12.8	50.5	18.2
Halo device[a]	4.0	4.0	1.0
Halo device[b]	11.7	8.4	2.4
Minerva body jacket[c]	14.0	15.5	0

[a]Data from Johnson RM, Hart DL, Simmons EF, et al. Cervical orthoses: a study comparing their effectiveness in restricting cervical motion in normal subjects. *J Bone Joint Surg Am.* 1977;59:332.
[b]Data from Lysell E. Motion in the cervical spine, thesis. *Acta Orthop Scand.* 1969;(Suppl 123):1.
[c]Data from Maiman D, Millington P, Novak S, et al. The effects of the thermoplastic Minerva body jacket on cervical spine motion. *Neurosurgery.* 1989;25:363-368.
Adapted from Norbury JW, Tilley E, Moore DP. Spinal orthoses. In Cifu DX, ed. *Braddom's Physical Medicine & Rehabilitation.* 5th ed. Philadelphia: Elsevier; 2016:277.

Table 27.3 Movement Restriction of Cervical and Cervicothoracic Orthoses

	Mean Residual Normal Motion (%)		
Orthosis	**Flexion or Extension**	**Lateral Bending**	**Rotation**
Normal[a]	100	100	100
Soft collar[a]	74.2	92.3	82.6
Philadelphia	28.9	66.4	43.7
Sternal occipital mandibular immobilizer	27.7	65.6	33.6
Four-poster	20.6	45.9	27.1
Yale cervicotho-racic brace	12.8	50.5	18.2
Halo[a]	4.0	4.0	1.0
Halo[b]Ŧ	11.7	8.4	2.4
Minervaŧ	14.0	15.5	0

[a]Data from Johnson RM, Hart DL, Simmons EF, et al. Cervical orthoses: a study comparing their effectiveness in restricting cervical motion in normal subjects. *J Bone Joint Surg Am.* 1977;59:332.
Ŧ[b]Data from Lysell E. Motion in the cervical spine, thesis. *Acta Orthop Scand.* 1969;(Suppl 123):1.
Norbury JW, Tilley E, Moore DP. Spinal orthoses. In Cifu DX, ed. *Braddom's Physical Medicine & Rehabilitation.* 5th ed. Philidelphia: Elsevier; 2016:275-287.

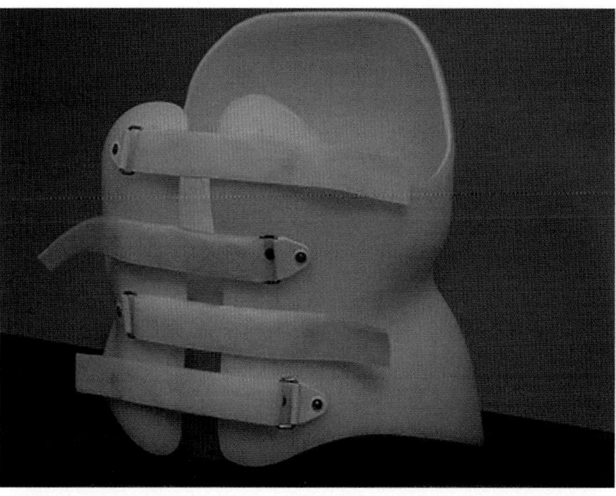

Fig. 27.6 Thoracolumbosacral Orthosis (custom-fabricated body jacket). (Adapted from Norbury JW, Tilley E, Moore DP. Spinal orthoses. In Cifu DX, ed. *Braddom's Physical Medicine & Rehabilitation*. 5th ed. Philidelphia: Elsevier; 2016:281.)

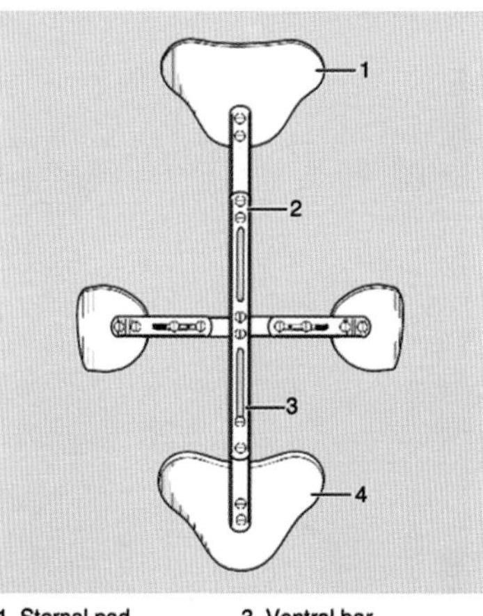

Fig. 27.7 Thoracolumbosacral orthosis: flexion control, CASH style. CASH brace components. (Adapted from: Fig 6.9 from Weppner JL, Alfano AP. Principles and Components of Spinal Orthoses. In: Webster JB, Murphy DP. *Atlas of Orthoses and Assistive Devices*. 5th Ed. Philadelphia: Elsevier; 2019. p. 73)

orthoses are Jewett or CASH. If loss of height >85%, orthoses alone may not prevent progression.[4,5]

Burst Fracture

Burst fractures are typically due to axial compression with sagittal flexion. Orthotic management is typically with a total contact-molded TLSO. Surgical intervention is generally indicated if the kyphotic curve is >25%, anterior height loss is >50%, or if there is subluxation, dislocation, or significant spinal canal compromise.[14]

Chance (Lap Belt) Fracture

This fracture type may be seen after flexion–distraction injuries. It may require surgery. Orthotic

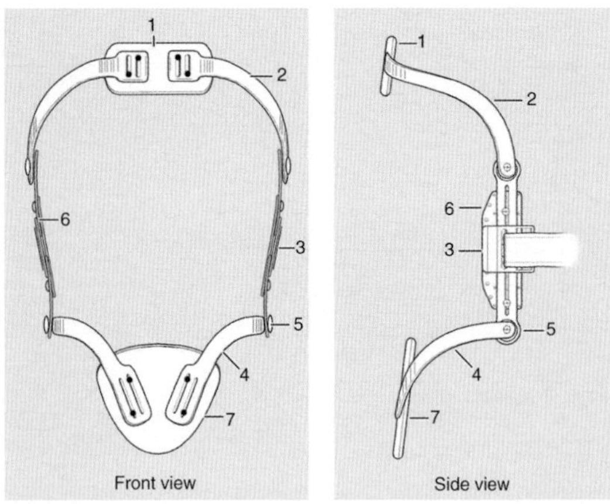

1. Sternal pad 2. Side rails 3. Quick-release closure lever 4. Pelvic band 5. Rotation connector 6. Adjustable lateral uprights 7. Suprapubic pad

Fig. 27.8 Thoracolumbosacral orthosis: flexion control, Jewett style. Jewett brace components. (Adapted from Weppner JL, Alfano AP. Principles and components of spinal orthoses. In: Webster JB, Murphy DP, eds. *Atlas of Orthoses and Assistive Devices*. 5th ed. Philadelphia: Elsevier; 2019:72.)

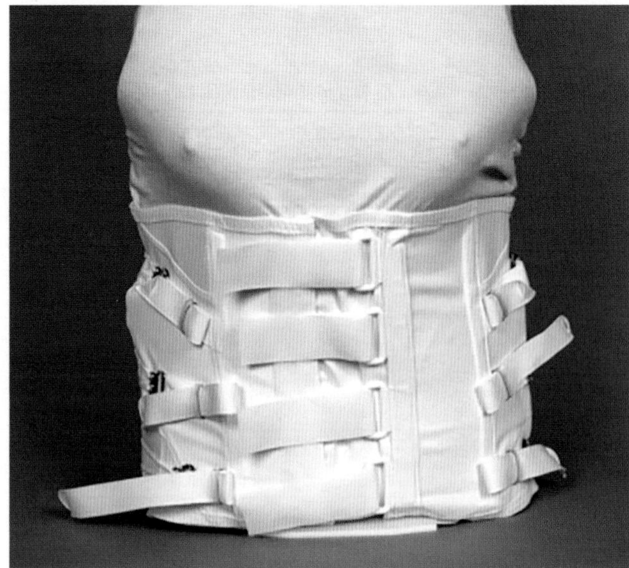

Fig. 27.10 Lumbosacral Corset. (Adapted from Norbury JW, Tilley E, Moore DP. Spinal orthoses. In Cifu DX, ed. *Braddom's Physical Medicine & Rehabilitation*. 5th ed. Philadelphia: Elsevier; 2016:282.)

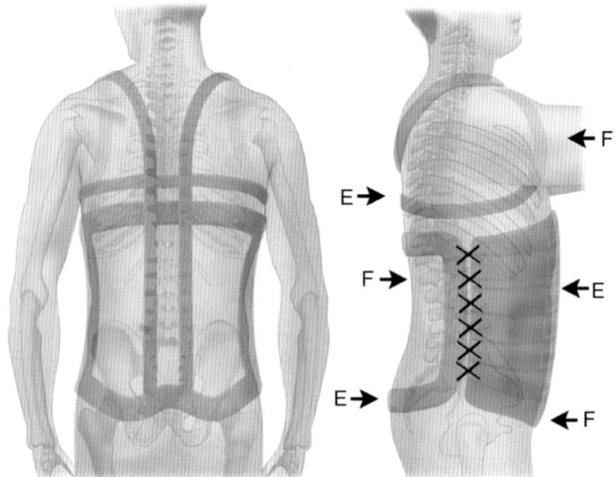

Fig. 27.9 Conventional thoracolumbosacral orthosis: sagittal-coronal control, Knight-Taylor style. With three-point pressure systems delineated. *E*, Extension control; *F*, flexion control. (B, Modified from American Academy of Orthopaedic Surgeons. *Atlas of Orthotics*. 2nd ed. St. Louis: CV Mosby; 1985. Adapted from Weppner JL, Alfano AP. Principles and components of spinal orthoses. In: Webster JB, Murphy DP, eds. *Atlas of Orthoses and Assistive Devices*. 5th ed. Philadelphia: Elsevier; 2019:74.)

management includes a TLSO w/anterior control or a total contact TLSO.

Lumbosacral Orthoses

Soft or Semirigid Corsets

The corset can provide some limited motion restriction, increase abdominal pressure, contribute to reduced axial load on vertebral bodies, and provide a kinesthetic reminder to control motion. Indications include mechanical low back pain, minor muscles spasms, muscle strain (Fig. 27.10).[11]

Lumbosacral (LSO-Chairback)

The LSO-chairback brace is composed of a thoracic band, pelvic band, and two paraspinal bars that control flexion/extension and some lateral flexion. Indications include degenerative disk disease, herniated disk, spondylolisthesis, mechanical back pain, and limited postoperative care for lumbar decompressions/fusions (Fig. 27.11).[10]

Lumbosacral (LSO-Knight)

This orthosis is the same as the chairback but includes lateral bars to reduce side motion along with flexion/extension. Indications include the same as those for chairback use.

Lumbosacral (LSO-Williams Flexion)

The LSO-Williams flexion brace is composed of a thoracic band, pelvic band, lateral bars, and oblique bars. Ultimately, it allows for flexion and restricts extension. Indications include low back pain, spondylolysis, and spondylolisthesis (Fig. 27.11).

Sacroiliac Orthoses

These orthoses can limit some pelvic flexion/extension as well as provide pelvic compression. They are largely prefabricated, soft, and adjustable. Indications include pelvis fractures, symphysis pubis fracture, or pain.[10]

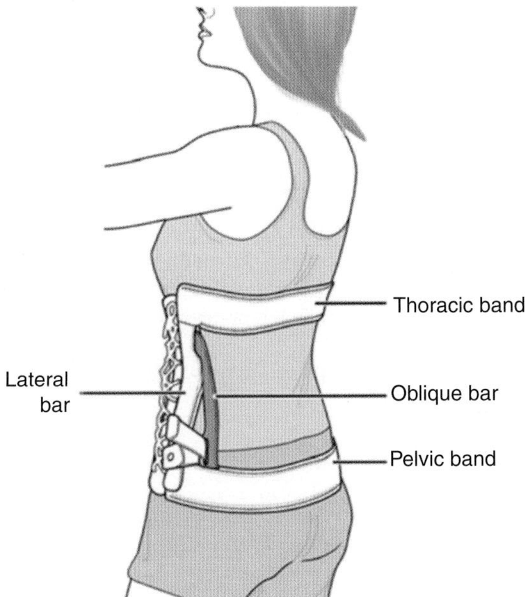

Fig. 27.11 Lumbosacral orthosis: extension–coronal control. The oblique bars of the Williams brace follow the body contour. The oblique bars provide structural integrity for the orthosis but do not contribute to motion control. Orthopaedic Surgeons. (Adapted from Weppner JL, Alfano AP. Principles and components of spinal orthoses. In: Webster JB, Murphy DP, eds. *Atlas of Orthoses and Assistive Devices*. 5th ed. Philadelphia: Elsevier; 2019: 72.)

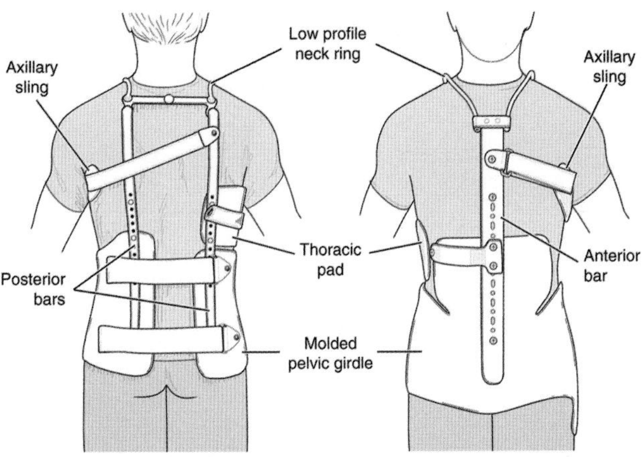

Fig. 27.12 Milwaukee Orthosis Components. (Adapted from Weppner JL, Alfano AP. Principles and components of spinal orthoses. In: Webster JB, Murphy DP, eds. *Atlas of Orthoses and Assistive Devices*. 5th ed. Philadelphia: Elsevier; 2019:82.)

Orthoses for Spinal Deformity

Orthoses can be an important treatment option for scoliosis and spinal deformities. Indications include idiopathic scoliosis; orthoses are indicated for children/adolescents who have curves of 25–40 degrees and at least 2 years of growth remaining.[15]

The Milwaukee brace is a commonly prescribed orthosis for treatment (Fig. 27.12). Additional custom-molded orthoses include the Boston Brace, Rosenberger, Miami, and Wilmington braces.[16]

Review Questions

1. What are potential complications of spinal orthoses?
   a. Pain
   b. Pressure injury
   c. Muscle atrophy
   d. All of the above
2. In general, how many points of contact are needed for appropriate spinal immobilization?
   a. 2
   b. 3
   c. 4
   d. 5
3. Head–cervical orthoses (such as the Miami J or Aspen collar) are most effective at limiting
   a. Flexion/extension
   b. Lateral bending
   c. Rotation
   d. Axial load
4. Axial compressive loads on the spine are generated from
   a. Gravity
   b. External forces
   c. Physical activity
   d. Muscle tension
   e. All of the above
5. Single-level thoracolumbar compression fractures are typically treated with
   a. Flexion orthosis
   b. Extension orthosis
   c. Total contact TLSO
   d. Surgical repair

REFERENCES

1. Frost F, Najarian CR. Spinal orthoses. In: Kirshblum S, Campagnolo DI, eds. *Spinal Cord Medicine*. 2nd ed. Philadelphia: Lippincott Williams & Wilkins; 2011:359–370.
2. Rolin OY, Carter III WE. Biomechanics of the spine. In: Webster JB, Murphy DP, eds. *Atlas of Orthoses and Assistive Devices*. 5th ed. Philadelphia: Elsevier; 2019:64–69.
3. Izzo R. Stability and instability of the spine. In: Manfrè L, ed. *Spinal Instability, New Procedures in Spinal Interventional Neuroradiology*. Switzerland: Springer International Publishing; 2015.
4. Romanoski N, Schultz S, Gater Jr DR. Orthoses for spinal trauma and postoperative care. In: Webster JB, Murphy DP, eds. *Atlas of Orthoses and Assistive Devices*. 5th ed. Philadelphia: Elsevier; 2019:105–114.
5. Patwardhan AG, Li S, Gavin TM, et al. Orthotic stabilization of thoracolumbar injuries: a biomechanical analysis of the Jewett hyperextension orthosis. *Spine*. 1990;15:654–661.
6. White A, Panjabi M. *Clinical Biomechanics of the Spine*. 2nd ed. Philidelphia: Lippincott; 1990.

7. Denis F. Spinal instability as defined by the three-column spine concept in acute spinal trauma. *Clin Orthop Relat Res.* 1984;189:65–76.
8. Denis F. The three-column spine and its significance in the classification of acute thoracolumbar spinal injuries. *Spine.* 1983;8:817–831.
9. Johnson RM, Hart DL, Simmons EF, et al. Cervical orthoses. A study comparing their effectiveness in restricting cervical motion in normal subjects. *J Bone Joint Surg Am.* 1977;59(3):332–339.
10. Norbury JW, Tilley E, Moore DP. Spinal orthoses. In: Cifu DX, ed. *Braddom's Physical Medicine & Rehabilitation.* 5th ed. Philidelphia: Elsevier; 2016:275–287.
11. Weppner JL, Alfano AP. Principles and components of spinal orthoses. In: Webster JB, Murphy DP, eds. *Atlas of Orthoses and Assistive Devices.* 5th ed. Philadelphia: Elsevier; 2019:69–89.
12. Jewett E. Hyperextension back brace. *J Bone Joint Surg.* 1937;19:1128.
13. Raiser SN, Alfano AP. Orthoses for osteoporosis. In: Webster JB, Murphy DP, eds. *Atlas of Orthoses and Assistive Devices.* 5th ed. Philadelphia: Elsevier; 2019:115–125.
14. Chang V, Holly LT. Bracing for thoracolumbar fractures. *Neurosurg Focus.* 2014;37(1):E3.
15. Newton P, Wenger D, Yaszay B. Idiopathic scoliosis. In: Weinstein SL, Flynn JM, eds. *Lovell and Winter's Pediatric Orthopaedics.* 7th Ed. Philadelphia: Lippincott Williams & Wilkins; 2013.
16. Blount W, Moe J. *The Milwaukee Brace.* Baltimore: Williams & Wilkins; 1973.

Posttraumatic Syringomyelia

CHAPTER 28

Lance L. Goetz

OUTLINE

Introduction

Syringomyelia is a relatively uncommon but potentially devastating cause of myelopathy or worsening of preexisting myelopathy. It can be categorized as congenital or acquired (from infection, trauma, or tumor, or vascular malformations)[1] and as "communicating" (originating from the central canal) and "noncommunicating" (developing within the substance of the spinal cord). Communicating syringomyelia is more commonly associated with congenital conditions such as Chiari malformations. Posttraumatic syringomyelia (PTS) is generally noncommunicating.[2] PTS refers to the development and progression of a cyst filled with cerebrospinal fluid (CSF) within the spinal cord. Symptomatic PTS occurs in about 3%–8% of persons with traumatic spinal cord injury (SCI).[3] A larger percentage is found on imaging when persons with subtle or no symptoms are included. PTS is often characterized clinically by the insidious progression of pain and loss of sensorimotor function that may manifest many years after traumatic SCI. If left untreated, PTS can result in loss of function, chronic pain, respiratory failure, or death. A variety of terms exist in the literature to describe syringomyelia and related conditions, including posttraumatic syringomyelia, syringe, spinal cord injury, syrinx, spinal cyst, spinal cord cyst, syringomyelia symptoms, syringomyelia surgery, and posttraumatic spinal cord injury. As the word "syringe" suggests, a syrinx is often tubelike in shape.

Pathophysiology

The pathophysiology of PTS is not fully understood. Formation of a cavity within the spinal cord is common after traumatic SCI,[4] but this cavity formation alone is not considered PTS. The cavitation represents, to varying degrees, a progressive process over time that can occur quickly or, more often, slowly and insidiously. Factors related to initial cavity formation include liquefaction of intraparenchymal hematoma, ischemia due to tethering, arterial or venous obstruction, release of intracellular lysosomal enzymes and excitatory amino acids, and mechanical damage from cord compression. Posttraumatic spinal cord tethering often occurs due to scar tissue that forms adhesions of the meninges to the spinal cord.[5] Tethering can be associated with neurologic compromise even in the absence of a visible cavity.[5] In PTS, cavity formation is followed by enlargement and extension of the cystic cavity. Rostral or caudal cyst extension may occur due to turbulent CSF flow or a "one-way valve" phenomenon that allows CSF into, but not out of, the cyst cavity. Tethering of the spinal cord results in impaired CSF circulation around the traumatized segment, and occurs as a sequela of bleeding-induced arachnoiditis, scarring, spinal canal stenosis, or kyphotic deformity.[4] The "slosh-and-suck" theory[6] proposes that increased epidural venous flow occurs during activities that produce effects like the Valsalva maneuver (e.g., coughing, sneezing) and results in increased pressure around the spinal cord, which cannot be dissipated because of disruptions in CSF flow. This pressure may force CSF into the cyst, resulting in expansion and extension. Coughing and sneezing can elicit symptoms, but there is controversy regarding the role that coughing-induced CSF pressure impulses may play in causing or worsening syringomyelia.[7,8] In PTS, traumatic SCI with tethering of the spinal cord to the dura results in impaired CSF circulation. Incomplete spinal canal decompression may predispose the person to tethering and CSF obstruction.[2] These factors are thought to cause syrinx development. Chronic mechanical stress to the spinal cord increases the risk for development of syringomyelia.[9] Spinal instrumentation without decompression is also associated with earlier onset of syringomyelia.

Epidemiology

Approximately 3%–4% of persons with traumatic SCI develop clinically symptomatic PTS. A larger percentage of persons have clinically silent syrinx cavities diagnosed by imaging techniques.[1] No racial differences are known for development of PTS. The incidence of PTS is higher in men due to the increased frequency of SCI in males; however, there is no association of manifestations of the condition with the patient's sex. Development of PTS can occur at any age, and it has been reported as early as 2 months to as late as 30 years after SCI.[2]

History and Physical

- Pain is the most commonly reported symptom.

Typically, considered neuropathic in nature and coded as "neuralgia or neuritis".

  - May be localized or diffuse and commonly reported as a dull ache, burning, or stabbing sensation.
  - Dermatomal pain presents with skin that is hypersensitive to light touch or pressure and may feel like a bruise, although no ecchymosis is present.
- Ascending sensory level and sensory dissociation (selective loss of pain and temperature sensation) are classic findings in progressive PTS.
- Symptoms are classically aggravated by postural change or the effects of the Valsalva maneuver induced by coughing or sneezing.
- Decreased reflex micturition, progressive orthostasis, autonomic dysreflexia, and relatively painless joint deformity or swelling (Charcot joint) also may occur.
- Spasticity is often increased compared to findings noted in prior examinations.
- Deep tendon reflex changes, either increased or decreased, may be noted compared with findings from prior examinations, and loss of reflexes and atrophy often occur over time.
- Headaches and neck ache are common in cervical syringomyelia.
- Numbness may involve the face if the syrinx has ascended into the brainstem (Fig. 28.1).
- Progressive weakness and wasting can occur but may be a late finding.
- Other signs may include a complete or partial Horner syndrome or other evidence of dysautonomia (e.g., labile blood pressure, hyperhidrosis).
- Signs may be unilateral because ascension of syrinxes often occurs unilaterally.
- The natural history of untreated syringomyelia is variable, with stabilization of symptoms in some persons and slow, persistent progression in others. Some persons continue to demonstrate progression of the condition, despite surgical intervention. The exact percentage of persons with initially asymptomatic syrinx cavities who become symptomatic is not known.

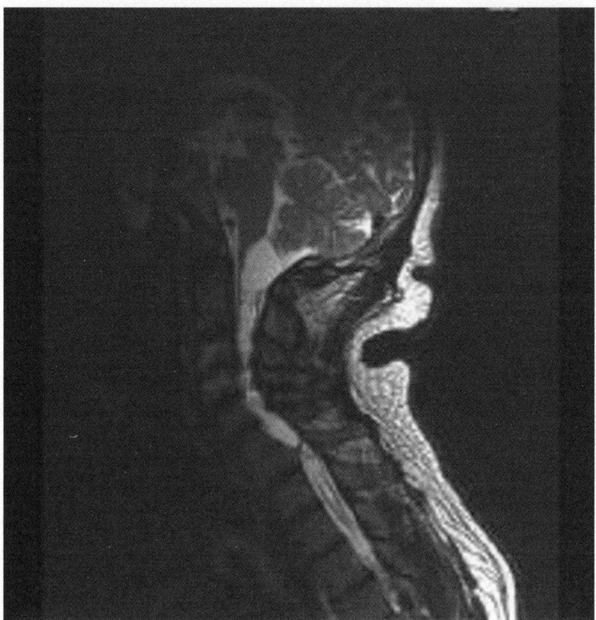

Fig. 28.1 T2-Weighted Sagittal Image of Large, Multiloculated Cervical Syrinx Extending Into Brainstem. Patient had preserved functional status.

Differential Diagnosis

Cervical, thoracic, or lumbar stenosis with myelopathy and/or radiculopathy, spinal cord tumor, spinal cord infarction, epidural abscess or hematoma, tethered cord syndrome, progressive noncystic myelopathy, and spinal instability should be considered.

Laboratory Studies

Pulmonary function tests, especially vital capacity, should be ordered on any patient with symptoms or suggested respiratory impairment. Serial studies are useful to document and monitor for progression of respiratory dysfunction. No specific laboratory blood studies have proven useful in the diagnosis or monitoring of PTS.

Imaging Studies

- Contrast-enhanced magnetic resonance imaging (MRI) is the imaging modality of choice for diagnosis of PTS.[5] Most PTS develops around the site of the original spinal cord lesion. T1 and T2 MRI sequences provide differentiation between CSF and normal spinal cord tissue and areas of spinal cord edema, myelomalacia, or gliosis. Serial examinations are necessary to evaluate for changes in cavity size over time.
- Clinical symptoms do not correlate with cavity size.[10]
- Contrast or myelography-enhanced computed tomography (CT-myelogram) can be useful to delineate the

extent of the syrinx cavity and localize CSF flow obstruction, arachnoid scarring, and tethering of the spinal cord.
- Plain radiographs of the spine delineate spinal deformities such as fractures, dislocations, and abnormal spinal kyphotic or lordotic changes. Flexion/extension views assist in evaluation of spinal stability.
- Ultrasonography may be used intraoperatively after laminectomy to visualize syrinx cavities and septations that may not be seen with other imaging modalities.[11,12]

Other Tests

- Serial quantitative strength measurements including pinch and grip tests or handheld myometry are useful in confirming progression of weakness.
- Calculation of the central motor conduction time using motor evoked potentials is useful in monitoring PTS over time. However, this technique is not widely available, and is currently most often utilized for intraoperative surgical monitoring of neural pathway integrity.
- Standard electromyographic techniques, including nerve conduction studies, F-wave latencies, and needle electromyography, may help identify other nerve lesions including radiculopathy, peripheral neuropathy, plexopathy, or motor neuron disease.[13]

Histologic Findings

- Pathologic section, cavitation of the gray matter within the spinal cord.
- May involve the central canal or may be located eccentrically.
- An inner layer of gliosis (scar) is usually present.
- Often involves the gray matter between the dorsal horns and posterior columns, possibly because of its relative avascularity and lack of connective tissue.
- Multiple cyst cavities, separated by complete or partial septae, are often present (Fig. 28.2).
- Cord edema is a risk factor for progression (Fig. 28.3).

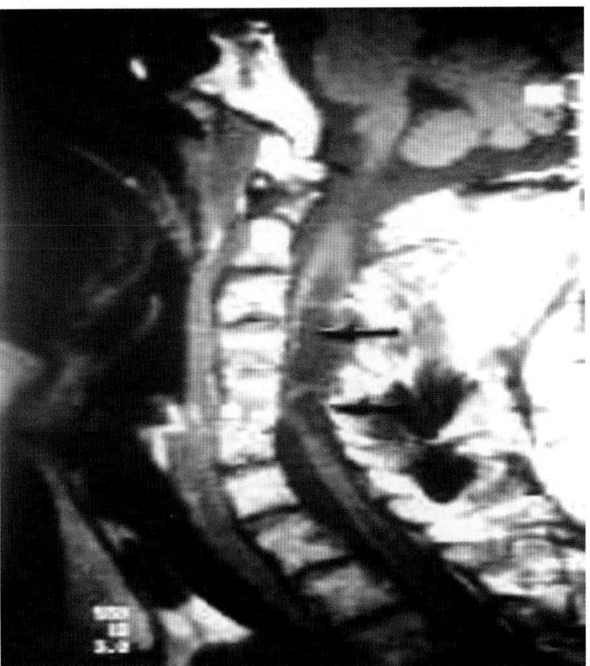

Fig. 28.2 T1-weighted cervical magnetic resonance imaging scan of multiple syrinx cavities *(arrows)* and thin secondary cavity extending into the thoracic spinal cord.

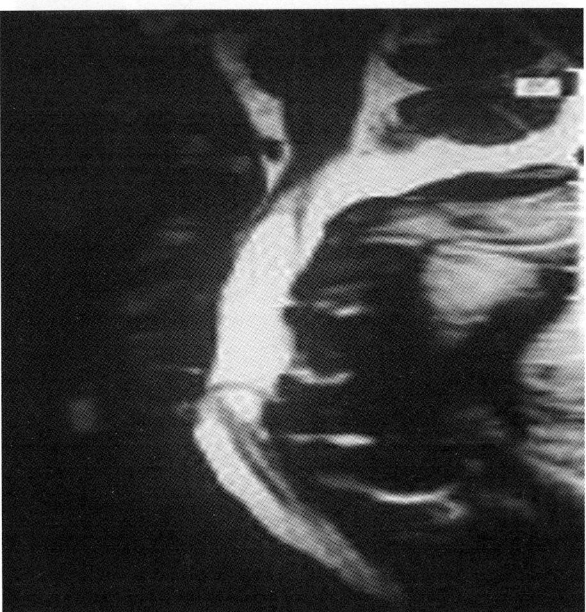

Fig 28.3 T2-weighted magnetic resonance imaging scan from the same individual as Fig. 28.2, which delineates the syrinx cavity. Note the spinal cord edema extending rostrally from the upper limit of the cavity.

Treatment

Physical and Occupational Therapy

- Preservation of range of motion and maintenance of function, including transfers, activities of daily living wheelchair mobility, and gait if applicable.
- Selection of appropriate assistive devices also is important.
- Physical therapy and kinesiotherapy are helpful in monitoring manual muscle strength, cardiovascular fitness, and joint function.
- Exercises and other mobilization activities that produce elevated intraabdominal pressure (i.e., like the Valsalva maneuver) should be avoided.

Other Services

- Psychologic support for adjustment to disability may be indicated.

- Cognitive or speech therapy may be needed in rare cases.

Medical Issues and Complications

- Increased weakness can result in functional loss, including transfers, wheelchair propulsion, gait, or self-care abilities.
- Functional losses, as well as impairments in sensation, predispose the patient to burns or skin breakdown. It is important to pay attention to changing seating needs if there is worsening sensorimotor function, balance, or changes in posture.
- Progressive impairments in respiratory function place patients at risk for atelectasis, pneumonia, or respiratory failure. Noninvasive or invasive mechanical ventilation may be required.
- Neuropathic arthropathy (Charcot joint) can occur as a result of lack of protective joint position sense.
- Morbidity is associated with weakness, loss of function, and chronic pain. Mortality can occur from involvement of brainstem respiratory centers or surgical complications.

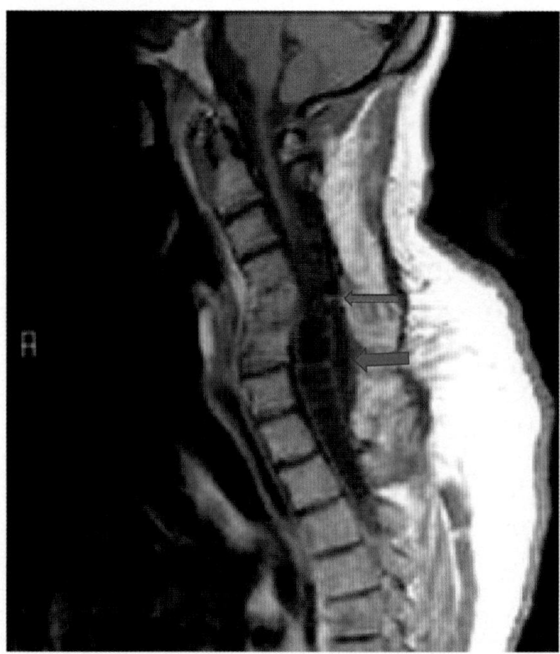

T1-weighted image demonstrating a large, multiloculated cervical syrinx cavity. This is a recurrent syrinx, which has come back despite an attempt at drainage utilizing shunting and expansile duraplasty.

Surgical Intervention

Surgery is frequently performed to prevent further expansion and collapse of syrinx cavities. Neurologic deterioration, pain, or autonomic dysreflexia may be indications for surgery. However, no surgical procedure has been uniformly successful in relief of symptoms or resolution of radiographic abnormalities. Surgical treatment has included simple drainage, a variety of shunting procedures, and decompressive laminectomy with expansion duraplasty. Cordectomy has also been performed.[9] The question of which persons to treat surgically is controversial. Ideally, surgery should be performed on persons with syrinx cavities that are enlarging but are not yet symptomatic or that only recently have become symptomatic. All surgical procedures potentially can cause loss of motor, sensory, reflex, or autonomic function.

- Historically, shunting of syrinx cavities, when performed alone, has been complicated by a high rate (up to 50%) of shunt failure or blockage and recurrent cyst expansion.[14]
- Duraplasty, dural grafting, and adhesiolysis (cutting of scar tissue adhesions) may be performed with the goal of reestablishing unrestricted subarachnoid CSF flow. An expansile duraplasty is felt by some to be a more physiologic way of treating a tethered spinal cord associated with syringomyelia.
- Percutaneous CT-guided drainage is not commonly used alone.
- Cordectomy is occasionally considered necessary to halt symptom progression.[5]

Medications

- Medical therapy is only for symptomatic control. Definitive treatment to date is surgical in nature.
- Centrally acting antispasticity agents such baclofen (Lioresal) or tizanidine (Zanaflex) are indicated when spasticity interferes with function, causes pain, or interferes with sleep.
- Tricyclic antidepressants were previously considered first-line treatment by specialists to treat neuropathic pain but are used less now due to risk of dysrhythmias. Doses used are generally lower than those required to treat depression.
- More recently, gabapentinoids, which are anticonvulsants, are commonly used by specialists to treat neuropathic pain. Gabapentin (Neurontin) has the advantage of reduced toxicity and side effects.
- Anticholinergics such as scopolamine (Transderm Scop) or hyoscyamine (Levsin) may help reduce gastrointestinal, salivary, and sudomotor (sweat gland) activity and can alleviate excess sweating in patients with PTS.
- Narcotic analgesics may be necessary in patients whose pain is not controlled with other agents. However, risks of respiratory depression, tolerance, and other side effects associated with this medication class limit their use.

Prognosis and Pitfalls

- Failure to recognize the symptoms of syringomyelia or attributing symptoms (pain, excess sweating, increased spasticity, numbness, or weakness) to other causes can result in morbidity, including neurologic deterioration. Clinicians should have a high index of suspicion for syringomyelia in any patient with SCI presenting with new onset or worsening of these symptoms.

- The presence of a peripheral nerve disorder can alter the signs of myelopathy, masking both the sensory loss and distal hyperreflexia. Worsening syringomyelia could be missed in this setting.

Review Questions

1. A 34-year-old man with T5 paraplegia for 14 years and known syringomyelia presents to your clinic with a stage 4 pressure injury under his right femur at the level of the trochanter. He has never had one before. He denies numbness or weakness in his arms. What should be considered?
   a. Motor evoked potentials of the upper extremities
   b. Dermatology consultation to evaluate for inflammatory skin disease
   c. Plain films of the spine to evaluate for scoliosis causing asymmetric sitting pressures
   d. Mental health evaluation
2. Which of the following is not a common finding in persons with posttraumatic syringomyelia?
   a. Headache
   b. Neuropathic pain
   c. Atrophy
   d. Rapid cognitive decline
3. Classic findings in progressive PTS include ascending sensory loss and:
   a. Asymmetric extensor plantar responses
   b. Fluctuating Hoffmann sign
   c. Sensory dissociation
   d. Painless weakness
4. The imaging study of choice in the diagnosis of PTS is:
   a. Intraoperative ultrasound
   b. CT-myelography
   c. Plain radiography
   d. Contrast-enhanced MRI
5. The most common presenting symptom in persons with PTS is:
   a. Autonomic dysreflexia
   b. Diffuse atrophy
   c. Focal weakness
   d. Pain

REFERENCES

1. Kleindienst A, Laut FM, Roeckelein V, Buchfelder M, Dodoo-Schittko F. Treatment of posttraumatic syringomyelia: evidence from a systematic review. *Acta Neurochir.* 2020;162(10):2541–2556.
2. Svircev J, Little JW. Syringomyelia. In: Kirshblum S, Campagnolo DI, Gorman P, eds. *Spinal Cord Medicine.* 2nd ed. New York: Demos Medical Publishing; 2011:569–573.
3. Rossier AB, Foo D, Shillito J, Dyro FM. Posttraumatic cervical syringomyelia. Incidence, clinical presentation, electrophysiological studies, syrinx protein and results of conservative and operative treatment. *Brain.* 1985;108(Pt 2):439–461.
4. Perrouin-Verbe B, Lenne-Aurier K, Robert R, et al. Post-traumatic syringomyelia and post-traumatic spinal canal stenosis: a direct relationship: review of 75 patients with a spinal cord injury. *Spinal Cord.* 1998;36(2):137–143.
5. Scelza W, Falci SP, Indeck C. Posttraumatic syringomyelia and spinal cord tethering. In: Kirshblum S, Lin VW, eds. *Spinal Cord Medicine.* 3rd ed. New York: Demos Medical Publishing; 2019:577–583.
6. Williams B. Pathogenesis of post-traumatic syringomyelia. *British Journal of Neurosurgery.* 1992;6(6):517–520.
7. Carpenter PW, Berkouk K, Lucey AD. Pressure wave propagation in fluid-filled co-axial elastic tubes. Part 2: mechanisms for the pathogenesis of syringomyelia. *J Biomech Eng.* 2003;125(6):857–863.
8. Elliott NSJ, Bertram CD, Martin BA, Brodbelt AR. Syringomyelia: a review of the biomechanics. *Journal of Fluids and Structures.* 2013;40:1–24.
9. Abel R, Gerner HJ, Smit C, Meiners T. Residual deformity of the spinal canal in patients with traumatic paraplegia and secondary changes of the spinal cord. *Spinal Cord.* 1999;37(1):14–19.
10. Goldstein B, Hammond MC, Stiens SA, Little JW. Posttraumatic syringomyelia: profound neuronal loss, yet preserved function. *Arch Phys Med Rehabil.* 1998;79(1):107–112.
11. Lee TT, Alameda GJ, Camilo E, Green BA. Surgical treatment of post-traumatic myelopathy associated with syringomyelia. *Spine (Phila Pa 1976).* 2001;26(24 Suppl):S119–S127.
12. Falci SP, Indeck C, Lammertse DP. Posttraumatic spinal cord tethering and syringomyelia: surgical treatment and long-term outcome. *J Neurosurg Spine.* 2009;11(4):445–460.
13. Little JW, Robinson LR. AAEM case report #24: electrodiagnosis in posttraumatic syringomyelia. *Muscle Nerve.* 1992;15(7):755–760.
14. Batzdorf U, Klekamp J, Johnson JP. A critical appraisal of syrinx cavity shunting procedures. *Journal of Neurosurgery.* 1998;89(3):382–388.

CHAPTER 29

Spasticity

Sean McAvoy and Derrick Miller

OUTLINE

Overview

Reflex arcs are suppressed by a combination of inhibitory upper and lower motor neuron pathways.[1] Spasticity from upper motor neuron (UMN) dysfunction, as in spinal cord injury (SCI), is likely caused by loss of descending inhibition that results in a net increase in the excitatory–inhibitory balance of reflexes and an increase in muscle tone and spasms.[1,2] Spasticity is estimated to affect between 29% and 68% of people following SCI.[3–8] Prompt management helps improve function, reduce discomfort, and reduce complications such as contractures, pain, fatigue, and pressure injuries. Proper management of spasticity is essential to maximizing the health and quality of life of people with SCI.

Definitions

Upper Motor Neuron Syndrome (UMNS)

A collection of motor control changes that occur following a UMN lesion. Some signs and symptoms include weakness, decreased motor control and dexterity, altered muscle tone, decreased endurance, exaggerated phasic (tendon jerks) and tonic (spastic) reflexes, and released flexor reflexes in the lower extremities. Spasticity is one part of the upper motor neuron syndrome (UMNS).

Spasticity

Defined as velocity-dependent increase in resistance to movement of a muscle group across a joint that results from hyperexcitability of the tonic stretch reflex. More broadly, spasticity is defined as disordered sensory-motor control, resulting from a UMN lesion, presenting as intermittent or sustained involuntary activation of muscles. Using the broader definition of spasticity encompasses multiple features of the UMN including clonus, spasms, spastic cocontraction, and weakness.

Muscle Tone

Resistance of a muscle to passive stretch.

Hypertonia

Abnormally elevated muscle tone.

Rigidity

Increased resistance to movement of a muscle group across a joint, independent of velocity.

Anatomy and Physiology

Normal Reflex

The anatomy and physiology of the reflex arc is complex, with reflexes controlled via multiple inhibitory and facilitatory pathways. All reflex arc pathways converge on the alpha motor neuron that innervates extrafusal muscle fibers, the cells responsible for muscular contraction, as the final common pathway (Fig. 29.1).[1] The predominant neurotransmitters involved in the regulation of reflex arcs are glutamate (excitatory), glycine (inhibitory), and gamma-aminobutyric acid (GABA) (inhibitory).[9] The sensory and integrating components of reflex physiology are even more complex than the motor unit.

The primary sensory organs are muscle spindles, Golgi tendon organs, and cutaneous nociceptive nerves. Muscle spindles sense stretch and muscle lengthening. They are composed of intrafusal fibers and are innervated by efferent gamma motor neurons and afferent

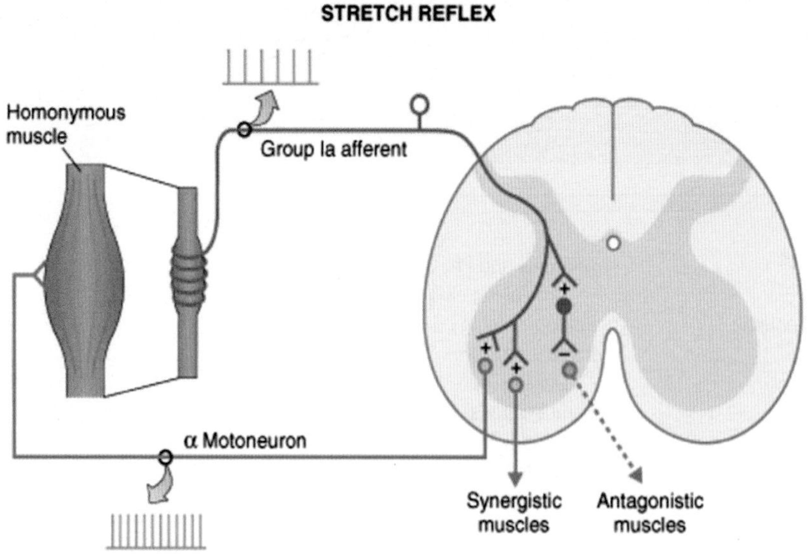

STRETCH REFLEX

Fig. 29.1 Stretch Reflex. (Adapted from Costanzo LS. *Physiology*. 3rd ed. Saunders Elsevier; 2006: 97-101.)

group II and Ia fibers.[1] The Golgi tendon organ, which detects changes in tension during both muscle lengthening and contraction, is innervated by group Ib nervous fibers.[1] In normal tonic reflex functioning, when a muscle is stretched, excitatory input is delivered from the Golgi tendon organ and muscle spindles to the motor unit, which triggers contraction and helps maintain muscular tone (Fig. 29.2). This excitatory process is offset by multiple inhibitory processes, both supraspinal and peripheral. In reciprocal inhibition, intrafusal fibers activate inhibitory neurons on antagonist muscles through Ia nerves.[1] In recurrent inhibition, a feedback loop is formed where an interneuron (the Renshaw cell) suppresses the alpha motor neurons that activate it.[1] In addition, sensory information from the Golgi tendon organs is transmitted via a Ib afferent nerve to inhibit alpha motor neurons.[1] This information from the peripheral nervous system is integrated with supraspinal input within the spinal cord to regulate phasic, tonic, monosynaptic, and polysynaptic reflexes (Fig. 29.3).

Note: Normal reflex physiology is controlled by supraspinal input, reciprocal inhibition, recurrent inhibition, a complex interneuron system, and the muscle spindle. Disruption of the net inhibitory effect on spinal reflexes is thought to be the etiology of spasticity.

Pathophysiology

Spasticity is a poorly understood and complex condition that can occur following damage to the spinal cord (vascular, infectious, neoplastic, traumatic). However, pathophysiology theories converge on the development of a net excitatory imbalance in the reflex arcs that activate the alpha motor neurons of the spinal cord.[1,2,10] Since the anatomy of the reflex arc is maintained, whereas supraspinal efferent connections are impaired following SCI, a leading theory for the etiology of reflex hyperexcitability is loss of descending inhibition. The initial flaccid phase after injury may suggest involvement of additional mechanisms. Some other theories of spasticity include loss of other inhibitory feedback on the reflexes including loss of disynaptic reciprocal Ia inhibition, loss of presynaptic inhibition of the Ia afferent terminal, and loss of nonreciprocal Ib inhibition.[1,11,12] Other theories include hyperexcitability of the alpha motor neuron excitability, receptor upregulation/denervation supersensitivity, axonal sprouting, and enhancements in cutaneous reflexes.[1,2,13]

Evaluation

General

There are a wide range of methods for evaluating spasticity. As the optimal management of spasticity involves accurate diagnosis, quantification of the severity of the spasticity, and the assessment and treatment of the underlying cause(s) when possible, it is important to use a standard and comprehensive approach to the initial evaluation. The diagnosis of spasticity in a patient with an UMN lesion is supported by the presence of positive and negative symptoms (Table 29.1). Following diagnosis, the severity can be quantified using a standardized scale. After the diagnosis is confirmed and the severity quantified, an evaluation of secondary (i.e., non-UMNS) potentiators should be performed. Noxious stimuli, such

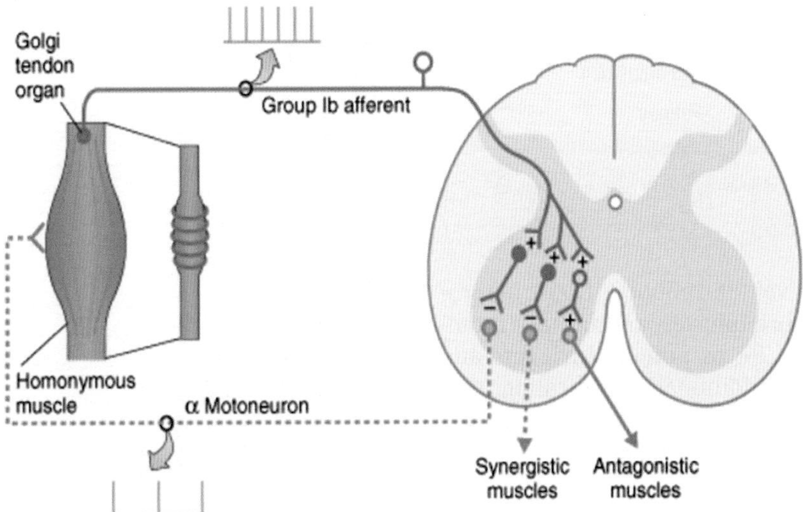

Fig. 29.2 Golgi Tendon Reflex. (Adapted from Costanzo LS. P*hysiology*. 3rd ed. Saunders Elsevier; 2006: 97-101.)

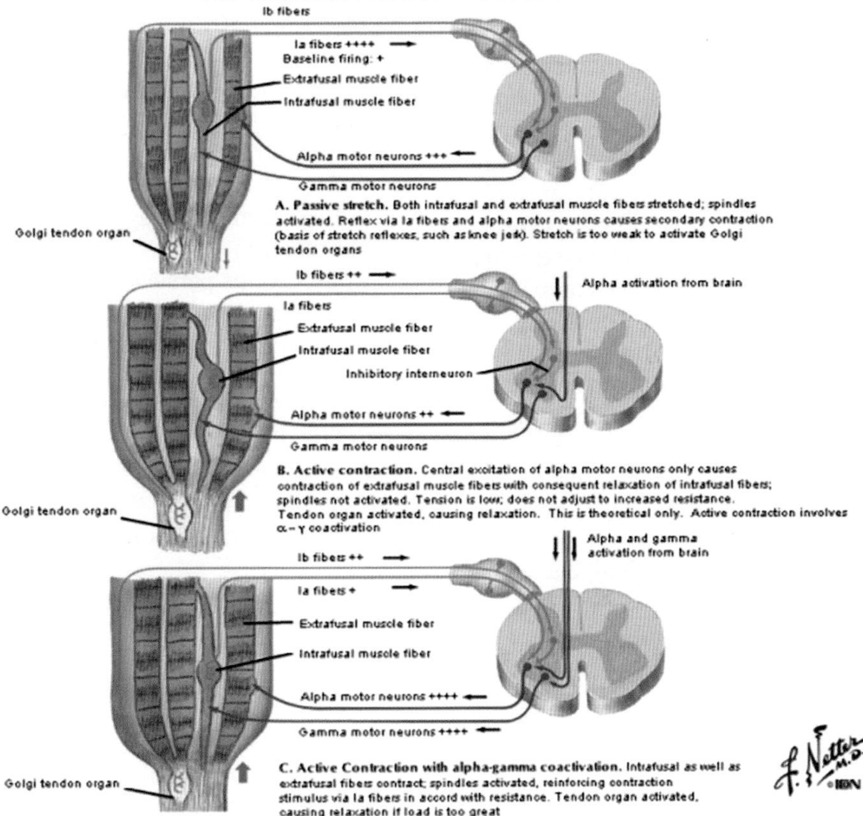

Fig. 29.3 Central Control of Muscle Stretch Reflex and Gamma Motor Neurons. (Adapted from Felten DL, O'Banion MK, Maida MS, eds. *Netter's Atlas of Neuroscience*. 4th ed. Fig. 10.14. Elsevier; 2022:239-253.)

Table 29.1 Positive and Negative Symptoms of Spasticity

Positive Symptoms	Negative Symptoms
Hyperreflexia	Weakness
Clonus	Incoordination
Spasms	Fatigue
Postural abnormalities	Pain

Positive symptoms are defined as abnormal behaviors, whereas negative symptoms are defined as performance deficits.

as infection, pain, deep vein thrombosis (DVT), heterotopic ossification, pressure injuries, and urinary retention, should be assessed for as potential triggers and potentiators of spasticity. Additionally, medications that may worsen spasticity, such as selective serotonin reuptake inhibitors, should be screened for.[14]

Spasticity Scales

Various scales are used for assessing spasticity, clinical and self-report. The spinal cord assessment tool for spastic reflexes (SCATS) has been shown to be both a valid and reliable clinical scale that includes electromyography (EMG) testing to measure clonus, flexor, and extensor spasms.[15,16] The spinal cord injury spasticity evaluation tool (SCI-SET) is a self-report scale that has been shown to be both valid and reliable in measuring problematic and beneficial components of spasticity in daily function.[17–19] The patient-reported impact of spasticity measure (PRISM) is another self-report scale that has been shown to be valid and reliable in measuring the impact of spasticity in veterans with SCI.[19,20] Multiple clinical scales often do not correlate well with each other or with patient-perceived levels of spasticity[3,21,22] and may measure different components of spasticity than do self-report scales. Therefore, it is best to use a consistent approach with both a clinical scale and a self-report scale.[23] Some older scales that may be less clinically reliable in SCI patients include the modified Ashworth scale, the modified Penn spasm frequency scale, the visual analogue scale, the Tardieu scale, and the pendulum test (Fig. 29.4).

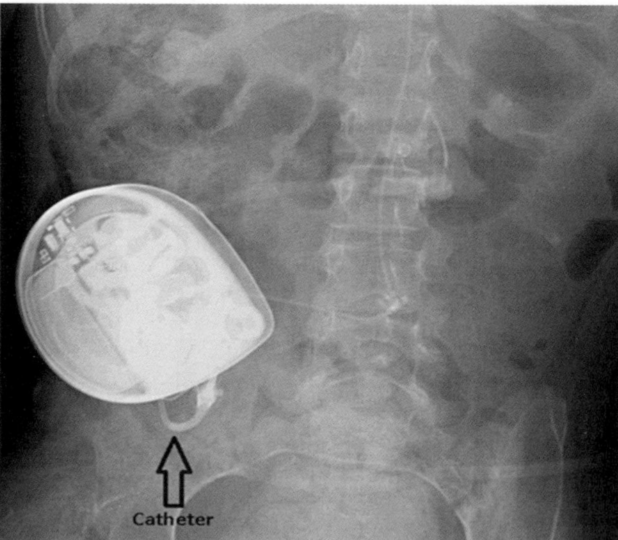

Fig. 29.4 An old abdominal X-ray of a patient reporting the sudden development of fever, itching, "heart beating out of their chest," and worsening of their spasticity.

Adapted Versions of the SCATS, SCI-SET, and PRISM Scales

Spinal Cord Assessment Tool for Spastic Reflexes (SCATS)[24]

Clonus. Duration of clonic bursts is timed following rapid passive dorsiflexion of the ankle.

1. No reaction
2. Mild: Clonus maintained for less than 3 seconds
3. Moderate: clonus maintained for 3–10 seconds
4. Severe: Clonus persists for longer than 10 seconds

Flexor Spasms. With the knee and hip extended to 0 degrees, extension of big toe, ankle dorsiflexion, and knee/hip flexion are visually observed following pinprick stimulus to the medial arch of the person's foot.

1. No reaction
2. Less than 10 degrees excursion of the knee and hip or excursion of the great toe
3. Moderate: 10–30 degrees of flexion at the knee and hip
4. Severe: 30 degrees or greater of flexion at the knee and hip

Extensor Spasms. Displacement of the patella is observed following hip and knee extension from 110 degrees and 90 degrees.

1. No reaction
2. Mild: Clonus persists for less than 3 seconds
3. Moderate: clonus lasting 3–10 seconds
4. Severe: Clonus persists for longer than 10 seconds

Spinal Cord Injury Spasticity Evaluation Tool (SCI-SET)[17]

Patients are asked to rate how their spasticity has impacted 18 areas of their life in the past 7 days. All questions are rated using the scale below.

−3 Extremely problematic
−2 Moderately problematic
−1 Somewhat problematic
0 No effect
1 Somewhat helpful
2 Moderately helpful
3 Extremely helpful
4 N/A

Patient Reported Impact of Spasticity Measure (PRISM)[20]

Patients are asked to rate the effects of spasticity on their life over a 7-day period.

1. Never true for me
2. Rarely true for me
3. Sometimes true for me
4. Often true for me
5. Very often true for me

Advanced Testing

Due to restricted resource availability, time constraints, expense, and limited clinical utility, advanced testing with EMG and biomechanical studies is best reserved for research purposes.[25] A commonly used biomechanical test is the pendulum test, in which various devices such as a handheld isokinetic dynamometer, an electrogoniometer, and a tachometer can be used to quantify spasticity at the knee or ankle following releasing the affected limb from an extended position.[26–28] EMG studies are often used to quantify reflex activity that is provoked by maneuvers including manual limb movement, tendon tap, flexion withdrawal reflexes, and with electrical stimulation to evoke responses. Advanced testing may be appropriate for monitoring response to drug therapies.[25,29] In addition, EMG can be used to localize spastic muscles for guiding neurolytic injections.

Complications

Spasticity affects many parts of a patient's life, and treatment decisions should consider the biopsychosocial model when managing the condition. Many complications are both serious and preventable and should be screened for on initial evaluation of any patient with spasticity. Direct functional impairment attributable to spasticity includes impacts and limitations on basic self-care, instrumental activities of daily living, and recreational activities. Some lifestyle impacts include effects on sleep, sexual function, mobility, and hygiene. Emotional ramifications can include difficulty with cosmesis, self-esteem, and mood. Health ramifications can range from joint contractures to development of pressure ulcers, bony fractures with potential malunion, heterotopic ossification, dislocation and/or subluxation of joints, acquired peripheral neuropathy, and pain.[30,31]

Benefits

Spasticity may offer benefits that both the caregiver and the patient can take advantage of.[3,20] On the PRISM scale, some patients report the positive effects of spasticity outweigh the negative effects.[20] Some medical benefits include help with maintenance of muscle bulk,[32] help with prevention of DVTs,[33–36] assistance in pressure ulcer prevention over bony prominences, and use of an early warning system for underlying disease processes. Some lifestyle benefits include assistance with ambulation, standing, and transferring.

Treatment of spasticity is aimed at minimizing pain and discomfort, maximizing function and quality of life, and prevention/treatment of complications. Common treatment options include preventive therapies, physical modalities/therapeutics, pharmacotherapy, injections/baclofen (Lioresal) pump, and surgery. Treatment is not necessary in all patients and should progress from least to most aggressive as necessary to improve outcomes and should begin early to prevent progression of spasticity and development of complications such as contractures. Multiple factors weigh into selecting the best therapy, including the distribution and positive/negative impacts of the spasticity, the patient's functional ability, and comorbidities or complications.

Treatment

Preventive Therapy

There are standard preventive strategies that should always be employed for new onset or worsening spasticity, including:

Proper bed positioning
Daily stretching and range of motion of all affected joints
Education on proper positioning, adequate bowel and bladder programs, daily skin inspections, etc.
Avoidance and treatment of exacerbators such as pain, noxious stimuli, syringomyelia,[37] and some medications such as selective serotonin reuptake inhibitors.

Physical Modalities

Temperature Modalities

Cold modalities such as cryotherapy may decrease tendon reflex excitability and clonus.[31] Heat therapeutics include deep heat with ultrasound and superficial heat with hot packs, fluid therapy, paraffin, and whirlpool. The effects of both cold and heat modalities vary[31,38] and may be of limited use in severe and chronic spasticity due to short duration of effect.

Stretching

Stretching is commonly used in clinical practice; however, it has been found to have no short- or long-term effects on joint mobility and the development of contractures.[39,40]

Splints, Casts, and Orthotics

Splints, casts, and orthotics can all be used to create prolonged stretch to spastic muscles. Some advantages include:

- Static splints allow for easy monitoring of skin and changes in range of motion due to being lightweight and removable.
- Dynamic splints: These can be adjusted during wear to increase range of motion, while allowing functional activities to be performed.
- Casting/serial casting may be beneficial by facilitating stretch as range of motion improves.

Other

Other physical modalities of varying benefit include:

- Transcutaneous electrical nerve stimulation
- Vibration
- Relaxation techniques
- Motor reeducation
- Biofeedback
- Acupuncture
- Massage
- Use of a tilt table or standing frame to create prolonged stretch

Pharmacotherapy

Pharmacotherapy is recommended only when preventive therapy and physical modalities fail to achieve desired results. Other causes of increased spasticity, such as urinary tract infection, should be treated if applicable prior to initiating pharmacotherapy. Nearly all medications have potentially serious side effects, and no single medication will have a beneficial effect in all patients. It is always advisable to start with the lowest possible dose, then titrate upward until the desired effect is achieved or the maximum dose is reached.

There are a range of medications used to manage spasticity, with the most common agents being baclofen, dantrolene sodium (Dantrium), tizanidine (Zanaflex), diazepam (Valium), and clonidine (Catapres) (Table 29.2). Other agents that may be considered in intractable spasticity include alpha agonists (phenothiazines), gabapentin (Neurontin), glycine, phenytoin (Dilantin), chlorpromazine (Thorazine), cyclobenzaprine (Flexeril), vincristine (Oncovin), cannabinoids, and morphine.

Invasive Techniques and Therapies

A variety of targeted therapies have been developed that vary significantly in invasiveness, side effect profile, complications, and indications. These therapies are generally recommended for patients who fail preventive and physical modalities. Surgery may be considered as a last resort for patients for whom all other treatments fail.

Local Anesthetics

Due to the short half-life of local anesthetics, they are mostly used to test for the potential efficacy of longer-acting agents such as phenol before initiating treatment. Drugs of this class such as lidocaine (Xylocaine) and bupivacaine (Marcaine) interfere with the increase in permeability of membrane to sodium during depolarization.[41]

Chemical Neurolytic

Phenol and ethyl alcohol are two commonly used chemical neurolytics. They are most useful in the treatment of localized spasticity, and induce nerve dysfunction by causing demyelination and axonal destruction/necrosis. Length of therapeutic effect varies from 2 months to 2 years.[42] Sensory and mixed nerves should be avoided when possible due to an increased risk of severe dysesthesias.[43,44] Care should be taken to avoid intravascular injection of phenol, which can cause seizures, cardiovascular collapse, and CNS compromise. The ideal concentration of phenol for neurolysis is not well-studied; limited studies support optimal concentration of phenol to use ranging from 3%–12%.[42] Concentrations of ethyl alcohol vary from 50%–100%.[45,46]

Neurotoxins

Spasticity caused by SCI is considered an off-label use for botulinum toxin. Botulinum toxin should be used for localized spasticity that is refractory to conservative management. There are eight antigenically distinguishable types (A–C1, C2–G) of botulinum toxin, all of which prevent muscle contraction by blocking acetylcholine release at the neuromuscular junction.[46] The weakness produced by botulinum toxin A usually lasts about 3 months.[46] Waiting at least 3 months between injections is recommended, as this is thought to reduce the risk of future treatment failure due to antibody formation to botulinum toxin.[47] The recommended dose varies per muscle being injected, with a maximum total dose (whole body combined) being 1500 units. Due to increased risk of dysphagia and breathing difficulties from systemic spread of the botulinum toxin, treatments should not exceed the maximum recommended dose, and should be used with extreme caution in patients with neuromuscular and respiratory diseases.

Intrathecal Medications and Pumps

Intrathecal therapy, delivered via a subcutaneous pump–catheter system in the intrathecal space, is reserved for spasticity that is refractory to more conservative management. Intrathecal pumps generally are more effective for lower limb spasticity than upper limb spasticity, though raising the tip of the catheter from the usual location (T10–L2) to the T6 level may help improve efficacy in the upper extremities.[48]

Table 29.2 Medications Commonly Used to Manage Spasticity

Agent	Contraindications	Side Effects	Monitoring Required	Mode of Action	Dosing (Adult)
Baclofen	Hypersensitivity	Pregnancy: – neonatal withdrawal can occur; causes fetal harm in animal models General: – drowsiness, sedation, dizziness, confusion, nausea, vomiting[15] – CNS effects may be additive to alcohol and other CNS depressants[15] – can cause worsening of psychotic disorders, confusional states, autonomic dysreflexia, seizure disorders	Renally excreted, alter dose in renal impairment[69] Hepatic: – no dose adjustments	Agonist of GABA-B	Initial dose 5 mg 1 to 3 times daily. Usual maximum dose 80 mg/day though some patients may require doses up to 120 mg/day[70,71] – Sudden withdrawal from baclofen can cause seizures, rhabdomyolysis, hallucinations, and death
Benzo-diazepines	Hypersensitivity Severe hepatic impairment	Weakness Sedation Drowsiness Hypotension Ataxia	Renal: – monitor, metabolized mostly by hepatic mechanism before excretion. – nondialyzable Hepatic: – use with caution as medication is hepatically metabolized. – oral tablets are contraindicated in severe hepatic impairment	Agonist of GABA-A receptor	Diazepam used most commonly due to long half-life Initial dosage: 2 mg twice daily or 5 mg at bedtime; increase gradually based on response and toleration, up to 40 to 60 mg/day in 3 to 4 divided doses – Sudden withdrawal from benzodiazepines can cause seizures, mental status changes, and hyperthermia
Alpha 2 Agonists					
Clonidine	Hypersensitivity	Hypotension Bradycardia Drowsiness Dizziness Fatigue Contact dermatitis Transient skin rash Upper abdominal pain[49,72,73]	Renal: – start at low dose and monitor closely Hepatic: – no dosage adjustment required	Alpha 2 agonist Inhibits excessive afferent sensory transmission below the level of injury[49]	0.05 mg 1×/day – Max dose 1.2 mg/day in divided doses total/day[74] – Taper dose gradually to reduce risk of rebound hypertension – Less frequently used as monotherapy due to variable benefit, significant SE profile, and risk of rebound hypertension during withdrawal[49]

Continued

Table 29.2 Medications Commonly Used to Manage Spasticity

Agent	Contraindications	Side Effects	Monitoring Required	Mode of Action	Dosing (Adult)
Tizanidine	Concomitant therapy with ciprofloxacin or fluvoxamine (potent CYP 1A2 inhibitors)[75,76] Hypersensitivity	Hypotension Syncope Sedation Visual hallucinations Drowsiness Dizziness Asthenia Bradycardia[75,76]	Hepatic impairment: – avoid use or reduce dose and monitor LFT's (baseline prior to starting and intermittently during use) Renal: – CrCL ≤25; use with caution – use with caution in elderly due to decreased renal clearance[75,76]	Alpha 2 agonist Increases polysynaptic inhibition that reduces facilitation of spinal motor neurons[75,76]	2 mg 1×/day at bedtime – > max dose 36 mg/day in 3 or 4 divided doses[77] – Taper dose gradually to reduce risk of rebound hypertension
Dantrolene	Hypersensitivity Hepatic failure, Cirrhosis	Weakness Headache Dizziness Somnolence Visual disturbances Elevated liver enzymes	Renal: – no dosing adjustments per manufacturer Hepatic: – contraindicated with active liver disease and cirrhosis	Acts directly on muscle preventing calcium release from sarcoplasmic reticulum	25 mg daily, max dose 400 mg/day in divided dosing
Cyproheptadine (off-label use)	– Use in newborns, infants, breastfeeding mothers Hypersensitivity – use in newborns, premature infants, breastfeeding mothers, elderly, debilitated patients – use in conditions such as stenosing peptic ulcer, acute angle closure glaucoma, etc.[78]	Polyphagia Weight gain CNS depression Beers criteria Concern for use in those with CV disease, increased IOP, respiratory disease, and thyroid dysfunction[79]	No hepatic or renal dose adjustments	Potent antihistamine and serotonin agonist with anticholinergic effects[80]	2–4 mg every 8 h –>8 mg every 8 h[70,81]

CNS, Central nervous system; *CrCL*, creatine clearance; *CV*, cardiovascular; *CYP*, cytochrome P450, *GABA*, gamma-aminobutyric acid; *IOP*, intraocular pressure; *LFTs*, liver function tests; *SE*, side effect.

Intrathecal Baclofen

Baclofen is the most commonly used intrathecal agent; however, morphine and clonidine can also be used.[49] Due to direct delivery of baclofen into the intrathecal space, the intrathecal baclofen (ITB) pump is associated with less systemic and CNS side effects such as sedation,[50] compared with the oral form of the medication. However, ITB also carries implantation risks such as bleeding/infection and has significantly higher costs. In addition, the effects of withdrawal and overdose are more severe.[51] Withdrawal symptoms include worsening spasticity, itching, tachycardia, hyperthermia, hypotension, mood changes, and, when severe, seizures, rhabdomyolysis, and multisystem organ failure. For this reason, patients should be provided with oral baclofen and education on indications for contacting their physician. In addition, "drug holidays," in which clonidine or morphine are alternated with baclofen, can be used to reduce dependency and withdrawal.[52]

Pump Insertion/Maintenance. Prior to ITB pump insertion, individuals with SCI should be tested for candidacy for pump insertion by injecting up to 150 μg of baclofen into the subarachnoid space using a lumbar puncture or an external catheter. A positive response indicates that the person is a good candidate for ITB pump insertion. One definition of a positive response is a reduction in the modified Ashworth scale by a minimum of one point in at least two muscle groups, and improvement reported by caregivers in the goals agreed upon with professionals.[49,53–68] Following insertion, the patient's pump should be adjusted to best control their symptoms, and the dose can be set to vary per time of the day as needed. The individual should return to the doctor at least once every 6 months for pump refills.

Surgical Treatment

Surgery is reserved as a last resort for patients who fail all other forms of management. There are many orthopedic and neurosurgical procedures available, with varying risk–benefit profiles, indications, and severity of side effects and complications.

Orthopedic Procedures

Help with restoring function, especially in the case of joint contractures and severe spasticity.

SPLATT: split anterior tibial tendon transfer
Tendon release
Tendon lengthening
Step-cut (Z-plasty) lengthening procedures
Tenotomy
Myotomy

Neurosurgical Procedures

Neurosurgical procedures vary significantly in destructive effect, with CNS procedures (i.e., cordotomy, etc.) being more destructive than the peripheral nervous system procedures (i.e., selective dorsal rhizotomy, etc.). Care should be taken to not further compromise function when choosing these surgeries.

Dorsal rhizotomy
Radiofrequency ablation
Peripheral neurectomy
Neuroablative procedures
Central electrical stimulators
Cordotomy
Cordectomy
Myelotomy

Summary

- 70% of patients who suffer from a SCI develop spasticity within 1 year. Spasticity affects many parts of a person's life (physical, social, emotional), and effective care requires a multidisciplinary team and holistic approach.
- Positive (abnormal behaviors) and negative (performance deficits) symptoms support the diagnosis of spasticity
- Spasticity is best graded using a combination of clinical and self-report scales. Some valid and reliable scales include the SCATS (clinical), the SCI-SET (self-report), and the PRISM (self-report). More advanced testing methods are often expensive, time consuming, unnecessary, and are mostly reserved for research.
- All patients with spasticity should be screened for complications. Many complications from spasticity are both severe and preventable (e.g., decubitus ulcer, infection)
- Goals of treatment should be geared at minimizing pain/discomfort, maximizing function and quality of life, and prevention/treatment of complications
- Spasticity can be a warning for an underlying disease process (noxious stimuli can trigger or exacerbate the process)
- Least invasive/safest treatments should be used first (preventive therapy → physical modalities → pharmacotherapy + injection techniques → intrathecal baclofen pump → surgery)
- Nearly all medications have potentially serious side effects, and no single medication is helpful for all patients
- Spasticity has benefits such as maintenance of muscle bulk, prevention of DVT, and benefit in activities such as ambulating, standing, and transferring

Review Questions

1. A 24-year-old male sustained an T10 AIS B SCI in a motor vehicle collision 6 months ago. He has developed worsening spasticity of the lower extremities that was resistant to conservative management and improved with 5 mg of baclofen three times a day. How might baclofen be improving this patient's spasticity?
   a. Increasing inhibitory feedback to spinal reflexes
   b. Inhibiting calcium release from the sarcoplasmic reticulum of muscle cells
   c. Direct inhibition of alpha motor neurons
   d. Inhibiting afferent sensory input to reflex arcs
   e. Increasing the firing rate of the Golgi tendon organ

2. You are performing a physical exam on a 40-year-old female patient who is 3 years status post T7 AIS A SCI. You notice that both legs have a smooth and consistent increase in tone on passive range of motion. With her knee partially flexed, you then quickly dorsiflex her foot and notice six to seven quick repeated plantarflexion movements. What types of reflexes contribute to these movements respectively?
   a. Phasic, tonic
   b. Tonic, clonic
   c. Phasic, clonic
   d. Tonic, phasic
   e. Not related to reflexes
3. A 40-year-old female patient with a medical history significant for systemic lupus erythematosus, hypertension, repeated urinary tract infections successfully treated with trimethoprim/sulfamethoxazole, and diabetes with a T6 ASIA C SCI sustained due to multiple sclerosis 20 years ago with right lower extremity spasticity that is well controlled on 5 mg baclofen oral three times daily suddenly develops worsening of her spasticity. In addition, she complains of recent burning with urination, and her urinalysis shows leukocytosis and >100,000 bacteria/mL. Her vitals are within normal limits, she has mild lower abdominal tenderness, no cardiovascular tenderness, and the remainder of her physical exam is normal. What is the best next step in management of this patient's spasticity?
   a. Switch medical management to clonidine
   b. Increase her dose of oral baclofen to 10 mg three times daily
   c. Start trimethoprim/sulfamethoxazole, and monitor for subsequent improvement in her spasticity
   d. Educate her on the importance of stretching for prevention of worsening of spasticity
   e. Consult neurology for management of potential multiple sclerosis flare
4. A 37-year-old patient with a history of essential hypertension and an T3 AIS A SCI developed 3 weeks ago is transferred to your service for inpatient rehabilitation. On physical examination you notice a "catch" around 40 and 45 degrees in the left and right legs, respectively, followed by a constant and mild increase in resistance to passive range of motion throughout the remainder of extension. What is the best first line of management for this patient?
   a. 5 mg oral baclofen three times daily
   b. Bilateral phenol femoral nerve blocks
   c. Serial casting
   d. Stretching three times per day and physical therapy
   e. 2 mg two times daily clonidine
5. A 55-year-old male with a medical history significant for type two diabetes, hypertension, and a T12 AIS C SCI due to small cell lung cancer presents to your office with worsening spasticity in his bilateral lower extremities that is refractory to conservative management with physical therapy and stretching. He has no known allergies, and recent laboratory work shows his kidney and liver function to be within normal limits. What is the best choice of initial pharmacotherapy for this patient?
   a. Baclofen 10 mg three times daily
   b. Baclofen 5 mg three times daily
   c. Tizanidine 4 mg four times daily
   d. Dantrolene 50 mg daily
   e. Proceed to phenol nerve block
6. You are called in to cover an inpatient rehabilitation service for a friend who is on sick leave. A patient calls the office reporting the sudden development of fever, itching, "heart beating out of their chest," and worsening of their spasticity. On chart-check, you notice an old abdominal X-ray (Fig. 29.4). What is the best next step in management?
   a. Tell the patient to go to the nearest emergency department and to take a dose of oral baclofen if available in case of pump failure, as this is a potentially life-threatening condition.
   b. Reassure the patient as this condition is normally mild and will resolve on its own
   c. Tell the patient to come to the office immediately so that you can assess them
   d. Tell the patient to take a dose of oral baclofen and reassure them that their symptoms will resolve
   e. Tell the patient that you will call them back after checking with the doctor who normally covers their service
7. A 25-year-old male patient with no significant medical history besides a C5 ASIA B traumatic SCI sustained in a motor vehicle collision at 6 years old comes to your office for management of four extremity spasticity. The spasticity is currently managed with a baclofen pump due to failure of conservative management (physical therapy, stretching), and intolerance/inefficacy of oral medications (baclofen, dantrolene, clonidine, and diazepam). He complains of worsening spasticity causing both pain and limited mobility of his wrist. He has modified Ashworth grade 4 spasticity in the wrist flexors functionally limiting tenodesis. The rest of his physical exam shows only mild spasticity of other muscle groups that he reports as not significantly painful or problematic. What is the most appropriate next step in management?
   a. Chemodenervation with botulinum toxin to the flexor carpi ulnaris and flexor carpi radialis
   b. Surgical management
   c. Physical/occupational therapy
   d. Increase the dose of intrathecal baclofen
   e. Switch from intrathecal baclofen to intrathecal morphine

REFERENCES

1. Mukherjee A, Chakravarty A. Spasticity mechanisms – for the clinician. *Frontiers in Neurology*. 2010;1:149.
2. Mayer NH. Clinicophysiologic concepts of spasticity and motor dysfunction in adults with an upper motoneuron lesion. *Muscle & Nerve*. 1997;6:S1–S14.
3. Maynard FM, Karunas RS, Waring 3rd WP. Epidemiology of spasticity following traumatic spinal cord injury. *Arch Phys Med Rehabil*. 1990;71(8):566–569.
4. Holtz KA, Lipson R, Noonan VK, Kwon BK, Mills PB. Prevalence and effect of problematic spasticity after traumatic spinal cord injury. *Arch Phys Med Rehabil*. 2017;98(6):1132–1138.
5. Sköld C, Levi R, Seiger A. Spasticity after traumatic spinal cord injury: nature, severity, and location. *Arch Phys Med Rehabil*. 1999;80(12):1548–1557.
6. Walter JS, Sacks J, Othman R, et al. A database of self-reported secondary medical problems among VA spinal cord injury patients: its role in clinical care and management. *Journal of Rehabilitation Research and Development*. 2002;39(1):53–61.
7. Johnson RL, Gerhart KA, McCray J, Menconi JC, Whiteneck GG. Secondary conditions following spinal cord injury in a population-based sample. *Spinal Cord*. 1998;36(1):45–50.
8. Levi R, Hultling C, Nash MS, Seiger A. The Stockholm spinal cord injury study: 1. medical problems in a regional SCI population. *Paraplegia.*. 1995;33(6):308–315.
9. Derderian C, Tadi P. Physiology, withdrawal response. [Updated 2020 Sep 11]. In: StatPearls [Internet]. Treasure Island (FL): StatPearls Publishing; 2020. https://www.ncbi.nlm.nih.gov/books/NBK544292/.
10. Sheean G. The pathophysiology of spasticity. *European Journal of Neurology*. 2002;9(S1):3–9.
11. Sehgal N, McGuire JR. Beyond Ashworth: electrophysiologic quantification of spasticity. *Physical Medicine and Rehabilitation Clinics of North America*. 1998;9(4):949–979.
12. Ivanhoe CB, Reistetter TA. Spasticity: the misunderstood part of the upper motor neuron syndrome. *American Journal of Physical Medicine & Rehabilitation*. 2004;83(10 Suppl):S3–S9.
13. Trompetto C, Marinelli L, Mori L, et al. Pathophysiology of spasticity: implications for neurorehabilitation. *BioMed Research International.*. 2014;2014:354906.
14. Stolp-Smith KA, Wainberg MC. Antidepressant exacerbation of spasticity. *Archives of Physical Medicine and Rehabilitation*. 1999;80(3):339–342.
15. Benz EN, Hornby TG, Bode RK, Scheidt RA, Schmit BD. A physiologically based clinical measure for spastic reflexes in spinal cord injury. *Archives of Physical Medicine and Rehabilitation*. 2005;86(1):52–59.
16. Akpinar P, Atici A, Ozkan FU, Aktas I, Kulcu DG, Kurt KN. Reliability of the spinal cord assessment tool for spastic reflexes. *Arch Phys Med Rehabil*. 2017;98(6):1113–1118.
17. Adams MM, Ginis KA, Hicks AL. The spinal cord injury spasticity evaluation tool: development and evaluation. *Arch Phys Med Rehabil*. 2007 Sep;88(9):1185–1192.
18. Ansari NN, Kashi M, Naghdi S. The spinal cord injury spasticity evaluation tool: a Persian adaptation and validation study. *J Spinal Cord Med*. 2017;40(4):380–388.
19. Ertzgaard P, Nene A, Kiekens C, Burns AS. A review and evaluation of patient-reported outcome measures for spasticity in persons with spinal cord damage: recommendations from the Ability Network – an international initiative. *J Spinal Cord Med*. 2020;43(6):813–823.
20. Cook KF, Teal CR, Engebretson JC, et al. Development and validation of patient reported impact of spasticity measure (PRISM). *J Rehabil Res Dev*. 2007;44(3):363–371.
21. Priebe MM, Sherwood AM, Thornby JI, Kharas NF, Markowski J. Clinical assessment of spasticity in spinal cord injury: a multidimensional problem. *Arch Phys Med Rehabil*. 1996 Jul;77(7):713–716.
22. Lechner HE, Frotzler A, Eser P. Relationship between self- and clinically rated spasticity in spinal cord injury. *Archives of Physical Medicine and Rehabilitation*. 2006;87(1):15–19.
23. Hsieh JTC, Wolfe DL, Miller WC, Curt A. Spasticity outcome measures in spinal cord injury: psychometric properties and clinical utility. *Spinal Cord*. 2008;46(2):86–95.
24. Rabchevsky AG, Kitzman PH. Latest approaches for the treatment of spasticity and autonomic dysreflexia in chronic spinal cord injury. *Neurotherapeutics: J American Society Experimental NeuroTherapeutics*. 2011;8(2):274–282.
25. Biering-Sørensen F, Nielsen J, Klinge K. Spasticity-assessment: a review. *Spinal Cord*. 2006;44:708–722.
26. Bajd T, Vodovnik L. Pendulum testing of spasticity. *Journal of Biomedical Engineering*. 1984;6(1):9–16.
27. Firoozbakhsh KK, Kunkel CF, Scremin AM, Moneim MS. Isokinetic dynamometric technique for spasticity assessment. *Am J Phys Med Rehabil*. 1993;72(6):379–385.
28. Lamontagne A, Malouin F, Richards CL, Dumas F. Evaluation of reflex- and nonreflex-induced muscle resistance to stretch in adults with spinal cord injury using hand-held and isokinetic dynamometry. *Phys Ther*. 1998;78(9):964–975. discussion 976-978.
29. Yablon SA, Stokic DS. Neurophysiologic evaluation of spastic hypertonia: implications for management of the patient with the intrathecal baclofen pump. *Am J Phys Med Rehabil*. 2004;83(10 Suppl):S10–S18.
30. Sun E, Hanyu-Deutmeyer AA. Heterotopic ossification. [Updated 2020 Aug 15]. In: StatPearls [Internet]. Treasure Island (FL): StatPearls Publishing; 2020 Jan. https://www.ncbi.nlm.nih.gov/books/NBK519029/.
31. Miglietta O. Action of cold on spasticity. *American Journal of Physical Medicine*. 1973;52(4):198–205.
32. Lofvenmark I, Werhagen L, Norrbrink C. Spasticity and bone density after a spinal cord injury. *Journal of Rehabilitation Medicine*. 2009;41(13):1080–1084.
33. Agarwal NK, Mathur N. Deep vein thrombosis in acute spinal cord injury. *Spinal Cord*. 2009;47(10):769–772.
34. Do JG, Kim DH, Sung DH. Incidence of deep vein thrombosis after spinal cord injury in Korean patients at acute rehabilitation unit. *Journal of Korean Medical Science*. 2013; 28(9):1382–1387.
35. Mackiewicz-Milewska M, Jung S, Kroszczyński AC, et al. Deep venous thrombosis in patients with chronic spinal cord injury. *The Journal of Spinal Cord Medicine*. 2016;39(4):400–404.
36. Kim SW, Charallel JT, Park KW, et al. Prevalence of deep venous thrombosis in patients with chronic spinal cord injury. *Archives of Physical Medicine and Rehabilitation*. 1994;75(9):965–968.
37. Goetz LL, De Jesus O, McAvoy SM. Posttraumatic syringomyelia. [Updated 2020 Nov 14]. In: StatPearls [Internet]. Treasure Island (FL): StatPearls Publishing; 2020 Jan. https://www.ncbi.nlm.nih.gov/books/NBK470405/.
38. Lehmann JF, Masock AJ, Warren CG, Koblanski JN. Effect of therapeutic temperatures on tendon extensibility. *Arch Phys Med Rehabil*. 1970;51(8):481–487.

39. Katalinic OM, Harvey LA, Herbert RD. Effectiveness of stretch for the treatment and prevention of contractures in people with neurological conditions: a systematic review. *Physical Therapy*. 2011;91(1):11–24.
40. Bovend'Eerdt TJ, Newman M, Barker K, Dawes H, Minelli C, Wade DT. The effects of stretching in spasticity: a systematic review. *Archives of Physical Medicine and Rehabilitation*. 2008;89(7):1395–1406.
41. Beecham GB, Bansal P, Nessel TA, et al. Lidocaine. [Updated 2020 Jul 10]. In: StatPearls [Internet]. Treasure Island (FL): StatPearls Publishing; 2020 Jan. https://www.ncbi.nlm.nih.gov/books/NBK539881/.
42. D'Souza RS, Warner NS. Phenol nerve block. [Updated 2020 Sep 2]. In: StatPearls [Internet]. Treasure Island (FL): StatPearls Publishing; 2020 Jan. https://www.ncbi.nlm.nih.gov/books/NBK525978/.
43. Tilton AH. Injectable neuromuscular blockade in the treatment of spasticity and movement disorders. *Journal of Child Neurology*. 2003;18(1_suppl):S50–S66.
44. Glenn MB, Elovic E. Chemical denervation for the treatment of hypertonia and related motor disorders: phenol and botulinum toxin. *The Journal of Head Trauma Rehabilitation*. 1997;12(6):40–62.
45. Ghai A, Sangwan SS, Hooda S, Kiran S, Garg N. Obturator neurolysis using 65% alcohol for adductor muscle spasticity. *Saudi Journal of Anaesthesia*. 2012;6(3):282–284.
46. Nigam PK, Nigam A. Botulinum toxin. *Indian Journal of Dermatology*. 2010;55(1):8–14.
47. Francisco G. Botulinum toxin: dosing and dilution. *American Journal of Physical Medicine & Rehabilitation*. 2004;83(10): S30–S37.
48. Burns AS, Meythaler JM. Intrathecal baclofen in tetraplegia of spinal origin:efficacy for upper extremity hypertonia. *Spinal Cord*. 2001;39(8):413–419.
49. Chang E, Ghosh N, Yanni D, Lee S, Alexandru D, Mozaffar T. A review of spasticity treatments: pharmacological and interventional approaches. *Crit Rev Phys Rehabil Med*. 2013;25(1-2):11–22.
50. Penn RD. Intrathecal baclofen for spasticity of spinal origin:seven years of experience. *Journal of Neurosurgery*. 1992;77(2):236–240.
51. McIntyre A, Mays R, Mehta S, et al. Examining the effectiveness of intrathecal baclofen on spasticity in individuals with chronic spinal cord injury: a systematic review. *The Journal of Spinal Cord Medicine*. 2014;37(1):11–18.
52. Heetla HW, Staal MJ, Kliphuis C, Van Laar T. The incidence and management of tolerance in intrathecal baclofen therapy. *Spinal Cord*. 2009;47(10):751–756.
53. Sayer C, Lumsden DE, Perides S, et al. Intrathecal baclofen trials: complications and positive yield in a pediatric cohort. *Journal of Neurosurgery. Pediatrics.*. 2016;17(2): 240–245.
54. Adams MM, Hicks AL. Spasticity after spinal cord injury. *Spinal Cord*. 2005;43(10):577–586.
55. Bohannon RW, Smith MB. Interrater reliability of a modified ashworth scale of muscle spasticity. *Physical Therapy*. 1987;67(2):206–207.
56. Mishra C, Ganesh GS. Inter-rater reliability of modified Ashworth scale in the assessment of plantar flexor muscle spasticity in patients with spinal cord injury. *Physiotherapy Research International.*. 2014;19(4):231–237.
57. Akpinar P, Atici A, Ozkan FU, et al. Reliability of the modified Ashworth scale and modified Tardieu scale in patients with spinal cord injuries. *Spinal Cord*. 2017;55(10):944–949.
58. Grippo A, Carrai R, Hawamdeh Z, et al. Biomechanical and electromyographic assessment of spastic hypertonus in motor complete traumatic spinal cord-injured individuals. *Spinal Cord*. 2011;49:142–148.
59. Lindberg PG, Gäverth J, Islam M, Fagergren A, Borg J, Forssberg H. Validation of a new biomechanical model to measure muscle tone in spastic muscles. *Neurorehabilitation and Neural Repair*. 2011;25(7):617–625.
60. Mayo M, DeForest BA, Castellanos M, Thomas CK. Characterization of involuntary contractions after spinal cord injury reveals associations between physiological and self-reported measures of spasticity. *Frontiers in Integrative Neuroscience*. 2017;11:2.
61. Fonseca LA, Grecco LAC, Politti F, et al. Use a portable device for measuring spasticity in individuals with cerebral palsy. *Journal of Physical Therapy Science*. 2013;25(3): 271–275.
62. Biering-Sørensen F, Hansen B, Lee BSB. Non-pharmacological treatment and prevention of bone loss after spinal cord injury: a systematic review. *Spinal Cord*. 2009;47(7): 508–518.
63. Khan F, Amatya B, Bensmail D, Yelnik A. Non-pharmacological interventions for spasticity in adults: an overview of systematic reviews. *Annals of Physical and Rehabilitation Medicine*. 2019;62(4):265–273.
64. Gündüz S, Kalyon TA, Dursun H, Möhür H, Bilgic F. Peripheral nerve block with phenol to treat spasticity in spinal cord injured patients. *Paraplegia.*. 1992;30(11):808–811.
65. Soni BM, Mani RM, Oo T, Vaidyanathan S. Treatment of spasticity in a spinal cord-injured patient with intrathecal morphine due to intrathecal baclofen tolerance: a case report and review of literature. *Spinal Cord*. 2003;41(10): 586–589.
66. Weingarden SI, Belen JG. Clonidine transdermal system for treatment of spasticity in spinal cord injury. *Arch Phys Med Rehabil*. 1992;73(9):876–877. PMID: 1514897.
67. Cyproheptadine hydrochloride tablets [prescribing information]. Nashville, TN: Westminster Pharmaceuticals, LLC; November 2019. https://dailymed.nlm.nih.gov/dailymed/fda/fdaDrugXsl.cfm?setid=526654c3-4c79-467e-ac73-01ae84ddbd78&type=display.
68. Cyproheptadine hydrochloride oral solution [safety data sheet]. East Brunswick, NJ InvaTech Pharma Solutions LLC; September 2018. https://imgcdn.mckesson.com/CumulusWeb/Click_and_learn/SDS_9QUAGN_CYPROHEPTADINE_HCL_SYRP_2MG_5ML.pdf.
69. Vlavonou R, Perreault MM, Barrière O, et al. Pharmacokinetic characterization of baclofen in patients with chronic kidney disease: dose adjustment recommendations. *J Clin Pharmacol*. 2014;54(5):584–592.
70. Galvez-Jimenez N. Symptom-based management of amyotrophic lateral sclerosis. UpToDate. http://www.uptodate.com. Accessed January 18, 2022.
71. Olek MJ, Narayan RN, Frohman EM, Frohman TC. Symptom management of multiple sclerosis in adults. UpToDate. http://www.uptodate.com. Accessed February 01, 2022.
72. Maynard FM. Early clinical experience with clonidine in spinal spasticity. *Paraplegia.*. 1986;24(3):175–182.

73. Manzon L, Nappe TM, DelMaestro C, Maguire NJ. Clonidine toxicity. In: StatPearls. StatPearls Publishing; 2020. [Updated June 30, 2020.] https://www.ncbi.nlm.nih.gov/books/NBK459374/.
74. Alstermark C, Amin K, Dinn SR, et al. Synthesis and pharmacological evaluation of novel gamma-aminobutyric acid type B (GABAB) receptor agonists as gastroesophageal reflux inhibitors. *J Med Chem*. 2008;51(14):4315–4320.
75. Corazza M, Mantovani L, Virgili A, Strumia R. Allergic contact dermatitis from a clonidine transdermal delivery system. *Contact Dermatitis*. 1995;32(4):246.
76. Tizanidine [prescribing information]. Chestnut Ridge, NY: Par Pharmaceutical; May 2017. https://www.parpharm.com/pdfs/catalog/generic/Tizandidne_PI_20200506.pdf.
77. Acorda Therapeutics. Zanaflex (Tizanidine hydrochloride). Ardsley, NY: Acorda Therapeutics; 2013. https://www.accessdata.fda.gov/drugsatfda_docs/label/2013/021447s011_020397s026lbl.pdf.
78. Cyproheptadine hydrochloride oral solution [prescribing information]. Largo, FL: VistaPharm, Inc; 2018.
79. Paton DM, Webster DR. Clinical pharmacokinetics of H1-receptor antagonists (the antihistamines). *Clin Pharmacokinet*. 1985;10(6):477–497.
80. Barbeau H, Richards CL, Bedard PJ. Action of cyproheptadine in spastic paraparetic patients. *J Neurol Neurosurg Psychiatry*. 1982;45(10):923–926.
81. Wainberg M, Barbeau H, Gauthier S. The effects of cyproheptadine on locomotion and on spasticity in patients with spinal cord injuries. *J Neurol Neurosurg Psychiatry*. 1990;53(9):754–763.

CHAPTER 30

Thermoregulation and Sweating

Brittni Micham

Autonomic dysregulation is a sequela of spinal cord injury (SCI) that is a potential cause of morbidity and mortality in persons with SCI. *Poikilothermia*, the inability to regulate body temperature, is a result of autonomic dysregulation in SCI.

Normal body temperature is defined as 95–101°F (35–38.4°C), and rectal temperature is generally considered the most accurate reflection of core temperature.[1] Normal thermoregulation occurs when afferent temperature signals travel from the skin and visceral organs through the spinal circuits to the hypothalamus, the body's central temperature regulator. When the hypothalamus determines the body temperature is abnormal, efferent signals are transmitted through the spinal cord to initiate appropriate temperature-regulating responses such as sweating and vasodilation or shivering and vasoconstriction. This relay system is interrupted in patients with SCI.

Preganglionic sympathetic neurons are located from T1–L2 in the spinal cord and regulate blood vessels and sweat glands.[2] Loss of supraspinal regulatory control results in overall reduced sympathetic activity below the level of injury (i.e., abnormal sweating, poor vasomotor response, and inability of skeletal muscle to shiver).[1–3] There is impaired thermoregulation and sweating below the level of injury. Patients with injuries above T8 frequently have poor regulation of body temperature (*mnemonic* = **T**emper-**8**-ture).[1] The higher the level of injury, the greater the body surface area affected; thus, patients with complete tetraplegia are particularly susceptible to hypothermia and hyperthermia.

Persons with complete tetraplegia generally have a core body temperature 1–2°F lower than persons without SCI.[3,4] Even when septic, a patient with complete tetraplegia may mount only a low-grade fever (99–100°F). Conversely, environmental factors (hot weather, excessive blankets) can lead to temperatures qualifying as a low-grade fever in these patients.[5] Careful clinical consideration of all involved factors is important when evaluating temperature in SCI to avoid misdiagnosis and potentially increased morbidity.

One particular phenomenon, known as neurogenic fever or "quad fever," is almost exclusively seen in patients with complete tetraplegia.[1] In approximately 4%–5% of individuals with complete tetraplegia, there will be an increase in body temperature without an identifiable cause such as infection or environmental factors.[6] In such cases, the fever etiology is a dysfunction of the central nervous system. It is important to remember that neurogenic fever is a diagnosis of exclusion, and other causes must absolutely be ruled out before deciding a patient has neurogenic fever.

An alternative cause of increased core temperature in persons with SCI is exercise-induced hyperthermia. Even exercising in cool or moderate temperatures may cause hyperthermia in a patient with a high thoracic or cervical level of injury.[7] Strategies for maintaining appropriate body temperature should be discussed with any patient or athlete before they undertake athletic activity. The patient should have a means of taking their temperature readily available. Site-specific cooling, such as cold towels or cooling vests, is usually the best initial approach.[8]

While reduced sweating below the level of injury is more commonly seen in persons with SCI, hyperhidrosis below the level of injury can also be a manifestation of autonomic dysfunction.[1–3] Excessive sweating can not only cause significant emotional distress, but moisture trapped against the skin by clothing or other barriers can lead to skin maceration and breakdown. Patients with hyperhidrosis should be educated to do frequent skin checks and use barrier creams, topical antiperspirants, or absorbent materials as needed to protect the skin.

Using culturally appropriate risk communication strategies, judicious education about thermal dysregulation should be provided to all persons with SCI, but particularly to those with a level of injury above T8. Clinicians should review with the patient signs of hypothermia (lethargy, confusion, decreased coordination, slowed breathing, etc.) and hyperthermia (confusion, tachypnea, nausea, dizziness, headache, etc.). The importance of vigilance during exercise or when exposed to extremes of temperature should be emphasized. Potential strategies for those patients who plan to engage in exercise or activities that risk exposure include space blankets, cooling sprays, and cooling vests.

Review Questions

1. Core body temperature is centrally regulated by the:
   a. Medulla
   b. Thalamus
   c. Hypothalamus
   d. Pituitary
2. Preganglionic sympathetic neurons located from T1–L2 in the spinal cord regulate all but the following:
   a. Sweat glands
   b. Vasomotor responses
   c. Skeletal muscle shivering
   d. Afferent skin temperature sensation
3. Patients with a level of injury above _____ are considered more at risk for poikilothermia and should be carefully educated about body temperature monitoring and regulation strategies.
   a. C4
   b. C6
   c. T6
   d. T8
4. Patients with complete tetraplegia generally have a core body temperature _____°F lower than persons without SCI.
   a. 0–1°F
   b. 1–2°F
   c. 2–3°F
   d. 1.5–2.5°F
5. Athletes with SCI may participate in activities involving extremes of temperature and are particularly vulnerable to both exercise-induced hyperthermia and exposure hypothermia. Temperature-regulating strategies could include all but the following:
   a. Ice bath/whole-body water immersion
   b. Cooling vest
   c. Cooling spray
   d. Thermal/space blankets

REFERENCES

1. Kirshblum S, Lin VW. *Spinal Cord Medicine.* 3rd ed. New York: Demos Medical; 2019.
2. Sabharwal S. *Essentials of Spinal Cord Medicine.* New York: Demos Medical; 2014.
3. Karlsson AK, Krassioukov A, Alexander MS, Donovan W, Biering-Sorenson F. International spinal cord injury skin and thermoregulation function basic data set. *Spinal Cord.* 2012;15(7):512–516.
4. Price MJ, Trbovich M. Thermoregulation following spinal cord injury. *Handb Clin Neurol.* 2018;157:799–820.
5. Mneimneh F, Moussalem C, Ghaddar N, Aboughali K, Omeis I. Influence of cervical spinal cord injury on thermoregulatory and cardiovascular responses in the human body: literature review. *J Clin Neurosci.* 2019;69:7–14.
6. Colachis SC, Otis SM. Occurrence of fever associated with thermoregulatory dysfunction after acute traumatic spinal cord injury. *Am J Phys Med Rehabil.* 1995;74:114–119.
7. Sawka MN, Latzka WA, Pandolf KB. Temperature regulation during upper body exercise: able-bodied and spinal cord injured. *Med Sci Sports Exerc.* 1989 Oct;21(5 Suppl):S132–S140.
8. Griggs KE, Price MJ, Goosey-Tolfrey VL. Cooling athletes with a spinal cord injury. *Sports Med.* 2015;45(1):9–21.

CHAPTER

31

Traumatic Brain Injury and Spinal Cord Injury

David H. Glazer and Daniel Krasna

OUTLINE

Introduction

The term *dual diagnosis* is used to describe the cooccurrence of traumatic spinal cord injury (SCI) and traumatic brain injury (TBI) as a result of a single event.[1] Given the added challenges of two acute neurologic conditions, SCI clinicians need to be aware of the incidence, common mechanisms of injury, diagnostic criteria, and unique management issues of cooccurring TBI in SCI.

Epidemiology

- Worldwide
  - TBI has a worldwide age-standardized prevalence of 759 per 100,000
  - SCI has an age-standardized prevalence of 368 per 100,000
  - Prevalence in 2016: 55 million individuals with TBI and 27 million with SCI[2]
- United States
  - Prevalence of TBI: 5.3 million individuals who are living with one or more TBIs
  - Incidence
    - 2.2 million emergency department visits
    - 280,000 hospitalizations
    - 50,000 deaths[3]

Etiology of Traumatic Brain Injury and Spinal Cord Injury

The most common causes for both SCI and TBI are motor vehicle collisions, falls, sport-related insults, and assaults.[4] These overlapping causes result in a high risk for a dual diagnosis in these two populations,[4] with incidences ranging from 40%–60%.[4,5] While studies in the United States have reported that mild TBI is common,[5] reports from other countries have found severe TBI to be the most common.[1] In patients diagnosed with severe TBI as the primary injury, 7%–8% of patients were found to have concomitant cervical spine injury.[1]

Given the significant rate of underdiagnosis of mild TBI in the general population and the added underdiagnosis of both mild and moderate TBI in the face of significant trauma, including SCI, particularly when the individual requires intubation and sedation on admission, the reported rates of combined SCI and TBI are likely significantly underreported. Thus, the rehabilitation clinicians may be the first to recognize the concomitant TBI.[6]

Mechanism of Injury

Although some studies have identified cervical level SCI to be associated with greater rates of TBI but not more severe injuries,[5] others have found cervical-and thoracic level injuries to be at similar high risk for dual diagnosis.[4] Motor vehicle collisions are the most common cause of dual diagnosis, followed by falls.

Pathophysiology

TBI is defined as an "alteration in function, or other evidence of brain pathology caused by an external force."[7] Brain injury severity is primarily based on the Glasgow Coma Scale, which categorizes acute severity into mild,[8–10] moderate,[11–14] or severe.[1–6] This designation is based on the best Glasgow coma score recorded within the first 24 hours following injury.[7] Severity can be further classified by duration of loss of consciousness and duration of posttraumatic amnesia (Table 31.1).[15,16]

The external force that results in TBI can occur as a result of direct impact against the skull or as acceleration and deceleration forces that transmit shear to axons.[7] Focal injuries are those that occur at the site of impact, whereas diffuse injuries are those that occur away from the site of impact. Primary injuries are those that occur at the time of the impact. In contrast, secondary injury develops later as a result of a signaling cascade initiated by the impact (Fig. 31.1).

Table 31.1 Criteria Used to Classify Traumatic Brain Injury Severity

Criterion	Mild	Moderate	Severe
Loss of consciousness	0–30 min	>30 min and <24 h	>24 h
Posttraumatic amnesia	<24 h	>24 h and <7 days	>7 days
Glasgow Coma Scale score	13–15	9–12	<9
Structural imaging	Normal	Normal or abnormal	Normal or abnormal

From Health K, Barcikowski J. Epidemiology and public health and prevention. In: Eapen BC, Cifu DX. *Brain Injury Medicine: Board Review.* Elsevier, 2021.

Focal injuries occur at the site of impact and include contusions and hemorrhages.[11] These lesions may cause predictable deficits in the functions controlled by specific anatomic areas.

Left Versus Right

- Most patients are left-side dominant, meaning their language center is in the left temporal lobe
- Very few left-handed individuals have a reverse
- Overall, there is a contralateral representation for motor and sensory functions

Different Lobes

- Frontal: anterior brain until central sulcus, lateral border is Sylvian fissure
  - Motor control in precentral sulcus
  - Premotor cortex anterior to this, connects with other areas and includes the Broca area as well as eye fields

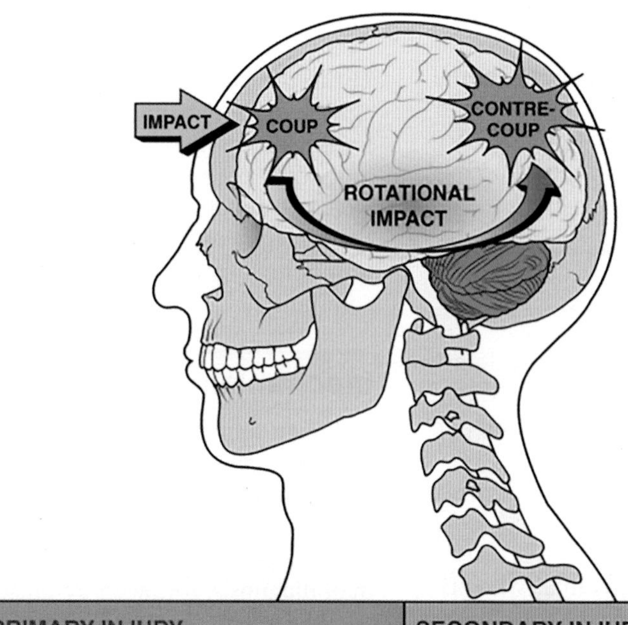

PRIMARY INJURY (at time of injury)	SECONDARY INJURY (hours, to days, to weeks)
• Due to force associated with mechanism - fall - motor vehicle accident - assault • Coup – Contrecoup - contusions • Shearing of blood vessels - epidural, subdural hematomas • Rotational forces causing axonal shearing - diffuse axonal injury	• Cellular mechanism and microenvironment changes of further dysfunction • Astrocyte foot swelling - breakdown of the blood–brain barrier • Gliosis • Glutamatergic release - activation of NMDA and AMPA receptors • cellular depolarization • excitotoxicity • mitochondrial dysfunction • caspace cascade

Fig. 31.1 Schematic of Primary and Secondary Injuries That Occur Due to Head Trauma. *AMPA*, α-amino-3-hydroxy-5-methyl-4-isoxazolepropionate; *NMDA*, N-methyl-D-aspartate. (From: Figure 25.1, Ellenbogen, Richard G., et al. *Principles of Neurological Surgery E-Book: Expert Consult-Online*, Elsevier, 2018.)

- Prefrontal cortex is the remainder
  - Dorsolateral prefrontal cortex: "executive functions such as working memory, decision making, problem solving and mental flexibility"[12]
  - Orbitofrontal cortex: social monitoring of behavior
  - Medial frontal/anterior cingulate: motivation, initiation, and reward[12,13]
- Temporal: language comprehension, object recognition
  - Medial temporal region: integration of emotional memory with current experience.
- Parietal
  - Postcentral gyrus: somatosensory cortex
  - Superior lobule: integrate sensory input
  - Inferior lobule: visuospatial integration, math[13]
- Occipital: visual cortex and processing of visual stimuli

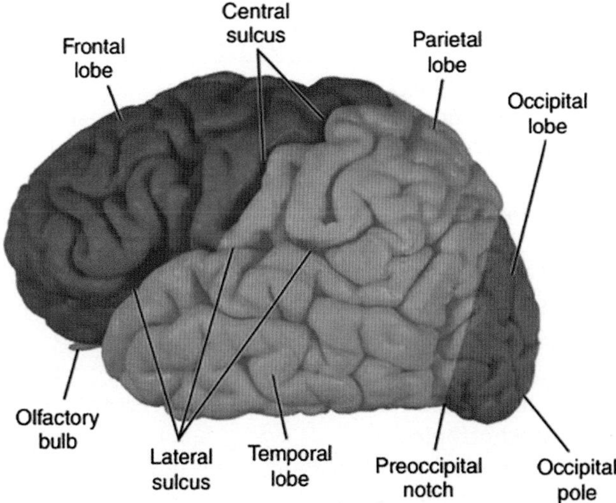

Fig. 31.2 Lobes of the Cerebral Hemisphere With Major Sulci. (From Gross anatomy and general organization of the central nervous system. In: Vanderah TW, Gould DJ. *Nolte's the Human Brain: An Introduction to Its Functional Anatomy*. 7th ed. Philadelphia: Elsevier; 2016:61. Fig. 3.8.)

Subcortical Structures

- Thalamus: relay station for somatosensory, arousal, visual, and auditory information as well as connections with limbic structures
- Hypothalamus: hormonal regulation, sleep
- Basal ganglia: motor, cognitive, and emotional modulation processing
- "The frontal-subcortical circuits responsible for these critical domains of higher intellectual function and empathic, motivated, nuanced human behavior are highly vulnerable to injury in the typical TBI"[12] (Fig. 31.2).

Primary Diffuse

Initial diffuse injuries can be extensive and cause dysfunction in any system that has white matter tracts passing through the area that suffered shearing from acceleration and deceleration during injury. The term *diffuse axonal injury* is used to describe this form of injury and can be graded based on the extent of the injury. It is more commonly seen after severe injury. These injuries are often not evident on initial imaging and are overall difficult to visualize on computed tomography (CT). Diffuse tensor imaging modality on magnetic resonance imaging (MRI) provides the best chance for visualizing macroscopic lesions.[14]

Secondary Injury

Secondary injury occurs both focally and diffusely, based on the disruption of cell membranes and subsequent neurochemical changes. The alteration of cell membranes leads to a drastic increase in glutamate release. This then causes "ionic disequilibrium" with potassium exiting and sodium and calcium entering at synaptic terminals, prompting the sodium–potassium pumps to consume more adenosine triphosphate in an attempt to correct the imbalance. This leads to consumption of energy. In addition, the influx of calcium triggers increased uptake of calcium into the mitochondria, which leads to impaired mitochondrial function via oxidative stress.[8] Additionally, secondary injury can refer to progression of focal swelling or ischemia, which may worsen deficits that are more localizable to specific anatomical structures as mentioned previously under primary focal injury.

Diagnosis

- Moderate and severe TBI are typically diagnosed with initial imaging obtained in the emergency department
- Due to the emergent needs of SCI, a diagnosis of mild TBI is often overlooked at the time of the initial trauma
  - Head CT scans of patients who have sustained mild TBI can be unrevealing of pathology
  - Despite a negative head CT, a patient could have sustained a TBI
  - A thorough history focused on mild TBI symptoms must be obtained
- Mild TBI symptoms can often be revealed during inpatient rehabilitation
  - Symptoms include headaches, dizziness, insomnia, balance impairment, emotional irritability/lability, depression/anxiety, impaired memory, executive dysfunction, behavioral manifestations, visual impairments, impaired communication[6]

Treatment and Management

- Agitation and aggression
  - Assess and control for external factors, such as pain from poor body positioning, occult fracture, tight clothing, kinked catheter, constipation, infection, and environmental stimuli, such as numerous people in room, bright lights, loud noises
  - Consider use of medications such as propranolol (Inderal), valproic acid, trazodone, quetiapine (Seroquel)
- Psychological changes
  - Use of mood stabilizers, antidepressants, and psychotropics
    - Atypical antipsychotics have fewer effects on dopamine and are better tolerated in TBI
    - Selective serotonin reuptake inhibitors have fewer side effects than other antidepressants
  - Counseling
- Cognitive and communication impairment
  - Neuropsychology evaluation
  - Speech therapy evaluation and treatment
  - Consider use of external resources such as alarms, computer applications, notebooks, and other assistive devices
  - Consider use of medications such as methylphenidate (Ritalin) for improving processing speed
- Sleep disturbance
  - Promote good sleep hygiene
  - Consider sleep apnea as a diagnosis and possible need for devices such as continuous positive airway pressure
  - Consider medications such as trazodone
  - "Z-drugs" such as zolpidem can cause further cognitive impairment or paradoxical increase in arousal
- Paroxysmal sympathetic hyperactivity
  - More common acutely, but can be seen years later
  - Symptoms include elevated blood pressure, tachycardia, sweating, muscle overactivity
  - Treat by reducing noxious stimuli; similar to dysreflexia episodes in SCI
  - Medications
    - Propranolol and gabapentin (Neurontin) for baseline control
    - Opiates for pain control during episode[11]
- Seizure prophylaxis
  - Immediate (within 24 hours), early (1–7 days), late (over 7 days)
  - Give 1 week of antiepileptics to prevent early seizures
  - May need long-term course if an early seizure occurs or if more severe injury in a location known to be a seizure focus
  - Initial studies done on phenytoin (Dilantin), but this can slow neurorecovery[9]
- Headache
  - First line: consider nonopiate analgesics
  - Determine type of headache
    - Cervicogenic pain can often cause headache, myofascial release in therapy
    - Migraine: pain, nausea, possible visual changes (aura)
    - Tension: bandlike, squeezing pain
    - Cluster: pain behind one eye
- Visual impairment
  - Evaluation by neurooptometry
  - Vision therapy
  - Consideration for eye lubricant
  - Possible need for new eyeglass prescription to include prism and/or tints
- Cranial nerve injury
  - Alterations of taste and smell due to olfactory nerve damage
    - Anatomy of cranial nerve one puts it at high risk for shear injury
    - Impaired olfaction can impact appetite
- Spasticity
  - Stretching
  - Medications
    - Baclofen (Lioresal)
    - Dantrolene (Dantrium)
    - Tizanidine (Zanaflex)
  - Chemodenervation with botulinum toxin
  - Nerve blocks with phenol or alcohol

Outcomes of Dual Diagnosis

Individuals who sustain both a TBI and an SCI have an increased length of stay in acute care and rehabilitation with lower discharge scores on the functional independence measure, more behavioral incidents, an increased need for nursing care hours, and have higher costs.[10]

Review Questions

1. A patient has been diagnosed with a T10 ASI B spinal cord injury after a car accident. Upon admission to the rehabilitation hospital, the attending physician discovers the patient has had a headache off and on since the accident. Acetaminophen has not decreased the pain. It is worsened when sleeping at night. What is a likely cause of the headache?
   a. Cervicogenic
   b. Tension
   c. Migraine
   d. Cluster
2. A 23-year-old male sustained a SCI and moderate TBI. He continues to have agitation and difficulty sleeping. Patient reports that pain is well controlled. He then recalls that prior to his injury he was

experiencing similar insomnia and agitation symptoms in addition to periods of sad mood. What is an appropriate next choice of medication?
   a. Escitalopram
   b. Valproic acid
   c. Quetiapine
   d. Propranolol
3. A 25-year-old male with a new traumatic spinal cord injury (T2 ASI A) sustained in a motor vehicle collision 3 weeks ago is having difficulty with carryover in therapy sessions at inpatient rehabilitation. His CT head scan on admission to the acute care hospital showed no intracranial abnormalities. What is the best initial step to help narrow the differential diagnosis?
   a. Repeat CT head
   b. Obtain MRI brain
   c. Neuropsychological testing
   d. Obtain further history from family
4. The physician notices that a new patient with traumatic spinal cord injury (T10 ASI A) is unable to propel the wheelchair in a straight line. The patient is often bumping into people and the wall. In addition, the patient always requests for the lights in the room to be dimmed and asks for Tylenol frequently. What is the likely cause?
   a. Migraine headache
   b. Vestibular disorder
   c. Vision impairment
   d. Weak left arm
5. A new patient at the rehabilitation hospital who sustained a moderate TBI is not maintaining sufficient caloric oral intake to allow for proper healing. The physician and dietician realize the likely cause is:
   a. Patient being a picky eater
   b. Constipation
   c. Olfactory nerve injury
   d. Elevated anxiety

REFERENCES

1. Pinto SM, Galang G. Concurrent SCI and TBI: epidemiology, shared pathophysiology, assessment, and prognostication. *Curr Phys Med Rehabil Rep.* 2016;4:71–79.
2. GBD 2016 Traumatic Brain Injury and Spinal Cord Injury Collaborators. Global, regional, and national burden of traumatic brain injury and spinal cord injury, 1990–2016: a systematic analysis for the Global Burden of Disease Study 2016. *Lancet Neurol.* 2019;18(1):56–87.
3. Traumatic Brain Injury in the United States: Epidemiology and Rehabilitation Centers for Disease Control and Prevention. (2015). Report to Congress on Traumatic Brain Injury in the United States: Epidemiology and Rehabilitation. National Center for Injury Prevention and Control; Division of Unintentional Injury Prevention. Atlanta, GA.
4. Budisin B, Bradbury CC, Sharma B, et al. Traumatic brain injury in spinal cord injury: frequency and risk factors. *J Head Trauma Rehabil.* 2016;31(4):E33–E42.
5. Macciocchi S, Seel RT, Thompson N, Byams R, Bowman B. Spinal cord injury and co-occurring traumatic brain injury: assessment and incidence. *Arch Phys Med Rehabil.* 2008;89(7):1350–1357.
6. Kushner DS, Alvarez G. Dual diagnosis: traumatic brain injury with spinal cord injury. *Phys Med Rehabil Clin N Am.* 2014;25(3):681–696, ix-x.
7. Wagner AK, et al. Traumatic brain injury. In: Cifu DX, ed. *Braddom's Physical Medicine and Rehabilitation.* 5th ed. Elsevier; 2016:961–998.
8. Prins M, Greco T, Alexander D, Giza CC. The pathophysiology of traumatic brain injury at a glance. *Dis Model Mech.* 2013;6(6):1307–1315.
9. Temkin NR, Dikmen SS, Wilensky AJ, Keihm J, Chabal S, Winn HR. A randomized, double-blind study of phenytoin for the prevention of post-traumatic seizures. *N Engl J Med.* 1990;323(8):497–502.
10. Bradbury CL, Wodchis WP, Mikulis DJ, et al. Traumatic brain injury in patients with traumatic spinal cord injury: clinical and economic consequences. *Arch Phys Med Rehabil.* 2008;89(12 Suppl):S77–S84.
11. Zasler ND, Katz DI, Zafonte RD. *Brain Injury Medicine Principles and Practice.* 2nd ed. Demos Medical; 2013.
12. McAllister TW. Neurobiological consequences of traumatic brain injury. *Dialogues Clin Neurosci.* 2011;13(3):287–300.
13. Eapen BC, Cifu DX. *Brain Injury Medicine: Board Review.* Philadelphia: Elsevier; 2021.
14. Mefsin FB, Gupta N, Hays Shapshak A, Taylor RS. Diffuse axonal injury. [Updated 2020 Jun 23]. In: StatPearls [Internet]. Treasure Island (FL): StatPearls Publishing; 2020 Jan. https://www.ncbi.nlm.nih.gov/books/NBK448102/.
15. O'Neil ME, Carlson K, Storzbach D, et al. Complications of Mild Traumatic Brain Injury in Veterans and Military Personnel: A Systematic Review [Internet]. Washington (DC): Department of Veterans Affairs (US); 2013 Jan. Table A-1, Classification of TBI Severity. https://www.ncbi.nlm.nih.gov/books/NBK189784/table/appc.t1.
16. Ellenbogen RG, Sekhar LN, Kitchen N. *Principles of Neurological Surgery E-Book: Expert Consult - Online.* 4th ed. Elsevier; 2018.

CHAPTER

32

Neuromodulatory and Disease-Modifying Agents

William McKinley and Steven Peretiatko

OUTLINE

Background

Damage to the spinal cord results in disrupted neuronal connections leading to impaired body function. Technological advances have led to the development of functional electrical stimulation (FES) systems that restore function in spinal cord injury (SCI) and disease-modifying agents that treat multiple sclerosis (MS).

Physiology of Functional Electrical Stimulation

FES applies electrical currents to neural tissues in a synchronized fashion for the purpose of restoring control over impaired or lost body function. FES systems allow individuals with SCI to utilize paralyzed limbs for functional motor activities and regain control of respiratory, bladder, bowel, and sexual function. Additionally, FES is used to prevent and treat pressure injuries, reduce pain, and improve muscular and cardiovascular fitness.[1] In order for FES to be effective, the lower motor neuron (LMN) pathway, including the anterior horn cell, spinal root, peripheral nerve, and neuromuscular junction (NMJ), must be spared from injury. With FES, nerves can be stimulated anywhere from origin to the motor point via electrodes. Electrical stimulation causes the neuronal transmembrane potential to reach threshold, resulting in propagation of an action potential along the LMN pathway to the NMJ, causing muscle contraction. Electrical stimulation has several parameters that modulate muscle contraction, including amplitude, duration, frequency, and pulse shape. The amplitude and duration determine the number of nerve fibers activated and thus force of contraction. Large nerve fibers are more easily stimulated and are recruited first. The pulse frequency determines the quality of muscle contraction. Each pulse with proper amplitude and duration produces a muscle twitch. With increasing frequency, the force produced by each twitch is summated, ultimately resulting in a sustained forceful contraction producing a smooth movement. Sensory fibers within the peripheral nerve are also stimulated, which can be painful if sensation is preserved. To reduce tissue damage from electrical stimulation, nerves rather than muscle are preferentially targeted by electrodes and a balanced asymmetric biphasic pulse shape is used.[2,3]

Functional Electrical Stimulation Components

Basic FES system components include:

- Power source: typically a portable battery
- Command control unit: supplies power to channels, processes sensor information, and outputs commands
- Controller: allows the individual to control when stimulation takes place via various methods (joystick, switches, breath force, electromyography [EMG] signals, voice recognition, or motion sensors)
- Stimulator: supplies electrical stimulation via lead wires to electrodes, which can be transcutaneous, percutaneous, or implanted
- Sensors: provide feedback[4–6]

If a system uses sensors to provide feedback, it is categorized as a *closed system*. Feedback signals from limbs can be obtained from externally placed goniometers that measure joint position and/or potentiometers that measure joint motion, placed at various joints. This allows the command control unit to calculate the velocity and acceleration of movement and adjust output commands in real time. This contrasts with an *open system*, which uses a set stimulation pattern to produce a coordinated action.[7]

There are advantages and disadvantages with each electrode type.

1. Transcutaneous electrodes are placed on the skin over desired nerves. They are inexpensive and adequate for therapeutic and short-term use. Some disadvantages include difficulty isolating nerves, difficulty stimulating deep structures, pain associated with stimulation of cutaneous nerves, and poor cosmesis.[6]
2. Percutaneous electrodes are placed intramuscularly and have been used in development but have not been approved for clinical use. This approach allows electrodes to be placed closer to desired targets. Some disadvantages include infection associated with cutaneous barrier disruption and granuloma formation.[6,8]
3. Implanted electrodes are surgically placed adjacent to a nerve (epineural), around a nerve via cuff, at the motor point on the muscle surface (epimysial), or within the muscle itself (intramuscular). Typically, the lead wires and stimulator are also implanted, whereas the control unit and power source are external. The stimulator receives commands and power through radiofrequency. This electrode type is ideal for long-term use and allows for stimulation of specific muscles, providing good muscle recruitment with low current requirements. Some disadvantages are increased system complexity and risks associated with surgery.[5,9]

Common Uses of Functional Electrical Stimulation

Upper Extremity Neuroprostheses

Upper extremity neuroprostheses provide hand/thumb grasp and release for individuals with cervical SCI. Transcutaneous or implanted electrodes are placed over forearm muscles, and a coordinated stimulation pattern is used to activate muscles in sequence to produce lateral pinch and palmar prehension.[10] Individuals control neuroprostheses using their preserved function via a push button or joint movement. The Handmaster (NESS H200) is a commercially available transcutaneous system that offers an adjustable hand wrist orthosis controlled by push button.[11] The Freehand System uses eight epimysial or intramuscular electrodes and is controlled with movement of the contralateral shoulder[12,13]; however, this system is not commercially available. To maximize function, neuroprostheses can be paired with surgical reconstruction. Transfer of the brachioradialis tendon can provide C5 or C6 tetraplegics with voluntary wrist extension, allowing for a tenodesis grasp. Likewise, transfer of the posterior deltoid tendon to triceps can allow an individual with C6 tetraplegia to have voluntary elbow extension.[14] Current research is focused on adding additional function by stimulation of more muscle groups, new methods of control, and the development of neuroprostheses for C4 and higher-level SCI.[1]

Lower Extremity Neuroprostheses

Lower extremity neuroprostheses allow individuals with incomplete and complete paraplegia to achieve postural control, stand, and ambulate. Transcutaneous or implanted electrodes are used to stimulate lumbar erector spinae and gluteal muscles bilaterally during sitting, allowing for trunk control. Stimulation of the knee, hip, and trunk extensors allow for the sit-to-stand transition.[2,4] One method to provide ambulation is stimulation of the quadriceps and peroneal nerves in specific sequences, as seen in the Parastep system.[15] In general, FES systems for the lower extremity are multichannel, typically requiring an orthosis (trunk or lower extremity support, such as an ankle-foot orthosis) and an assistive device, such as a walker. With these components, numerous devices have been developed and tested in clinical trials, and some have been made commercially available over the years. The Parastep is an example of a transcutaneous system; users control the system with push buttons built into a walker that allows for standing and ambulation.[16] The Case Western Reserve University Neuroprosthesis is an implanted system that allows for standing and ambulation. This system uses a total of 16 implanted electrodes in lower extremity muscles, including erector spinae, gluteus maximus, adductor magnus, semimembranosus, tibialis anterior, tensor fasciae latae, quadriceps, and sartorius.[17] Lower extremity FES devices have also been developed to target specific deficits, such as foot drop. Currently available devices include the Bioness L300 and WalkAide, which use transcutaneous electrodes targeting the common peroneal nerve.[18,19] Furthermore, hybrid systems combine FES with bracing or motorized exoskeletons to provide improved stability and to reduce energy expenditure.[20–22] Another method of neuromodulation is epidural electrical stimulation, which activates motor neurons and has been used with body weight-supported treadmill training to facilitate functional ambulation.[23] Importantly, lower extremity FES research has shown favorable exercise-related physiologic effects for cardiovascular and muscular conditioning leading to the development of FES leg cycle ergometers that are widely used in rehabilitation today.[24,25]

undermining, tunneling, wound bed description, wound edges, periwound skin, volume, and character of exudate.[32] Digital photography has been used to enhance wound assessment and documentation and to provide visual assessment of wounds over time. A major benefit of wound photo documentation is the potential use in telemedicine, which can increase patient access to expert wound care and management.[33]

The Spinal Cord Injury Pressure Ulcer Monitoring Tool is a tool that was designed for wound assessment specific to the SCI population.[34–40] This tool was designed to assess pressure ulcers/injuries and healing in the SCI population and consists of seven variables: wound surface area, depth, edges, tunneling, undermining, exudate type, and necrotic tissue amount. The tool was developed to monitor the rate of wound healing and identify when a wound does not make progress over several weeks. Using objective data, the interdisciplinary team can make decisions to alter the plan of care based on weekly measurements and a total score.[41]

Pressure Ulcer/Injury Staging

PI staging provides a way to communicate the degree of tissue damage in pressure ulcers. The staging system was defined by Shea in 1975 and provides a name to the amount of anatomical tissue loss. In April 2016, the National Pressure Ulcer Advisory Panel revised their pressure ulcer staging to include new "pressure injury" terminology to replace "pressure ulcer" terms, and "suspected" was deleted from deep tissue injury classification.[26] PIs are never back-staged, meaning once a wound is identified as a stage 3 PI, it is never referred to as a stage 1 or 2. Rather, the wound would be referred to as a healing stage 3 PI. In addition, only PI are staged. Diabetic foot ulcers may be graded (such as Wagner grades), but no other wounds are staged (Fig. 33.2).[26]

Deep Tissue Injury

Purple or maroon localized area of discolored but intact skin or blood-filled blister due to damage of underlying soft tissue from pressure and or shear.

Stage 1

Intact skin with nonblanchable redness of a localized area, which may appear differently in darkly pigmented skin. Usually over a bony prominence.

Stage 2

Partial-thickness loss of dermis presenting as a shallow open pressure injury with a red, pink wound bed without slough. May also present as an intact or open/ruptured serum-filled blister. Adipose is not visible and deeper tissues are not visible. There is no granulation, slough, or eschar.

Stage 3

Full-thickness tissue loss. Subcutaneous fat may be visible, but bone, tendon, or muscle are not exposed. Slough or eschar may be present but does not obscure the depth of tissue loss. May include undermining, tunneling, and epibole (rolled edges).

Stage 4

Full-thickness tissue loss with exposed bone, tendon, or muscle. Slough or eschar may be present on some parts of the wound bed. Undermining, tunneling, and epibole may be present. Depth varies by anatomical location.

Unstageable

Full-thickness tissue loss in which the actual depth of the injury is completely obscured by slough (yellow, tan, gray, green, or brown) and/or eschar (tan, brown, or black). If the eschar or slough is removed, a stage 3 or stage 4 pressure injury will be revealed.

Medical Device–Related Pressure Injury

(This describes the wound etiology.) The resultant pressure injury generally conforms to the pattern or shape of the device. The injury should be staged using the staging system.

Mucosal Membrane Pressure Injury

Mucosal membrane pressure injury is found on mucous membranes with a history of a medical device in use at the location of the injury. Due to the anatomy of the tissue, these injuries cannot be staged.[4]

Management/Treatment

PI treatment is one of the most challenging clinical problems in hospital.[29] The management of pressure is interdisciplinary, including primary care physicians, dermatologists, infectious disease consultants, social workers, psychologists, dietitians, podiatrists, home and wound-care nurses, rehabilitation professionals, and surgeons. Once a patient has developed a PI, immediate treatment is recommended, including local wound care, adjunctive treatments, and/or surgical management.[25] One of the treatment priorities once a PI is diagnosed is to eliminate the pressure to the wound, and as the SCI population spends extended times sitting, this often means bedrest to unload ischial or sacrum/coccyx pressure injuries.[25] There are two types of wounds—acute and chronic—and the primary difference between the two types is the rate of healing. An acute wound heals in an orderly, timely, and durable manner and does not require long-term follow-up. Acute wounds have an identifiable mechanism of injury such as trauma or surgery. Some sources suggest the trajectory for acute wound healing is complete within 4 weeks.[42] Chronic wounds do not progress through healing in an orderly

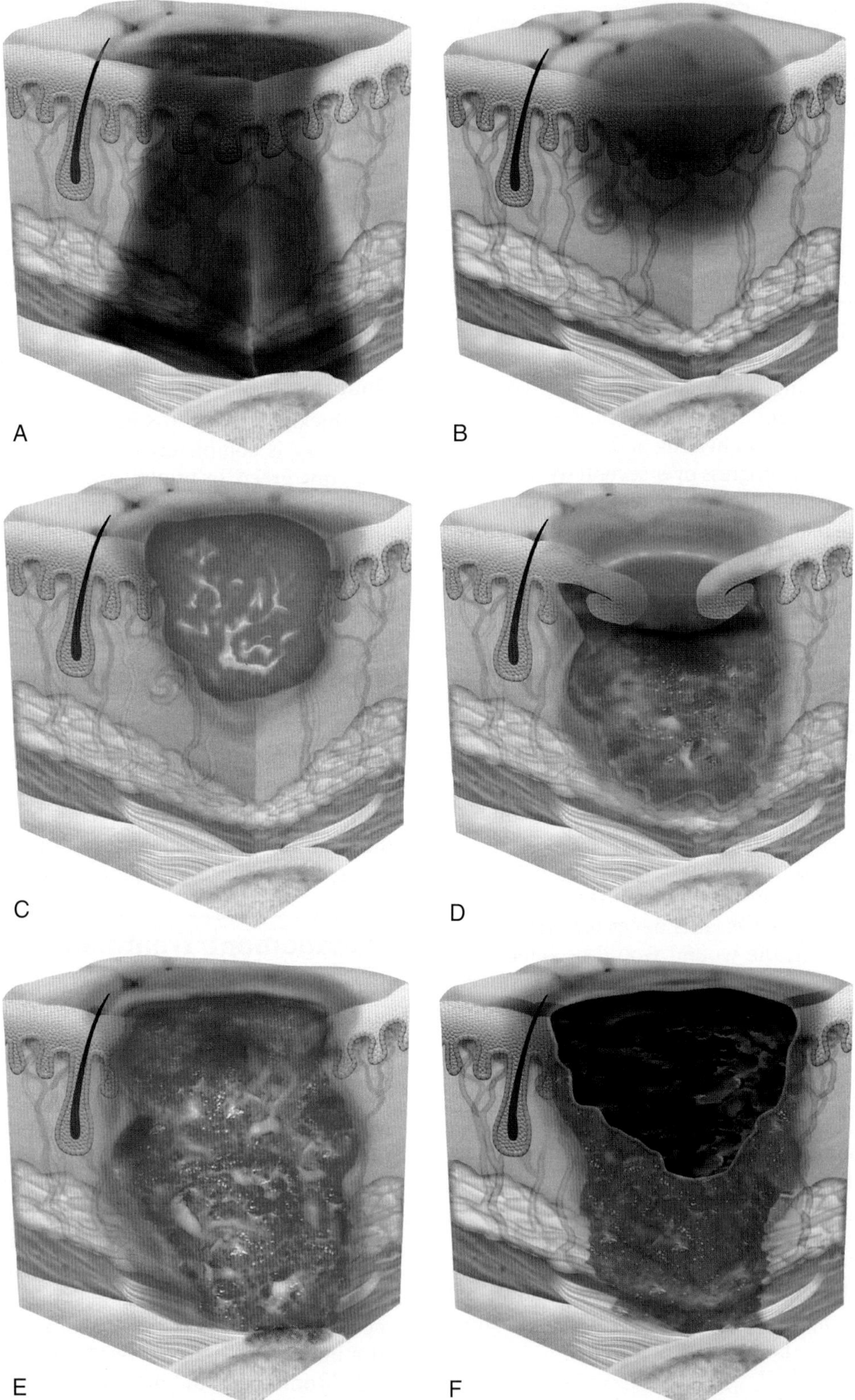

Fig. 33.2 Pressure Injury: Risk Assessment and Prevention. (A) Deep tissue pressure injury: persistent nonblanchable deep red, maroon, or purple discoloration. (B) Stage 1: nonblanchable erythema of intact skin. (C) Stage 2: partial-thickness skin loss with exposed dermis. (D) Stage 3: full-thickness skin loss. (E) Stage 4: full-thickness skin and tissue loss. (F) Unstageable pressure injury: obscured full-thickness skin and tissue loss. From Yeager JJ. Integumentary function. In: Meiner S, Yeager J, eds. *Gerontologic Nursing*. 6th ed. St. Louis: Elsevier; 2019:279–310.

manner; they commonly plateau or stall at some point due to various pathologic conditions; consequently, predictable tissue repair does not occur.[42] Common features of chronic wounds include a prolonged or excessive inflammatory phase due to large volumes of necrotic tissue or high bacterial loads, persistent or recurrent infections, the formation of bacterial biofilms and/or the failure of fibroblasts, endothelial cells, and keratinocytes to produce the new vessels and tissues required for durable closure of the defect.[42]

PI treatment involves management of local infections, removal of necrotic tissue, maintenance of a moist environment for wound healing, and possibly surgery. Debridement is indicated when necrotic tissue is present. Urgent sharp debridement should be performed if advancing cellulitis or sepsis occurs. Necrotic tissue promotes bacterial growth and impairs wound healing, and it should be debrided until eschar is removed and granulation tissue is present. Debridement, however, is not recommended for heel PI that have stable, dry eschar without edema, erythema, fluctuance, or drainage.[2,29] Anticoagulation is a relative contraindication for sharp debridement.[1,29] Mechanical, enzymatic, and autolytic debridement methods are nonurgent treatments. Wound cleansing, preferably with normal saline and appropriate dressings, is a mainstay of treatment for clean PI and after debridement. Bacterial load can be managed with cleansing. Topical antibiotics should be considered if there is no improvement in healing after 14 days. Systemic antibiotics are used in patients with advancing cellulitis, osteomyelitis, or systemic infection.[1,29]

Adjunctive treatments may include electrical stimulation, hyperbaric oxygen, negative-pressure wound therapy (NPWT), growth factors, and skin equivalents.[34] Electrical stimulation (direct electric current delivered through the wound bed using surface electrodes) is used to improve pressure injury healing.[3,29] In electrical stimulation, high-volt pulse current should be used, as it penetrates deeper and has a lower risk of burns. Daily 1-hour sessions are commonly used. Contraindications include cancer (could stimulate cancerous cells) or osteomyelitis (may cause premature closure) or patients that have demand-type pacemakers.[29,32]

NPWT is adjunctive treatment that promotes healing by applying controlled localized negative pressure to the wound bed.[34] The use of NPWT promotes granulation tissue growth due to increased local blood flow, removal of chronic edema, and reduced bacterial counts. NPWT is contraindicated over vital structures, thick exudates, necrotic material, or significant purulence that would render the therapy ineffective or lead to bleeding complications.[30]

Dressings that maintain a moist wound environment facilitate healing and can be used for autolytic debridement.[1,29] Dressings include transparent films, hydrogels, alginates, foams, and hydrocolloids. Transparent films effectively retain moisture and may be used alone or with hydrogels. Hydrogels can be used for deep wounds with light exudate. Alginates and foams are highly absorbent and are useful for moderate to heavy exudate. Dressing selection is dictated by clinical judgment and wound characteristics; currently no moist dressing (including saline-moistened gauze) is superior.[1,29]

Urinary catheters or fecal management systems may be needed to prevent bacterial contamination, as wounds are often colonized with bacteria. A trial of topical antimicrobials should be used for up to 2 weeks for clean PI that are not healing properly after 2–4 weeks of optimal wound care. Quantitative bacteria tissue cultures (swab/tissue biopsy) should be performed for nonhealing PI or for signs of infection. Systemic antibiotics are not recommended unless there is evidence of advancing cellulitis, osteomyelitis, and bacteremia.[1,29]

PIs are difficult to resolve. More than 70% of stage 2 PI heal after 6 months of treatment; only 50% of stage 3 PI and 30% of stage 4 PI heal within this period. Surgical consultation should be obtained for patients with stage 3 or 4 PI that do not respond to optimal care or when rapid closure is needed for quality of life. Surgical approaches include direct closure; skin grafts; and skin, musculocutaneous, and free flaps.[15,29] Advantages of surgical management include wound debridement with soft tissue coverage, improved healing from underlying osteomyelitis, and restoration of tissue to resist shear, friction, and pressure.[30] Disadvantages of surgical intervention include complications (sepsis, dehiscence, hematoma, partial/total flap loss) with complication rates ranging from 6.6% to 53%.[30] Patients must take responsibility for following acute and long-term postflap protocols. The behaviors that contributed to the wound must be modified or the wound will reoccur. The patient is not considered a candidate if these criteria cannot be met.[15]

Conclusions

Wounds in persons with SCI are quick to develop, slow to heal, and prone to complications. These wounds can negatively impact physical, psychological, emotional, and financial status, as well as quality of life. Physiological changes that occur in SCI render the tissues below the level of injury markedly different from innervated tissues and slower to respond to healing modalities.[15] Care of the SCI person with wounds requires an interdisciplinary team approach, good family/caregiver and adequate social support. It is imperative that the patient maintain a healthy lifestyle, change behaviors that resulted in the wound, and is compliant in pressure relief and wound care for optimal healing to occur. If these behaviors cannot be achieved, palliative wound care should be considered. The patient can live with a chronic wound and have quality of life that does not require restricted bed rest that would not result in wound closure in the long term.

Review Questions

1. Pressure injuries are:
   a. chronic wounds
   b. acute wounds
   c. partial-thickness injury
   d. full-thickness injury
2. A way to assess a patient's risk for the development of pressure ulcers/injuries is to:
   a. Do a complete skin assessment
   b. Complete a body system review
   c. Use pressure ulcer/injury staging system
   d. Use the Braden risk assessment tool
3. What is a pressure ulcer/injury?
   a. Area of localized injury to the skin and/or underlying soft tissue
   b. An acute wound from friction
   c. Localized damage to the skin and underlying soft tissue
   d. Wound located on the lower leg
4. Once a patient has developed a pressure ulcer/injury, what should the first intervention be?
   a. Get patient up in chair as much as possible
   b. Remove the source of pressure
   c. Consult dietician
   d. Meticulous skin care
5. Where is the pressure ulcer/injury most likely to occur?
   a. Lower legs
   b. Over a bony prominence
   c. Occipital area
   d. Ears

REFERENCES

1. Ratliff C, Droste L. *Wound, Ostomy and Continence Nurses Society. Guideline for Prevention and Management of Pressure Ulcers (Injuries). WOCN Clinical Practice Guideline Series 2.* Mt. Laurel, NJ: Author. WOCN; 2016.
2. Agency for Healthcare Research and Quality. Preventing Pressure Ulcers in Hospitals: A Tool Kit for Improving Quality of Care. https://www.ahrq.gov/patient-safety/settings/hospital/resource/pressureulcer/tool/index.html.
3. National Pressure Ulcer Advisory Panel, European Pressure Ulcer Advisory Panel, & Pan Pacific Pressure Injury Alliance *Prevention and Treatment of Pressure Ulcers: Clinical Practice Guideline*. Western Australia: Cambridge Media: Osborne Park; 2014.
4. NPIAP2016B. National Pressure Injury Advisory Panel [Internet]. NPIAP Pressure Injury Staging and Pictures. 2016. https://npiap.com/page/PressureInjuryStages.
5. Stechmiller JK, Cowan LJ, Oomens CWJ. Bottom-up (pressure hear) injuries. In: Doughty DB, McNichol L, eds. *Wound Ostomy and Continence Society Core Curriculum: Wound Management.* Baltimore: Wolters Kluwer; 2015:313–332.
6. Brem H, Maggi J, Nierman D, et al. High cost of stage IV pressure ulcers. *Am J Surg.* 2010;200(4):473–477.
7. Russo CA, Steiner C, Spector W. Hospitalizations Related to Pressure Ulcers Among Adults 18 Years and Older, 2006: Statistical Brief #64. In: Healthcare Cost and Utilization Project (HCUP) Statistical Briefs Internet]. Rockville (MD): Agency for Healthcare Research and Quality (US); 2006]. https://www.ncbi.nlm.nih.gov/books/NBK54557/.
8. Cowan LJ, Ahn H, Flores M, et al. Pressure ulcer prevalence by level of paralysis in patients with spinal cord injury in long-term care. *Adv Skin Wound Care.* 2019;32(3):122–130.
9. National Spinal Cord Injury Statistical Center [Internet]. https://www.nscisc.uab.edu/Public/2018%20Annual%20Report%20-%20Complete%20Public%20Version.pdf.
10. Krishnan S. Factors Associated With Occurrence and Early Detection of Pressure Ulcers Following Spinal Cord Injury. [Internet]. Doctoral Dissertation. http://d-scholarship.pitt.edu/21223/1/Krishnan_S_.pdf.
11. Jaul E, Calderon-Margalit R. Systemic factors and mortality in elderly patients with pressure ulcers. *Int Wound J.* 2015;12(3):254–259. https://onlinelibrary.wiley.com/doi/epdf/10.1111/iwj.12086.
12. Kottner J, Balzer K, Dassen T, Heinze S. Pressure ulcers: a critical review of definitions and classifications. *Ostomy Wound Manage.* 2009;55(9):22–29.
13. Pieper BA. Pressure ulcers: impact, etiology, and classification. In: Bryant R, Nix D, eds. *Acute and Chronic Wounds: Current Management Concepts.* 5th ed. : Mosby; 2016:124–139.
14. Groah SL, Schladen M, Pineda CG, Hsieh C-HJ. Prevention of pressure ulcers among people with spinal cord injury: a systematic review. *PM&R.* 2015 Jun;7(6):613–636.
15. Rappl L, Brienza D. Skin and wound care for the spinal cord injured patient. In: Doughty DD, McNichol LL. *Wound Ostomy and Continence Nurses Society Core Curriculum: Wound Management.* Baltimore: Wolters Kluwer; 2015:253–270.
16. Banks MD, Graves N, Bauer JD, Ash S. Cost effectiveness of nutrition support in the prevention of pressure ulcer in hospitals. *Eur J Clin Nutrition.* 2013;67(1):42–46.
17. Salzberg CA, Byrne DW, Cayten CG, van Niewerburgh P, Murphy JG, Viehbeck M. A new pressure ulcer risk assessment scale for individuals with spinal cord injury. *Am J Phys Med Rehabil.* 1996;75(2):96–104.
18. Peerless JR, Davies A, Klein D, Yu D. Skin complications in the intensive care unit. *Clin Chest Med.* 1999;20(2):453–467. x.
19. Reddy M, Gill SS, Rochon PA. Preventing pressure ulcers: a systematic review. *JAMA.* 2006;296(8):974–984.
20. Teasell RW, Arnold JM, Krassioukov A, Delaney GA. Cardiovascular consequences of loss of supraspinal control of the sympathetic nervous system after spinal cord injury. *Arch Phys Med Rehabil.* 2000;81(4):506–516.
21. Thijssen DHJ, Maiorana AJ, O'Driscoll G, Cable NT, Hopman MTE, Green DJ. Impact of inactivity and exercise on the vasculature in humans. *Eur J Appl Physiol.* 2010;108(5):845–875.
22. Castro MJ, Apple DF, Staron RS, Campos GE, Dudley GA. Influence of complete spinal cord injury on skeletal muscle within 6 months of injury. *J Appl Physiology Bethesda Md 1985.* 1999;86(1):350–358.
23. Gefen A. Tissue changes in patients following spinal cord injury and implications for wheelchair cushions and tissue loading: a literature review. *Ostomy Wound Manage.* 2014;60(2):34–45.

24. Rittweger J, Gerrits K, Altenburg T, Reeves N, Maganaris CN, de Haan A. Bone adaptation to altered loading after spinal cord injury: a study of bone and muscle strength. *J Musculoskeletal Neuronal Interact.* 2006;6(3):269–276.
25. Alverzo JP, Rosenberg JH, Sorensen CA, DeLeon SS. Nursing care and education for patients with spinal cord injury. In: Sisto SA, Druin E, Macht Sliwinski M, eds. *Spinal Cord Injuries [Internet].* Elsevier; 2009:37–68. https://linkinghub.elsevier.com/retrieve/pii/B9780323006996100036.
26. Cowan L. Wound Series Part 3: Pressure Ulcers and Injuries-Risk Factors, Diagnosis, Staging, Management (ceufast.com). https://ceufast.com/course/wound-series-part-3-pressure-ulcers-risk-factors-diagnosis-staging-management.
27. Bates-Jensen B. Assessment of the patient with a wound. In: Doughty DB, McNichol LL. *Wound Ostomy and Continence Nurses Society Core Curriculum.* Baltimore: Wolters Kluwer; 2015:38–68.
28. Bergstrom N, Braden B. A prospective study of pressure sore risk among institutionalized elderly. *J Am Geriatric Soc.* 1992;40(8):747–758.
29. Bluestein D, Javaheri A. Pressure ulcers: prevention, evaluation, and management. *Am Fam Physician.* 2008;78(10): 1187–1194.
30. Kruger EA, Pires M, Ngann Y, Sterling M, Rubayi S. Comprehensive management of pressure ulcers in spinal cord injury: current concepts and future trends. *J Spinal Cord Med.* 2013;36(6):572–585.
31. Raetz J, Wick K. Common questions about pressure ulcers. *Am Fam Physician.* 2015;92(10):888–894.
32. Sussman C, Bates-Jensen B. Pressure ulcers: pathophysiology, detection and prevention. In: Sussman C, Bates-Jensen B, eds. *Wound Care: A Collaborative Practice Manual for Health Professionals.* Philadelphia: Wolters Kluwer Lippincott Williams & Wilkins; 2012.
33. Bryant RA, Nix DP. *Acute and Chronic Wounds: Current Management Concepts.* St. Louis, MO: CV Mosby; 2016.
34. Lyder CH, Ayello EA. Pressure ulcers: a patient safety issue. In: Hughes RG, ed. *Patient Safety and Quality: An Evidence-Based Handbook for Nurses [Internet].* Rockville, MD: Agency for Healthcare Research and Quality (US); 2008.
35. Brienza D, Antokal S, Herbert L, et al. Friction-induced skin injuries—are they pressure ulcers? An updated NPUAP white paper. *J Wound Ostomy Continence Nursing.* 2015;42(1):62–64.
36. DeLisa JA, Mikulic MA. Pressure ulcers. What to do if preventive management fails. *Postgrad Med.* 1985;77(6): 209–212. 218-220.
37. McKinley WO, Tewksbury MA, Godbout CJ. Comparison of medical complications following nontraumatic and traumatic spinal cord injury. *J Spinal Cord Med.* 2002;25(2): 88–93.
38. Maklebust J, Magnam M. Pressure ulcer prevention: specific measures and agency-wide strategies. In: Doughty DB, McNichol LL. *Wound Ostomy and Continence Nurses Soceity Core Curriculum: Wound Managment.* Wolters Kluwer; 2015:333–361.
39. Wilborn W. Pressure ulcer prevention strategies. *Nursing Made Incredibly Easy.* 2015;13(6):10–12.
40. Consortium for Spinal Cord Medicine, Paralyzed Veterans of America. *Pressure ulcer prevention and treatment following spinal cord injury: a clinical practice guideline for health-care providers.* Washington, DC: Consortium for Spinal Cord Medicine; 2014.
41. Thomason SS, Luther SL, Powell-Cope GM, Harrow JJ, Palacios P. Validity and reliability of a pressure ulcer monitoring tool for persons with spinal cord impairment. *J Spinal Cord Med.* 2014;37(3):317–327.
42. Beitz J. Wound healing. In: Doughty DB, McNichol LL, eds. *Wound Ostomy and Continence Nurses Society Core Curriculum.* Baltimore: Wolters Kluwer; 2016:38–68.

CHAPTER 34

Nutritional and Body Composition Assessments After Spinal Cord Injury

Milissa L. Janisko, David R. Dolbow, and Ashraf S. Gorgey

OUTLINE

Background

Dynamic changes in body composition parameters impact several life time comorbidities after spinal cord injury (SCI).[1] Understanding these changes can facilitate better healthcare, improve quality of life, and reduce socioeconomic burdens after SCI. The outcome of the body composition profile after SCI is a complex interaction of several pathological factors that are likely to be accentuated by level and severity of the injury. Although the percentage contribution of each factor can be estimated from research,[1–3] these estimates will vary greatly from one person to another based on the chronicity, severity, level of SCI, and existing comorbidities (Fig. 34.1).

Nutrition and Initial Body Composition Changes During Critical Response

In the acute stage after SCI, nutritional needs can be difficult to estimate due to the hypermetabolic state and expected body composition changes that occur with a decrease in lean body mass and an increase in fat mass below the level of injury.[4] Immediately following SCI, a critical illness response includes uncontrolled catabolism of proteins, resistance to anabolic signals, and relative preservation of fat tissue.[5] The various stress-triggered mechanisms result in a loss of muscle mass up to 5% per day.[5] The systemic loss of skeletal muscle is highlighted by an accelerated loss of skeletal muscle below the level of injury, 18%–46% of the cross-sectional area within the first 6 weeks and 45%–80% within the first 24 weeks.[1,6–8] Fat-free mass composed of metabolically active muscle, bone, and body organs account for the majority of the basal metabolic rate (BMR), with muscle mass providing 85% of the influence of fat-free mass on energy expenditure.[9–11] After SCI, muscle mass loss results in a greater than 50% decrease in total daily expenditure,[11–13] which is seen at rest and during physical activity.[14] These factors, along with a decreased physical activity rate that is 40% lower than individuals without a SCI,[15] result in an obesity rate of 66%–97%.[16–19] Similar to muscle mass, bone mass also decreases at an accelerated rate, with as much as 33% of bone mass lost in the trabecular-rich areas of the legs during the first 3–4 months after injury.[20–23]

Energy Expenditure, Body Composition, and Weight Management

Energy expenditure can be broken down into three components: BMR, dietary-induced thermogenesis, and activity energy expenditure. BMR is the energy required to maintain homeostasis and metabolic activities of cells at rest and is the largest component of daily energy expenditure.[2] In the acute stage of SCI, depending on injury level, individuals may require nutrition support to meet nutritional needs, which can be more closely monitored and adjusted for weight management control until oral intake is safe and appropriate to resume. As individuals with SCI progress from the acute to the chronic stage, the change in body composition will decrease the resting metabolic rate (RMR).[4,24] This is likely explained by the relative loss in lean body mass. There is no definitive time frame as to when this change

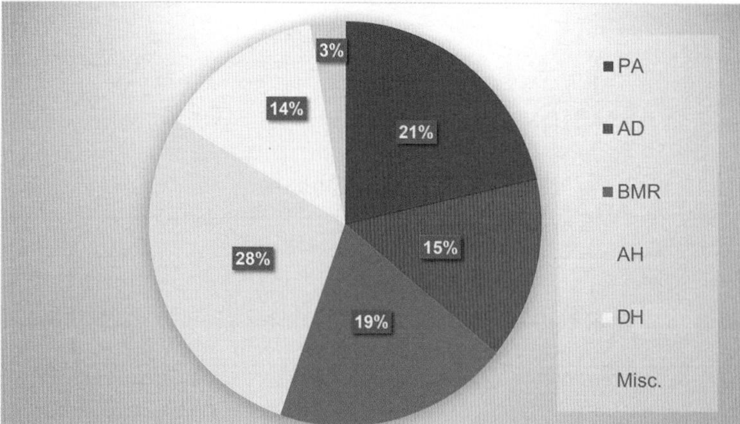

Fig. 34.1 Body Composition Profile After Spinal Cord Injury. Factors that may contribute to body composition changes in persons with spinal cord injury, including level of physical activity *(PA)*, autonomic dysfunction *(AD)*, basal metabolic rate *(BMR)*, anabolic hormone *(AH)*, poor dietary habits *(DH)*, and miscellaneous factors *(Misc)*.

occurs, and the time variations appear to depend on the individual and complications that may occur postinjury. Once the hypermetabolic acute state ceases, the BMR and resting energy expenditure begin to decrease. Some individuals may never recover the ability to consume oral intake and will continue to require nutrition support, which, as stated above, will be easier to adjust to meet nutritional needs for weight management. However, for individuals who meet their nutritional needs via oral intake, weight management becomes a challenge.

Although many calculations are used to determine RMR, these may not be accurate, and typically overestimate nutritional needs in individuals with SCI. Measured energy expenditure has been shown to be at least 10% and can be as much as 54% below predicted levels.[2,24,25] Indirect calorimetry is the gold standard for determining the nutritional requirements for individuals with SCI. However, this option is frequently not available to clinicians in the clinical setting, and the procedure for obtaining an accurate BMR is often impractical.[2] In the chronic rehabilitation stage, frequently kcal/kg is used to determine estimated energy needs with 22.7 kcal/kg for tetraplegia and 27.9 kcal/kg for paraplegia, although acuteness of injury, gender, and physical activity level should be taken into consideration.[24] Recent research has shown that it is possible to use an SCI population-specific BMR prediction equation by using anthropometric measurements (i.e., circumferences and/or diameters), which would not cause a significant workload on the clinician.[2] If energy intake exceeds the RMR, weight gain will result and may progress to neurogenic obesity, which can then progress to metabolic syndrome: central obesity, vascular inflammation, hypertension, dyslipidemia, and glucose intolerance.[12] Individuals may also have had these medical conditions prior to their SCI or there may be a genetic component that increases their risk of developing them in the future. The Undesired weight gain and obesity are usually seen more often in those with oral intake and dietary restrictions may be necessary to meet caloric needs for weight management.

Body mass index (BMI) is commonly calculated to determine weight status: using the formula: weight (kg)/height (m^2) in which a BMI greater than or equal to 25 kg/m^2 and 30 kg/m^2 is considered overweight and obese, respectively. However, multiple studies have shown that BMI–criteria is not accurate or reliable in individuals with SCI due to the changes in body composition.[1,26] Others have shown that a BMI of 22 kg/m^2 or higher can be used to assess weight recommendation for individuals with SCI,[27] but additional research is still needed. Waist circumference can be an easy method to indicate obesity, specifically abdominal visceral fat, and recent studies have shown that measured waist circumferences in males with SCI of ≥89.1 cm when seated and ≥86.5 cm when supine should be classified as having central obesity.[28,29]

Dietary Interventions and Macronutrients

Protein Requirements

In the acute stage of SCI, a negative nitrogen balance may persist for 7 weeks or longer as nitrogen excretion increases with the change in body weight and lean body mass loss.[24] Attempting to achieve a positive nitrogen balance with aggressive nutrition support is generally unsuccessful and can result in overfeeding, so usually up to 2 g protein/kg ideal body weight is adequate to prevent substrate overload.[24] In the chronic/rehabilitation stage, baseline maintenance protein needs are 1.0–1.2 g/kg to assure adequate protein intake while maintaining skin integrity with adjustments as necessary based on medical needs (i.e., kidney disease, pressure injuries, etc.).[24] As pressure injuries are often a common complication seen in individuals with SCI, protein intake recommendations for those with stage 1–2 pressure injuries are 1.2–1.5 g/kg and stage 3–4 pressure injuries are 1.5–2 g/kg.[30] Unless medically contraindicated, a daily multivitamin with minerals would be recommended to assure all wound healing micronutrients are addressed. There has also been additional research showing that a vitamin combination of cyanocobalamin/pyridoxine/folic acid can promote wound healing in individuals with diabetes as well as those with elevated homocysteine levels.[31]

Fluid Requirements and Dietary Interventions for Neurogenic Bowel and Bladder Dysfunction

SCI will usually result in some type of neurogenic bowel and bladder dysfunction.[32] Individuals with a neurogenic bowel may have an increase in colonic transit time resulting in hard stools, which, when complicated by the frequent use of opioid pain medications that contribute to constipation,[24] may require medications and dietary adjustments. While a healthy, high-fiber diet that includes fruits, vegetables, whole grains, legumes, and adequate fluid intake can help improve constipation management, an unhealthy diet of high-fat foods, spicy foods, caffeine, and other stimulants can change gut function and cause fecal incontinence.[4] Depending on the bladder management plan, fluid restriction may be required where all fluids and high-water content foods should be documented to prevent exceeding daily restrictions. In general, 1 mL of fluid per calorie plus an additional 500 mL/day is a baseline recommendation to assure adequate hydration with adjustments for constipation or diarrhea as necessary.[24] For individuals who are using intermittent catheterization for bladder management, a fluid restriction of approximately 2000 mL/day is often used.

Dietary Interventions and Medical Concerns

Studies have shown that individuals with SCI tend to consume the appropriate amount of caloric energy for their estimated needs but, unfortunately, tend to have an excess of protein, carbohydrate, dietary fat, and saturated fat intake, and a deficit in fiber, vitamins A, pantothenic acid (B5), biotin, (B7), C, D, E, and minerals such as calcium, magnesium, and potassium.[4] Gorgey et al. studied the percentage of macronutrients and their relative contribution or relationship to BMR and body composition.[33] They noted that persons with SCI consume a higher percentage fat in their diet, and this accounted for 29%–34% of the changes seen in whole body fat mass.[33] The authors also noted that the total caloric intake as reported by daily dietary intake was lower than both their BMR and total caloric intake,[33] but this malnourishment status may lead to slowing of the metabolism and increase of the circulating cortisol and state of hypercatabolism.

A distinctive part of dietary intake with SCI may be the challenge of intact brain mechanisms that address appetite and satiety but reduced or absent physiological cues that suppress appetite.[4] A recent case report clearly highlighted percentage fat mass and visceral adiposity decreased in a person with SCI after caloric intake was limited by 25% and the macronutrient composition altered. The person managed to rely on less dietary fat and increased their dietary intake from protein and fibers over a 16-week period.[34] Additional research has shown improvement in overall nutritional status when macronutrients are adjusted with a lower carbohydrate intake consisting of whole grains, fruits, and low-fat dairy products; a higher protein intake of low-fat meats and fish, eggs, legumes, and nuts; and limiting red meat and fat intake to <30% total calories with <6% from saturated fats.[4] Individuals with SCI are at a greater risk for cardiovascular disease (CVD), atherogenesis, and elevated lipid levels likely due to immobilization, as well as a potential family history of CVD.[24] Modifiable risk factors that should be addressed to manage CVD are obesity, the ability for exercise based on level of injury, dietary factors, and smoking.[24] Standard dietary interventions can be incorporated to improve lipid profiles. Individuals with SCI are also at greater risk of developing osteopenia and osteoporosis due to neurogenic hormonal changes along with the lack of bone protective mechanical stresses provided by weight-bearing and vigorous muscle contractions.[20,21,35] Additional risk factors include individuals with long-term use of glucocorticoids and with diets lacking in calcium and vitamin D.

On physical examination, abdominal fat is usually seen in individuals with SCI. The increase in both waist and abdominal circumferences reflects an increase in visceral adiposity.[36] Visceral adiposity is characterized by ectopic infiltration of fat mass surrounding the internal gut organs and is especially troubling due to its link to metabolic and cardiovascular diseases.[1,37–41] Adipose tissue in those with SCI is reported to be 58% greater in cross-sectional area than in age, sex, and waist circumference matched non-SCI individuals.[38] Additional consequences are glucose intolerance and insulin resistance (50%–75% prevalence) with a two to three times greater risk of diabetes mellitus II.[1,42] In persons with SCI, the association between visceral adiposity and altered metabolic profile has been established.[39] Believed that visceral adiposity is likely to storm the circulation with a spectrum of inflammatory cytokines.[17,28]

Body Composition Assessment Techniques

There are numerous methods for calculating body composition with varying degrees of accuracy, difficulty, and expense. The criterion standard for measuring total body fat and body fat percentage (BF%) is the four-compartment model (4CM).[19] The four compartments and measuring techniques include[19]:

- body density (hydrostatic weighing)
- bone (dual-energy X-ray absorptiometry [DXA])
- water (isotope dilution using deuterium oxide)
- fat (remaining tissue minus the other components)

There has only been one large cohort study using the 4CM to determine body composition for those with SCI (both paraplegia and tetraplegia).[19] Using BF% >22 for men and >35 for women, 97% of the 72 participants were determined to be obese, with a mean BF% of 42.4% +/- 8.6%. This provides strong evidence that supports the belief that obesity is an epidemic in the SCI population.[19] This method's shortcomings are that it is expensive, time-consuming, labor-intensive, and most healthcare providers do not have adequate facilities to perform the required comprehensive testing.

Dual-Energy X-Ray Absorptiometry

A DXA scan measurement is based on the attenuation of the number of photons in two separate X-ray beams at different energy levels. The greater the tissue density, the greater the attenuation of photons.[21] DXA is considered the gold standard for measuring bone mineral density and is one component of the 4CM. Measurement via DXA scanning has been shown to slightly underestimate BF% compared with the 4CM, which may be due to soft tissue being blocked from the scan by the overlying bone density.[19] This method does require high-cost DXA scanners, the need for a trained densitometry technician, and the need to transfer and correctly position the individual with SCI. We have recently determined the precision of using DXA in measuring regional and total body composition in persons with SCI.

Hydrostatic Weighing

Hydrostatic weighing measures body density through water displacement when submerged and has long been accepted as an accurate measurement technique when trained technicians are used; however, it is a time- and labor-intensive procedure and is not readily available to most clinicians. Also, individuals need to be submerged underwater multiple times during the weighing process, which can produce anxiety and deter participation, especially in those with paralysis.[19]

Air Displacement Plethysmography (Bod Pod)

The Bod Pod measures body composition through the air displacement in a sealed container once entered by the individual. Like other measuring devices, the Bod Pod is expensive and rarely available in the clinical setting. One aspect of the testing procedure that can be troublesome for those with SCI is the total lung volume test, which accounts for the lungs' residual air after expiration. Weakness or paralysis of expiratory muscles disrupts the ability to efficiently force air out of the lungs, skewing the results.[19]

Bioelectrical Impedance Analysis

Bioelectrical impedance analysis (BIA) sends a weak electric current through the body with the voltage measured to calculate the impedance of the body. Body composition is estimated based on the idea that muscle contains a high percentage of total body water, so the more muscle, the less impedance. Fat, on the other hand, has poor conductance of electrical current. Although BIA is less costly and less labor-intensive, the BF% is significantly underestimated.[19]

Skinfold Thickness Measurements

Skinfold thickness measured with a skinfold caliper determines the thickness of a double layer of skin and underlying fat deposits. Because skin thickness varies minimally from person to person, this procedure gives a reasonable estimation of the subcutaneous fat thickness.[43] However, for individuals with paralysis, skinfold measures for estimating BF% were found to be unreliable[44] and resulted in the underestimation of BF%.[45] Additional studies comparing skinfold thickness measurements with the 4CM have supported these results.[19] Skinfold thickness measurements are less expensive than the more technologically based procedures, but there is a time commitment, as each site must undergo multiple caliper measures by a trained technician. Several regression formulas for anthropometrics measures based on the 4CM have been created with one simple and accurate formula using age, sex, weight, and abdominal skinfold.[19]

Magnetic Resonance Imaging

The use of magnetic resonance imaging (MRI) is considered the most precise and accurate way of measuring body composition in persons with SCI.[7,46] The caveat is that MRI technology is expensive and requires a high level of technical expertise. Our group has continuously used MRI to measure muscle cross-sectional area in response to disuse, spasticity, and exercise training and the changes in visceral adiposity and other ectopic bone marrow adiposity.[47–49] Most of the research studies that have errors incorporated with MRI do not exceed 5%.[7,40] In an attempt to translate applications of MRI to the clinical field, we have developed a number of anthropodermic equations that can be easily applied by clinicians to estimate regional body composition changes after SCI.[46,50]

Review Questions

1. A 25-year-old male suffered an automobile accident resulting in a C5 motor complete SCI. He is now 1 year postinjury. What body composition changes would we expect to have occurred over the past year?
   a. Dramatic loss of muscle mass, bone mass, total body fat mass, and visceral fat with only minimally increased intramuscular fat in the paralyzed legs.
   b. Dramatic loss in muscle mass, whereas bone is essentially unchanged. A significant increase in total body fat mass and visceral fat with only minimally increased intramuscular fat in the paralyzed legs.
   c. Dramatic loss in muscle mass and bone mass. A significant increase in total body fat mass and with only minimally increased visceral fat and intramuscular fat in the legs.
   d. Dramatic loss of muscle mass and bone mass with a significant increase in total body fat, visceral fat, and intramuscular fat in the paralyzed legs.
2. What are the three compartments that make up energy expenditure?
   a. Basal metabolic rate, dietary-induced thermogenesis, activity energy expenditure
   b. Homeostasis, energy expenditure, metabolic activities
   c. Body composition, metabolic rate, lean body mass
   d. Inflammation, body composition, activity energy expenditure
3. A 47-year-old male with C6 AIS A tetraplegia has a stage 4 sacral pressure injury. How much protein per kilogram should he consume for wound closure?
   a. 0.8–1 g/kg
   b. 1.2–1.5 g/kg
   c. 1.5–2 g/kg
   d. No increased protein needs
4. The ideal macronutrient diet composition for individuals with an SCI would be:
   a. High carbohydrate, high protein, and low fat and saturated fat
   b. Low carbohydrate, low protein, and high fat and saturated fat
   c. Low carbohydrate, high protein, and low fat and saturated fat
   d. High carbohydrate, low protein, and high fat and saturated fat

REFERENCES

1. Gorgey AS, Dolbow DR, Dolbow JD, Gater DR. Effects of spinal cord injury on body composition and metabolic profile-part I. *Journal of Spinal Cord Medicine.* 2014;37(6): 693–702.
2. Nightengale TE, Gorgey AS. Predicting basal metabolic rate in men with motor complete spinal cord injury. *Med Sci Sports Exerc.* 2018;50(6):1305–1312.
3. Abilmona SM, Sumrell RM, Gill RS, Adler RA, Gorgey AS. Serum testosterone levels may influence body composition and cardiometabolic health in men with spinal cord injury. *Spinal Cord.* 2019;57(3):229–239.
4. Gater DR, Bauman C, Cowan R. A primary care provider's guide to diet and nutrition after spinal cord injury. *Top Spinal Cord Inj Rehabil.* 2020;26(3):197–202.
5. Preiser JC, Ichai C, Orhan JC, Groeneveld ABJ. Metabolism response to the stress of critical illness. *British Journal of Anaesthesia.* 2014;113(6):945–954.
6. Castro MJ, Apple Jr. DF, Hillegass EA, Dudley GA. Influence of complete spinal cord injury on skeletal muscle cross-sectional area within the first 6 months of injury. *European Journal of Applied Physiology and Occupational Physiology.* 1999;80(4):373–378.
7. Gorgey AS, Dudley GA. Skeletal muscle atrophy and increased intramuscular fat after incomplete spinal cord injury. *Spinal Cord.* 2007;45(4):304–309.
8. Shah PK, Steven JE, Gregory CM, et al. Lower-extremity muscle cross-sectional area after incomplete spinal cord injury. *Arch Phys Med Rehabil.* 2006;87(6):772–778.
9. Buchholz AC, McGillivray CF, Penchcarz PB. Differences in resting metabolic rate between paraplegia and able-bodied subjects are explained by differences in body composition. *American Journal Clinical Nutrition.* 2003;77(2):371–378.
10. Chun SM, Kim HR, Shin HI. Estimating the basal metabolic rate from fat free mass in individuals with motor complete spinal cord injury. *Spinal Cord.* 2017;55:844–847.
11. Farkas GJ, Gater DR. Energy expenditure and nutrition in neurogenic obesity following spinal cord injury. *J Phys Med Rehabil.* 2020;2(1):11–13.
12. Farkas GJ, Gorgey AS, Dolbow DR, Gater DR. Caloric intake relative to total daily energy expenditure using a spinal cord injury-specific correction factor: an analysis by level of injury. *Am J Phys Med Rehabil.* 2019;98(11):947–952.
13. Farkas GJ, Pitot MA, Berg AS, Gater DR. Nutritional status in chronic spinal cord injury: a systematic review and meta-analysis. *Spinal Cord.* 2019;57:3–17.
14. Shea BL, Leiter J, Cowley KC. Energy expenditure as a function of activity level after spinal cord injury: the need for tetraplegia-specific energy balance guidelines. *Frontiers in Physiology.* 2018:9 Article 1286.
15. Berg-Emons Van den, Bussmann JB, Stam HJ. Accelerometry based activity spectrum in persons with chronic physical conditions. *Arch Phys Med Rehabil.* 2010;91: 1856–1861.
16. Dolbow DR, Credeur D, Lemacks JL, et al. Electrically induced cycling and nutritional counseling for counteracting obesity after spinal cord injury: a pilot study. *J Spinal Cord Med.* 2021;44(4):533–540.
17. Farkas GJ, Gater DR. Neurogenic obesity and systematic inflammation following spinal cord injury: a review. *J Spinal Cord Med.* 2018;41(4):378–387.

18. Han SH, Lee BS, Choi HS, et al. Comparison of fat mass percentage and body mass index in Koreans with spinal cord injury according to the severity and duration of motor paralysis. *Annals of Rehabilitation Medicine*. 2015;39(3):384–392.
19. Gater DR, Farkas GJ, Dolbow DR, Berg A, Gorgey AS. Body composition assessment after motor complete spinal cord injury: development of a clinically relevant equation to estimate body fat. *Topics in Spinal Cord Injury Rehabil.* 2021;27(1):11–22.
20. Dolbow DR, Gorgey AS, Daniels JA, Adler RR, Gater Jr. DR. The effects of spinal cord injury and exercise on bone mass: a literature review. *NeuroRehabilitation*. 2011;29(3): 261–269.
21. Dolbow DR, Gorgey AS. Non-pharmacological management of osteoporosis. *Clinical Kinesiology*. 2013;67(2):6–9.
22. Garland DE, Stewart CA, Adkins RH, et al. Osteoporosis after spinal cord injury. *Journal of Orthop Res*. 1992;10(3):371–378.
23. Eser P, Frotzler A, Zehnder Y. Fracture threshold in the femur and tibia of people with spinal cord injury as determined by peripheral quantitative computed tomography. *Arch Phys Med Rehabil.* 2005;86(3):498–504.
24. Academy of Nutrition and Dietetics [Internet]. Evidence Analysis Library. https://www.eatright.org.
25. Sisto SA, Druin E, Macht Sliwinski M. *Spinal Cord Injuries: Management and Rehabilitation*. St Louis: Mosby Elsevier; 2009.
26. Spungen AM, Adkins RH, Stewart CA, et al. Factors influencing body composition in persons with spinal cord injury: a cross-sectional study. *J Appl Physiol (1985)*. 2003;95(6):2398–2407.
27. Laughton GE, Buchholz AC, Martin Ginis KA, Goy RE, Group SSR. Lower body mass index cutoffs better identifies obese persons with spinal cord injury. *Spinal Cord*. 2009;47(10): 757–762.
28. Sumrell RM, Nightingale TE, McCauley LS, Gorgey AS. Anthropometric cutoffs and associations with visceral adiposity and metabolic biomarkers after spinal cord injury. *PLOS ONE*. 2018;13(8):e0203049.
29. Gill S, Sumrell RM, Sima A, Cifu DX, Gorgey AS. Waist circumference cutoff identifying risks of obesity, metabolic syndrome, and cardiovascular disease in men with spinal cord injury. *PLoS One*. 2020;15(7):e0236752.
30. National Pressure Injury Advisory Panel 2019 [Internet]. https://www.npiap.com.
31. Boykin Jr JV, Baylis C. Homocysteine – A stealth mediator of impaired wound healing: a preliminary study. *Wounds*. 2006;18(4):101–116.
32. Sezer N, Akkus S, Ugurlu FG. Chronic complications of spinal cord injury. *World J Orthop*. 2015(1):24–33.
33. Gorgey AS, Caudill C, Sistrun S, et al. Frequency of dietary recalls, nutritional assessment, and body composition assessment in men with chronic spinal cord injury. *Arch Phys Med Rehabil.* 2015;96(9):1646–1653.
34. Gorgey AS, Lester RM, Ghatas MP, Sistrun SN, Lavis T. Dietary manipulation and testosterone replacement therapy may explain changes in body composition after spinal cord injury: a retrospective case report. *World J Clin Cases*. 2019;7(17):2427–2437.
35. Rittweger J, Jerris K, Altenburg T, et al. Bone adaptation to altered loading after spinal cord injury: a study of bone and muscle strength. *Journal of Musculoskeletal Neuronal Interact.* 2006;6(3):269–276.
36. Gorgey AS, Ennasr AN, Farkas G, Gater DR. Anthropometric prediction of visceral adiposity in persons with spinal cord injury. *Top Spinal Cord Inj Rehabil.* 2021;27(1):23–35.
37. Despres JP, Lemieux I. Abdominal obesity and metabolic syndrome. *Nature*. 2006;444:881–887.
38. Edwards LA, Bugaresti JM, Buchholz AC. Visceral adipose tissue and the ratio of visceral to subcutaneous adipose tissue are greater in adults with than those without spinal cord injury, despite matching waist circumferences. *American Journal of Clinical Nutrition*. 2008;87:600–607.
39. Gorgey AS, Mather KJ, Gater DR. Central adiposity associations to carbohydrate and lipid metabolism in individuals with complete motor spinal cord injury. *Metabolism*. 2011;60(6):843–851.
40. Gorgey AS, Gater DR. Regional and relative adiposity patterns in relation to carbohydrate and lipid metabolism in men with spinal cord injury. *Appl Physiol Nutr Metab*. 2011;36(1):107–114.
41. Gorgey AS, Farkas BS, Dolbow DR, Khalil RE, Gater DR. Gender dimorphism in central adiposity may explain metabolic dysfunction after spinal cord injury. *Am Academy of Phys Med & Rehabil.* 2017:1–11.
42. Cragg JJ, Noonan VK, Dvorak M, Krassioukov A, Mancini J, Borisoff JF. Spinal cord injury and type 2 diabetes. *Neurology*. 2013;81(21):1864–1868.
43. Pollack ME, Schmidt DH, Jackson AS. Measurement of cardiorespiratory fitness and body composition in the clinical setting. *Comprehensive Therapy*. 1980;6(9):12–27.
44. Dolbow DR. Skinfold thickness and circumference measurements of subjects with hemiplegia. *Amer Corr Ther J.* 1985;39(1):20–24.
45. Muggiano M, Bertoli S, Margonato V, Veicsteinas A, Testolin G. Body composition assessment in spinal cord injury. *Acta Diabetol.* 2003;40(Suppl 1):S183–S186.
46. Wade RC, Gorgey AS. Anthropometric prediction of skeletal muscle cross-sectional area in persons with spinal cord injury. *J Appl Physiol (1985)*. 2017;122(5):1255–1261.
47. Gorgey AS, Dudley GA. Spasticity may defend skeletal muscle size and composition after incomplete spinal cord injury. *Spinal Cord*. 2008;46(2):96–102.
48. Gorgey AS, Mather KJ, Cupp HR, Gater DR. Effects of resistance training on adiposity and metabolism after spinal cord injury. *Med Sci Sports Exerc*. 2012;44(1):165–174.
49. Gorgey AS, Khalil RE, Gill R, Gater DR, Lavis TD, Cardozo CP, Adler RA. Low-dose testosterone and evoked resistance exercise after spinal cord injury on cardio-metabolic risk factors: an open-label randomized clinical trial. *J Neurotrauma*. 2019;36(18):2631–2645.
50. McCauley LS, Sumrell RM, Gorgey AS. Anthropometric prediction of visceral adipose tissue in persons with motor complete spinal cord injury. *PM R*. 2018;10(8): 817–825. e2.

CHAPTER 35

Endocrine/Metabolic

Tommy Sutor, Jacob Goldsmith, and Ashraf S. Gorgey

OUTLINE

Introduction

Fundamentally, *metabolism* is a term describing all chemical reactions in the body that involve the breakdown of organic compounds or bodily tissues (i.e., catabolism) and synthesis of new molecules or tissues (i.e., anabolism).[1] Overall health is optimal when the balance between catabolism and anabolism is maintained to ensure normal physiological homeostasis of the surviving cells. However, spinal cord injury (SCI) disrupts this balance and results in a sequelae of metabolic disorders. After SCI, reduced physical activity is compounded by reduced anabolic hormone activity, disrupted autonomic nervous system function, and a number of major changes in body composition that are characterized by 50% loss in sublesion muscle mass (i.e., disuse muscle atrophy) and increased ectopic adiposity similar to intramuscular fat and visceral adiposity. This may lead to improper storage and utilization of energy substrates (carbohydrates and lipids) and metabolic inflexibility. Failure to partition as well as to utilize energy resources may in turn cause a cascade of secondary health complications such as impaired glucose tolerance, insulin resistance, dyslipidemia, obesity, and development of type 2 diabetes mellitus.

This chapter will give an overview of the changes to metabolic and endocrine activity after SCI. Particular focus will be given to post-SCI changes in glucose metabolism, lipid metabolism, testosterone, growth hormone, and insulin growth factors, as well as inflammatory biomarkers such as interleukin 6 (IL-6), tumor necrosis factor-alpha (TNF-α), and c-reactive protein (CRP). Secondary health effects of these changes will also be discussed, such as obesity and type 2 diabetes mellitus,[2–6] which are summarily referred to as *cardiometabolic syndrome*. The complex interactions of metabolic and endocrine changes with spasticity will also be considered. The effects of exercise and diet to combat these metabolic consequences will be discussed throughout these sections.

The following table provides a list of metabolic variables that are likely to be impacted following SCI (Fig. 35.1; Table 35.1).

Decreased Basal Metabolic Rate After Spinal Cord Injury

Key Points

- SCI results in reduced physical activity, contributing to reduced basal metabolic rate and lean mass.
- These factors in turn lead to increased adiposity and worsened cardiometabolic function.
- Increasing fat-free mass, energy expenditure, and reducing caloric intake can combat these effects.[7]

Basal metabolic rate (BMR) is the energy required to maintain bodily metabolic activity at rest, and accounts for up to 70% of total daily energy expenditure in inactive individuals after SCI.[8] BMR declines after SCI to 1200–1400 kcal/day, largely due to decreased lean mass.[9] These changes in body composition contribute to a significant decrease in total daily energy expenditure and the accumulation of fat mass (i.e., neurogenic obesity).[10] Indirect calorimetry is considered the best method to measure BMR or its surrogate, resting metabolic rate. However, indirect calorimetry requires specific training and is not readily clinically accessible. To

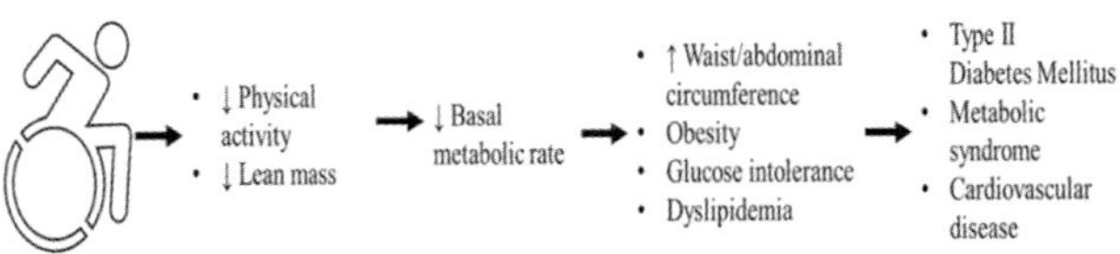

Fig. 35.1 Schematic of the Sequence of Events and Factors Leading to Negative Metabolic Outcomes After Spinal Cord Injury.

Table 35.1 List of Metabolic Variables That Are Likely to Be Impacted Following Spinal Cord Injury

Metabolic Profile Component	Healthy Value/ Range	Changes After Spinal Cord Injury
Basal metabolic rate (kcal/ day)	1800–2200	1200–1400
Glucose tolerance	Fasting glucose levels: <100 mg/dL	Impaired glucose tolerance: >100 mg/dL Indicative of diabetes: >140 mg/dL
Lipid metabolism/ storage	Triglycerides: <150 mg/dL LDL-C: <100 mg/dL HDL-C: >40 mg/dL	Triglycerides: ≥150 mg/dL LDL-C: >160 mg/dL HDL-C: <40 mg/dL (men) or <50 mg/dL (women)

HDL-C, High-density lipoprotein cholesterol; *LDL-C*, low-density lipoprotein cholesterol.

Table 35.2 Spinal Cord Injury–Specific Body Composition and Anthropometric Equations to Estimate Basal Metabolic Rate

Components Used to Estimate Basal Metabolic Rate	Formula	Accurate to Within:
FFM and anthropometrics	19.789 × FFM (kg) + 5.156 × weight (kg) + 8.09 × height (cm) − 15.301 × calf circumference (cm) − 850.55	± 84 kcal/day
Anthropometrics alone	13.202 × height (cm) + 11.329 × weight (kg) − 16.729 × TAD (cm) − 1185.45	± 112 kcal/day

FFM, Fat-free mass derived from dual X-ray absorptiometry; *TAD*, transverse abdominal diameter.

address these limitations, SCI-specific body composition and anthropometric equations exist to allow clinicians to reliably estimate BMR (Table 35-2).[11]

BMR can then be multiplied by the SCI-specific factor of 1.15 to predict total daily energy expenditure.[12] Importantly, this correction factor has been tested when true BMR is obtained via indirect calorimetry; thus, the accuracy of predicting total daily energy expenditure by multiplying *predicted* basal metabolic rate by 1.15 has not been confirmed. It is important to note that in the able-bodied population, total daily energy expenditure can be predicted by multiplying basal metabolic rate by 1.2; however, using this factor instead of the SCI-specific factor of 1.15 can over estimate the energy needs of a person with SCI, potentially leading to gains in fat mass of up to 3.2 kg (7 lbs.) per year.[12]

Glucose and Lipid Metabolism; Insulin Resistance and Dyslipidemia

Key Points

- Glucose and lipid metabolism worsen after SCI, causing a multitude of metabolic consequences.
- Reasons for the dysregulated metabolism extend beyond physical inactivity to factors such as dysregulated autonomic function.
- Aerobic or resistance training exercise are both options to combat dysfunctional glucose and lipid metabolism.
- Metformin monotherapy is a standard medication used to treat hyperglycemia/diabetes mellitus in SCI.[13]
- Statins (10–20 mg/day)[13] or dose-titrated extended-release niacin[14] are medication options for treating dyslipidemia.

Current estimates state that glucose intolerance and insulin resistance occur in as many as 62% of persons with SCI, though true prevalence may be even higher, but it is not captured by current research designs.[5,15–17] Importantly, glucose intolerance, which can be determined with an oral glucose tolerance test, is not directly indicative of insulin resistance, as research has shown a higher prevalence of glucose intolerance than outright diabetes mellitus in persons with SCI.[18] The main reason for this change in glucose metabolism likely is the loss of overall lean body mass, particularly skeletal muscle that occurs after SCI.[19,20] Persons with SCI also may have significantly more intramuscular fat than noninjured individuals, a factor also associated with impaired glucose tolerance.[20,21] Additionally, while direction of causality has not been established, visceral adipose tissue (VAT) has been positively correlated with fasting plasma glucose and negatively correlated with fasting plasma insulin, indicating that VAT is likely a marker or consequence of dysregulated glucose metabolism after SCI.[22] Studies have shown that restoring lean mass as well decreasing ectopic adiposity is likely to be associated with enhanced glucose metabolism after SCI.[23–25] Lower extremity functional electrical cycling may restore lean mass and improve insulin sensitivity, and reduce circulating glucose and insulin levels.[26,27] Other forms of exercise such as seated aerobic exercise at high intensities may positively alter glucose metabolism and insulin resistance after SCI.[28]

Persons with SCI have a high prevalence of decreased high-density lipoprotein cholesterol (HDL-C), and/or increased triglycerides (TG) and low-density lipoprotein cholesterol (LDL-C).[7,12,29] Approximately 39% of persons with SCI have elevated total cholesterol, 76% have low HDL-C, 34% have elevated TG, and 58% have an elevated TG:HDL-C ratio.[29] Strong associations have been established between these factors and markers of obesity such as abdominal circumference, trunk fat mass, and total-body fat mass.[30–33] Similar to glucose metabolism, VAT increases disproportionately after SCI, and is positively related to the total-cholesterol:HDL-C ratio after SCI.[22] Increased waist circumference values in persons with SCI also seem to be correlated with VAT to a greater extent than uninjured controls.[34]

Interestingly, sympathetic nervous system innervation to the liver and VAT appear to play a dual role after SCI. Both detrimental TG and very low-density lipoprotein, and beneficial HDL levels are reduced in those with injuries higher than T4 (assumed to have dysfunctional sympathetic regulation) vs. lower than T5 level injuries (assumed to have sympathetic function closer to normal). These differences even persist when controlling for VAT volume.[35] Therefore, reduced sympathetic function and increased VAT mass negatively affect cardiometabolic profile following SCI.

Mitigating dyslipidemia may be possible through medication or exercise interventions. Niacin monotherapy can increase HDL-C levels while decreasing LDL-C and total cholesterol levels.[14] Fenofibrate (Tricor) monotherapy may also decrease total cholesterol and LDL-C while increasing HDL-C.[36] Circuit resistance training, neuromuscular electrical stimulation resistance training with diet changes, and aerobic exercise can also positively change lipid profiles in persons with SCI.[24,28,37] Upper extremity cycling and circuit resistance training can favorably alter health parameters following SCI[38,39]; however, targeting the larger muscles of the lower extremities may be superior for increased muscle hypertrophy and cardiometabolic health.[40–42]

Anabolic Hormones

Key Points

- Testosterone, growth hormone (GH), insulin-like growth factor 1 (IGF-1), and other anabolic hormones are reduced after SCI, and are associated with increased fat and decreased lean mass.
- Baclofen (Lioresal), a common antispasticity drug, may increase IGF-1.
- Neuromuscular electrical stimulation (NMES) resistance training may improve anabolic hormones and mitigate negative consequences of deficient levels.
- Testosterone replacement therapy patches (2–6 mg/day) are shown to be safe in men with SCI, and effects are augmented if combined with resistance training exercise.[23]

Reduced anabolic hormone levels after SCI precipitate the loss of skeletal muscle and lean tissue mass.[43–50] Testosterone deficiency, defined as serum testosterone levels <325 ng/dL, is present in about 43% of males with SCI.[50] Importantly, prevalence of testosterone reduction appears to be associated with injury severity, as the prevalence of low testosterone is approximately 60% in men with motor complete SCI compared to 17% in those with motor incomplete injuries.[50] Consequences of reduced testosterone include greater chances of increased VAT volume, total fat mass, and associated factors such as increased fasting insulin, glucose, and TG.[51] Moreover, persons with SCI experience cardiovascular disease, osteoporosis, and reduced lean mass earlier in life and at higher rates compared with age-matched able-bodied individuals.[52]

Reduced GH, often measured using its surrogate IGF-1 as a marker, is associated with reduced lean mass and increased fat mass after SCI.[45,48] It is difficult to determine whether the SCI itself vs. secondary consequences like obesity and inactivity contribute to reduced GH production. In one study, persons with SCI had significantly more body fat as well as significantly less stimulated GH production than their monozygotic twins.[53] In the same study, however, the release of GH was correlated with baseline GH levels only in the twin with SCI, and not the uninjured twin. In rat and human models, reductions in IGF-1 have been associated with skeletal muscle atrophy and increased fat mass accumulation.[7,48,54] Regardless of causation, reductions in these hormones contribute to negative changes in body composition; they can also be considered an indirect contributor to the metabolic changes that occur after SCI.

Studies have shown that GH and IGF-1 can be modulated either pharmacologically or after exercise. Bauman et al. showed that a low dose of the antispasmodic drug baclofen likely increases serum-circulating IGF-1.[48] IGF-1 has also been shown to be elevated in persons with SCI who have greater spasticity.[55] Spasticity may actually attenuate the decline in muscle mass and affect body composition in persons with SCI.[56,57] Previous research has demonstrated that spasticity is negatively related to android and trunk fat mass and positively related to lean mass, which may act to maintain metabolic rate in persons with SCI.[17] This significant relationship between spasticity and body composition was attributed to the role of insulin growth factors in men with SCI.[55] Moreover, 12 weeks of NMES resistance training resulted in a 35% increase in IGF-1, which is negatively associated with increases in VAT.[24] However, a follow-up study found that 16 weeks of NMES resistance training combined with transdermal testosterone replacement yielded declined serum IGF-1 and increased insulin-like growth factor binding protein 3 (IGFBP-3).[23] Elevated IGFBP-3 may also bind IGF-1 in serum and prevent its degradation, thus preserving the function of IGF-1.[58] Additionally, IGFBP-3 can inhibit insulin-stimulated glucose uptake in VAT, and therefore may exert favorable effects on adiposity.[59]

Inflammation After Spinal Cord Injury

Key Points

- Inflammation (measured by biomarkers such as TNF-α, IL-6, or CRP) is elevated by SCI.
- These inflammatory factors likely interact to have overall negative consequences for glucose and lipid metabolism.
- Exercise may reduce adiposity, which consequently reduces inflammation, or may reduce inflammation directly.

SCI, independent of other factors is associated with chronic, systemic low-grade inflammation.[60,61] Similarly, obesity is associated with increased systemic inflammation in the general population.[62,63] Thus, persons with SCI can be considered to have an elevated risk of increased systemic inflammation as well as its consequences.

TNF-α is one adipokine (a cell-signaling protein secreted by adipose tissue) that can trigger systemic inflammation and initiates downstream effects linked to glucose and lipid metabolism.[64–66] Plasma and adipose tissue concentrations of TNF-α are higher in persons with SCI.[67] Particularly, VAT cross-sectional area, VAT volume, liver adiposity, abdominal circumference, and waist circumference are all significantly related to circulating TNF-α levels.[67,68] TNF-α is thought to play a role in inducing insulin resistance[69] and decreasing levels of HDL-C in persons with SCI,[67] thereby having negative consequences for both glucose and lipid metabolism.

IL-6 is another inflammatory protein secreted by both adipose and nonadipose tissue. Circulating levels of IL-6 are associated with waist circumference in the general population[70,71] and are positively correlated with fasting insulin levels in persons with SCI.[61] Elevated IL-6 is also associated with circulating TG levels,[72] indicating an effect on lipid metabolism. Furthermore, in persons with SCI, both IL-6 and TNF-α are associated with high-sensitivity CRP, which is a marker of systemic inflammation originating from the liver.[10,73] Importantly, IL-6 production appears to be linked to TNF-α activity.[74,75] Thus, it must be remembered that separate markers of inflammation cannot necessarily be considered independently when characterizing the overall role of inflammation on metabolic dysfunction in persons with SCI.

In the general population, reducing adipose tissue mass reduces overall inflammation,[76] but exercise may also affect inflammation independent of adiposity.[77] Lower extremity functional electrical stimulation cycling has been shown to reduce inflammatory biomarkers in persons with SCI.[26] As little as 30 minutes of seated aerobic exercise can acutely reduce TNF-α, with reductions being sustained at least 1 hour postexercise.[78] Previous research has also demonstrated a chronic impact on inflammation with significantly reduced levels of IL-6, TNF-α, and CRP as well as blood glucose and insulin levels in participants with SCI after 10 weeks of functional electrical stimulation cycling. These results suggest that functional electrical stimulation is an effective mode for reducing inflammation and cardiovascular risk following SCI.[26]

Disorders of Metabolic and Endocrine Consequences

Key Points

- Obesity and diabetes mellitus rates are elevated in the SCI population, regardless of diagnostic criteria.
- Increased obesity and diabetes mellitus rates result from aforementioned metabolic and hormonal factors, and thus can be treated with medication or exercise.

Obesity

Two-thirds of individuals with SCI are likely to be obese and at risk for cardiometabolic complications related to obesity.[79,80] Recent recommendations suggest that a body mass index of ≥22 kg/m^2 in someone with a SCI is associated with body fat levels considered obese in the general population; thus, the standard of body fat is thought to be a better cut-off of obesity in the SCI population.[5,81,82] Using this cut-off value, the prevalence of obesity in people with SCI is estimated to be 76.7%. Waist circumference is thought to be more sensitive than body mass index to determine obese vs. nonobese status, and has an SCI-specific cut-off value of 86.5 cm. When using this cut-off value, it is estimated that approximately 36% of individuals with SCI are obese.[83]

Diabetes Mellitus and Cardiometabolic Syndrome

Cardiometabolic syndrome affects as many as 59% of persons with SCI,[84] and estimates on the prevalence of diabetes mellitus in persons with SCI vary from 20%–50%.[5,54] Although this is a wide range, even the lowest estimates indicate that diabetes mellitus is at least three times more prevalent in people with SCI than in the general population. This is characterized by increased levels of fasting plasma glucose and hyperinsulinemia.[85]

Type 2 diabetes mellitus has been associated with numerous comorbidities that escalate in an age-dependent manner.[86] It is interesting to note that increasing waist circumference and VAT have been considered as predeterminant or predictive factors for developing type 2 diabetes.[83] Both aerobic[87,88] and resistance exercise training[89,90] have been shown to enhance glucose effectiveness and insulin sensitivity following SCI by increasing glucose transporter type 4 expression and activity in skeletal muscle. Glucose transporter type 4 plays a vital role in regulating glucose metabolism by transporting glucose into the cell for utilization.[87,91]

Conclusion

Many interrelated factors that affect one another may occur simultaneously and lead to metabolic dysfunction after SCI. These include decreased physical activity, which can simultaneously lead to glucose intolerance, insulin resistance, decreased lean mass, and increased fat mass, all of which increase the risk of conditions such as obesity and type 2 diabetes. A combination of a more active lifestyle and nutritional management are the best tools available to combat these factors that lead to metabolic dysfunction. Structured exercise interventions that can specifically induce muscle hypertrophy to consequently increase lean mass and decrease fat mass, such as the use of neuromuscular or functional electrical stimulation, should be considered as a component of a more active lifestyle whenever possible.

Review Questions

1. Which of the following are biomarkers associated with inflammation?
   a. Testosterone, GH, IGF-1
   b. LDL-C, HDL-C, IGFBP-3
   c. TNF-α, IL-6, CRP
2. How might spasticity offer metabolic benefits for a person with SCI?
   a. Spasticity is a precursor to restored voluntary function, which can be utilized to increase physical activity.
   b. Spasticity may help maintain lean mass and/or reduce fat mass, which is beneficial for overall metabolism.
   c. Spasms release proteins that affect lipid metabolism.
3. Which of the following combinations of factors can be combined into formulas to predict BMR? Choose all that apply.
   a. Fat mass (kg), weight, age, thigh circumference
   b. Percent body fat, weight, height, forearm circumference
   c. Height, weight, transverse abdominal diameter
   d. Fat-free mass (kg), weight, height, calf circumference
4. Which of the following is one of the main reasons glucose metabolism is altered after SCI?
   a. Reduced lean body mass, in particular skeletal muscle mass
   b. Increased basal metabolic rate
   c. Spasticity
   d. Reduced growth hormone and IGF-1
5. Which of the following interventions can result in hypertrophy of paralyzed muscles and improve metabolic profile, even after motor complete SCI?
   a. Upper body aerobic training
   b. Neuromuscular electrical stimulation or functional electrical stimulation
   c. Dietary changes
   d. Baclofen

REFERENCES

1. Blanco A, Blanco G. Metabolism. In: Blanco A, Blanco G, eds. *Medical Biochemistry [Internet]*. New York: Academic Press; 2017:275–281. https://www.sciencedirect.com/science/article/pii/B9780128035504000136.
2. Grundy SM, Brewer HB, Cleeman JI, Smith SC, Lenfant C. Definition of metabolic syndrome. *Arterioscler Thromb Vasc Biol.* 2004;24(2):e13–e18.
3. Grundy SM. Obesity, metabolic syndrome, and cardiovascular disease. *J Clin Endocrinol Metab.* 2004 Jun;89(6):2595–2600.
4. Gater D, Pai A. Metabolic disorders. In: Campagnolo D, Kirshblum S, Nash M, Heary R, Gorman P, eds. *Spinal Cord Medicine.* 2nd ed. Lippincott: Williams & Wilkins; 2011:185–210.
5. Gater DR, Farkas GJ, Berg AS, Castillo C. Prevalence of metabolic syndrome in veterans with spinal cord injury. *J Spinal Cord Med.* 2019 Jan;42(1):86–93.
6. Holt RIG. International Diabetes Federation re-defines the metabolic syndrome. *Diabetes Obes Metab.* 2005 Sep;7(5):618–620.
7. Gorgey AS, Dolbow DR, Dolbow JD, Khalil RK, Castillo C, Gater DR. Effects of spinal cord injury on body composition and metabolic profile—part I. *J Spinal Cord Med.* 2014 Nov;37(6):693–702.
8. Nightingale TE, Williams S, Thompson D, Bilzon JLJ. Energy balance components in persons with paraplegia: daily variation and appropriate measurement duration. *Int J Behav Nutr Phys Act [Internet].* 2017 Sep:14. https://www.ncbi.nlm.nih.gov/pmc/articles/PMC5615439/.
9. Buchholz AC, McGillivray CF, Pencharz PB. Differences in resting metabolic rate between paraplegic and able-bodied subjects are explained by differences in body composition. *Am J Clin Nutr.* 2003 Feb;77(2):371–378.
10. Farkas GJ, Gater DR. Neurogenic obesity and systemic inflammation following spinal cord injury: a review. *J Spinal Cord Med.* 2018 Jul;41(4):378–387.
11. Nightingale TE, Gorgey AS. Predicting basal metabolic rate in men with motor complete spinal cord injury. *Med Sci Sports Exerc.* 2018 Jun;50(6):1305–1312.
12. Farkas GJ, Gorgey AS, Dolbow DR, Berg AS, Gater DR. Caloric intake relative to total daily energy expenditure using a spinal cord injury-specific correction factor: an analysis by

level of injury. *Am J Phys Med Rehabil.* 2019 Nov;98(11): 947–952.
13. Nash M, Groah S, Gater D, et al. Identification and management of cardiometabolic risk after spinal cord injury: clinical practice guideline for health care providers. *Top Spinal Cord Inj Rehabil.* 2018;Fall;24(4):379–423.
14. Nash MS, Lewis JE, Dyson-Hudson TA, et al. Safety, tolerance, and efficacy of extended-release niacin monotherapy for treating dyslipidemia risks in persons with chronic tetraplegia: a randomized multicenter controlled trial. *Arch Phys Med Rehabil.* 2011 Mar;92(3):399–410.
15. Olle MM, Pivarnik JM, Klish WJ, Morrow JR. Body composition of sedentary and physically active spinal cord injured individuals estimated from total body electrical conductivity. *Arch Phys Med Rehabil.* 1993 Jul;74(7):706–710.
16. Sedlock DA, Laventure SJ. Body composition and resting energy expenditure in long term spinal cord injury. *Spinal Cord.* 1990 Sep;28(7):448–454.
17. Gorgey AS, Chiodo AE, Zemper ED, Hornyak JE, Rodriguez GM, Gater DR. Relationship of spasticity to soft tissue body composition and the metabolic profile in persons with chronic motor complete spinal cord injury. *J Spinal Cord Med.* 2010 Feb;33(1):6–15.
18. Bauman WA, Adkins RH, Spungen AM, Waters RL. The effect of residual neurological deficit on oral glucose tolerance in persons with chronic spinal cord injury. *Spinal Cord.* 1999 Nov;37(11):765–771.
19. Aksnes AK, Hjeltnes N, Wahlstrom EO, Katz A, Zierath JR, Wallberg-Henriksson H. Intact glucose transport in morphologically altered denervated skeletal muscle from quadriplegic patients. *Am J Physiol-Endocrinol Metab.* 1996 Sep 1; 271(3):E593–600.
20. Gorgey AS, Dudley GA. Skeletal muscle atrophy and increased intramuscular fat after incomplete spinal cord injury. *Spinal Cord.* 2007 Apr;45(4):304–309.
21. Elder CP, Apple DF, Bickel CS, Meyer RA, Dudley GA. Intramuscular fat and glucose tolerance after spinal cord injury–a cross-sectional study. *Spinal Cord.* 2004 Dec;42(12):711–716.
22. Gorgey AS, Mather KJ, Gater DR. Central adiposity associations to carbohydrate and lipid metabolism in individuals with complete motor spinal cord injury. *Metabolism..* 2011 Jun;60(6):843–851.
23. Gorgey AS, Khalil RE, Gill R, et al. Low-dose testosterone and evoked resistance exercise after spinal cord injury on cardio-metabolic risk factors: an open-label randomized clinical trial. *J Neurotrauma.* 2019 Sep;36(18):2631–2645.
24. Gorgey AS, Mather KJ, Cupp HR, Gater DR. Effects of resistance training on adiposity and metabolism after spinal cord injury. *Med Sci Sports Exerc.* 2012 Jan;44(1):165–174.
25. Mahoney ET, Bickel CS, Elder C, et al. Changes in skeletal muscle size and glucose tolerance with electrically stimulated resistance training in subjects with chronic spinal cord injury. *Arch Phys Med Rehabil.* 2005 Jul;86(7):1502–1504.
26. Griffin L, Decker MJ, Hwang JY, et al. Functional electrical stimulation cycling improves body composition, metabolic and neural factors in persons with spinal cord injury. *J Electromyogr Kinesiol Off J Int Soc Electrophysiol Kinesiol.* 2009 Aug;19(4):614–622.
27. Mohr T, Dela F, Handberg A, Biering-Sørensen F, Galbo H, Kjaer M. Insulin action and long-term electrically induced training in individuals with spinal cord injuries. *Med Sci Sports Exerc.* 2001 Aug;33(8):1247–1252.
28. de Groot PCE, Hjeltnes N, Heijboer AC, Stal W, Birkeland K. Effect of training intensity on physical capacity, lipid profile and insulin sensitivity in early rehabilitation of spinal cord injured individuals. *Spinal Cord.* 2003 Dec;41(12):673–679.
29. Nash MS, Mendez AJ. A guideline-driven assessment of need for cardiovascular disease risk intervention in persons with chronic paraplegia. *Arch Phys Med Rehabil.* 2007 Jun;88(6):751–757.
30. Wilmet E, Ismail AA, Heilporn A, Welraeds D, Bergmann P. Longitudinal study of the bone mineral content and of soft tissue composition after spinal cord section. *Paraplegia..* 1995 Nov;33(11):674–677.
31. Gorgey AS, Mather KJ, Poarch HJ, Gater DR. Influence of motor complete spinal cord injury on visceral and subcutaneous adipose tissue measured by multi-axial magnetic resonance imaging. *J Spinal Cord Med.* 2011;34(1):99–109.
32. Gorgey AS, Gater DR. A preliminary report on the effects of the level of spinal cord injury on the association between central adiposity and metabolic profile. *PM&R..* 2011; 3(5):440–446.
33. Kemp BJ, Spungen AM, Adkins RH, Krause JS, Bauman WA. The relationships among serum lipid levels, adiposity, and depressive symptomatology in persons aging with spinal cord injury. *J Spinal Cord Med.* 2000;23(4):216–220.
34. Emmons RR, Garber CE, Cirnigliaro CM, Kirshblum SC, Spungen AM, Bauman WA. Assessment of measures for abdominal adiposity in persons with spinal cord injury. *Ultrasound Med Biol.* 2011 May;37(5):734–741.
35. Fountaine MFL, Cirnigliaro CM, Kirshblum SC, McKenna C, Bauman WA. Effect of functional sympathetic nervous system impairment of the liver and abdominal visceral adipose tissue on circulating triglyceride-rich lipoproteins. *PLoS ONE.* 2017 Mar;12(3). e0173934.
36. La Fountaine MF, Cirnigliaro CM, Hobson JC, et al. A four month randomized controlled trial on the efficacy of once-daily fenofibrate monotherapy in persons with spinal cord injury. *Sci Rep..* 2019 Nov;9(1):17166.
37. Nash MS, Jacobs PL, Mendez AJ, Goldberg RB. Circuit resistance training improves the atherogenic lipid profiles of persons with chronic paraplegia. *J Spinal Cord Med.* 2001;24(1):2–9.
38. Widman LM, McDonald CM, Abresch RT. Effectiveness of an upper extremity exercise device integrated with computer gaming for aerobic training in adolescents with spinal cord dysfunction. *J Spinal Cord Med.* 2006;29(4):363–370.
39. Jacobs PL, Nash MS, Rusinowski JW. Circuit training provides cardiorespiratory and strength benefits in persons with paraplegia. *Med Sci Sports Exerc.* 2001 May;33(5):711–717.
40. Taylor JA, Picard G, Widrick JJ. Aerobic capacity with hybrid fes rowing in spinal cord injury: comparison with arms-only exercise and preliminary findings with regular training. *PM&R..* 2011;3(9):817–824.
41. Glaser RM. Arm exercise training for wheelchair users. *Med Sci Sports Exerc [Internet].* 1989 Oct;21(5 Suppl):S149–S157.
42. Hasnan N, Ektas N, Tanhoffer AIP, et al. Exercise responses during functional electrical stimulation cycling in individuals with spinal cord injury. *Med Sci Sports Exerc.* 2013 Jun;45(6):1131–1138.
43. Bauman WA, Spungen AM, Flanagan S, Zhong YG, Alexander LR, Tsitouras PD. Blunted growth hormone response to intravenous arginine in subjects with a spinal cord injury. *Horm*

Metab Res Horm Stoffwechselforschung Horm Metab. 1994 Mar;26(3):152–156.

44. Halstead LS, Groah SL, Libin A, Hamm LF, Priestley L. The effects of an anabolic agent on body composition and pulmonary function in tetraplegia: a pilot study. *Spinal Cord.* 2010 Jan;48(1):55–59.
45. Gregory CM, Vandenborne K, Huang HFS, Ottenweller JE, Dudley GA. Effects of testosterone replacement therapy on skeletal muscle after spinal cord injury. *Spinal Cord.* 2003 Jan;41(1):23–28.
46. Groah S, Kehn M. The state of aging and public health for people with spinal cord injury: lost in transition? *Top Spinal Cord Inj Rehabil.* 2010 Feb 24;15(3):1–10.
47. Zmuda JM, Thompson PD, Winters SJ. Exercise increases serum testosterone and sex hormone-binding globulin levels in older men. *Metabolism.*. 1996 Aug;45(8):935–939.
48. Bauman WA, Kirshblum SC, Morrison NG, Cirnigliaro CM, Zhang R-L, Spungen AM. Effect of low-dose baclofen administration on plasma insulin-like growth factor-I in persons with spinal cord injury. *J Clin Pharmacol.* 2006 Apr;46(4):476–482.
49. Florini JR, Ewton DZ, Coolican SA. Growth hormone and the insulin-like growth factor system in myogenesis. *Endocr Rev.* 1996 Oct;17(5):481–517.
50. Durga A, Sepahpanah F, Regozzi M, Hastings J, Crane DA. Prevalence of testosterone deficiency after spinal cord injury. *PM R.*. 2011 Oct;3(10):929–932.
51. Abilmona SM, Sumrell RM, Gill RS, Adler RA, Gorgey AS. Serum testosterone levels may influence body composition and cardiometabolic health in men with spinal cord injury. *Spinal Cord.* 2019 Mar;57(3):229–239.
52. Bauman WA, La Fountaine MF, Spungen AM. Age-related prevalence of low testosterone in men with spinal cord injury. *J Spinal Cord Med.* 2014 Jan;37(1):32–39.
53. Bauman WA, Zhang RL, Spungen AM. Provocative stimulation of growth hormone: a monozygotic twin study discordant for spinal cord injury. *J Spinal Cord Med.* 2007;30(5):467–472.
54. Guasconi V, Puri PL. Epigenetic drugs in the treatment of skeletal muscle atrophy. *Curr Opin Clin Nutr Metab Care.* 2008 May;11(3):233–241.
55. Gorgey AS, Gater DR. Insulin growth factors may explain relationship between spasticity and skeletal muscle size in men with spinal cord injury. *J Rehabil Res Dev.* 2012;49(3):373–380.
56. Gorgey AS, Dudley GA. Spasticity may defend skeletal muscle size and composition after incomplete spinal cord injury. *Spinal Cord.* 2008 Feb;46(2):96–102.
57. Gorgey AS, Chiodo AE, Gater DR. Oral baclofen administration in persons with chronic spinal cord injury does not prevent the protective effects of spasticity on body composition and glucose homeostasis. *Spinal Cord.* 2010 Feb;48(2):160–165.
58. Ranke MB. Insulin-like growth factor binding-protein-3 (IGFBP-3). *Best Pract Res Clin Endocrinol Metab.* 2015 Oct;29(5):701–711.
59. Haywood NJ, Slater TA, Matthews CJ, Wheatcroft SB. The insulin like growth factor and binding protein family: novel therapeutic targets in obesity & diabetes. *Mol Metab.*. 2018 Oct;19:86–96.
60. Diaz D, Lopez-Dolado E, Haro S, et al. Systemic inflammation and the breakdown of intestinal homeostasis are key events in chronic spinal cord injury patients. *Int J Mol Sci.* 2021 Jan;22(2):744.
61. Wang T-D, Wang Y-H, Huang T-S, Su T-C, Pan S-L, Chen S-Y. Circulating levels of markers of inflammation and endothelial activation are increased in men with chronic spinal cord injury. *J Formos Med Assoc.* 2007 Nov;106(11):919–928.
62. Illán-Gómez F, Gonzálvez-Ortega M, Orea-Soler I, et al. Obesity and inflammation: change in adiponectin, c-reactive protein, tumour necrosis factor-alpha and interleukin-6 after bariatric surgery. *Obes Surg.* 2012 Jun;22(6):950–955.
63. Sopasakis VR, Sandqvist M, Gustafson B, et al. High local concentrations and effects on differentiation implicate interleukin-6 as a paracrine regulator. *Obes Res.* 2004;12(3):454–460.
64. Chen G, Goeddel DV. TNF-R1 signaling: a beautiful pathway. *Science.*. 2002 May;296(5573):1634–1635.
65. Hotamisligil GS, Shargill NS, Spiegelman BM. Adipose expression of tumor necrosis factor-alpha: direct role in obesity-linked insulin resistance. *Science.*. 1993 Jan; 259(5091):87–91.
66. Cawthorn WP, Sethi JK. TNF-α and adipocyte biology. *FEBS Lett.* 2008;582(1):117–131.
67. Sumrell RM, Nightingale TE, McCauley LS, Gorgey AS. Anthropometric cutoffs and associations with visceral adiposity and metabolic biomarkers after spinal cord injury. *PLoS ONE.* 2018 Aug;13(8):e0203049.
68. Rankin KC, O'Brien LC, Segal L, Khan MR, Gorgey AS. Liver adiposity and metabolic profile in individuals with chronic spinal cord injury. *BioMed Res Int. Aug;2017.* 2017: e1364818.
69. Grant RW, Stephens JM. Fat in flames: influence of cytokines and pattern recognition receptors on adipocyte lipolysis. *Am J Physiol-Endocrinol Metab.* 2015 Jun;309(3):E205–E213.
70. Kern PA, Ranganathan S, Li C, Wood L, Ranganathan G. Adipose tissue tumor necrosis factor and interleukin-6 expression in human obesity and insulin resistance. *Am J Physiol-Endocrinol Metab.* 2001 May;280(5): E745–E751.
71. Vozarova B, Weyer C, Hanson K, Tataranni PA, Bogardus C, Pratley RE. Circulating interleukin-6 in relation to adiposity, insulin action, and insulin secretion. *Obes Res.* 2001;9(7):414–417.
72. van Hall G, Steensberg A, Sacchetti M, et al. Interleukin-6 stimulates lipolysis and fat oxidation in humans. *J Clin Endocrinol Metab.* 2003 Jul;88(7):3005–3010.
73. Gibson AE, Buchholz AC, Martin Ginis KA. C-reactive protein in adults with chronic spinal cord injury: increased chronic inflammation in tetraplegia vs paraplegia. *Spinal Cord.* 2008 Sep;46(9):616–621.
74. Senn JJ, Klover PJ, Nowak IA, et al. Suppressor of Cytokine Signaling-3 (SOCS-3), a potential mediator of interleukin-6-dependent insulin resistance in hepatocytes. *J Biol Chem.* 2003 Apr;278(16):13740–13746.
75. Rotter V, Nagaev I, Smith U. Interleukin-6 (IL-6) induces insulin resistance in 3T3-L1 adipocytes and is, like IL-8 and tumor necrosis factor-α, overexpressed in human fat cells from insulin-resistant subjects. *J Biol Chem.* 2003 Nov;278(46):45777–45784.
76. Selvin E, Paynter NP, Erlinger TP. The effect of weight loss on c-reactive protein: a systematic review. *Arch Intern Med.* 2007 Jan;167(1):31–39.

77. Plaisance EP, Grandjean PW. Physical activity and high-sensitivity c-reactive protein. *Sports Med Auckl NZ.* 2006;36(5):443–458.
78. Donia SA, Allison DJ, Gammage KL, Ditor DS. The effects of acute aerobic exercise on mood and inflammation in individuals with multiple sclerosis and incomplete spinal cord injury. *NeuroRehabilitation.*. 2019;45(1):117–124.
79. Gorgey AS, Gater DR. Prevalence of obesity after spinal cord injury. *Top Spinal Cord Inj Rehabil.* 2007;12(4):1–7.
80. Wahman K, Nash MS, Westgren N, Lewis JE, Seiger A, Levi R. Cardiovascular disease risk factors in persons with paraplegia: the Stockholm spinal cord injury study. *J Rehabil Med.* 2010 Mar;42(3):272–278.
81. Laughton GE, Buchholz AC, Martin Ginis KA, Goy RE. Lowering body mass index cutoffs better identifies obese persons with spinal cord injury. *Spinal Cord.* 2009 Oct;47(10):757–762.
82. de Groot S, Post MWM, Postma K, Sluis TA, van der Woude LHV. Prospective analysis of body mass index during and up to 5 years after discharge from inpatient spinal cord injury rehabilitation. *J Rehabil Med.* 2010 Nov;42(10):922–928.
83. Gill S, Sumrell RM, Sima A, Cifu DX, Gorgey AS. Waist circumference cutoff identifying risks of obesity, metabolic syndrome, and cardiovascular disease in men with spinal cord injury. *PLoS ONE.* 2020 Jul;15(7):e0236752.
84. Dopler Nelson M, Widman LM, Abresch RT, et al. Metabolic syndrome in adolescents with spinal cord dysfunction. *J Spinal Cord Med.* 2007;30(Suppl 1):S127–139.
85. Bauman WA, Spungen AM. Disorders of carbohydrate and lipid metabolism in veterans with paraplegia or quadriplegia: a model of premature aging. *Metabolism.*. 1994 Jun;43(6):749–756.
86. LaVela SL, Weaver FM, Goldstein B, et al. Diabetes mellitus in individuals with spinal cord injury or disorder. *J Spinal Cord Med.* 2006;29(4):387–395.
87. Gorgey AS, Graham ZA, Bauman WA, Cardozo C, Gater DR. Abundance in proteins expressed after functional electrical stimulation cycling or arm cycling ergometry training in persons with chronic spinal cord injury. *J Spinal Cord Med.* 2017 Jul;40(4):439–448.
88. Phillips SM, Stewart BG, Mahoney DJ, et al. Body-weight-support treadmill training improves blood glucose regulation in persons with incomplete spinal cord injury. *J Appl Physiol.* 2004 Aug;97(2):716–724.
89. Gorgey AS, Graham ZA, Chen Q, et al. Sixteen weeks of testosterone with or without evoked resistance training on protein expression, fiber hypertrophy and mitochondrial health after spinal cord injury. *J Appl Physiol.* 2020 Apr;128(6):1487–1496.
90. Ryan TE, Brizendine JT, Backus D, McCully KK. Electrically induced resistance training in individuals with motor complete spinal cord injury. *Arch Phys Med Rehabil.* 2013 Nov;94(11):2166–2173.
91. Tremblay F, Dubois M-J, Marette A. Regulation of GLUT4 traffic and function by insulin and contraction in skeletal muscle. *Front Biosci J Virtual Libr.* 2003 Sep;8:d1072–1084.

CHAPTER 36

Infections With Spinal Cord Injury

Kyle Jisa and William Carter

OUTLINE

Infections in Patients With Spinal Cord Injury

Predisposing Factors to Infection

Spinal cord injury (SCI) leads to an increased risk for infectious processes through multiple mechanisms. Administration of glucocorticoids, increased stress, malnutrition, and prolonged hospitalization after injury can all lead to immunosuppression. Neurogenic bladder leads to bladder stasis and disruption to the naturally protective effect of normal voiding along with bladder catheterization. Additionally, ineffective cough and retained pulmonary secretions can predispose to subsequent pneumonia. Higher levels of proinflammatory cytokines are often seen after SCI and may also be a result of occult infection.[1]

Evaluation for Infection and Antibiotic Treatment

Establishing a diagnosis of infection in individuals with SCI can be challenging. New-onset or increased referred or neurogenic pain is a common initial symptom, which can be challenging to localize in the face of altered or absent sensation.[2] Fever may not necessarily be infectious in nature but can instead be the result of poikilothermia—the inability to regulate body temperature between heat production and heat loss. Up to 20% of fevers may be due to autonomic dysfunction in individuals with injury above T6. Autonomic dysreflexia may also present with fever; the presence of bradycardia can help differentiate from infection with expected tachycardia. Elevated temperature within those with acute tetraplegia may last for several months without any identifiable infectious etiology, often leading to excess diagnostic workup and antibiotic administration.

Physiologic changes that occur after injury should be considered when providing treatment with antibiotics. Loss of mobility leads to muscle atrophy and an associated increase in subclinical extracellular edema, which can lead to underdosing of antibiotics due to a larger volume of distribution in comparison to able-bodied persons. Antibiotic concentration can be partially corrected for by overestimating creatinine clearance, for example using the Cockcroft-Gault equation that was developed based upon able-bodied persons. A 24-hour urine collection can also be utilized to better determine true renal function.[2,3]

Urinary Tract Infection

Urinary tract infections (UTI) are the most common infection to occur in individuals with SCI, with an estimated 2.5 infections per patient annually. Bacteriuria is highly prevalent in individuals with SCI and neurogenic bladder, occurring in approximately 70% in those who use intermittent straight catheterization and nearly 100% in those with chronic indwelling urinary systems.[4] Vesicoureteral reflux, increased postvoid residuals, bladder outlet obstruction, and urolithiasis are all complications of neurogenic bladder that lead to increased UTI risk.[5] Clinically, individuals with SCI rarely present with dysuria or urinary urgency but rather with changes in typical voiding habits, increased postvoid residuals, foul urine, worsening spasticity, or autonomic dysreflexia. Importantly, pyelonephritis may develop without back pain due to altered sensation.

Utilization of pyuria on urinalysis is a frequent marker for helping to determine UTI; however, the presence of pyuria does not solely indicate UTI, particularly in patients who utilize urinary catheterization.[6] Pyuria may be present secondary to urothelium inflammation associated with indwelling urinary catheters, urolithiasis, and interstitial nephritis. When urine culture is obtained to guide UTI treatment, organisms isolated are typically gram-negative bacilli and enterococci. If *Proteus* is cultured, it should always be treated because it indicates the presence of urease that splits urea to form ammonia and carbon dioxide and may secondarily cause increased urine pH and precipitation of ions and urolithiasis formation.[7] Isolation of multiple organisms may not represent contamination as commonly seen in able-bodied persons, but rather a prior UTI that did not have appropriate antimicrobial coverage for all pathogens. When it is unclear which cultured organisms are colonization versus pathogenic, it is reasonable to treat all microorganisms. Microorganisms that are cultured in both urine and blood cultures confirm the pathogenicity of the urine culture result.

Techniques to prevent UTIs have been employed with varying efficacy. If possible, switching to intermittent catheterization or condom catheter systems from indwelling catheters is preferred to reduce both UTI and urolithiasis risk. Antimicrobial catheters have demonstrated evidence to reduce UTIs.[8,9] Limited evidence exists to support cranberry as a supplement to prevent UTI, which is theorized to inhibit bacteria (particularly *Escherichia coli*) from adhering to the uroepithelium.[10] Conversely, evidence exists to support deliberate colonization with *E. coli* 83972 to prevent UTI.[11] Injection of botulinum toxin into the detrusor muscle may reduce UTIs through reduction of bladder pressure and ureteral reflux.[12]

Pneumonia

Pneumonia is the most common cause of death in both acute and chronic SCI at a rate of 30%–50%.[13,14] During the acute stage after injury, intubation at hospitalization increases the risk for ventilator-associated pneumonia. Furthermore, many patients will have ongoing difficulty with retained pulmonary secretions and ineffective cough. Clinical presentation of pneumonia may include tachypnea, tachycardia, fever, and leukocytosis. In individuals with altered perception of dyspnea and developing respiratory muscle fatigue, respiratory failure may develop without clinical symptoms. It is recommended that arterial blood gases be monitored when treating pneumonia.

Several commonly occurring conditions may be confused for, or even complicate, acute pneumonia. Atelectasis may mimic pneumonia and present with low-grade fever and leukocytosis. The left lung is preferentially affected by both atelectasis and pneumonia due to the left main stem bronchus branching at a more acute angle, which also results in greater difficulty suctioning during pulmonary toilet. Pulmonary embolism, which occurs in approximately 5% of individuals with an acute SCI, can also be mistaken for pneumonia. Chemical pneumonitis may develop after aspiration of gastric contents and can be differentiated from aspiration pneumonia with an adequate respiratory secretion sample.

When pneumonia is diagnosed, consideration of the most likely pathogen should be performed and pursued. As seen in the general population, community-acquired pneumonia in SCI is typically due to *Streptococcus pneumoniae, Haemophilus influenzae*, or *Branhamella catarrhalis*. For patients who are ventilator-dependent, the three most common etiologies include methicillin-resistant *Staphylococcus aureus* (MRSA), *Pseudomonas aeruginosa*, and *Acinetobacter baumannii*. Aspiration pneumonia is typically due to gram-negative or anaerobic bacteria.

Recommended antibiotic treatment duration for a diagnosis of pneumonia is typically 10 to 14 days.[4] In the case of community-acquired pneumonia, empiric treatment can be performed with a respiratory fluoroquinolone or combination macrolide and cephalosporin antibiotics. For patients with respiratory devices, the treatment regimen should include coverage of *MRSA* and *P. aeruginosa*.

Pressure Injury Infection

Development of a pressure injury occurs with the disruption to the integrity of the skin barrier that can then proceed to bacterial colonization and infection.[15] Risk factors for pressure injury development include paresis secondary to SCI, decreased activity while hospitalized, diabetes mellitus, malnutrition, altered sensation, incontinence, and prolonged hospitalization.[16,17] The sites most commonly affected by pressure injuries include the ischium, sacrum, and greater trochanter.[18] Clinically, an infection of a pressure injury may present with fever, erythema, edema, warmth, and purulence.

When clinical suspicion for infection is high, it is important to recognize that pressure injuries are universally colonized by bacteria. Due to this, swab culture samples should not be routinely obtained unless infection is clinically apparent. Swab cultures may mislead the practitioner toward unnecessary antibiotics, leading to multidrug-resistant organism (MDRO) colonization. Rather, deep tissue biopsy is the most reliable diagnostic method for guiding treatment. Implicated pathogens most commonly include *Staphylococcus, Streptococcus*, gram-negative, and anaerobic bacteria. A combination of nuclear scintigraphy and magnetic resonance imaging may also be considered for determining the presence of underlying abscess or osteomyelitis, in addition to infected pressure injuries.

Treatment of pressure injury infections often requires a combined medical and surgical approach for resolution. Involvement of surgery is utilized to both debride and drain nonviable tissue. Infections that do not appear to improve warrant reevaluation of antibiotic regimen for appropriate coverage and consideration of undiagnosed fistula or abscess. The utilization of negative-pressure vacuum devices should also be considered.[19]

Osteomyelitis

The development of osteomyelitis is most commonly below pressure injuries but can be difficult to diagnose. Other, less common causes of osteomyelitis include hematogenous, prosthesis-related, postoperative, and vertebral osteomyelitis. It is important to recognize that clinical evaluation does not correlate well in diagnosing osteomyelitis. This includes duration of nonhealing pressure injury, presence of purulence, exposure of bone, fever, leukocytosis, elevation of inflammatory markers (e.g., c-reactive protein/erythrocyte sedimentation rate), plain radiographs, and nuclear scintigraphy. Rather, when clinical suspicion is high, the gold standard for accurate diagnosis is a bone biopsy; however, the high sensitivity of nuclear imaging study avoids the need for bone biopsy when the study is negative. When osteomyelitis is present below pressure injuries, it is often due to two or more pathogens; gram-positive cocci (*S. aureus and Streptococcus*), gram-negative bacilli (*P. aeruginosa* and *Enterobacteriaceae*), anaerobes (*Bacteroides* and *Fusobacterium*), and, rarely, *Candida* are commonly implicated.[20]

Treatment of osteomyelitis is typically with antibiotics for at least 6 weeks, although ideal duration of therapy is unclear. Parenteral therapy is typically utilized, but patients may be transitioned to oral regimens if they are highly bioavailable. Surgical intervention is typically most successful when there is a combination of debridement and muscle flap surgery. The transposition of healthy vascular muscle helps improve removal of nonviable tissue, improve infection resistance, and increase vascular supply for bone healing.[21,22]

Bloodstream Infection

Bacteremia in SCI is most commonly secondary to UTI, pneumonia, pressure injuries, and vascular line infections. In comparison to the general population, individuals with SCI are at higher risk for gram-negative bacteremia with vascular line infection. Therefore, it is recommended that the empiric antibiotic regimen be expanded to account for this. For patients without an apparent source after workup, an undiagnosed abscess should be considered.[23–25]

Intraabdominal Infection

Biliary tract infections are the most frequent intraabdominal infection. This occurs due to cholelithiasis more commonly than in able-bodied persons. In individuals with high spinal cord lesions, altered sensation may alter the clinical presentation, which may then include abdominal distension, abdominal wall spasms, and abdominal rigidity without localized pain.[26] Patients are also at higher risk of developing *C. difficile* infection due to frequent infections and prolonged antibiotic administration. At times, active *C. difficile* infection can remain undetectable due to altered sensation until the development of the most severe complications, such as toxic megacolon or bowel perforation.

Multidrug-Resistant Organism

As a complication of prolonged hospitalization and frequent administration of antibiotics, development of MDROs in rehabilitation units and long-term care units is common. Cultured organisms may include MRSA, vancomycin-resistant *Enterococcus* (VRE), and extended-spectrum beta-lactamase gram-negative bacteria. VRE is typically cultured from urine in patients with chronic indwelling urinary catheters, whereas MRSA can colonize multiple areas of the body. The presence of VRE in the urine is often representative of asymptomatic bacteriuria but creates inherently higher risk for subsequent bacteremia.[27]

Review Questions

1. The most common cause of death in SCI is:
   a. Urosepsis
   b. Pneumonia
   c. Autonomic dysreflexia
   d. Intraabdominal infections
2. The gold standard for diagnosing osteomyelitis is:
   a. Nuclear scintigraphy
   b. Swab culture of exposed bone
   c. Bone biopsy
   d. Magnetic resonance imaging
3. Vascular line infections in SCI patients are at higher risk for what type of pathogen in comparison with the general population?
   a. Gram-negative bacteria
   b. MRSA
   c. *Candida*
   d. Anaerobic bacteria
4. A patient develops symptoms concerning for sepsis and is found to have *S. aureus* on two of two blood cultures after being started on broad-spectrum antibiotics. Workup is unremarkable for UTI, pneumonia, pressure injuries, osteomyelitis, and gastrointestinal infection. The next best step in management is to:
   a. Attribute findings to contamination and discontinue antibiotics immediately
   b. Discontinue antibiotics after 7 to 10 days of treatment

c. Continue antibiotics and repeat blood cultures every 48 hours until negative
d. Evaluate for an occult abscess

5. Which of the following bacteria is recommended to be always treated if found to grow on urine culture in SCI patients?
a. Vancomycin-resistant *Enterococcus* (VRE)
b. *E. coli*
c. *Proteus*
d. *Klebsiella*

REFERENCES

1. Davies AL, Hayes KC, Dekaban GA. Clinical correlates of elevated serum concentrations of cytokines and autoantibodies in patients with spinal cord injury. *Arch Phys Med Rehabil.* 2007;88(11):1384–1393.
2. Garcia-Arguello LY, O'Horo JC, Farrell A, et al. Infections in the spinal cord-injured population: a systematic review. *Spinal Cord.* 2017;55(6):526–534.
3. DeJong G, Groah SL. Advancing SCI health care to avert rehospitalization. *J Spinal Cord Med.* 2015;38(6):696–699.
4. Darouiche RO, Green BG, Donovan WH, et al. Multicenter randomized controlled trial of bacterial interference for prevention of urinary tract infection in patients with neurogenic bladder. *Urology.*. 2011;78(2):341–346.
5. García Leoni ME, Esclarín De Ruz A. Management of urinary tract infection in patients with spinal cord injuries. *Clin Microbiol Infect.* 2003;9(8):780–785.
6. Hooton TM, Bradley SF, Cardenas DD, et al. Diagnosis, prevention, and treatment of catheter-associated urinary tract infection in adults: 2009 International Clinical Practice Guidelines from the Infectious Diseases Society of America. *Clin Infect Dis.* 2010;50(5):625–663.
7. Hung EW, Darouiche RO, Trautner BW. Proteus bacteriuria is associated with significant morbidity in spinal cord injury. *Spinal Cord.* 2007;45(9):616–620.
8. Li L, Ye W, Ruan H, Yang B, Zhang S, Li L. Impact of hydrophilic catheters on urinary tract infections in people with spinal cord injury: systematic review and meta-analysis of randomized controlled trials. *Arch Phys Med Rehabil.* 2013;94(4):782–787.
9. Bermingham SL, Hodgkinson S, Wright S, Hayter E, Spinks J, Pellowe C. Intermittent self catheterisation with hydrophilic, gel reservoir, and non-coated catheters: a systematic review and cost effectiveness analysis. *BMJ.*. 2013;346:e8639.
10. Hess MJ, Hess PE, Sullivan MR, Nee M, Yalla SV. Evaluation of cranberry tablets for the prevention of urinary tract infections in spinal cord injured patients with neurogenic bladder. *Spinal Cord.* 2008;46(9):622–626.
11. Darouiche RO, Riosa S, Hull RA. Comparison of *Escherichia coli* strains as agents for bacterial interference. *Infect Control Hosp Epidemiol.* 2010;31(6):659–661.
12. Jia C, Liao L-M, Chen G, Sui Y. Detrusor botulinum toxin A injection significantly decreased urinary tract infection in patients with traumatic spinal cord injury. *Spinal Cord.* 2013;51(6):487–490.
13. Kopp MA, Watzlawick R, Martus P, et al. Long-term functional outcome in patients with acquired infections after acute spinal cord injury. *Neurology.*. 2017;88(9):892–900.
14. Burns SP. Acute respiratory infections in persons with spinal cord injury. *Phys Med Rehabil Clin N Am.* 2007;18(2):203–216. v-2.
15. Joseph C, Nilsson Wikmar L. Prevalence of secondary medical complications and risk factors for pressure ulcers after traumatic spinal cord injury during acute care in South Africa. *Spinal Cord.* 2016;54(7):535–539.
16. Salzberg CA, Byrne DW, Cayten CG, van Niewerburgh P, Murphy JG, Viehbeck M. A new pressure ulcer risk assessment scale for individuals with spinal cord injury. *Am J Phys Med Rehabil.* 1996;75(2):96–104.
17. Hoff JM, Bjerke LW, Gravem PE, Hagen EM, Rekand T. [Pressure ulcers after spinal cord injury]. *Tidsskr Nor Laegeforen.* 2012;132(7):838–839. (In Norwegian).
18. Brienza D, Krishnan S, Karg P, Sowa G, Allegretti AL. Predictors of pressure ulcer incidence following traumatic spinal cord injury: a secondary analysis of a prospective longitudinal study. *Spinal Cord.* 2018;56(1):28–34.
19. Sunn G. Spinal cord injury pressure ulcer treatment: an experience-based approach. *Phys Med Rehabil Clin N Am.* 2014;25(3):671–680. ix.
20. Brunel A-S, Lamy B, Cyteval C, et al. Diagnosing pelvic osteomyelitis beneath pressure ulcers in spinal cord injured patients: a prospective study. *Clin Microbiol Infect.* 2016;22(3):267 e1-8.
21. Marriott R, Rubayi S. Successful truncated osteomyelitis treatment for chronic osteomyelitis secondary to pressure ulcers in spinal cord injury patients. *Ann Plast Surg.* 2008 Oct;61(4):425–429.
22. Berbari EF, Kanj SS, Kowalski TJ, et al. 2015 Infectious Diseases Society of America (IDSA) Clinical Practice Guidelines for the Diagnosis and Treatment of Native Vertebral Osteomyelitis in Adults. *Clin Infect Dis.* 2015;61(6):e26–e46.
23. Evans CT, Burns SP, Chin A, Weaver FM, Hershow RC. Predictors and outcomes of antibiotic adequacy for bloodstream infections in veterans with spinal cord injury. *Arch Phys Med Rehabil.* 2009;90(8):1364–1370.
24. Dinh A, Saliba M, Saadeh D, et al. Blood stream infections due to multidrug-resistant organisms among spinal cord-injured patients, epidemiology over 16 years and associated risks: a comparative study. *Spinal Cord.* 2016;54(9):720–725.
25. Wall BM, Mangold T, Huch KM, Corbett C, Cooke CR. Bacteremia in the chronic spinal cord injury population: risk factors for mortality. *J Spinal Cord Med.* 2003;26(3):248–253.
26. Apisarnthanarak A, Bailey TC, Fraser VJ. Duration of stool colonization in patients infected with extended-spectrum beta-lactamase-producing *Escherichia coli* and *Klebsiella pneumoniae*. *Clin Infect Dis.* 2008;46(8):1322–1323.
27. Kappel C, Widmer A, Geng V, et al. Successful control of methicillin-resistant *Staphylococcus aureus* in a spinal cord injury center: a 10-year prospective study including molecular typing. *Spinal Cord.* 2008;46(6):438–444.

CHAPTER 37

Evaluation and Management of Pain After Spinal Cord Injury

Robert J. Trainer and Denise D. Lester

OUTLINE

Introduction

Pain after spinal cord injury (SCI) is common and, when unmanaged, can have deleterious effects on patients' emotional, physical, social function, independence, financial earning potential, and overall quality of life. Understanding the underlying mechanisms for your patient's SCI pain will assist in directing specific therapeutic interventions and prevent delayed rehabilitation.

Prevalence and Etiology

Current screening tools have identified an overall prevalence of SCI pain of 70%–80%, and in community-dwelling individuals who are 12 or more months after SCI, 44% have pain that interferes with daily activities (Fig. 37.1). Central pain can occur after spinal cord lesions from various etiologies, including traumatic injury, syringomyelia, infarction, and myelitis, or from cerebral lesions of nonvascular origin, such as multiple sclerosis, tumor. Regardless of the nature of the lesion and its localization in the central nervous system, aberrant neural activity in deafferented circuits and an imbalance between facilitatory and inhibitory neural pathways cause neuropathic central pain.[1–5] In a large cohort of SCI patients, musculoskeletal pain was the most common type of pain experienced and was present in 59% of patients. At-level neuropathic pain was present in 41%, below-level neuropathic pain was present in 34%, and visceral pain was present in 5%. Below-level pain is seen in 23%–52% and described as the "most severe or excruciating" of all SCI pain reported.[6,7] A delayed time to onset of pain is often seen, and it is important for the patient to understand and have expectations that it will occur. In one study, the mean time to onset of SCI pain was 1.6 years; the shortest onset times included at-level pain (1.2 years) and pain above the level of injury or musculoskeletal pain (1.3 years). Below-level neuropathic pain (1.8 years) and visceral pain (4.2 years) developed later.[3] Delayed SCI pain must be distinguished from a new medical problem, such as a syrinx. Patients, especially with motor incomplete lesions, may also have onset of postlaminectomy pain syndrome. This is characterized by epidural fibrosis and advanced adjacent level deterioration years after spinal fusion. The International Spinal Cord Injury Pain classification was created in 2012.[8,9]

Chronic Pain Classification (Table 37.1)

Musculoskeletal Pain

Back and neck pain are common in persons with SCI with an incidence similar to the 60% seen in the general population. Individuals with SCI may have had spine fusions, adjacent level deterioration, advanced facet arthritis, sacroiliitis, and epidural fibrosis.[10] This can lead to postlaminectomy pain syndrome or failed back surgery syndrome,[11,12] for which there exists an algorithm of care.[6,13–15] People with incomplete SCI are vulnerable to back pain, especially if they are able to walk but still have weakness. Spasticity, if present, can worsen musculoskeletal pain. Secondary pain in patients with SCI may need activity modification as well as modification of transfer aides including wheelchair height, home, and industrial hygiene.[16–19] Upper limb (shoulder, elbow, and hand) pain can make it difficult to transfer safely and perform other activities of daily living and, although it is often undertreated, requires prompt attention and intervention.[20]

Nociceptive Pain Types

The International Association for the Study of Pain defines nociceptive pain as pain arising from activation of nociceptors, where a nociceptor is defined as a

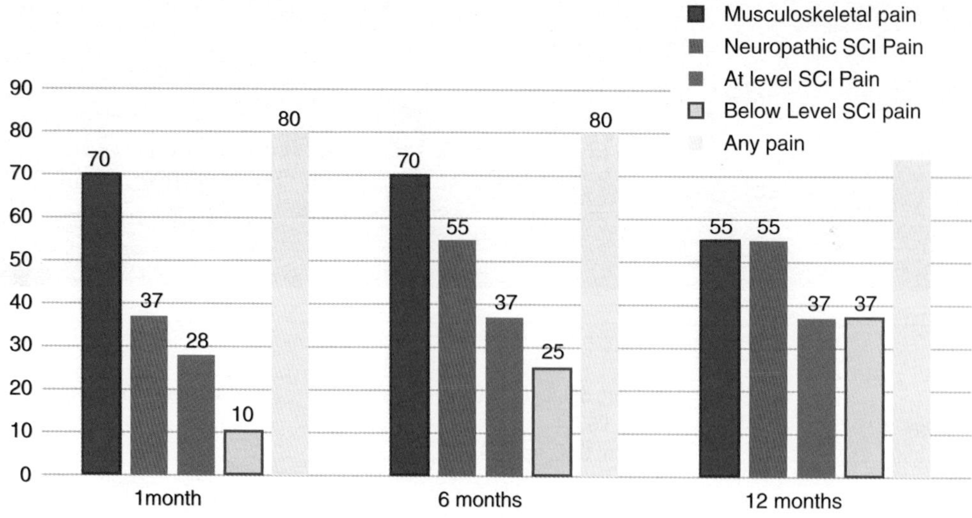

Fig. 37.1 Data Representing the Prevalence of Spinal Cord Injury Related Pain.

Table 37.1 Chronic SCI Related Pain Classification

Broad Type (Tier One) Pain Type	Broad System (Tier Two) Pain Subtype	Specific Structures and Pathology (Tier Three) Primary Pain Source and/or Pathology
Nociceptive	Musculoskeletal pain	Bone, joint, muscle trauma, or inflammation Mechanical instability Muscle spasm Secondary overuse syndromes
	Visceral pain	Renal calculus, bowel dysfunction, and sphincter dysfunction
	Other nociceptive pain	Autonomic dysreflexia headache, migraine headache, surgical skin incision
Neuropathic	At-level of spinal cord injury pain	Nerve root compression (including cauda equina) Syringomyelia Spinal cord trauma/ischemia Dual level cord and root trauma
	Below-level of spinal cord injury pain	Spinal cord trauma/ischemia
	Other neuropathic pain	Compressive mononeuropathies
Other pain		Fibromyalgia Complex regional pain syndrome type 1 Interstitial cystitis Irritable bowel syndrome

peripheral nerve ending on a sensory receptor that is capable of transducing and encoding noxious stimuli. It is usually divided into musculoskeletal, neuropathic, and visceral pain. Neuropathic pain is caused by a lesion or disease of the somatosensory system. At-level SCI pain is neuropathic pain when the SCI lesion is the source of the pain. At-level SCI pain can be attributed to SCI or peripheral nerve root injury and is characterized by sensory deficits, neuropathic allodynia, hyperalgesia, hyperpathia, and dysesthesias such as burning, stinging, and shocking descriptors. An example of at-level pain would be syringomyelia.[21] Below-level pain is more common and believed to be due to reorganization of the nervous system, especially when an SCI is complete.

Definitions

- Allodynia is the perception of pain from a stimulus that in a healthy organism is not painful.
- Hyperalgesia is an enhanced perception of pain from a stimulus that does evoke pain in a healthy organism but to a lesser extent.
- Primary sensitization is an enhanced sensation and related enhanced neuronal transmission within and around the site of injury likely due to reorganization of neuronal signaling directly from the injury.
- Secondary sensitization is an enhanced sensation and neural transmission at body sites removed from the site of injury. Changes in spinal cord neurons lead to increased excitability. This likely involves wide dynamic range neurons (WDR).

- Supraspinal sensitization is assumed to change the cortical elements involved in pain perception. These in turn would modulate the spinal cord processing of afferent nociceptive input through descending modulatory pathways.

Assessing Spinal Cord Injury–Related Pain

Physical exam and history taking for SCI pain start with determining (1) the type of pain present (above, at, below, visceral); (2) the symptomatic experience (burning, lancinating, aching); (3) the most similar neuropathic pain equivalent; and (4) presence of any type of abnormal pain (hyperalgesia, allodynia). The three main areas of focus for pain transmission have been the (1) anterior spinothalamic tract (STT) (the pathway for crude touch, pain, temperature, and pressure); (2) the dorsal columns (fasciculus gracilis and fasciculus cuneatus) that carry conscious proprioception and discriminative touch; and (3) the somatosensory cortex, where pathways converge and perception of pain resides. Modern-day realization of the *balance* of these systems is helping our understanding of the complexity of SCI pain. Residual STT function together with neuronal hyperexcitability, likely due to a lesion of inhibitory Interneuron (IN) at the rostral end of injury, are hypothesized to develop central pain.[22] Hyperexcitable WDR neurons that cause evoked pain may be involved in the pathogenesis of central pain.[23–25]

Treatment Options

A pain ladder for optimal therapy for SCI pain should be used in order of invasiveness and risk. A typical SCI pain therapeutic ladder would include (in increasing order of invasiveness and risk) physical agents, psychological approaches, medications, noninvasive neuromodulation, interventional diagnostic and therapeutic spine procedures, intrathecal pump therapy, neurosurgical destructive lesioning, and implanted neuromodulation devices in the brain.

Physical and Psychological Management

The standard rehabilitation approaches to pain using physical modalities and psychological interventions can have a profound and meaningful effect on SCI pain and wellbeing.

Pharmacologic Management

Nonsteroidal antiinflammatory drugs (NSAIDS) such as aspirin, ibuprofen (Advil), and naproxen (Aleve) are most commonly used to treat musculoskeletal pain, with side effects including stomach upset or bleeding problems. Antiseizure medications such as gabapentin (Neurontin) and pregabalin (Lyrica) are used to treat neuropathic pain with some benefit specifically in SCI pain,[26,27] with side effects including dizziness, sleepiness, and leg swelling. Antidepressants commonly used for SCI-related pain management include selective serotonin norepinephrine reuptake inhibitors (SNRI), such as venlafaxine (Effexor) and duloxetine (Cymbalta), and tricyclics, such as amitriptyline (Elavil) and desipramine (Norpramin). Opiates, including morphine, codeine, hydrocodone (Vicodin), and oxycodone (OxyContin), may be used to treat neuropathic and musculoskeletal pain, although side effects and potential for habit formation make their use less desirable long-term. Muscle relaxants and antispasticity medications, such as diazepam (Valium), baclofen (Lioresal), and tizanidine (Zanaflex), are used to treat spasm-related, musculoskeletal pain. Topical local anesthetics such as a lidocaine patch may be used to treat pain allodynia. In clinical practice, evidence exists for gabapentinoids, tricyclic antidepressants, SNRI, tramadol (Ultram), and, for partial injuries, lamotrigine (Lamictal).[25] Specifically for neuropathic SCI pain, the following medication approach has been recommended: First-line agents include gabapentin, pregabalin, tricyclic antidepressants, and SNRIs (e.g., duloxetine, venlafaxine.). Second-line agents include capsaicin 8% patches, lidocaine patches, and tramadol. Third-line agents include strong opioids and botulinum toxin A (Botox). Additionally, there is a weak recommendation against the use of cannabinoids and valproate (Depakote), and a strong recommendation against the use of levetiracetam (Keppra) and mexiletine (Mexitil).

Noninvasive Therapies in Evolution

Ketamine (Ketalar), a dissociative anesthetic, produces analgesia and amnesia and has a novel antidepressant effect. Early doses of 1.0–2.0 mg/kg proved effective for pain but with undesirable psychic side effects. Later, combining the drug with benzodiazepines allowed more rationale and safer use.[28] Dose and protocols vary, with 0.5 mg/kg given over 30–45 min used to produce minimal-duration analgesia that is effective for depression.[29–33] Treating patients with a 100-hour infusion of S-ketamine (dose titrated up to 20–30 mg h^{-1}) results in long-term pain relief lasting up to 3 months following treatment.[34]

Intrathecal pump usage for chronic pain was first published for continuous application of morphine in 1985,[35] and many revisions for optimal patient selection and trialing have been made.[36–38] Penn and Kroin were the first to describe the treatment of severe spasticity using intrathecal baclofen in 1984.[39] The Food and Drug Administration approval of the modern intrathecal drug delivery system in 1991 has yielded three agents approved as medications for intrathecal use: two for pain (morphine and ziconotide [Prialt]) and one for spasticity (baclofen). A number of other agents, including bupivacaine (Marcaine), clonidine (Catapres), and fentanyl, are commonly used. Summaries of these approaches are available.[38–84]

Conclusions

Understanding and managing SCI-related pain is time intensive and complex. Although formalized training in SCI and pain training programs are limited, the significant prevalence of a range of pain issues in individuals with acute and chronic SCI necessitates that all skilled practitioners enhance their knowledge and apply the integrative, team-based principles outlined. The four-pronged approach to capture the individual with SCI-related pain experience includes assessing (1) the type of pain present (above, at, below, visceral); (2) the symptomatic experience (burning, lancinating, aching); (3) the most similar neuropathic pain equivalent will be the goal of the physical exam and history; and (4) presence of any type of abnormal pain (hyperalgesia, allodynia). Proper management of chronic SCI pain requires an understanding of the neuroanatomy of the lesion, the plasticity of the nervous system, and the available options for therapy.

Review Questions

1. Which SCI condition is most likely to result in the most severe form of SCI pain?
   a. Complete SCI
   b. Incomplete SCI with preservation of the STT and absence of the dorsal column
   c. Incomplete SCI with preservation of the dorsal column and absence of the STT
   d. Incomplete SCI with presence of both dorsal column and STT
2. What is the most common form of neuropathic SCI pain?
   a. Musculoskeletal pain
   b. Above the level pain
   c. Below the level pain
   d. Visceral pain
3. What is the most severe form of neuropathic SCI pain?
   a. Musculoskeletal pain
   b. Above the level pain
   c. Below the level pain
   d. Visceral pain
   e. c and d
4. What are the two classes of medications with efficacy for neuropathic SCI pain?
   a. Muscle relaxants and NSAIDS
   b. SNRI and NSAIDS
   c. Tricyclic antidepressants and gabapentinoids
   d. N-methyl-D-aspartate receptor antagonists and SSRI
5. Which subset of the population of patients with SCI pain might benefit the most from assisted ambulation therapy?
   a. Those with spasticity as a major complaint
   b. Those with motor incomplete lesions and allodynia
   c. Those with postlaminectomy pain
   d. All of the above
6. Which condition is most likely to respond to interventional targeted transforaminal epidural steroid injections?
   a. Above the level musculoskeletal pain
   b. Below the level neuropathic pain
   c. At the level neuropathic pain
   d. Visceral pain
7. Which pathway is responsible for transmitting crude touch, pain, temperature, and pressure to the somatosensory cortex?
   a. Corticospinal tracts
   b. Dorsal columns
   c. Reticulospinal tracts
   d. Spinocerebellar tracts
8. What is the average time to onset of below-the-level pain after SCI?
   a. Immediate
   b. 3–6 months
   c. 6–12 months
   d. >12 months
9. Following delayed onset of neuropathic pain, what two conditions can reasonably be excluded?
   a. Wheelchair ergonomics
   b. Postlaminectomy pain syndrome
   c. Infection
   d. Syrinx
   e. All of the above
   f. b and d
10. What unifying mechanism might explain both spasticity and pain after SCI?
    a. Supraspinal sensitization
    b. Dorsal column and corticospinal tract imbalance
    c. Loss of inhibitory interneurons
    d. Somatosensory cortex reorganization

REFERENCES

1. Finnerup NB, Johannesen IL, Sindrup SH, Bach FW, Jensen TS. Pain and dysesthesia in patients with spinal cord injury: a postal survey. *Spinal Cord.* 2001;39(5):256–262.
2. Finnerup NB, Johannesen IL, Bach FW, Jensen TS. Sensory function above lesion level in spinal cord injury patients with and without pain. *Somatosens Mot Res.* 2003;20(1):71–76.
3. Finnerup NB. Pain in patients with spinal cord injury. *Pain.* 2013;154(Suppl 1):S71–S76.
4. Kim HY, Lee HJ, Kim TL, et al. Prevalence and characteristics of neuropathic pain in patients with spinal cord injury referred to a rehabilitation center. *Ann Rehabil Med.* 2020;44(6):438–449.

5. Nepomuceno C, Fine PR, Richards JS, et al. Pain in patients with spinal cord injury. *Arch Phys Med Rehabil.* 1979;60(12):605–609.
6. Siddall PJ, Loeser JD. Pain following spinal cord injury. *Spinal Cord.* 2001;39(2):63–73.
7. Barrett H, McClelland JM, Rutkowski SB, Siddall PJ. Pain characteristics in patients admitted to hospital with complications after spinal cord injury. *Arch Phys Med Rehabil.* 2003;84(6):789–795.
8. Dijkers MP, Bryce TN. Introducing the International Spinal Cord Injury Pain (ISCIP) Classification. *Pain Manag.* 2012;2(4):311–314.
9. Bryce TN, Biering-Sorensen F, Finnerup NB, et al. International Spinal Cord Injury Pain (ISCIP) Classification: Part 2. Initial validation using vignettes. *Spinal Cord.* 2012;50(6): 404–412.
10. Slipman CW, Shin CH, Patel RK, et al. Etiologies of failed back surgery syndrome. *Pain Med.* 2002;3(3):200–214. discussion 214–217.
11. Bailey JC, Kurklinsky S, Sletten CD, Osborne MD. The effectiveness of an intensive interdisciplinary pain rehabilitation program in the treatment of post-laminectomy syndrome in patients who have failed spinal cord stimulation. *Pain Med.* 2018;19(2):385–392.
12. Schaller B. Controversies in failed back surgery syndrome. *Eur Spine J.* 2005;14(10):1037–1038. author reply 1039.
13. Ganty P, Sharma M. Failed back surgery syndrome: a suggested algorithm of care. *Br J Pain.* 2012;6(4):153–161.
14. Siddall PJ, McClelland JM, Rutkowski SB, Cousins MJ. A longitudinal study of the prevalence and characteristics of pain in the first 5 years following spinal cord injury. *Pain.* 2003;103(3):249–257.
15. North RB, Kumar K, Wallace MS, et al. Spinal cord stimulation versus re-operation in patients with failed back surgery syndrome: an international multicenter randomized controlled trial (EVIDENCE study). *Neuromodulation.* 2011; 14(4):330–335. discussion 335-336.
16. Finley MA, McQuade KJ, Rodgers MM. Scapular kinematics during transfers in manual wheelchair users with and without shoulder impingement. *Clin Biomech.* 2005;20(1):32–40.
17. Tsai CY, Boninger ML, Hastings J, Cooper RA, Rice L, Koontz AM. Immediate biomechanical implications of transfer component skills training on independent wheelchair transfers. *Arch Phys Med Rehabil.* 2016;97(10):1785–1792.
18. Toro ML, Koontz AM, Cooper RA. The impact of transfer setup on the performance of independent wheelchair transfers. *Hum Factors.* 2013;55(3):567–580.
19. Barbareschi G, Holloway C. Understanding independent wheelchair transfers. Perspectives from stakeholders. *Disabil Rehabil Assist Technol.* 2020;15(5):545–552.
20. Dalyan M, Cardenas DD, Gerard B. Upper extremity pain after spinal cord injury. *Spinal Cord.* 1999;37(3):191–195.
21. Jensen TS, Baron R, Haanpaa M, et al. A new definition of neuropathic pain. *Pain.* 2011;152(10):2204–2205.
22. Cohen MJ, Song ZK, Schandler SL, Ho WH, Vulpe M. Sensory detection and pain thresholds in spinal cord injury patients with and without dysesthetic pain, and in chronic low back pain patients. *Somatosens Mot Res.* 1996;13(1):29–37.
23. Eide PK, Jorum E, Stenehjem AE. Somatosensory findings in patients with spinal cord injury and central dysaesthesia pain. *J Neurol Neurosurg Psychiatry.* 1996;60(4):411–415.
24. Haanpaa M. Assessment and mechanisms of mechanical allodynia. *Scand J Pain.* 2011;2(1):7–8.
25. Haanpaa M. Are neuropathic pain screening tools useful for patients with spinal cord injury? *Pain.* 2011;152(4): 715–716.
26. Cardenas DD, Nieshoff EC, Suda K, et al. A randomized trial of pregabalin in patients with neuropathic pain due to spinal cord injury. *Neurology.* 2013;80(6):533–539.
27. Cardenas DD, Emir B, Parsons B. Examining the time to therapeutic effect of pregabalin in spinal cord injury patients with neuropathic pain. *Clin Ther.* 2015;37(5):1081–1090.
28. Coppel DL, Bovill JG, Dundee JW. The taming of ketamine. *Anaesthesia.* 1973;28(3):293–296.
29. Green SM, Krauss B. The taming of ketamine – 40 years later. *Ann Emerg Med.* 2011;57(2):115–116.
30. Domino EF. Taming the ketamine tiger. 1965. *Anesthesiology.* 2010;113(3):678–684.
31. Morris LS, Costi S, Tan A, Stern ER, Charney DS, Murrough JW. Ketamine normalizes subgenual cingulate cortex hyper-activity in depression. *Neuropsychopharmacology.* 2020;45(6):975–981.
32. Christensen A, Pruskowski J. The role of ketamine in depression #384. *J Palliat Med.* 2020;23(1):136–138.
33. Fava M, Freeman MP, Flynn M, et al. Double-blind, placebo-controlled, dose-ranging trial of intravenous ketamine as adjunctive therapy in treatment-resistant depression (TRD). *Mol Psychiatry.* 2020;25(7):1592–1603.
34. Collins S, Sigtermans MJ, Dahan A, Zuurmond WW, Perez RS. NMDA receptor antagonists for the treatment of neuropathic pain. *Pain Med.* 2010;11(11):1726–1742.
35. Wang JK. Intrathecal morphine for intractable pain secondary to cancer of pelvic organs. *Pain.* 1985;21(1):99–102.
36. Hamza M, Doleys DM, Saleh IA, Medvedovsky A, Verdolin MH, Hamza M. A prospective, randomized, single-blinded, head-to-head long-term outcome study, comparing intrathecal (IT) boluses with continuous infusion trialing techniques prior to implantation of drug delivery systems (DDS) for the treatment of severe intractable chronic nonmalignant pain. *Neuromodulation.* 2015;18(7):636–648. discussion 649.
37. Doleys DM, Hamza M. Intrathecal therapy: broadening the perspective. *Pain Med.* 2015;16(1):23–24.
38. Deer TR, Hayek SM, Pope JE, et al. The Polyanalgesic Consensus Conference (PACC): recommendations for trialing of intrathecal drug delivery infusion therapy. *Neuromodulation.* 2017;20(2):133–154.
39. Penn RD, Kroin JS. Intrathecal baclofen alleviates spinal cord spasticity. *Lancet.* 1984;1(8385):1078.
40. Davidoff G, Roth E, Guarracini M, Sliwa J, Yarkony G. Function-limiting dysesthetic pain syndrome among traumatic spinal cord injury patients: a cross-sectional study. *Pain.* 1987;29(1):39–48.
41. Formento E, Minassian K, Wagner F, et al. Electrical spinal cord stimulation must preserve proprioception to enable locomotion in humans with spinal cord injury. *Nat Neurosci.* 2018;21(12):1728–1741.
42. Drew GM, Siddall PJ, Duggan AW. Responses of spinal neurones to cutaneous and dorsal root stimuli in rats with mechanical allodynia after contusive spinal cord injury. *Brain Res.* 2001;893(1-2):59–69.
43. Harden RN. Chronic neuropathic pain. Mechanisms, diagnosis, and treatment. *Neurologist.* 2005;11(2):111–122.

44. Hains BC, Klein JP, Saab CY, Craner MJ, Black JA, Waxman SG. Upregulation of sodium channel Nav1.3 and functional involvement in neuronal hyperexcitability associated with central neuropathic pain after spinal cord injury. *J Neurosci.* 2003;23(26):8881–8892.
45. Craner MJ, Hains BC, Lo AC, Black JA, Waxman SG. Co-localization of sodium channel Nav1.6 and the sodium-calcium exchanger at sites of axonal injury in the spinal cord in EAE. *Brain.* 2004;127(Pt 2):294–303.
46. Lampert A, Hains BC, Waxman SG. Upregulation of persistent and ramp sodium current in dorsal horn neurons after spinal cord injury. *Exp Brain Res.* 2006;174(4):660–666.
47. Jang SH, Lee J, Yeo SS. Central post-stroke pain due to injury of the spinothalamic tract in patients with cerebral infarction: a diffusion tensor tractography imaging study. *Neural Regen Res.* 2017;12(12):2021–2024.
48. Jang JY, Lee SH, Kim M, Ryu JS. Characteristics of neuropathic pain in patients with spinal cord injury. *Ann Rehabil Med.* 2014;38(3):327–334.
49. Mailis A, Bennett GJ. Dissociation between cutaneous and deep sensibility in central post-stroke pain (CPSP). *Pain.* 2002;98(3):331–334.
50. Greenspan DJ, Ohara S, Sarlani E, Lenz AF. Allodynia in patients with post-stroke central pain (CPSP) studied by statistical quantitative sensory testing within individuals. *Pain.* 2004;109(3):357–366.
51. Watson PNC, Evans RJ, Watt VR, Birkett N. Post-herpetic neuralgia: 208 cases. *Pain.* 1988;35(3):289–297.
52. Watson PNC, Evans RJ, Watt VR. Post-herpetic neuralgia and topical capsaicin. *Pain.* 1988;33(3):333–340.
53. Watson CPN, Deck JH, Morshead C, Van der Kooy D, Evans RJ. Post-herpetic neuralgia: further post-mortem studies of cases with and without pain. *Pain.* 1991;44(2):105–117.
54. Nurmikko T, Wells C, Bowsher D. Pain and allodynia in postherpetic neuralgia: role of somatic and sympathetic nervous systems. *Acta Neurol Scand.* 1991;84(2):146–152.
55. Sakai T, Tomiyasu S, Yamada H, Sumikawa K. Evaluation of allodynia and pain associated with postherpetic neuralgia using current perception threshold testing. *Clin J Pain.* 2006;22(4):359–362.
56. Lazaro C, Caseras X, Banos JE, Catalonian Group for the Study of Postherpetic Neuralgia Postherpetic neuralgia: a descriptive analysis of patients seen in pain clinics. *Reg Anesth Pain Med.* 2003;28(4):315–320.
57. Sjoqvist O. The conduction of pain in the fifth nerve and its bearing on the treatment of trigeminal neuralgia. *Yale J Biol Med.* 1939;11(6):593–600.
58. Polan M. Pain control: trigeminal neuralgia--a review of etiology and treatment. *Zahntechnik (Zur).* 1966;24(1):229–234.
59. Brisman R. Constant face pain in typical trigeminal neuralgia and response to gamma knife radiosurgery. *Stereotact Funct Neurosurg.* 2013;91(2):122–128.
60. Campbell RL, Trentacosti CD, Eschenroeder TA, Harkins SW. An evaluation of sensory changes and pain relief in trigeminal neuralgia following intracranial microvascular decompression and/or trigeminal glycerol rhizotomy. *J Oral Maxillofac Surg.* 1990;48(10):1057–1062.
61. Ramachandran VS, Rogers-Ramachandran D, Cobb S. Touching the phantom limb. *Nature.* 1995;377(6549):489–490.
62. Ramachandran VS, Rogers-Ramachandran D. Phantom limbs and neural plasticity. *Arch Neurol.* 2000;57(3):317–320.
63. Ramachandran VS, Brang D, McGeoch PD. Dynamic reorganization of referred sensations by movements of phantom limbs. *Neuroreport.* 2010;21(10):727–730.
64. Ramachandran V, Chunharas C, Marcus Z, Furnish T, Lin A. Relief from intractable phantom pain by combining psilocybin and mirror visual-feedback (MVF). *Neurocase.* 2018;24(2):105–110.
65. Seo CH, Park CH, Jung MH, et al. Increased white matter diffusivity associated with phantom limb pain. *Korean J Pain.* 2019;32(4):271–279.
66. Cheung A, Podgorny P, Martinez JA, Chan C, Toth C. Epidermal axonal swellings in painful and painless diabetic peripheral neuropathy. *Muscle Nerve.* 2015;51(4):505–513.
67. Snedecor SJ, Sudharshan L, Cappelleri JC, Sadosky A, Mehta S, Botteman M. Systematic review and meta-analysis of pharmacological therapies for painful diabetic peripheral neuropathy. *Pain Pract.* 2014;14(2):167–184.
68. Best TJ, Best CA, Best AA, Fera LA. Surgical peripheral nerve decompression for the treatment of painful diabetic neuropathy of the foot – a level 1 pragmatic randomized controlled trial. *Diabetes Res Clin Pract.* 2019;147:149–156.
69. Ding Y, Yao P, Li H, Zhao R, Zhao G. Evaluation of combined radiofrequency and chemical blockade of multi-segmental lumbar sympathetic ganglia in painful diabetic peripheral neuropathy. *J Pain Res.* 2018;11:1375–1382.
70. Richter RW, Portenoy R, Sharma U, Lamoreaux L, Bockbrader H, Knapp LE. Relief of painful diabetic peripheral neuropathy with pregabalin: a randomized, placebo-controlled trial. *J Pain.* 2005;6(4):253–260.
71. Carroll DG, Kline KM, Malnar KF. Role of topiramate for the treatment of painful diabetic peripheral neuropathy. *Pharmacotherapy.* 2004;24(9):1186–1193.
72. Slangen R, Pluijms WA, Faber CG, Dirksen CD, Kessels AG, van Kleef M. Sustained effect of spinal cord stimulation on pain and quality of life in painful diabetic peripheral neuropathy. *Br J Anaesth.* 2013;111(6):1030–1031.
73. Hein M, Ji G, Tidwell D, et al. Kappa opioid receptor activation in the amygdala disinhibits CRF neurons to generate pain-like behaviors. *Neuropharmacology.* 2021;185:108456.
74. Lewis GN, Wartolowska KA, Parker RS, et al. A higher grey matter density in the amygdala and midbrain is associated with persistent pain following total knee arthroplasty. *Pain Med.* 2020;21(12):3393–3400.
75. Narita M, Kaneko C, Miyoshi K, et al. Chronic pain induces anxiety with concomitant changes in opioidergic function in the amygdala. *Neuropsychopharmacology.* 2006;31(4):739–750.
76. Simons LE, Moulton EA, Linnman C, Carpino E, Becerra L, Borsook D. The human amygdala and pain: evidence from neuroimaging. *Hum Brain Mapp.* 2014;35(2):527–538.
77. Kutch JJ, Ichesco E, Hampson JP, et al. Brain signature and functional impact of centralized pain: a multidisciplinary approach to the study of chronic pelvic pain (MAPP) network study. *Pain.* 2017;158(10):1979–1991.
78. Megnin J. Commissural myelotomy in neoplastic abdomino-pelvic pain. *Bull Alger Carcinol.* 1948;1:47–53.
79. Gildenberg PL. Myelotomy and percutaneous cervical cordotomy for the treatment of cancer pain. *Appl Neurophysiol.* 1984;47(4-6):208–215.

80. Vedantam A, Koyyalagunta D, Bruel BM, Dougherty PM, Viswanathan A. Limited midline myelotomy for intractable visceral pain: surgical techniques and outcomes. *Neurosurgery*. 2018;83(4):783–789.
81. Lee SP, Dinglasan V, Duong A, Totten R, Smith JA. Individuals with recurrent low back pain exhibit significant changes in paraspinal muscle strength after intramuscular fine wire electrode insertion. *PM R*. 2020;12(8):775–782.
82. Schilder JC, Sigtermans MJ, Schouten AC, et al. Pain relief is associated with improvement in motor function in complex regional pain syndrome type 1: secondary analysis of a placebo-controlled study on the effects of ketamine. *J Pain*. 2013;14(11):1514–1521.
83. Yoo M, D'Silva LJ, Martin K, et al. Pilot study of exercise therapy on painful diabetic peripheral neuropathy. *Pain Med*. 2015;16(8):1482–1489.
84. Wang Q, Guo ZL, Yu YB, Yang WQ, Zhang L. Two-point discrimination predicts pain relief after lower limb nerve decompression for painful diabetic peripheral neuropathy. *Plast Reconstr Surg*. 2018;141(3):397e–403e.

Psychological Aspects of Spinal Cord Injury

CHAPTER 38

Caitlin P. Campbell and Brian Mutcher

OUTLINE

Individuals who experience spinal cord injury (SCI) may experience a variety of emotional reactions to their injury and change in physical functioning. Fortunately, a majority of individuals with SCI experience positive adjustment and minimal lasting mental health concerns. For individuals with SCI who are experiencing emotional concerns, it is encouraged that medical providers collaborate with the various specialists on the treatment team to help address the concerns.

Affective Disorders

Depressive Disorder

Depression is the most studied mental health concern after an SCI. The prevalence rate for major depressive disorder in the SCI population is 22%.[1] Major depressive disorder is often not a reaction to SCI, but may be exacerbated by the SCI. Depression is associated with increased pain, cardiovascular disease, pressure injuries, urinary tract infections, repeated hospital admissions, unemployment, poor quality of life, and minimal life participation and community engagement.[2] Risk factors for depression include: being female, unemployed at time of injury, current unemployment, other mental illness diagnoses, current alcohol or substance abuse, changes in body image, shame, and loss of independence.[3] The medical team can also unintentionally contribute to depression due to biased beliefs of quality of life for someone living with SCI. Negative mood states can increase the risk of medical complications, longer hospitalizations, decreased self-care independence, spending more time in bed and fewer days off the medical unit, and difficulties with transportation. Protective factors include increased social engagement, physical activity, and greater time since injury.[4]

When completing differential diagnosis, ensure to rule out the possibility of symptoms being caused by effects of a medical condition, medications, drugs, environment, or other factors. The combination of psychotherapy and pharmacotherapy is more effective than either modality alone.[4,5] If medication is indicated for helping manage depressive symptoms, be mindful of possible medication interactions and side effects (e.g., fluoxetine [Prozac] may increase spasticity; possibility of serotonin syndrome if using other serotonergic agonists; anticholinergic side effects).[4] Due to frequent polypharmacy, consider obtaining an electrocardiogram for QTc prolongation prior to starting a serotonergic agent, particularly citalopram (Celexa) or other medication with a proarrhythmic risk (e.g., prochlorperazine [Compazine] or methadone [Dolophine]).[4] When starting antidepressant medications, the initial dosage should be half of the typical starting dose, and up-titration should occur at about half the rate of that typically used in non–medically ill populations; time to achieve full therapeutic effect is similar to that in the non-SCI population.[4] To help reduce pill burden, consider medications that might provide coverage for multiple issues (e.g., venlafaxine [Effexor] for depression and nociceptive pain). Also address other comorbid conditions that may exacerbate depression (e.g., pain, obstructive sleep apnea).

Anxiety Disorder

Anxiety is a common emotional reaction after SCI; when anxiety negatively impacts daily functioning, it rises to the level of a disorder. The prevalence rate for anxiety disorders in the SCI population is 27%.[4] Generalized anxiety disorder and panic disorder are common in the SCI population. Anxiety disorders are associated with greater pain and poorer functioning.[4] When assessing for anxiety, be sure to rule out symptoms that are better explained by the effects of a medical condition, medications, drugs, environment, or other factors.

Medication and behavioral interventions for anxiety are roughly equal[4]; base treatment decisions on patient preference, polypharmacy, medication interactions, side effects, and availability of mental health providers. Selective serotonin reuptake inhibitors (SSRIs) and serotonin and norepinephrine reuptake inhibitors are first-line medications to treat anxiety; clinical improvement can be expected within 4 weeks, but can be observed between 2–6 weeks of initiating medication.[4] Benzodiazepines have fallen out of favor for treating anxiety due to potential of tolerance and dependence; however, they may be indicated in cases of acute severe anxiety or panic. For panic disorder, SSRIs are first-line medications.[4] Similarly to using medication to treat depression, be mindful of potential medication interactions and side effects.

Trauma-Related Disorders

People who sustain SCIs often experience traumatic events that led to their injury (e.g., car accident, fall, acts of violence). Five to twenty percent of people who experienced a traumatic SCI experience symptoms of acute stress disorder (ASD) in the first 3–30 days after their accident[4,6]; ASD is considered a severe stress reaction that warrants clinical intervention. ASD is a poor predictor for posttraumatic stress disorder (PTSD), and most individuals who develop PTSD did not have an ASD diagnosis.[7] Prevalence rate of PTSD in individuals with SCI ranges from 7%–60%; individuals with minority racial-ethnic identities report higher levels of PTSD than non-Hispanic Whites.[8] Risk factors that increase chance of developing PTSD include: depression, lower levels of acceptance or adjustment, psychological distress, anxiety, negative appraisals, neuroticism, and pain.[4] Women are more likely to report more severe PTSD symptoms.[4] PTSD is related to lower social participation, hopelessness/helplessness, and low self-efficacy.[4]

First-line treatment for ASD is trauma-focused psychotherapy; there is insufficient evidence that medication is effective.[4] Psychotherapy should also be offered for individuals with symptoms of PTSD, if available. Some patients may prefer pharmacotherapy to manage symptoms. Benzodiazepines may be helpful for managing acute anxiety, agitation, or sleep disruption in the immediate period following the traumatic event; be mindful of long-term use, as this can negatively impact adaptation, which could increase risk for developing PTSD.[4] Sertraline (Zoloft), paroxetine (Paxil), and fluoxetine (Prozac) are front-line antidepressants for PTSD.[9–12]

Suicide

Individuals with SCI are three to five times more likely to die by suicide than the general population.[4] The risk for suicide is greatest in the first 6 years postinjury.[4] It is important to assess early during initial hospitalization or rehabilitation, soon after discharge home, and at least annually; repeat assessment for risk at any time to reassess symptoms or if there has been a change in the patient's status.

When a patient displays either direct (e.g., giving away possessions, seeking access to lethal means) or indirect (e.g., social withdrawal, increased substance use, increased feelings of hopelessness) signs of suicide, it is imperative the patient's mental health status and safety are assessed. Asking direct, nonjudgmental questions increases the likelihood of receiving honest responses; directly asking about suicide will not increase the risk for suicide.[4] If the patient is deemed to be at high acute risk for suicide, hospitalization can help maintain safety; a 1:1 sitter is indicated if patient has to be on SCI unit due to care needs (Table 38.1). Aggressively address any modifiable factors and optimize treatment for any coexisting mental health conditions. If a patient at risk for suicide is also prescribed antidepressants or other medications with a high-risk profile, it is prudent to prescribe medications with low risk of lethal overdose and to limit the amount of medication dispensed at a time, use blister packs, etc.[4].

Substance Use Disorders

Substance use and substance use disorders (SUDs) are a common comorbidity in the SCI population. As many as 19% report heavy drinking, with 14% endorsing significant alcohol related problems.[13] Tobacco smoking has been estimated at 35.3%[14] and is associated with poor health and increased mortality.[15,16] Nicotine (2 mg) is associated with increased severity of neuropathic pain in smokers.[17] Prevalence estimates for other drugs have ranged as high as 14%.[18]

Daily opioid use may be as high as 35.2% in individuals with SCI, while 17.6%–25.8% self-report significant misuse of pain medications.[19,20] Unfortunately, prescription pain medication use itself has been associated with higher mortality in the SCI population.[20,21]

SUDs can be chronic and relapsing. As such, these biopsychosocial conditions may require episodic or continuous care, similar to that required for other chronic diseases such as diabetes.[22] Rehabilitation physicians

Table 38.1 Factors Associated With Increased Risk for Suicide

Non-Hispanic Whites	Posttraumatic Stress Disorder
Paraplegia	Schizophrenia
T1–S3 AIS A, B, or C	Bipolar disorder
History of or current substance abuse	Posttraumatic stress disorder
Past suicide attempts	Traumatic brain injury
Major depressive disorder	Chronic pain

Adapted from Paralyzed Veterans of America. Clinical practice guidelines: management of mental health disorders, substance use disorders, and suicide in adults with spinal cord injury clinical practice guideline for health care providers. 2020.
AIS, American Spinal Injury Association (ASIA) Impairment Scale.

and psychologists have recognized these conditions affect patient outcomes and are prepared to integrate assessment and treatment within the rehabilitation setting.[23,24] A recent review of electronic health records in the United States found an SCI diagnosis was moderately associated with alcohol and nicotine use disorders, and strongly associated with cannabis and opioid use disorders, in comparison with controls.[25] The Paralyzed Veterans of America's clinical practice guidelines for spinal cord medicine recommend screening all SCI patients during rehabilitation with appropriate referrals for diagnosis and treatment.[4]

Although there is no SCI-specific SUDs treatment, some basic practices should be considered. This includes patient education regarding the risks associated with substance use (i.e., recommended alcohol limits), including those specific to SCI and its common secondary conditions, such as respiratory ailments. Medication interactions with substances are another significant area for education, as effects on psychosocial well-being.

The ability to implement nonpharmacological and/or medication-assisted treatments will vary with regard to any particular rehabilitation setting. At a minimum, brief counseling from treatment providers has been shown to improve outcomes for alcohol and tobacco and can be integrated into screening procedures.[26,27,28] The rehabilitation team can punctuate and reinforce patient behaviors consistent with efforts at abstinence, moderation, and harm reduction, as appropriate. Patient factors to consider in treatment planning include medical stability, clinical presentation, length of stay, family involvement, and personal preference. Setting factors will include expertise among the rehabilitation team (i.e., psychologists, social workers, pharmacists), as well as additional inpatient referral sources, such as a dedicated substance abuse treatment or tobacco cessation program. Upon completion of SCI rehabilitation, appropriate referrals for further mental health intervention, substance abuse treatment programs, and/or community-based self-help, such as 12-step programs, should be considered, especially for individuals with severe SUDs.

Cognitive Impairment

Cognitive impairment can be common in individuals with SCI, with up to 60% displaying some degree of cognitive decline. People with SCI are 13 times more likely to experience cognitive impairment compared to non-SCI populations.[29] Cognitive deficits are associated with diminished functional gains in rehabilitation programs, increased aggressive behaviors, higher likelihood of rehospitalizations, limited learning of novel living skills for successful reintegration into the community, poor self-perceptions, and lower quality of life.[29]

Traumatic brain injuries (TBI) often co-occur with SCI, with 16%–59% of cases having a concomitant TBI[30–32]; however, the level of cognitive impairment that is observed in the SCI population is beyond the incidence rate TBI could explain.[33] Other contributing factors to cognitive impairment include: secondary trauma as result of cerebral edema, hypoxic and anoxic events, cardiovascular and cerebrovascular dysfunction, sleep apnea, core body temperature dysregulation, medication side effects, neurogenic lower urinary tract dysfunction, and pain.[31,32,34] An accelerated cognitive aging process has also been found in the SCI population.[35,36] Cognitive impairment can lead to depression, decreased ability to complete instrumental activities of daily living, reduced health-related quality of life, and decreased independence.[29,37]

Conversion Disorder (Functional Neurological Symptom Disorder)

When a patient presents to the SCI rehabilitation facility with clinical findings clearly incompatible with neurological disease, a conversion disorder or functional neurological symptom disorder (CD-FNSD) must be considered. Examples of such findings include: Hoover sign; normal strength present in the affected hip's extension with contralateral hip flexion against resistance[38]; weak ankle plantar flexion during supine examination in a patient able to walk on tiptoes; and tremors that change when the individual is distracted, such as in the tremor entrainment test.[39] Associated features of a patient's history include recent stress or trauma (physical or psychological) that may have temporal relevance to onset,[38] biological vulnerabilities, childhood trauma, conditioning through reinforcement of physical disability, and cultural norms that stigmatize psychological suffering. Precise prevalence is unknown, with many symptoms being transient; however, such symptoms are present in approximately 5% of referrals to neurology clinics.[40]

A mental disorder diagnosis cannot be made solely due to unexplained medical symptoms, although it is a key feature here, precisely because it is possible to demonstrate definitive inconsistence with medical pathophysiology. Diagnostic criteria include: (1) one or more symptoms of altered voluntary sensory or motor function; (2) incompatibility between the clinical symptoms and recognized neurological or medical conditions; (3) symptoms or impairment not better explained by another mental or medical condition; (4) the symptom of deficit causes clinically significant distress or impairment in social, occupational, or other important areas of functioning or warrants medical evaluation.[40] The diagnosis can be specified further by type (i.e., with weakness or paralysis, with abnormal movements, with anesthesia or sensory loss, etc.) duration (acute or persistent), and with or without psychological stressors. Favorable prognostic factors include acceptance of the diagnosis and short duration of the symptoms. Negative prognostic factors include maladaptive personality traits, the comorbid physical disease (including neurological conditions), and the receipt of disability benefits.[41]

Diagnostic criteria have evolved to exclude unreliable judgments regarding conscious intent and include definitive signs of pathophysiological incompatibility. However, with definitive evidence of feigning, such as drastic performance differences across settings, one must consider the diagnosis of a factitious disorder with an apparent intent to assume a dependent/sick role, or malingering with an apparent attempt to obtain incentives, such as money or relief from circumstances.[40]

Treatment of CD-FNSD in the rehabilitation setting is recommended and should be symptom-focused accordingly (i.e., patients with symptoms of paraplegia in a SCI rehabilitation unit).[42] A helpful framework for the patient and the team is to view treatment as a means of improving the way the brain processes information by disrupting established emotional and physical patterns that sustain the symptoms. Mental health professionals can assist the patient with cognitive-behavioral therapy methods, whereas physical therapists can assist with restoring normal movements and completing activities of daily living.[43–45] Currently, there is no gold standard of treatment, but treatment research and case study suggests functioning can be improved through interdisciplinary rehabilitation.

Review Questions

1. Which of the following is considered a first-line medication for the treatment of generalized anxiety disorder?
   a. Diazepam (Valium)
   b. Sertraline (Zoloft)
   c. Propranolol (Inderal)
   d. Alprazolam (Xanax)
2. All of the following are risk factors for suicide EXCEPT:
   a. Chronic pain
   b. Major depressive disorder
   c. Substance abuse
   d. Hospitalization
3. What is considered the first-line treatment for acute stress disorder?
   a. Trauma-focused psychotherapy
   b. Sertraline (Zoloft)
   c. Venlafaxine (Effexor)
   d. Citalopram (Celexa)
4. Which of the following has shown the best efficacy for treatment of major depressive disorder?
   a. Psychotherapy
   b. Psychotherapy and pharmacotherapy
   c. Pharmacotherapy
   d. Electroconvulsive therapy
5. Substance use disorders can be chronic and relapsing conditions that:
   a. Should be avoided during the active phase of physical rehabilitation
   b. Require screening among all rehabilitation patients
   c. Can benefit from brief episodic counseling
   d. Are not serious conditions affecting the SCI population due to disability
6. Patients suspected of a conversion disorder (functional neurological symptom disorder) with motor paralysis:
   a. Find relief when they realize symptoms are "all in my head"
   b. Benefit from the interdisciplinary assessment and treatment of inpatient rehabilitation
   c. Are most effectively treated in a mental health setting
   d. Function at baseline when medical staff are not observing

REFERENCES

1. Williams R, Murray A. Prevalence of depression after spinal cord injury: a meta-analysis. *Arch Phys Med Rehabil.* 2015;96(1):133–140.
2. Craig A, Tran Y, Middleton J. Psychological morbidity and spinal cord injury: a systemic review. *Spinal Cord.* 2009;47:108–114.
3. van Gorp S, Kessels AG, Joosten EA, van Kleef M, Patijn J. Pain prevalence and its determinants after spinal cord injury: a systematic review. *Eur J Pain.* 2015;19(1):5–14.
4. Paralyzed Veterans of America. Clinical practice guidelines: management of mental health disorders, substance use disorders, and suicide in adults with spinal cord injury clinical practice guideline for health care providers. 2020
5. Cuijpers P, van Straten A, Warmerdam L, Andersson G. Psychotherapy versus the combination of psychotherapy and pharmacotherapy in the treatment of depression: a meta-analysis. *Depress Anxiety.* 2009;26(3):279–288.
6. Sandroff BM, DeLuca J. Will behavioral treatments for cognitive impairment in multiple sclerosis become standards-of-care? *Int J Psychophysiology.* 2020;154:67–69.
7. Bryant RA. Acute stress disorder as a predictor of posttraumatic stress disorder: a systematic review. *J Clin Psychiatry.* 2011;72(2):233–239.
8. Cao Y, Li C, Newman S, Lucas J, Charlifue S, Krause JS. Posttraumatic stress disorder after spinal cord injury. *Rehab Psych.* 2017;62(2):178–185.
9. Brady K, Pearlstein T, Asnis GM, et al. Efficacy and safety of sertraline treatment of posttraumatic stress disorder: a randomized controlled trial. *Journal of the American Medical Association.* 2000;283:1837–1844.
10. Marshall RD, Beebe KL, Oldham M, Zaninelli R. Efficacy and safety of paroxetine treatment for chronic PTSD: a fixed-dose, placebo-controlled study. *American Journal of Psychiatry.* 2001;158:1982–1988.

11. Watts BV, Schnurr PP, Mayo L, Young-Xu Y, Weeks WB, Friedman MJ. Meta-analysis of the efficacy of treatments for posttraumatic stress disorder. *J Clin Psychiatry.* 2013;74(6):e541–e550.
12. Lee DJ, Schnitzlein CW, Wolf JP, Vythilingam M, Rasmusson AM, Hoge CW. Psychotherapy versus pharmacotherapy for posttraumatic stress disorder: systemic review and meta-analyses to determine first-line treatments. *Depress Anxiety.* 2016;33(9):792–806.
13. Gerhart KA, Johnson RL, Whiteneck GG. Health and psychosocial issues of individuals with incomplete and resolving spinal cord injuries. *Paraplegia.* 1992;30(4):282–287.
14. Geyh S, Nick E, Stirnimann D, Ehrat S, Muller R, Michel F. Biopsychosocial outcomes in individuals with and without spinal cord injury: a Swiss comparative study. *Spinal Cord.* 2012;50(8):614–622.
15. Griffiths T, Myers D, Talbot A. A study of the validity of the scaled version of the General Health Questionnaire in paralysed spinally injured out-patients. *Psychological Medicine.* 1993;23(2):497–504.
16. Avluk OC, Gurcay E, Gurcay AG, Karaahmet OZ, Tamkan U, Cakci A. Effects of chronic pain on function, depression, and sleep among patients with traumatic spinal cord injury. *Ann Saudi Med.* 2014;34(3):211–216.
17. Guest R, Craig A, Perry KN, et al. Resilience following spinal cord injury: a prospective controlled study investigating the influence of the provision of group cognitive behavior therapy during inpatient rehabilitation. *Rehabilitation Psychology.* 2015;60(4):311–321.
18. Geyh S, Kunz S, Muller R, Peter C, SwiSCI Study Group. Describing functioning and health after spinal cord injury in the light of psychological-personal factors. *J Rehab Medicine.* 2016;48(2):219–234.
19. Glass CA. Psychological intervention in physical disability–with special reference to spinal cord injury. *J Mental Health.* 1994;3(4):467–476.
20. Goldman RL, Radnitz CL, McGrath RE. Posttraumatic stress disorder and major depression in veterans with spinal cord injury. *Rehabil Psychology.* 2008;53(2):162–170.
21. Borsbo B, Gerdle B, Peolsson M. Impact of the interaction between self-efficacy, symptoms and catastrophising on disability, quality of life and health in with chronic pain patients. *Disabil Rehabil.* 2010;32(17):1387–1396.
22. Harper LA, Coleman JA, Perrin PB, et al. Comparison of mental health between individuals with spinal cord injury and able-bodied controls in Neiva, Colombia. *J Rehabil Research Dev.* 2014;51(1):127–136.
23. Heinemann A, Williams RT, Wilson CS, et al. Evaluating the psychometric properties of depression measures in persons with SCI and major depressive disorder. *Archives of Physical Medicine and Rehabilitation.* 94(10):e20-e21.
24. Heinemann AW, Doll MD, Armstrong KJ, Schnoll S, Yarkony GM. Substance use and receipt of treatment by persons with long-term spinal cord injuries. *Arch Phys Med Rehabil.* 1991;72(7):482–487.
25. Graupensperger S, Corey JJ, Turrisi RJ, Evans MB. Individuals with spinal cord injury have greater odds of substance use disorders than non-SCI comparisons. *Drug and Alcohol Dependence.* 2019;205(1):107608.
26. Centers for Disease Control and Prevention. https://www.cdc.gov.
27. Centers for Disease Control and Prevention. Planning and Implementing Screening and Brief Intervention for Risky Alcohol Use: A Step-by-Step Guide for Primary Care Practices. Atlanta, Georgia: Centers for Disease Control and Prevention, National Center on Birth Defects and Developmental Disabilities, 2014. https://www.cdc.gov/ncbddd/fasd/alcohol-screening.html.
28. Tobacco Use and Dependence Guideline Panel. *Treating Tobacco Use and Dependence: 2008 Update.* Rockville (MD): US Department of Health and Human Services; 2008. https://www.ncbi.nlm.nih.gov/books/NBK63952/.
29. Sachdeva R, Gao F, Chan CCH, Krassioukov AV. Cognitive function after spinal cord injury: a systematic review. *Neurology.* 2018;91(13):611–621.
30. Craig A, Guest R, Tran Y, Middleton J. Cognitive impairment and mood states after spinal cord injury. *J Neurotrauma.* 2016;34(6):1156–1163.
31. Nott MT, Baguley IJ, Heriseanu R, et al. Effects of concomitant spinal cord injury and brain injury on medical and functional outcomes and community participation. *Top Spinal Cord Inj Rehabil.* 2014;20:225–235.
32. Macciocchi S, Seel RT, Thompson N, Byams R, Bowman B. Spinal cord injury and cooccurring traumatic brain injury: assessment and incidence. *Arch Phys Med Rehabil.* 2008;89:1350–1357.
33. Michael DB, Guyot DR, Darmody WR. Coincidence of head and cervical spine injury. *J Neurotrauma.* 1989;6:177–189.
34. Kennedy P, Evans MJ. Evaluation of post-traumatic distress in the first 6 months following SCI. *Spinal Cord.* 2001;39:381–386.
35. Bombardier CH, Lee DC, Tan DL, Barber JK, Hoffman JM. Comorbid traumatic brain injury and spinal cord injury: screening validity and effect on outcomes. *Arch Phys Med Rehabil.* 2016;97(10):1628–1634.
36. Chiaravalloti ND, Weber E, Wylie G, Dyson-Hudson T, Wecht JM. Patterns of cognitive deficits in persons with spinal cord injury as compared with both age-matched and older individuals without spinal cord injury. *J Spinal Cord Med.* 2018;43:1–10.
37. Molina B, Segura A, Serrano JP, et al. Cognitive performance of people with traumatic spinal cord injury: a cross-sectional study comparing people with subacute and chronic injuries. *Spinal Cord.* 2018;56(8):796–805.
38. Stone J, LaFrance Jr WC, Brown R, Spiegel D, Levenson JL, Sharpe M. Conversion disorder: current problems and potential solutions for DSM-5. *J Psychosom Res.* 2011;71(6):369–376.
39. Edwards MJ, Bhatia KP. Functional (psychogenic) movement disorders: merging mind and brain. *Lancet Neurol.* 2012;11(3):250–260.
40. American Psychiatric Association *Somatic symptoms and related disorders. Diagnostic and Statistical Manual of Mental Disorders.* 5th ed. Washington, DC: APA Publishing; 2013.
41. Crimlisk HL, Bhatia K, Cope H, David A, Marsden CD, Ron MA. Slater revisited: 6 year follow up study of patients with medically unexplained motor symptoms. *BMJ.* 1998;316(7131):582–586.
42. Heruti RJ, Levy A, Adunski A, Ohry A. Conversion motor paralysis disorder: overview and rehabilitation model. *Spinal Cord.* 2002;40:327–334.

43. O'Neal MA, Baslet G. Treatment of patients with a functional neurological disorder (conversion disorder): an integrated approach. *American J Psychiatry*. 2018;175(4):307–314.
44. Nielsen G, Buszewicz M, Stevenson F, et al. Randomised feasibility study of physiotherapy for patients with functional motor symptoms. *J Neurology, Neurosurgery & Psychiatry*. 2017;88(6):484–490.
45. Krebs J, Scheel-Sailer A, Oertli R, Pannek J. The effects of antimuscarinic treatment on the cognition of spinal cord injured individuals with neurogenic lower urinary tract dysfunction: a prospective controlled before-and-after study. *Spinal Cord*. 2018;56(1):22–27.

CHAPTER 39

Traumatic Myelopathy

Lavina Jethani, Mahmut T. Kaner, and Isaac Hernandez Jimenez

OUTLINE

Cervical Traumatic Myelopathy

Descriptions/Definitions

- Spinal cord injury (SCI) occurs after an insult to the spinal cord; it can be traumatic or atraumatic, presenting clinically with disturbances in the motor, sensory, or autonomic nervous system(s).
- Traumatic cervical SCI is defined by the stability of injury, location, and/or mechanism of injury.[1]
- *Spondylosis* refers to the degeneration of the vertebral discs and bodies. This process often leads to spinal stenosis. If the cervical spinal cord is compressed at a certain level, it develops cervical spinal myelopathy.
- Spinal canal stenosis is a major premorbid risk factor for traumatic cervical myelopathy in the elderly population.
- They can impact respiratory function.

Epidemiology

- Most commonly caused by motor vehicle accidents (MVAs) → falls → violence (gunshot wounds [GSW]) → sports (diving accidents).
- C5–C6 is the most common level of injury.
- Tetraplegia: incomplete (40.6%) → complete (18%).[2]

Pathophysiology

- The cervical spine is the most commonly injured part of the cord due to its exposed location above the torso and its high flexibility.
- Mechanism of injuries
  - *Transection*: penetrating (GSW, stabbing, etc.) or massive blunt trauma, displaced bony fragments into the spinal canal or herniated disc.
  - *Compression*: hypertrophied ligamentum flavum compresses the cord in elderly patients upon forced extension injuries or hematomas in trauma.
  - *Contusion*: bony dislocations, subluxations, or fracture fragments.
  - *Vascular compromise:* anterior spinal artery compression by bony dislocation (Table 39.1).[3]
- Congenital cervical spinal canal stenosis is shown to be a major predisposing factor to myelopathy.
  - Normal cervical spinal canal is ~17 mm.
  - Relative stenosis 10–13 mm.
  - Absolute stenosis <10mm.[4]
- In elderly patients, the ligament flavum buckling, ossification/hypertrophy of the posterior longitudinal ligament, and osteophyte overgrowth can cause cord compression resulting in myelopathy after a fall or trauma.[5]
- Cervical disc bulging can lead to myelopathy and/or radiculopathy, depending on the disc material's direction, compromising the nervous system.

Initial Management

- Cervical spine immobilization with a rigid cervical collar, lateral head supports with a backboard should be initiated in trauma patients in the settings of MVA, assault, fall from height, or sports-related injury (possible adverse effects: e.g., pressure ulcers and aspiration).
- Cervical spine immobilization should be maintained until unstable SCI is excluded with necessary diagnostic imaging.
- Oteir et al. reported the importance of transferring the patient from the board to a stretcher to prevent emergency department complications.[6]
- Cervical SCI from GSWs often results in severe neurologic deficits. Beaty et al. reported that 30% of 144

Table 39.1 Mechanisms of Injury Classification

Mechanisms of Spinal Injury	Stability
Flexion	
Anterior wedge fracture	Stable
Flexion teardrop fracture	Extremely unstable
Clay shoveler fracture	Stable
Subluxation	Potentially unstable
Bilateral facet dislocation	Always unstable
Atlantooccipital dislocation	Unstable
Anterior atlantoaxial dislocation with or without fracture	Unstable
Odontoid fracture with lateral displacement	Unstable
Fracture of transverse process	Stable
Flexion–Rotation	
Unilateral facet dislocation	Stable
Rotary atlantoaxial dislocation	Unstable
Extension	
Posterior neural arch fracture (C1)	Unstable
Hangman fracture (C2)	Unstable
Extension teardrop fracture	Usually stable in flexion; unstable in extension
Posterior atlantoaxial dislocation with or without fracture	Unstable
Vertical Compression	
Burst fracture of vertebral body	Stable
Jefferson fracture (C1)	Extremely unstable
Isolated fractures of articular pillar and vertebral body	Stable

From Kaji AH, Hockberger RS. Chaper 36: Spinal Injuries. In: *Rosen's Emergency Medicine: Concepts and Clinical Practice.* 9th ed. Elsevier; 2018.

cervical GSW injuries required surgery due to instability.[7]
- Higher cervical cord injuries (above C3) may cause immediate respiratory paralysis due to lack of diaphragmatic innervation.

Symptoms and Signs of Traumatic Cervical Spinal Cord Injury

- Neurologic:
  - Altered mental status
  - Abnormal motor examination
  - Abnormal sensory examination
  - Abnormal or absent reflexes
  - Autonomic dysfunction
  - Hypothermia or hyperthermia
- Musculoskeletal:
  - Neck pain at rest or with isometric neck motion
  - Decreased cervical range of motion
  - Posterior midline cervical tenderness
  - Muscle spasm of cervical muscles
- Cardiovascular:
  - Hypotension with bradycardia (neurogenic shock)
- Respiratory:
  - Diaphragmatic breathing without retractions

Diagnosis

- Plain radiographs can be sought as an initial approach. They depict bony structures and detect fractures, alignment of the spinal column, vertebral height, and chronic findings such as disc space narrowing, osteophytes, loss of cervical lordosis, and overall degeneration of the cervical spine.
  - Sagittal views help physicians assess alignment, which can help determine the approach for any possible surgical intervention.[8]
- Magnetic resonance imaging (MRI) is the gold standard that must be obtained in patients with signs/symptoms of cervical myelopathy.
- Computed tomography (CT) imaging is superior to MRI to demonstrate bony changes and foraminal stenosis.
- CT myelography is used if there are any contraindications to obtaining an MRI in patients with cardiac pacemakers, metallic fragments in the body, or any other contraindications for an MRI.

Spinal Cord Injury without Radiographic Abnormality (SCIWORA) is defined as the presence of a neurologic deficit in the absence of evidence of bony injury on plain radiograph or CT.

Treatment

Treatment depends primarily upon spinal stability and concomitant injuries.

Conservative Treatment

- If CT demonstrates minor spinal fracture pattern (stable injury) without neurogenic deficit, conservative treatment should be the initial approach.
- Conservative treatment of a cervical fracture involves closed reduction under fluoroscopic guidance and halo-vest immobilization.
- Halo vest is the most restrictive immobilization method used in unstable cervical, upper thoracic fractures, and dislocations as low as T3. Halo fixation complications include local infection, pressure injury, scarring, or pin loosening.[9]
- For stable cervical spinal column injuries, the objectives of conservative treatment are pain management, maintaining/improving function, and protecting the cervical spine to prevent the pathology's progression in patients with cervical spondylosis (Table 39.2).
- Physical therapy, including gait and balance training, strengthening, and gait aide assessment and

prescription, is recommended for patients with clinical sign/symptoms of cervical myelopathy.

- Cervical immobilization with soft collar or brace should be recommended to patients with radiographic findings of severe cervical stenosis with mild/moderate cervical spinal myelopathy to prevent further injuries from a possible injury such as falls, MVA, or vigorous activities such as heavy lifting, or sports accidents.[8]
- It is crucial to educate patients about seeking medical attention in the presence of developing bowel/bladder incontinence, worsening motor weakness and sensory loss, and worsening gait abnormality. Repeat imaging is required in case patients develop any of these issues.[10–13]

Surgical Treatment

- Goals for surgical intervention in traumatic cervical spine injury with SCI include reducing dislocations and decompression of neural elements and stabilizing the spinal column.
- Most penetrating injuries require surgical exploration to detect any possible material in the tissue and clean the wound to prevent infection.
- Early surgical intervention is effective in International Standards for Neurological Classification of SCI (ISNCSCI) motor scores in early surgery patients (<24 hours after SCI).[14]
- Different surgical approaches exist to treat traumatic and nontraumatic cervical myelopathy as follows:
  - *Laminectomy* refers to removing bone from the back of the cervical spine with a dorsal approach.
  - *Laminectomy with fusion* prevents the instability or kyphosis after laminectomy surgeries alone.
  - *Laminoplasty* is the surgical method that enlarges the spinal canal without fusion or to removing the laminae to reduce late failures.
  - *Anterior/ventral approach surgeries* remove ventral osteophytes.
  - Combined dorsal and ventral approach can be used in patients with significant cervical kyphotic deformity and three or more corpectomies are needed.
  - Anterior cervical diskectomy and fusion (ACDF)
  - Posterior spinal fusion
- It is important to assess patients for possible brachial plexus or other peripheral nerve stretch injuries due to prolonged positioning during such surgeries and/or secondary to the original trauma (Figs. 39.1 and 39.2)

Table 39.2 Summary of Pain Management

Analgesic Medications	NSAIDs, Opioids, Muscle Relaxants
Neuromodulating Agents	Gabapentin, pregabalin, tricyclic agents (amitriptyline or nortriptyline), and duloxetine

From Cuccurullo S. *Physical Medicine and Rehabilitation Board Review.* 3rd ed. Springer; 2014.

- Cervical collars can be used postoperatively, depending on the surgeon's preference. The use of collars after surgeries lacks objective data in the recent literature.[15]
- Common complications postoperatively include *dysphagia* (especially after ACDF) and *C5 nerve root palsies* (both from dorsal and ventral approach surgeries).
- Edwards et al. reported a 31% rate of developing persistent dysphagia or dysphonia after ventral approach surgeries.[16]
- *Postoperative neck pain* and *decreased range of motion of the neck* might occur regardless of dorsal vs. ventral approach, which affects the patient's quality of life and/or function.
- Progressive kyphotic deformity after cervical laminectomy can take place, leading to clinical deterioration and poor outcomes.[17]

Conclusion

- Traumatic cervical SCI occurs most commonly due to MVA, falls, assault, and sport-related injuries.
- Elderly patients with cervical spondylosis are in a high-risk group to develop myelopathy even after a simple fall.
- Spinal immobilization with a rigid cervical collar, lateral head supports, and backboard should be maintained until cervical SCI is excluded.
- Cervical trauma can cause stable or unstable SCI from flexion, flexion–rotation, extension, or compression.
- Initially, plain radiographs or CT should be ordered to assess bony structures for spinal column alignment; an MRI should be ordered if imaging suggests ligamentous injury and/or SCI.
- High-level cervical SCI may cause immediate respiratory paralysis. Conservative treatment of cervical fractures is closed reduction under fluoroscopic guidance and halo-vest immobilization.
- If imaging demonstrates an unstable injury, surgery is indicated.
- Goals for surgical intervention include reducing dislocations and decompression of neural elements and stabilizing the spinal column.

Thoracolumbar Traumatic Myelopathy

Descriptions/Definitions

- Traumatic thoracic and lumbar SCIs affect the lower extremities and, depending on the level, can affect muscles responsible for respiration and trunk control.
- The upper extremities and diaphragm are unaffected.
- The autonomic nervous system may be affected most commonly in injuries above T6.

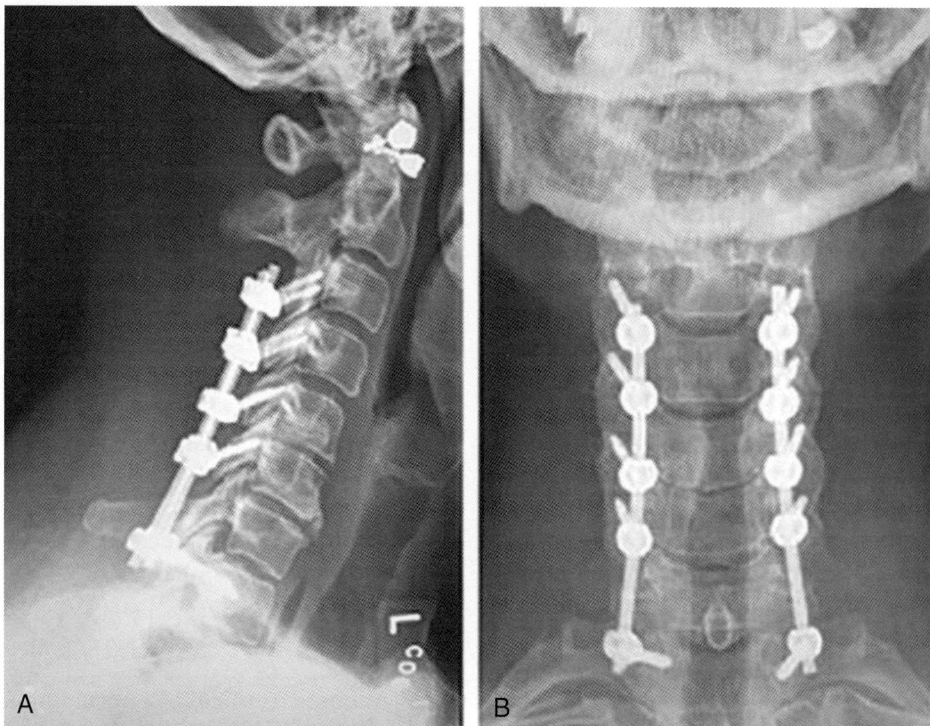

Fig. 39.1 (A) Lateral and (B) anteroposterior radiographs depicting C3–T1 instrumented laminectomy and fusion. C3–C6 received lateral mass screw fixation, C7 was skipped due to small lateral masses, and T1 received pedicle screw instrumentation. (From Koreckij TD. Intraoperative spinal cord and nerve root injuries. In: Garfin S, Eismont F, Bell G, Bono C, Fischgrund J. *Rothman-Simeone and Herkowitz's The Spine*. 7th ed. Elsevier; 2018.)

- The bowel, bladder, and pelvic organs are also affected.
- The injury may be complete or incomplete.
- Lower lumbar vertebral injuries can result in conus medullaris syndrome (CMS) or cauda equina syndrome (CES). CMS may occur from injury to the T12–L2 vertebral levels (rarely T11), and CES may occur from injury to the L3–L5 vertebral levels (rarely L2).[18]

Epidemiology

- T12 is the most common level of paraplegia.[2]
- Of all SCI patients,
  - 18.7% have incomplete paraplegia
  - 11.6% have complete paraplegia.[2]
- In about 10%–38% of thoracolumbar injuries, the conus medullaris or cauda equina is involved.[19]

Etiology/Pathogenesis

The top four causes of spinal cord injury in the United States are MVAs, falls, violence (mostly GSWs), and sports (mostly diving).[2] Falls and sports are more likely to result in cervical SCI. Therefore, *most traumatic thoracolumbar injuries are caused by MVAs and GSWs*.

The thoracolumbar junction (T10–L2) is the most common area of injury in the thoracic and lumbar spine due to the stress caused by the intersecting of two areas of the spine with different characteristics. SCI occurs as a result of 10%–25% of fractures in this area. At this junction lies the conus medullaris, and a mixed CMS-CES injury is likely.[20]

Clinical Characteristics

- CMS occurs from injury to the conus, which generally lies at L1–L2 and results in areflexic bowel, bladder, and lower limbs. The bulbocavernosus reflex (BCR) and micturition reflexes are often impaired but may be preserved in high conus lesions.[2] Saddle anesthesia and sexual dysfunction are usually present with or without weakness in the lower extremities (LE).[18]
- CES results from injury below the conus and results in lower motor neuron (LMN) injury with motor weakness, atrophy, and areflexia of the LE (L2–S2); areflexic bowel and bladder (S2–S4), impotence, and sexual dysfunction. The BCR is absent. *Prognosis for motor function recovery is better than upper motor neuron injuries*[2] (Fig. 39.3).
- More proximal thoracolumbar injuries are likely to result in spastic bladder or detrusor sphincter dyssynergia. Patients with neurogenic bladder likely require an indwelling catheter or intermittent catheterization.

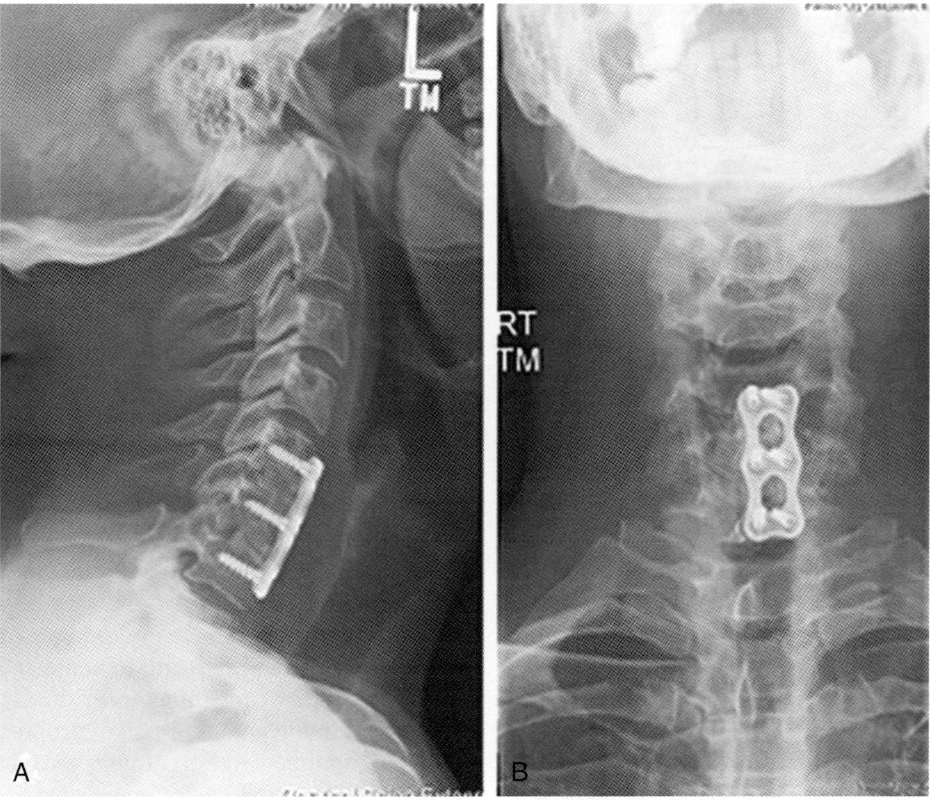

Fig. 39.2 (A) Lateral and (B) anteroposterior radiographs depicting two-level instrumented anterior cervical discectomy and fusion through the standard Smith-Robinson approach. (From Koreckij TD. Intraoperative spinal cord and nerve root injuries. In: Garfin S, Eismont F, Bell G, Bono C, Fischgrund J. *Rothman-Simeone and Herkowitz's The Spine*. 7th ed. Elsevier; 2018.)

- Proximal thoracolumbar injured patients have slowed gut motility, decreased rectal sensation, and decreased ability to evacuate the rectum. They benefit from bowel programs involving digital stimulation. Meanwhile, those with an LMN bowel from CMS or CES will have slowed motility distally and a flaccid anal sphincter, putting them at risk for incontinence. Classically, they benefit from stool bulking and manual evacuation.
- Autonomic dysreflexia should be expected in those with lesions above T6 and can occur with lesions as low as T10.[2,8]
- Orthostatic hypotension can occur in patients with any level of injury.
- Respiratory dysfunction due to impaired cough can occur in patients with lesions up to L1, as the abdominal muscles aid in expiration. The internal intercostals (expiration) and external intercostals (inspiration) are affected in injuries up to T11.[8]

Diagnosis and Exam

- CT and MRI may be used to diagnose traumatic SCI. CT is used when an emergent situation warrants and does not allow time for an MRI. Cord signal abnormality is better visualized on *MRI, the gold standard for imaging of a SCI* (Fig. 39.4).[21]
- MRI is also better for visualizing the posterior ligament complex (PLC) , intervertebral discs, and the spinal cord, compared with a CT scan.[8,19] It is the modality of choice to visualize spinal ligaments, space-occupying spinal canal lesions, and compression of neurologic structures that are nonosseous sources of impingement, such as disc herniation epidural hematoma.[20]
- X-rays can detect vertebral injuries such as fracture and displacement but will not show cord injury.[22] X-ray can detect the mechanism of injury (morphology), including compression, distraction, and translation/rotation[23] (Fig. 39.5).
- Upright X-rays are beneficial for detecting instability.
- Initial exam with weakness and abnormal sensation of the legs is suggestive of paraplegia.[8]
- Physical exam may also reveal a palpable gap or step-off on the spine's palpation, progressive neurological deficits, or progressive kyphosis.
- Sacral sparing in the ISNCSCI exam is present if any of the following are preserved: S4–S5 light touch sensation or pinprick sensation on either side, deep anal pressure sensation, or voluntary anal contraction. Sacral sparing is diagnostic on an incomplete injury. The absence of sacral sparing can be due to complete SCI, CMS, CES, or spinal shock.[2]

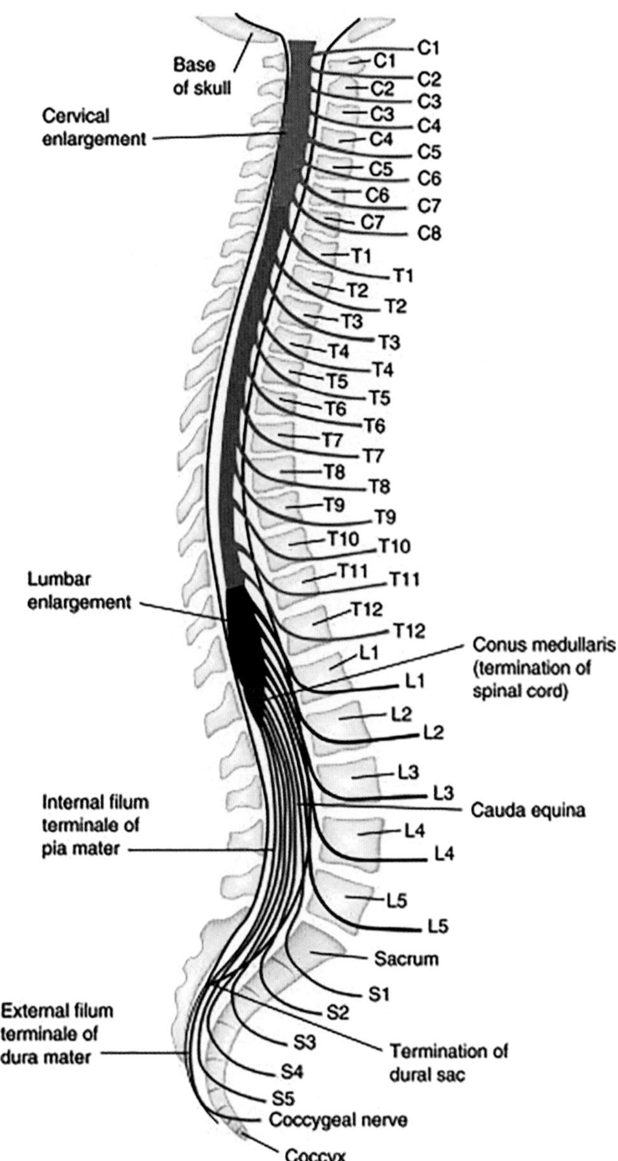

Fig. 39.3 Spinal Cord and Cauda Equina. (From Joshua M. Rosenow. Anatomy of the Nervous system. In: Krames ES, Peckham PH, Rezai AR, Editors. Neuromodulation: Comprehensive Textbook of Principles, Technologies, and Therapies, Second Edition. London: Elsevier; 2018. pp. 25–29.)

- Spinal shock classically lasts for about a month but may be significantly shorter or longer. The first sign of emerging from spinal shock is a delayed upgoing great toe with Babinski reflex testing followed in about 24 hours by the BCR/anal wink reflex. If not present within 24 hours, LMN injury is likely. LE reflexes may return in 2–3 weeks or after up to 3 months.[2]

Treatment

Injury to the thoracolumbar spine is unstable when two of the three columns of the spine are involved. The anterior column comprises the anterior vertebral body, the anterior longitudinal ligament, and the anterior half of the annulus fibrosus. The middle column is made up of the posterior vertebral body, the posterior longitudinal ligament, and the posterior half of the annulus fibrosus. The posterior column includes all of the posterior elements (including the pedicles).[8] Either posterior column injury or injury to any two columns indicates the need for surgery.[24] All dislocation injuries require surgery (Fig. 39.6).

The severity of the injury is graded by the thoracolumbar injury classification and severity score (TLICS) as per the AOSpine Spine Trauma Study Group and is a newer system to determine if surgery is needed.[24,25] The integrity of the PLC, injury morphology, and neurological status are graded on a scale of 1–3 or 4. A total score of less than or equal to 3 indicates that surgery is unnecessary, whereas a score of greater than or equal to 5 indicates necessary surgery. A score of 4 indicates that surgery may or may not be recommended depending on the case and surgeon's discretion.[23]

Due to SCI necessarily involving neurological deficits, patients will often have undergone clinically necessary surgery before presenting to acute rehabilitation.[20]

In neurologically intact individuals without posterior element involvement or risk of progressive spinal instability, nonoperative treatment may be pursued. Compression fractures can often be treated by bracing alone (i.e., Jewett brace), and burst fractures may be treated with a thoracolumbosacral orthosis.[25]

Traction to restore or maintain alignment of the spine may be applied prior to surgery.

Anterior, posterior, or a combined approach can be taken if surgery is recommended. A systematic review found that the posterior approach was associated with significantly better outcomes concerning canal decompression, operative times, and perioperative blood loss.[26]

With pedicle screw instrumentation, a posterior approach allows for three-column fixation and decompression of anteriorly compressive pathologies.[24]

Symptomatic thoracic disc herniation (TDH) is a pathology that requires special consideration, as it is both rare (incidence of 1 in 1,000,000) and difficult to treat surgically due to proximity to the spinal cord. It most often occurs at T8–L1, at ages 30–50 years, and only up to one-third of cases are preceded by trauma. Surgical indications include intractable back or radicular pain, neurological deficits, and myelopathy signs. Giant calcified TDH (> 40% spinal canal occupation) is frequently associated with myelopathy, intradural extension, and postoperative complications. Midline calcified hernias are approached from a transthoracic incision, whereas lateralized soft hernias can be approached from a posterolateral incision. A posterolateral approach is preferred to avoid lung injury. TDH is rare and technically difficult, and surgery may require intraoperative CT. Neurological deterioration, dural tear, and subarachnoid–pleural fistula are the most severe complications.[27,28]

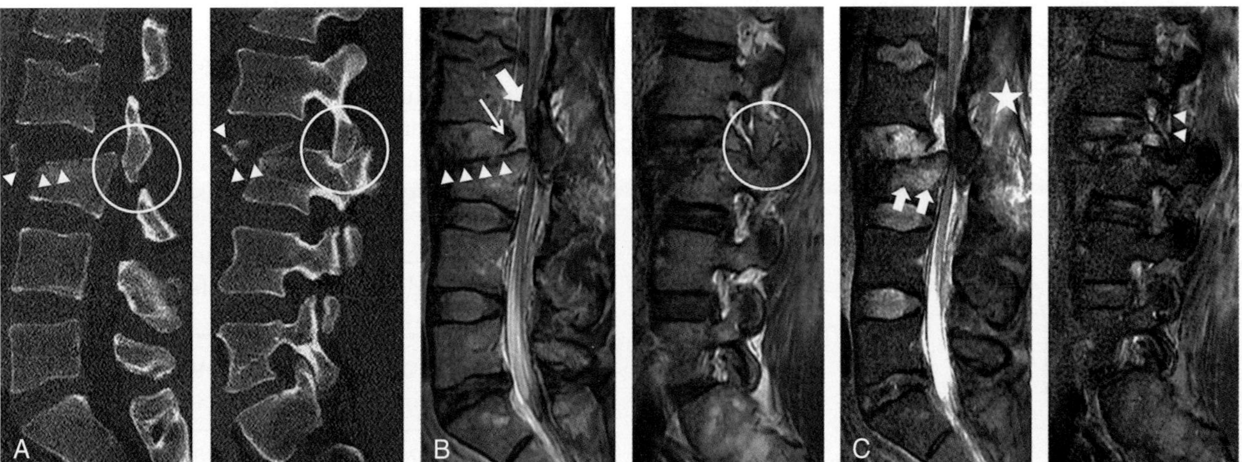

Fig. 39.4 Jumped facet of the lumbar spine with cord transection: 49-year-old man presents with paraplegia after MVA. (A) Sagittal CT image demonstrates compression fracture of the L2 with jumped L2 facet on the left *(circle left)* and rotation of the right L2 facet into the spinal canal *(circle right)*. Compression L3 fracture is also present *(arrowheads)*. The canal appears completely occluded. (B) Sagittal T2WI demonstrates widening of the disc space with increased fluid signal *(arrowheads)*, disruption of the posterior longitudinal ligament *(thin arrow)*, and abrupt discontinuity of the conus terminalis and cauda equina above the level of the fracture *(thick arrow)*. Perched left facet is evident *(circle)*. (C) T2WI-FS demonstrates increased marrow signal at site of L3 compression fracture *(arrows)* and linear fluid signal within the left L2 articular facet *(arrowheads)* corresponding to hairline fracture also faintly evident with extensive increased signal posteriorly *(star)* is consistent with ligamentous injury. (From Kawakyu-O'Connor D, Bordia R, Nicola R. Magnetic resonance imaging of spinal emergencies. *Mag Reson Imaging Clin of N*. 2016;24(2):325-344.)

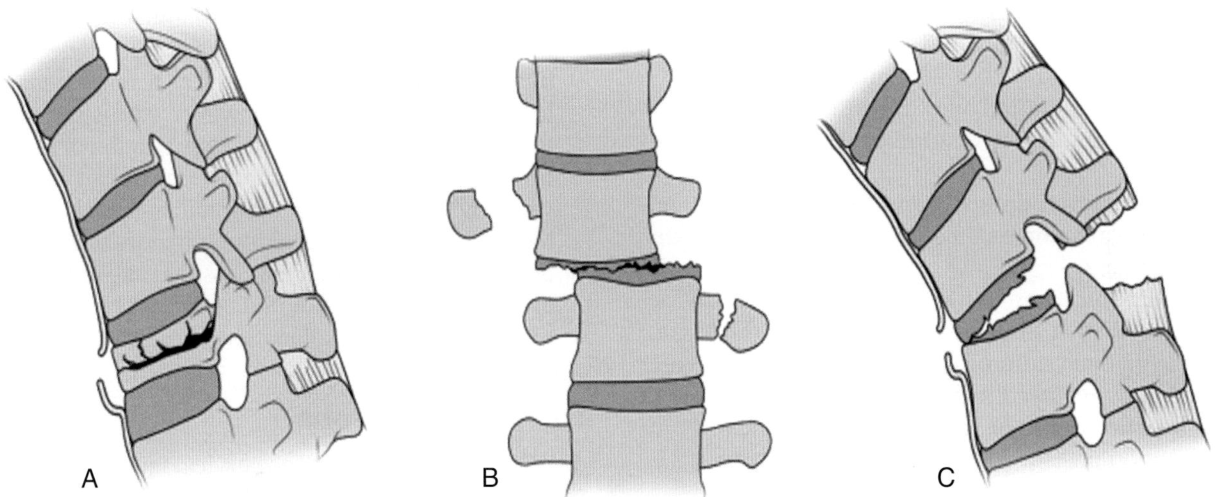

Fig. 39.5 Simplified drawings depicting injury morphology used in the Thoracolumbar Injury Classification and Severity Score (TLICSS). (A) Compression morphology. The vertebral body buckles under load to produce a compression or burst fracture. (B) Translation/rotation morphology. The vertebral column is subjected to shear or torsional forces that cause the rostral part of the spinal column to translate or rotate with respect to the caudal part. (C) Distraction morphology. The rostral spinal column becomes separated from the caudal segment due to distractive forces. Combinations of these morphologic patterns may occur. (Riascos R, Bonfante E. Chapter 28: Spinal Trauma. In: Haaga JR, Boll DT, eds. *CT and MRI of the Whole Body*. 6th ed. Elsevier; 2017 [Fig. 28–30].)

Fusion is recommended in multilevel herniation cases in the context of Scheuermann disease, when more than 50% of bone is resected from the vertebral body, in patients with preoperative back pain or herniation at the thoracolumbar junction.[27,29,30]

The use of methylprednisolone following SCI is not recommended based on several studies that showed no benefit and adverse effects.[20,31]

Prognosis

In a study of 53 patients with thoracolumbar SCI by Skeers et al., the overall mean maximal spinal cord compression was 40% +/− 21%. Those determined to be ASIA Impairment Scale (AIS) A exhibited greater compression than grade C and D patients ($P<0.05$).[32]

Several retrospective studies suggest that early surgery for acute thoracolumbar SCI, either within 24

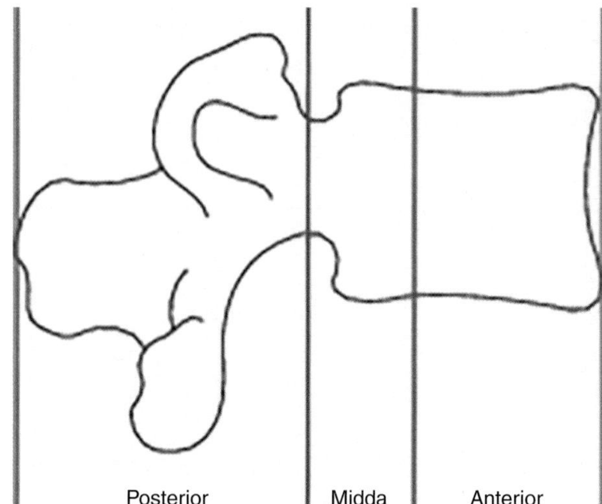

Fig. 39.6 The Three-Column Concept of Spinal Anatomy. (Ferguson RL, Allen BL Jr: A mechanistic classification of thoracolumbar spine fractures, Clin Orthop 189:77–88, 1984, with permission.)

hours or 48 hours instead of after, leads to a more favorable outcome.[33–40] Only one of these trials was prospective, but it was not randomized.[40]

A couple of studies have found no difference, though one concluded that there was no difference in severe injury, and the other compared emergency management to management still within 24 hours.[41,42]

The prognoses of CMS and CES postsurgery are generally favorable, with some noticeable improvement.[43–46]

Longer symptom duration and history of back and leg pain indicate worse CES outcomes, especially bilateral sciatica.[20,47]

Note that in certain patient cases, a patient may be better served by fusion surgery to stabilize the spine, especially if they suffered a polytrauma, have severe pain, or may not need a brace after surgery. In such cases, a patient may be better able to participate in rehabilitation postsurgery than without surgery.

Prevention

Prevention of MVA and GSW injuries is paramount in preventing thoracolumbar spinal cord injuries. Fall prevention is also important, though most spinal cord injuries resulting from falls occur at the cervical levels.[48]

Conclusions

- Traumatic thoracolumbar myelopathies can cause autonomic dysfunction if they are above T6, respiratory dysfunction above T12, and neurogenic bowel and bladder, in addition to motor and sensory deficits. They also include CMS and CES, which can occur as high as the T11 vertebral level.
- MRI is the gold standard for imaging the spinal cord.
- Spinal shock classically lasts for about 1 month.
- The need for surgery can be determined by (1) using the three-column model of the spine, where surgery is recommended for injury to any two columns or just the posterior column; and (2) the TLICS, which assesses the type of injury and severity of neurological deficits.
- Studies suggest that earlier rather than later surgery, when needed, leads to a more favorable prognosis.

Unspecified and Multilevel Myelopathy

- Patients who have an unknown multilevel SCI can suffer complications at any SCI level, from those listed earlier in high cervical level tetraplegics to those with injuries at the level of the cauda equina.
- Treatment for multilevel noncontiguous spinal fractures should, in general, follow the guidelines for the treatment of each region of injury. Treatment should be individualized.[49]
- A patient may have a mixed picture of upper motor neuron and LMN neurogenic bowel and bladder.[50] Close monitoring, medication adjustments, and urodynamic studies will be instrumental.
- In most cases, it is possible to be able to determine sensory and motor levels as well as a single neurological level of injury (NLI); however, this is not always the case when performing the classification of the ASIA Impairment Scale (AIS)and the Zone of Partial Preservation (ZPP). ASIA's International Standards Committee recommends that in cases with more than one SCI, an AIS and a ZPP should be classified as Not Determinable (ND); additionally, the comment box should be used to give a full explanation of the findings.[51]

Review Questions

1. What is the most common cervical level for traumatic cervical spinal cord injury?
   a. C3
   b. C4
   c. C5
   d. C6
2. Which one of the cervical spinal column injuries is always unstable?
   a. Anterior wedge fracture
   b. Burst fracture of vertebral body
   c. Unilateral facet dislocation
   d. Bilateral facet dislocation
3. Which of the following cervical immobilizer is the most restrictive?
   a. Philadelphia collar
   b. Aspen collar
   c. SOMI immobilizer
   d. Halo

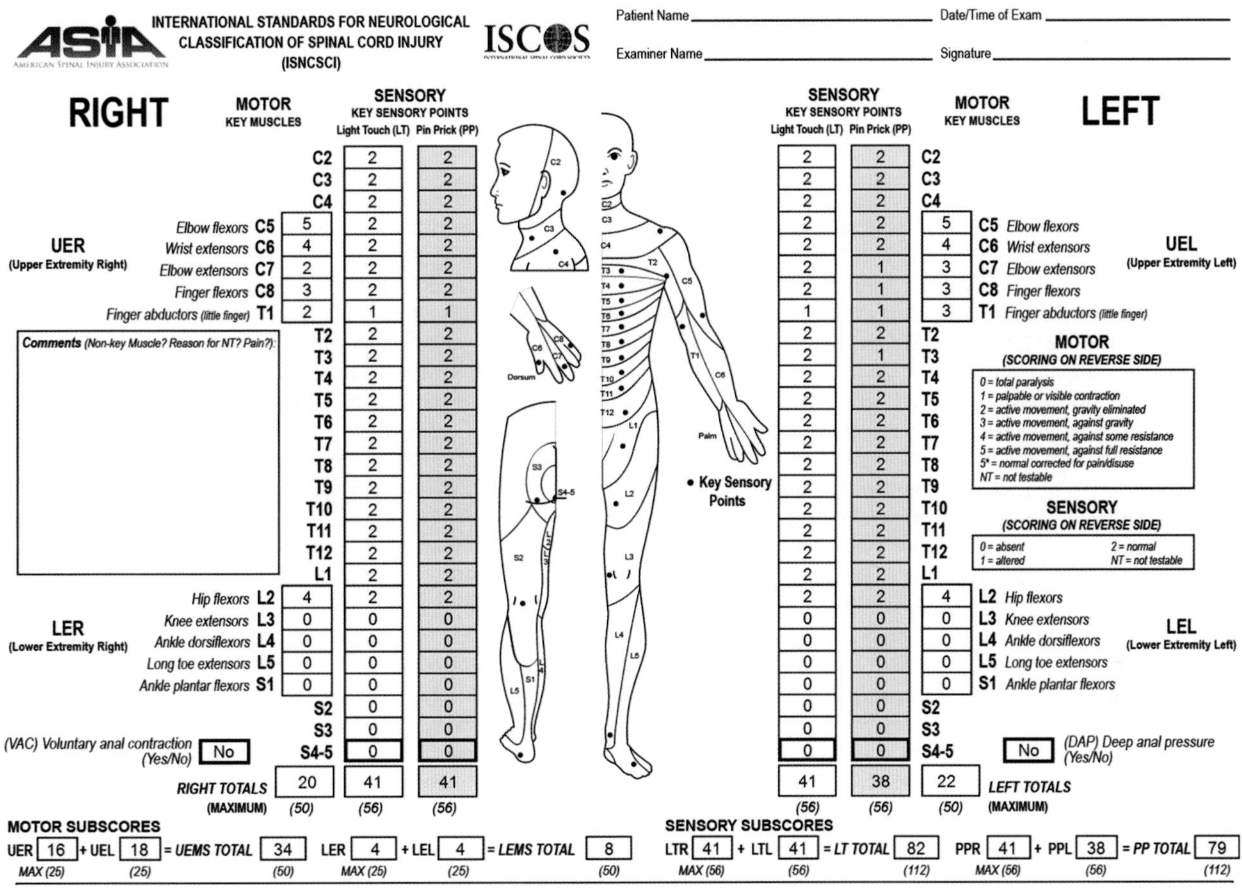

ASIA (American Spinal Injury Association) — INTERNATIONAL STANDARDS FOR NEUROLOGICAL CLASSIFICATION OF SPINAL CORD INJURY (ISNCSCI) — ISCOS

Patient Name ____________ Date/Time of Exam ____________

Examiner Name ____________ Signature ____________

RIGHT MOTOR KEY MUSCLES	Level	RIGHT Motor	RIGHT Light Touch (LT)	RIGHT Pin Prick (PP)	LEFT Light Touch (LT)	LEFT Pin Prick (PP)	LEFT Motor	Level	LEFT MOTOR KEY MUSCLES
	C2		2	2	2	2		C2	
	C3		2	2	2	2		C3	
	C4		2	2	2	2		C4	
Elbow flexors	C5	5	2	2	2	2	5	C5	Elbow flexors
Wrist extensors	C6	4	2	2	2	2	4	C6	Wrist extensors
Elbow extensors	C7	2	2	2	2	1	3	C7	Elbow extensors
Finger flexors	C8	3	2	2	2	1	3	C8	Finger flexors
Finger abductors (little finger)	T1	2	1	1	1	1	3	T1	Finger abductors (little finger)
	T2		2	2	2	2		T2	
	T3		2	2	2	1		T3	
	T4		2	2	2	2		T4	
	T5		2	2	2	2		T5	
	T6		2	2	2	2		T6	
	T7		2	2	2	2		T7	
	T8		2	2	2	2		T8	
	T9		2	2	2	2		T9	
	T10		2	2	2	2		T10	
	T11		2	2	2	2		T11	
	T12		2	2	2	2		T12	
	L1		2	2	2	2		L1	
Hip flexors	L2	4	2	2	2	2	4	L2	Hip flexors
Knee extensors	L3	0	0	0	0	0	0	L3	Knee extensors
Ankle dorsiflexors	L4	0	0	0	0	0	0	L4	Ankle dorsiflexors
Long toe extensors	L5	0	0	0	0	0	0	L5	Long toe extensors
Ankle plantar flexors	S1	0	0	0	0	0	0	S1	Ankle plantar flexors
	S2		0	0	0	0		S2	
	S3		0	0	0	0		S3	
	S4-5		0	0	0	0		S4-5	
RIGHT TOTALS (MAXIMUM)		20 (50)	41 (56)	41 (56)	41 (56)	38 (56)	22 (50)		LEFT TOTALS (MAXIMUM)

UER (Upper Extremity Right); LER (Lower Extremity Right); UEL (Upper Extremity Left); LEL (Lower Extremity Left)

Comments (Non-key Muscle? Reason for NT? Pain?):

(VAC) Voluntary anal contraction (Yes/No): No

(DAP) Deep anal pressure (Yes/No): No

MOTOR (SCORING ON REVERSE SIDE)
0 = total paralysis
1 = palpable or visible contraction
2 = active movement, gravity eliminated
3 = active movement, against gravity
4 = active movement, against some resistance
5 = active movement, against full resistance
5* = normal corrected for pain/disuse
NT = not testable

SENSORY (SCORING ON REVERSE SIDE)
0 = absent; 1 = altered; 2 = normal; NT = not testable

• Key Sensory Points

MOTOR SUBSCORES: UER 16 + UEL 18 = UEMS TOTAL 34; LER 4 + LEL 4 = LEMS TOTAL 8 (MAX (25), (25), (50); MAX (25), (25), (50))

SENSORY SUBSCORES: LTR 41 + LTL 41 = LT TOTAL 82; PPR 41 + PPL 38 = PP TOTAL 79 (MAX (56), (56), (112); MAX (56), (56), (112))

Fig. 39.7 International Standards for Neurological Classification for Spinal Cord Injury. (American Spinal Injury Association: International Standards for Neurological Classification of Spinal Cord Injury, revised 2019; Richmond, VA.)

4. An injury to the T12 vertebra is most likely to be caused by what kind of spinal cord injury?
   a. A T12 traumatic SCI
   b. A lumbar spinal cord injury
   c. CMS
   d. CES
5. Which is the earliest sign of emerging from spinal shock?
   a. Motor return
   b. Sensory return
   c. A delayed Babinski reflex
   d. Neurogenic bowel starts to develop
6. A 25-year-old man suffers cervical and lumbar vertebral fractures requiring fusion surgery following an MVA. His examination on arrival to an inpatient rehabilitation unit is as shown in Fig. 39.7.

How would this exam be scored?
   a. C6 AIS A
   b. C6 AIS D plus a L2 AIS A
   c. L2 AIS A
   d. C6 AIS ND

REFERENCES

1. Maroon JC, Abla AA. Classification of acute spinal cord injury, neurological evaluation, and neurosurgical considerations. *Crit Care Clin.* 1987;3(3):655–677.
2. Cuccurullo S. Physical Medicine and Rehabilitation Board Review. 3rd ed. Springer Publishing Company; 2014.
3. Spragg M, Wagner M. 5th ed.Marx JA, Hockberger RS, Walls RM, eds. *Rosen's Emergency Medicine: Concepts and Clinical Practice.* 1–3 St. Louis: Mosby; 2002.
4. Gaillard F. Cervical canal stenosis. Reference Article, Radiopaedia.org [Internet]. https://radiopaedia.org/articles/cervical-canal-stenosis?lang=us.
5. Bohlman HH, Emery SE. The pathophysiology of cervical spondylosis and myelopathy. *Spine Phila Pa 1976.* 1988;13(7):843–846.
6. Oteir AO, Smith K, Stoelwinder JU, Middleton J, Jennings PA. Should suspected cervical spinal cord injury be immobilised? a systematic review. *Injury.* 2015;46(4):528–535.
7. Beaty N, Slavin J, Diaz C, Zeleznick K, Ibrahimi D, Sansur CA. Cervical spine injury from gunshot wounds. *J Neurosurg Spine.* 2014;21(3):442–449.
8. Kirshblum S, Lin VW. *Spinal Cord Medicine.* DemosMEDICAL; 2019.
9. Botte M, Byrne T, Abrams R, Garfin S. Halo skeletal fixation: techniques of application and prevention of complications. *J Am Acad Orthop Surg.* 1996;4(1):44–53.
10. Levin K. Cervical spondylotic myelopathy. In: UpToDate, Post, TW (Ed), UpToDate, Waltham, MA, 2020.
11. Toledano M, Bartleson JD. Cervical spondylotic myelopathy. *Neurol Clin.* 2013;31(1):287–305.
12. Yoshimatsu H, Nagata K, Goto H, et al. Conservative treatment for cervical spondylotic myelopathy. Prediction of

treatment effects by multivariate analysis. *Spine J*. 2001;1(4):269–273.
13. Kadanka Z, Bednarík J, Vohánka S, et al. Conservative treatment versus surgery in spondylotic cervical myelopathy: a prospective randomised study. *Eur Spine J*. 2000;9(6): 538–544.
14. Wilson JR, Singh A, Craven C, et al. Early versus late surgery for traumatic spinal cord injury: the results of a prospective Canadian cohort study. *Spinal Cord*. 2012;50(11):840–843.
15. Heary RF, Agarwal N, Ghogawala Z, Amankulor N. Spondylotic and myelopathic myelopathies. In: Kirshblum S, Lin VW, eds. *Spinal Cord Medicine*. 3rd ed. New York: Springer Publishing Company; 2018.
16. Edwards CCI, Karpitskaya Y, Cha C, et al. Accurate identification of adverse outcomes after cervical spine surgery. *JBJS*. 2004;86(2):251–256.
17. Yonenobu K, Okada K, Fuji T, Fujiwara K, Yamashita K, Ono K. Causes of neurologic deterioration following surgical treatment of cervical myelopathy. *Spine*. 1986;11(8):818–823.
18. Brouwers E, van de Meent H, Curt A, Starremans B, Hosman A, Bartels R. Definitions of traumatic conus medullaris and cauda equina syndrome: a systematic literature review. *Spinal Cord*. 2017;55(10):886–890.
19. Looby S, Flanders A. Spine trauma. *Radiol Clin North Am*. 2011;49(1):129–163.
20. Radcliff KE, Kepler CK, Delasotta LA, et al. Current management review of thoracolumbar cord syndromes. *Spine J*. 2011;11(9):884–892.
21. Bozzo A, Marcoux J, Radhakrishna M, Pelletier J, Goulet B. The role of magnetic resonance imaging in the management of acute spinal cord injury. *J Neurotrauma*. 2011;28(8):1401–1411.
22. Parizel PM, van der Zijden T, Gaudino S, et al. Trauma of the spine and spinal cord: imaging strategies. *Eur Spine J*. 2010;19(Suppl 1):S8–S17.
23. Vaccaro AR, Lehman RA, Hurlbert RJ, et al. A new classification of thoracolumbar injuries: the importance of injury morphology, the integrity of the posterior ligamentous complex, and neurologic status. *Spine*. 2005;30(20):2325–2333.
24. Ghobrial GM, Jallo J. Thoracolumbar spine trauma: review of the evidence. *J Neurosurg Sci*. 2013;57(2):115–122.
25. Vaccaro AR, Oner C, Kepler CK, et al. AOSpine thoracolumbar spine injury classification system: fracture description, neurological status, and key modifiers. *Spine*. 2013;38(23):2028–2037.
26. Zhu Q, Shi F, Cai W, Bai J, Fan J, Yang H. Comparison of anterior versus posterior approach in the treatment of thoracolumbar fractures: a systematic review. *Int Surg*. 2015;100(6):1124–1133.
27. Bouthors C, Benzakour A, Court C. Surgical treatment of thoracic disc herniation: an overview. *Int Orthop*. 2019;43(4):807–816.
28. Court C, Mansour E, Bouthors C. Thoracic disc herniation: surgical treatment. *Orthop Traumatol Surg Res*. 2018;104(1S):S31–S40.
29. Vanichkachorn JS, Vaccaro AR. Thoracic disk disease: diagnosis and treatment. *J Am Acad Orthop Surg*. 2000;8(3):159–169.
30. Krauss WE, Edwards DA, Cohen-Gadol AA. Transthoracic discectomy without interbody fusion. *Surg Neurol*. 2005;63(5):403–408. discussion 408–409.
31. Coleman WP, Benzel D, Cahill DW, et al. A critical appraisal of the reporting of the National Acute Spinal Cord Injury Studies (II and III) of methylprednisolone in acute spinal cord injury. *J Spinal Disord*. 2000;13(3):185–199.
32. Skeers P, Battistuzzo CR, Clark JM, Bernard S, Freeman BJC, Batchelor PE. Acute thoracolumbar spinal cord injury: relationship of cord compression to neurological outcome. *J Bone Joint Surg Am*. 2018;100(4):305–315.
33. Schaeffer HR. Cauda equina compression resulting from massive lumbar disc extrusion. *Aust N Z J Surg*. 1966;35(4):300–306.
34. Delamarter RB, Sherman J, Carr JB. Pathophysiology of spinal cord injury. Recovery after immediate and delayed decompression. *J Bone Joint Surg Am*. 1995;77(7):1042–1049.
35. Shapiro S. Medical realities of cauda equina syndrome secondary to lumbar disc herniation. *Spine*. 2000;25(3):348–351. discussion 352.
36. Jerwood D, Todd NV. Reanalysis of the timing of cauda equina surgery. *Br J Neurosurg*. 2006;20(3):178–179.
37. Todd NV. Cauda equina syndrome: the timing of surgery probably does influence outcome. *Br J Neurosurg*. 2005;19(4):301–306. discussion 307–308.
38. Ahn UM, Ahn NU, Buchowski JM, Garrett ES, Sieber AN, Kostuik JP. Cauda equina syndrome secondary to lumbar disc herniation: a meta-analysis of surgical outcomes. *Spine*. 2000;25(12):1515–1522.
39. DeLong WB, Polissar N, Neradilek B. Timing of surgery in cauda equina syndrome with urinary retention: meta-analysis of observational studies. *J Neurosurg Spine*. 2008;8(4):305–320.
40. Fehlings MG, Vaccaro A, Wilson JR, et al. Early versus delayed decompression for traumatic cervical spinal cord injury: results of the Surgical Timing in Acute Spinal Cord Injury Study (STASCIS). *PLoS One*. 2012;7(2):e32037.
41. Gleave JRW, Macfarlane R. Cauda equina syndrome: what is the relationship between timing of surgery and outcome? *Br J Neurosurg*. 2002;16(4):325–328.
42. Crocker M, Fraser G, Boyd E, Wilson J, Chitnavis BP, Thomas NW. The value of interhospital transfer and emergency MRI for suspected cauda equina syndrome: a 2-year retrospective study. *Ann R Coll Surg Engl*. 2008;90(6):513–516.
43. Rahimi-Movaghar V, Vaccaro AR, Mohammadi M. Efficacy of surgical decompression in regard to motor recovery in the setting of conus medullaris injury. *J Spinal Cord Med*. 2006;29(1):32–38.
44. Transfeldt EE, White D, Bradford DS, Roche B. Delayed anterior decompression in patients with spinal cord and cauda equina injuries of the thoracolumbar spine. *Spine*. 1990;15(9):953–957.
45. Chou D, Hartl R, Sonntag VKH. Conus medullaris syndrome without lower-extremity involvement in L-1 burst fractures: report of four cases. *J Neurosurg Spine*. 2006;4(3): 265–269.
46. Buchner M, Schiltenwolf M. Cauda equina syndrome caused by intervertebral lumbar disk prolapse: mid-term results of 22 patients and literature review. *Orthopedics*. 2002;25(7). 727–231.
47. Kennedy JG, Soffe KE, McGrath A, Stephens MM, Walsh MG, McManus F. Predictors of outcome in cauda equina syndrome. *Eur Spine J*. 1999;8(4):317–322.
48. Bellon K, Kolakowsky-Hayner SA, Chen D, McDowell S, Bitterman B, Klaas SJ. Evidence-based practice in primary prevention of spinal cord injury. *Top Spinal Cord Inj Rehabil*. 2013;19(1):25–30.

49. Lian XF, Zhao J, Hou TS, Yuan JD, Jin GY, Li ZH. The treatment for multilevel noncontiguous spinal fractures. *Int Orthop*. 2007;31(5):647–652.
50. Calenoff L, Chessare JW, Rogers LF, Toerge J, Rosen JS. Multiple level spinal injuries: importance of early recognition. *Am J Roentgenol*. 1978 Apr;130(4):665–669.
51. Kirshblum S, Snider B, Rupp R, Read MS, International Standards Committee of ASIA and ISCoS. Updates of the International Standards for Neurologic Classification of Spinal Cord Injury: 2015 and 2019. *Phys Med Rehabil Clin N Am*. 2020;31(3):319–330.

CHAPTER

40 Nontraumatic Myelopathies

Joanne M. Delgado-Lebron, Eduardo Nadal-Ortiz, and Andres Gutierrez

OUTLINE

Motor Neuron Diseases[1]

Motor neuron diseases include amyotrophic lateral sclerosis (ALS), progressive muscular atrophy, progressive bulbar palsy, and primary lateral sclerosis (PLS). ALS and PLS involve the upper motor neuron (UMN) and will be discussed here.

Amyotrophic Lateral Sclerosis

ALS affects adults of all ages (mean: 58-years), and has a male predominance. Clinical presentation usually begins with focal weakness; onset occurs in one limb in at least half of the cases, followed by a combination of UMN (weakness, spasticity, hyperreflexia, pathologic reflexes, and pseudobulbar features) and lower motor neuron (LMN) signs (weakness, muscle atrophy, and fasciculations). Bulbar involvement is common, including dysarthria, tongue atrophy, fasciculations, hyperactive gag and jaw reflexes, and pseudobulbar palsy. The sensory nervous system is clinically spared. Diagnosis is clinical and should include both UMN and LMN findings. Electromyogram and nerve conduction studies are frequently used to support LMN findings and confirm the diagnosis with different levels of certainty based on El Escorial Criteria (Box 40.1).[2,3] Treatment is mostly supportive. Some medications, including riluzole (Rilutek) and endaravone, (Radicava) have been shown to prolong survival for several months and halt ALS progression during early stages, respectively.[4] Survival is poor, with respiratory failure the most common cause of death. Some metabolic and toxic disorders can mimic motor neuron disease, including hyperthyroidism, hyperparathyroidism, adult GM2 gangliosidosis, and lead and mercury toxicity.

Primary Lateral Sclerosis

PLS is a slowly progressive, symmetric spastic paraparesis that commonly presents in the early fifth decade or later. Symptoms are limited to corticospinal tract dysfunction involving extremities and the bulbar region. It occurs sporadically with no family history.[1]

Cervical Myelopathy

Cervical myelopathy is caused by a combination of factors, including external compression from spondylotic canal stenosis, biomechanical stretch injury, and vascular factors.[5] The incidence increases with advancing age and is higher in men.[6] Symptoms include progressive gait dysfunction, muscle weakness, loss of hand dexterity (with muscle wasting), and later, as disease progresses, bladder dysfunction. There is a mixed picture of corticospinal tract findings and flaccid weakness in the affected segments due to anterior horn cell impingement.[7] Diagnosis is made with magnetic resonance imaging (MRI) (Fig. 40.1). Poorer prognosis is associated with longer disease duration, severe symptoms, and older age. Conservative treatment is appropriate for patients with mild disease or those with contraindications for surgery. Surgical management should be considered for those with moderate to severe disease or rapidly progressive symptoms to prevent the progression of neurological deficits.

Infectious Myelopathies

Infectious myelopathies are caused by an abscess within the spinal cord due to expansion of local infection or hematogenous spread, typically on

■ **Box 40.1** Revised El Escorial Criteria With Awaji Modification

1. Principles

The diagnosis of amyotrophic lateral sclerosis (ALS) requires:

(a) The presence of

i. Evidence of *lower motor neuron (LMN) degeneration* by clinical, electrophysiologic, or neuropathologic examination

ii. Evidence of *upper motor neuron (UMN) degeneration* by clinical examination

iii. *Progressive spread of symptoms or signs* within a region or to other regions, as determined by history, physical examination, or electrophysiologic tests

Together with:

(b) The absence of

i. *Electrophysiologic or pathologic evidence of other disease process* that might explain the signs of LMN and/or UMN degeneration

ii. *Neuroimaging evidence of other disease process* that might explain the observed clinical and electrophysiologic signs

2. Diagnostic Categories

Clinically definite ALS is defined by *clinical or electrophysiologic* evidence by the presence of LMN as well as UMN signs in the bulbar region and at least two spinal regions or the presence of LMN and UMN signs in three spinal regions.

Clinically probable ALS is defined on *clinical or electrophysiologic* evidence by LMN and UMN signs in at least two regions with some UMN signs necessarily rostral to (above) the LMN sign.

Clinically possible ALS is defined when *clinical or electrophysiologic* signs of UMN and LMN dysfunction are found in only one region; or UMN signs are found alone in two or more regions; or LMN signs are found rostral to UMN signs. Neuroimaging and clinical laboratory studies will have been performed and other diagnoses must have been excluded.

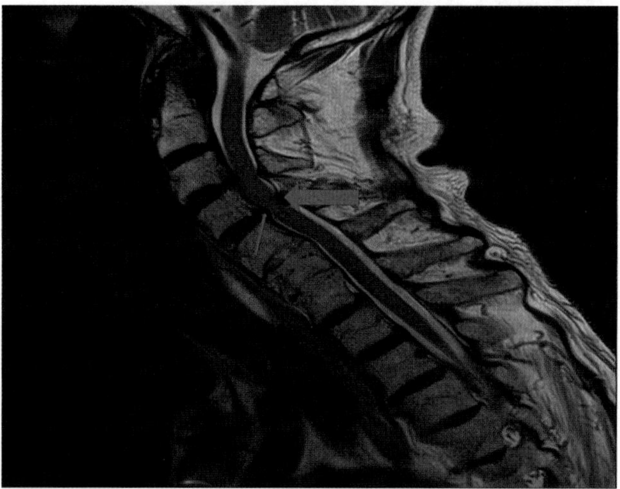

Fig. 40.1 Case of 89-year-old male admitted due to numbness and impaired balance, with good motor strength preservation. Cervical Spine MRI Sagittal T2 C4/C5 level: shows degenerative desiccation and herniation of the intervertebral disc *(small arrow)*. There is evidence of calcification of the posterior spinal and posterior compression by the ligamentum flavum *(large arrow)*. Findings result in severe spinal cord compression.

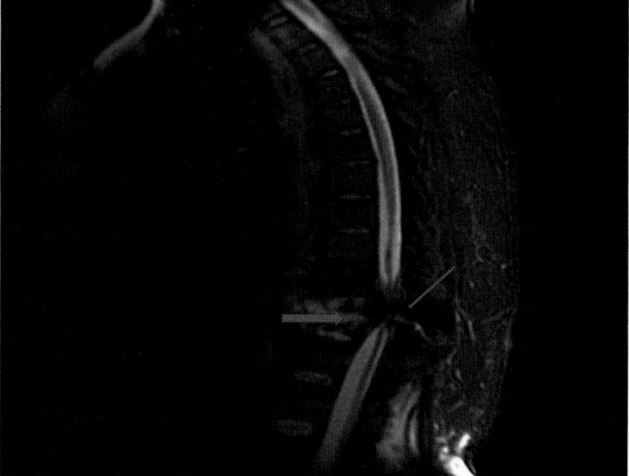

Fig. 40.2 Case of 51-year-old male with history of diabetes mellitus, obesity, and infectious spondylitis at T11–T12 level. T2 Thoracic Spine MRI sagittal view showing an irregular fluid collection occupying the T10 and T11 vertebral bodies *(large arrow)*, which are felt to be collapsed with posterior displacement and stenosis of the canal at this level *(thin arrow)*.

immunocompromised patients (bacterial endocarditis, intravenous drug abuser, urinary tract infection). The most common etiologic agents are gram-positive cocci such as *Staphylococcus* or *Streptococcus* species, but other microorganisms need to be considered based on risk factors such as a history of spine surgery, penetrating trauma, injected drug use, alcoholism, suppressed immune system, and diabetes mellitus.[8] Infectious myelopathies commonly present with fever and severe pain in the affected area, and may evolve to include sensory and motor deficits. Diagnosis is through MRI with gadolinium, and treatment consists of antibiotics and surgical excision. Prognosis is dependent on the time of decompression with complete resolution of symptoms of those treated early. (Fig. 40.2)

Tuberculin Osteomyelitis (Pott Disease)

Tuberculin osteomyelitis is caused by *Mycobacteria tuberculosis* and usually affects the thoracic vertebrae, resulting in myelopathy due to direct compression from the bony involvement.[8] Symptoms include chills, night sweats, weight loss, and localized axial pain. Diagnosis is through MRI of the spine and confirmed by a polymerase chain reaction of biopsied tissue.

Neurosyphilis

Neurosyphilis is caused by *Treponema pallidum*. It is more common in men and those who are HIV-positive. Late infection (tabes dorsalis) causes loss of posterior columns. Most commonly, inflammation involving the meninges and periphery of the spinal cord with accompanying atrophy is present, whereas vasculitis infarct, pachymeningeal inflammation, and dorsal column atrophy are less common.[9] Neurosyphilis is typically seen at the cervical and thoracic cord. Treatment consists of antibiotics, usually penicillin.

West Nile Virus

West Nile virus affects the spinal nerve roots and anterior horn cells. It presents in adults as acute, painless, asymmetric weakness, sometimes of a single limb, and resembles poliomyelitis.[8] Diagnosis is through electromyogram and nerve conduction showing anterior horn cell and axonal motor involvement.

Vacuolar Myelopathy

Vacuolar myelopathy can be seen in late stages of AIDS when CD4 counts are very low. It often occurs in conjunction with dementia and peripheral neuropathies. It typically involves the thoracic spinal cord and presents with progressive, painless leg weakness, stiffness, sensory loss, imbalance, and sphincter dysfunction in the absence of sensory level.[9] Biopsy shows white matter destruction of the dorsal columns and corticospinal tracts similar to vitamin B12 deficiency myelopathy.[8]

Tropical Spastic Paraplegia

Tropical spastic paraplegia is transmitted sexually or through exposure to contaminated blood. It appears as slowly progressive leg weakness and gait ataxia. The clinical course is similar to primary progressive multiple sclerosis in which gait impairment leads to wheelchair mobility 5 to 10 years after onset.[10] It is caused by human T-lymphocytic virus Type 1.

Immune-Mediated and Inflammatory Myelopathies

Generally, immune-mediated and inflammatory myelopathies have different etiologies. However, as a group, they are called transverse myelitis. Transverse myelitis can be idiopathic or secondary to a broader neurologic or systemic condition.[11] On initial presentation, it may be difficult to distinguish among the different causes, and that is where a comprehensive history and physical examination are important.[12] General transverse myelitis presents with weakness, sensory loss, pain, and bladder/bowel dysfunction, or a combination of these symptoms.[11,12] Neurological symptoms usually progress over a few hours, days, or weeks, and reach a nadir under 4 weeks if untreated.[11,12] One characteristic finding of transverse myelitis is the recognizable sensory level on physical examination.[11,13] Diagnosing the specific cause of transverse myelitis requires an extensive workup in most cases before it can be called idiopathic transverse myelitis. Diagnostic workup includes whole spine and brain MRI with gadolinium showing

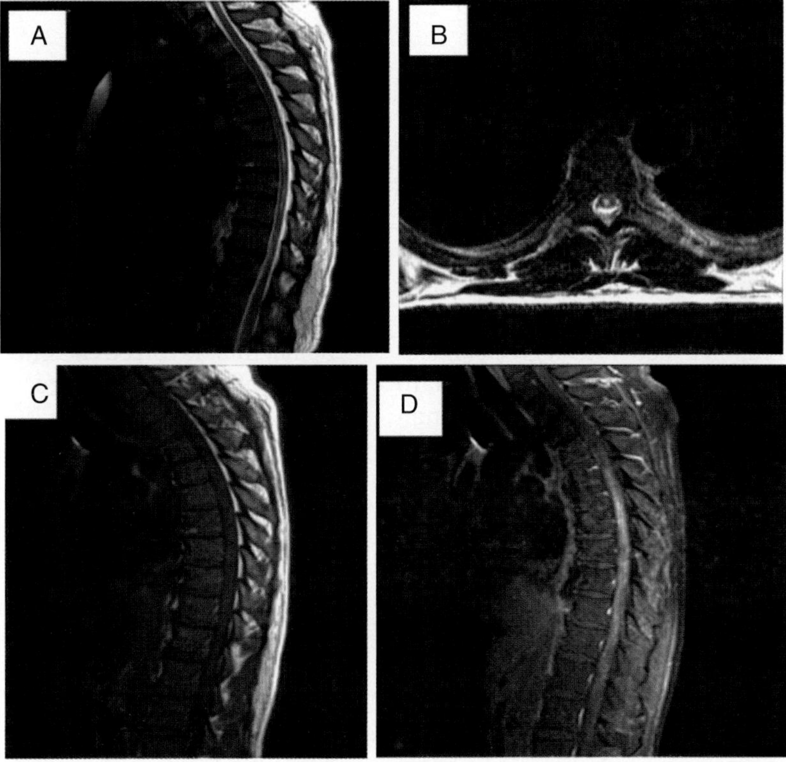

Fig. 40.3 (A) Sagittal T2 and (B) axial T2 showing longitudinally extensive transverse myelitis with hyperintensity seen in the central aspect of the cord. (C) Sagittal T1 precontrast and (D) sagittal T1 postcontrast showing enhancement of the cord in acute presentation.

Table 40.1 Characteristics of Most Common Etiologies of Transverse Myelitis

Multiple Sclerosis	Neuromyelitis Optica	Connective Tissue Diseases (Systemic lupus erythematosus, Sjrogren syndrome)	Sarcoidosis	Postinfectious	Paraneoplastic
Short segment, <3 levels, unilateral	Longitudinally extensive (LE), >3 levels	Longitudinally extensive	Short or LE	LE	Rare
Initial isolated event in 20%–40%	Centrally located, cord swelling	+/− Extensive gray matter involvement in systemic lupus erythematosus	Meningeal inflammation in post gadolinium MRI	Viral, bacterial, fungal, and in rare cases parasitic	Antineuronal antibodies and paraneoplastic antibodies (antiamphiphysin and CRMP-5 associated with breast and lung cancer)
+Oligoclonal bands	Optic neuritis and brainstem involvement (intractable nausea/vomit)	Long-term immunosuppression	Elevated angiotensin-converting enzyme levels in blood and/or cerebral spinal fluid	Consider the ones that are treatable: syphilis, herpesviruses, HIV, and tuberculosis	Management: treat the underlying neoplasm, usually not responsive to corticosteroids
+Brain MRI with 2 or more demyelinating lesions	+AQP4 in most cases		Cerebral spinal fluid with significantly elevated protein, pleocytosis with polymorphonuclear leukocytes and low glucose		
	Long-term immunosuppression		May need anti-tumor necrosis factor therapy if no response to corticosteroids		

Greenberg BM, Frohman EM. Immune-mediated myelopathies. *CONTINUUM Lifelong Learning in Neurology.* 2015;21(1):121-131; West TW, Hess C, Cree BAC. Acute transverse myelitis: demyelinating, inflammatory, and infectious myelopathies. *Semin Neurol.* 2012;32(2):97-113.

gadolinium enhancement (Fig. 40.3), cerebral spinal fluid (CSF) analysis, and specific serum antibodies as indicated.[12] Treatment of transverse myelitis includes initial empiric high-dose corticosteroids, followed by plasma exchange or intravenous immune globulin in many cases.[11,12] If a specific etiology is identified, it is then treated accordingly. Prognostically, it is estimated that one-third of persons affected recover with little or no sequela, one-third retain a moderate degree of residual disability, and one-third will worsen or remain severely disabled.[12] Table 40.1 shows the most common etiologies of transverse myelitis.

Multiple Sclerosis

Multiple sclerosis is an immune-mediated disorder affecting the central nervous system through demyelination and degenerative processes. Women between the ages of 20 to 50 years may present with four phenotypes: relapse and remission, clinically isolated syndrome, secondary progression, and primary progressive. Common symptoms include optic neuritis, fatigue, gait impairment, weakness, numbness, and tingling. Diagnosis is made using MRI (McDonald Criteria: lesions dissemination in time and space). Treatment includes disease-modifying therapy (Fig. 40.4, Table 40.2).

Neoplastic Myelopathies

Spinal tumors can be classified as primary spinal tumors, metastases to spinal cord or vertebrae, and primary bone tumors in the spine.[14] They can be further subdivided into three classes corresponding to their anatomic location (shown in Table 40.1).[15] Clinical presentation can be variable, with pain being the most common, and often the presenting, symptom. Other symptoms that may develop include extremity weakness, sensory abnormalities, bowel and bladder dysfunction, sexual dysfunction, and gait abnormalities; if extensive compression occurs, then paraplegia or quadriplegia may also develop (Tables 40.3, 40.4). Specific characteristics of some of the most common tumors are discussed in Table 40.4.[14–17]

Spinal Cord Injury Secondary to Vascular Disease

Spinal Arteriovenous Malformation

Extramedullary spinal arteriovenous malformations arise from fistulas between an artery (high pressure) and a vein (low pressure) at the spinal cord, which shunts the blood, causing compression or "steal phenomenon."[9] It can occur at the nerve root, dorsal lower thoracic, or lumbar cord with symptoms of neurogenic claudication, leg weakness, sensory deficits, back pain, and/or neurogenic bladder. Most common symptoms are progressive. It is most common in middle-aged and older patients. The diagnosis is made by spinal angiography, and treatment is surgical or embolization of the fistula.

- Type I (dural arteriovenous fistulas) are the most common (85%)
- Type II intramedullary, true arteriovenous malformations nidus
- Type III juvenile, entire spinal canal
- Type IV intradural/extramedullary, rare

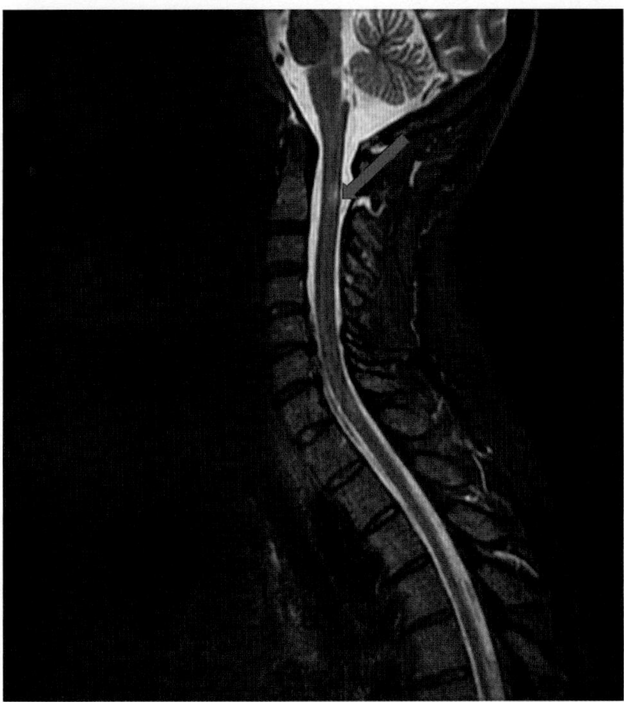

Fig. 40.4 Case of 48-year-old female patient with relapsing–remitting multiple sclerosis. Cervical spine MRI T2 sequence with a focal hyperintensities *(arrow)* at the level of C2–C3 and C5. Short Segment lesion <3 levels dorsally located.

Spinal Cord Stroke

A spinal cord stroke is caused by insufficient blood flow in the aorta or segmental arteries (usually preceded by hypotension), which reduces blood flow in the anterior spinal artery. Abdominal aorta disease and aortic

Table 40.2 Types of Multiple Sclerosis

Type	Presentation	
Relapsing–remitting	Acute attacks return to baseline 4–8 weeks	
Secondary progressive	Progressive neurologic deficits without returning to baseline	Common sequelae of relapsing–remitting (10–20 years onset)
Primary progressive	Continuous and progressive neurologic decline without attacks	Worst prognosis

Table 40.3 List of Most Common Spinal Tumors Classified by Anatomic Location

Intradural tumors (40%–45%)	Intradural intramedullary (15%–33%)	Ependymomas
		Astrocytomas
		Others: oligodendroglioma, hemangioblastomas, lipoma, metastases
	Intradural extramedullary (66%–75%)	Nerve sheath tumors (schwannomas, neurofibromas)
		Meningiomas
		Myxopapillary ependymoma
		Others: paragangliomas, drop metastases, epidermoid cysts
Extradural tumors (50%–55%)	Metastatic (90%–95%)	Lung, breast, prostate, lymphoma
	Primary spinal tumors	Plasma cell tumors
		Hemangiomas
		Primary bone tumors (i.e., Osteoid osteoma, osteochondroma, giant cell tumors, osteosarcomas)

Prevalence shown in parentheses.

Table 40.4 Characteristics of the Most Common Spinal Cord Tumors

Spinal Cord Tumors	Anatomical Classification	Most Common Location	Management/ Prognosis	Other Pearls	Histologic Features	MRI Findings
Ependymoma	Intradural intramedullary	Centrally located Cervical more than thoracic	GTR RT if STR Better prognosis if GTR compared with partial resection regardless of radiation therapy	Most common intramedullary tumor in adults in the 2nd to 4th decade	Perivascular pseudorosettes (spoke-wheel pattern)	Diffuse enhancement of mass with gadolinium. Cap sign noted at poles of tumor (hemosiderin deposition) in 1/3 of ependymomas Associated with syringomyelia
Astrocytoma	Intradural intramedullary	Peripherally Cervical	GTR RT if high-grade astrocytoma or progressive disease Poor prognosis with grade III or IV	Most common intramedullary tumor in children Grade 1 associated with NF1	Bipolar piloid cells Eosinophilic Rosenthal fibers	Cap sign usually absent Syringomyelia less frequently
Schwannomas	Intradural extramedullary	At the dorsal nerve roots. Cervical more often than cauda equina and conus more often than thoracic	Mostly benign GTR STR if near critical structures RT not recommended Good prognosis	Associated with NF2	Abundant fibrous tissue Prominent nerve fibers	Enhancing well circumscribed mass Dumbbell shape if extending through dura mater
Neurofibroma				Associated with NF1 (higher risk of malignant transformation)		
Meningioma	Intradural extramedullary	Ventrolateral Females 80% thoracic Males cervical equal to thoracic Ventrolateral location	Mostly benign Asymptomatic patients: followed clinically Mostly GTR 3%–6% recurrence RT if STR or recurrence	Multiple tumors associated with NF2	Formation of lobules separated by septa Psammoma bodies	Dural tail surrounding dural perimeter
Metastatic SC tumors	Extradural	Thoracic spine (60%)	SC compression: steroids and emergent decompression. Poor prognosis if delayed treatment RT urgent if surgery contraindicated or life expectancy <3 months	Lung, breast, prostate most common source		Contrast enhanced extra-dural mass

GTR, Gross total resection; *NF1*, neurofibromatosis type 1; *NF2*, neurofibromatosis type 2; *RT*, radiation therapy; *SC*, spinal cord; *STR*, Subtotal resection.

surgery are the most common causes of spinal cord infarction.[10] Clinical symptoms include muscle weakness and loss of pain/temperature below the level of injury with preservation of soft-touch and proprioception (anterior spinal artery cord syndrome), neurogenic bladder, and bowel. Diagnosis is through MRI, and treatment consists of improving cord perfusion. Prognosis is usually unfavorable for neurological recovery.

Intraspinal Hemorrhage

It can occur at the epidural or subdural space. Intraspinal hemorrhage is associated with trauma, tumors, vascular malformations, and patients with coagulopathy.[18] It presents as back or neck pain at the site of bleeding followed by weakness and sensory deficits below the affected area. Diagnosis is through MRI or CT and treatment is emergent evacuation (Fig. 40.5).

Radiation Myelopathy

Radiation myelopathy is a rare, slowly progressive myelopathy that primarily affects the white matter. Commonly there is a long latency between completion of radiation and symptom onset; it is seen mostly after 9 to 15 months of radiation.[9] Symptoms include motor and sensory deficits below the level of injury.

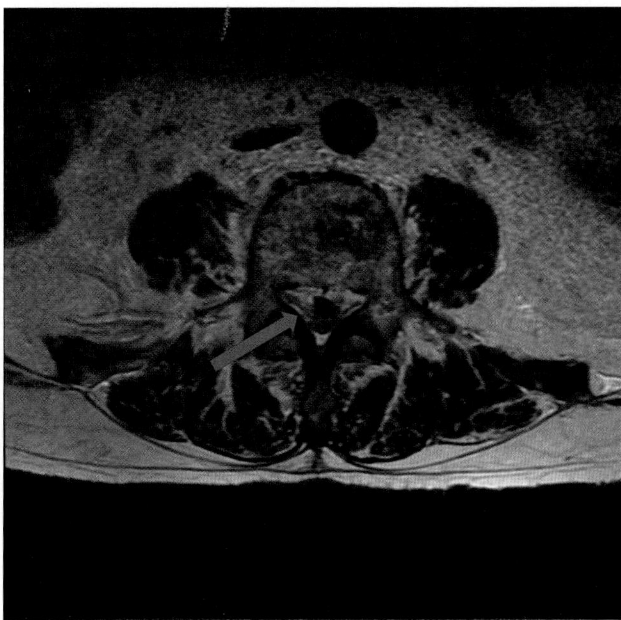

Fig. 40.5 Lumbar spine MRI T2 coronal view of an 87-year-old male chronic anticoagulation with acute compression fractures of L4 and L5 without significant retropulsion. Associated ventral epidural hematoma *(arrow)* resulting in severe spinal canal stenosis at the L3.

Nutritional and Toxic Myelopathies

Subacute Combined Degeneration

Subacute combined degeneration occurs secondary to vitamin B12 deficiency due to inadequate intake (vegan diet), malabsorption (i.e., pernicious anemia), or inactivation of vitamin B12 (i.e., nitrous oxide abuse). Vitamin B12 plays a role in the methylation of components for myelin synthesis. Subacute combined degeneration most commonly affects posterior columns of the spinal cord and lateral corticospinal tract and presents with weakness and impaired vibration and proprioception (Fig. 40.6). Diagnosis is made using blood tests that find decreased B12 levels in the blood and/or increased homocysteine and methylmalonic acid levels. Management involves supplementation of vitamin B12 with good prognosis of recovery.[19]

Spinocerebellar Degeneration

Spinocerebellar degeneration occurs secondary to vitamin E deficiency, most commonly in chronic malabsorption syndromes. Vitamin E protects against oxidative stress and inhibits membrane phospholipid fatty acid peroxidation. It affects dorsal root ganglia, spinocerebellar tracts, the cerebellar cortex, and anterior horn cells and presents with cerebellar ataxia, impaired vibration and proprioception, weakness, and ophthalmoplegia. Diagnosis is made through serum vitamin E levels. Treatment involves oral supplementation, which may improve symptoms.[20]

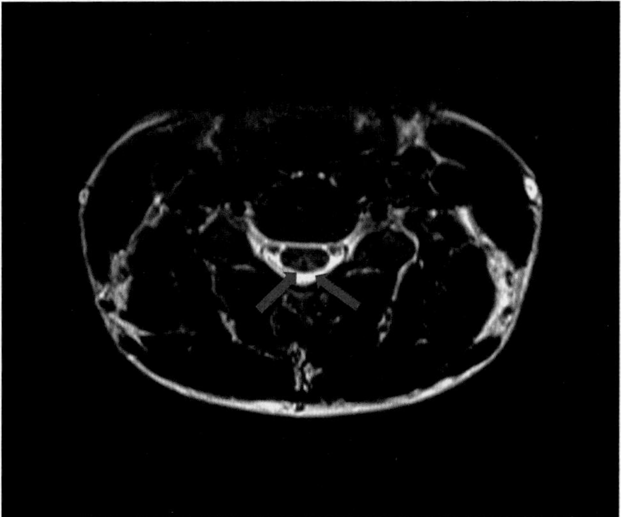

Fig. 40.6 27-year-old male with nitrous oxide abuse resulting in subacute combined degeneration. *Red arrows* indicate subtle T2 hyperintensities within the dorsal columns of the cervical cord.

Copper Deficiency

The most common cause of copper deficiency is a prior history of gastric surgery or excessive zinc ingestion that results in Wallerian degeneration and demyelination of the dorsal columns and brainstem. The clinical presentation consists of sensory ataxia and spastic gait. Diagnosis is made by decreasing serum copper or ceruloplasmin, decreasing 24-hour urinary copper excretion, or increasing zinc serum or urinary levels. Treatment consists of oral supplementation if deficient or discontinuation of excess zinc supplementation.[21]

Lathyrism

Lathyrism is seen after ingestion of *Lathyrus sativus* (legume; Indian peas). It causes an increase in oxidative stress and impairs the mitochondrial oxidative phosphorylation chain. It presents with spastic paraparesis with possible sphincter involvement. Diagnosis is made by history of exposure and serum thiocyanate levels. Deficits are usually permanent, and there are no specific treatments.[19–22]

Hereditary and Congenital Myelopathies

Hereditary Spastic Paraplegia

Hereditary spastic paraplegia (HSP) is associated with approximately 50 genes (including autosomal dominant, autosomal recessive, and X-linked), autosomal dominant accounts for 75%–80% of cases, and spastic paraplegia 4 that is caused by Spastin gene mutations is the most common type of autosomal dominant HSP. Age of onset is infancy through the seventh decade,[23] with an infantile onset often associated with delayed independent walking. HSP may be classified as pure or complicated.[23–25] The clinical hallmark of pure HSP is a gradual and progressive spastic weakness of the lower extremities, usually symmetric, with variable involvement of impaired vibration sensation and autonomic dysfunction and spasticity being much more prominent than weakness.[23] Complicated HSP includes symptoms of optic nerve atrophy, ataxia, dystonia, deafness retinitis pigmentosa, amyotrophy, peripheral neuropathy, pseudobulbar signs, mental retardation, and adult-onset dementia. Diagnosis is clinical and confirmed with genetic testing. Routine laboratory testing is commonly done to exclude other etiologies.[24] CSF and electromyogram and nerve conduction velocity are typically unremarkable.[24,25] MRI is usually grossly unremarkable, with thinning of the cervical and thoracic spinal cord reported on some occasions.[24] Treatment consists of symptomatic management.

Spinal Muscular Atrophy

Spinal muscular atrophy (SMA) is characterized by progressive flaccid weakness and muscle atrophy secondary to selective degeneration of the spinal cord LMNs. Autosomal recessive SMA is caused by mutations of *SMN1* (a telomeric gene) and accounts for approximately 95% of all cases. Morbidity and mortality are inversely correlated with age of onset. Four types of SMA exist (Table 40.5).

Bulbospinal Muscular Atrophy

Bulbospinal muscular atrophy, or Kennedy syndrome, is an X-linked form of SMA. It is the most frequent type of adult-onset SMA caused by a CAG expansion in the androgen receptor gene.[23] The average age of onset is the third decade with cramps and difficulty chewing due to masseter muscle weakness common. It is associated with proximal muscle weakness and other bulbar muscle involvement such as perioral and tongue fasciculations, tongue atrophy, dysphagia, and dysarthria. Nonneurological symptoms include gynecomastia, oligospermia, testicular atrophy, and erectile dysfunction.

Poliomyelitis and Postpolio Syndrome

Poliomyelitis is caused by poliovirus, of the enterovirus family, and can affect both children and adults.[26,27] The mode of infection is through the alimentary tract carried by sewage, polluted rivers, and flies, and contracted by ingestion of contaminated water or food and hand to mouth or fecal–oral transmission.[27] Early symptoms include fever, drowsiness, headache, nausea, vomiting, constipation, and sore throat, which can then progress to a major illness affecting the central nervous system that presents with headaches and back pain.[27,28] It targets the motor neurons of the anterior horn cells of the spinal cord and the brainstem, leading to an asymmetric muscular paralysis with varying severity, including autonomic disturbances and central respiratory depression.[26,27] After the acute phase, there is a progressive recovery phase associated with the reinnervation process of those muscle fibers denervated during the initial phase through axonal spouting,[26] which occurs through a long period of months to years.[28] Reinnervation is not complete and residual deficits are common.[26,27] Long-term effects of poliomyelitis include chronic pain (mainly due to degenerative joint disease), muscle weakness, and fatigue.[28] Treatment is supportive, including a focused rehabilitation program.[26]

Postpolio syndrome is defined as a clinical entity affecting polio survivors with the onset of new symptoms, several years after the initial polio attack, following a period of stability.[26] Postpolio syndrome is a

Table 40.5 Types of Spinal Muscular Atrophy

Type 1	Type 2	Type 3	Type 4
Werdnig-Hoffman Disease (WHD)	Chronic WHD	Kugelberg-Welander	
50% of cases	25% of cases	25% of cases	Very rare
Birth–6 months	6–18 months (chronic infantile form)	After 18 months (chronic juvenile form)	Adult onset
Diffuse weakness (proximal>distal) and severe hypotonia, poor feeding, respiratory failure (cause of death)	Delayed acquisition of major motor milestones. Survival 2 years, respiratory failure.	Slowly progressive proximal weakness, ambulatory but with difficulties standing up from a chair or using stairs	Benign course, normal life expectancy
SMN1 deletions with 2 copies of *SMN2*	*SMN1* point mutation with 3 or more copies of *SMN2*	*SMN1* point mutation gene with 3 or more *SMN2* copies	
Grouped muscle fiber atrophy with predominance type 1 fibers			

diagnosis of exclusion, and the following criteria must be met:[26,27,29]

- Confirmed prior medical history of poliomyelitis.
- Partial or almost complete neurological recovery after the acute period.
- Period of neurological stability usually lasting for at least 15 years.
- New sudden onset and quickly progressing muscle weakness with at least two new symptoms including:
  - Excessive fatigue
  - Muscle or joint pain
  - Muscle atrophy
  - Cold intolerance

The pathophysiology of postpolio syndrome is poorly understood and thought to be multifactorial,[26,27,29] including possible exhaustion of the denervation–reinnervation process that occurred after acute disease, a defect in neuromuscular conduction and exhaustion of acetylcholine stores, autoimmune inflammatory process, or reactivation of residual poliovirus.[26,30]

Review Questions

1. Which of the following patterns of the neurologic deficit would be most likely after a 75-year-old male had a hypotension episode during an aortic aneurysm repair surgery 8 weeks ago?
   a. Reduced proprioception in the lower extremities, with preserved motor function and pain/temperature sensation in all extremities
   b. Saddle anesthesia with bladder/bowel dysfunction
   c. Upper extremity weakness with preserved lower extremity strength
   d. Weakness and reduced pain/temperature sensation with preserved proprioception in the lower extremities
2. The most common cause of spasticity in patients >55-years-old is:
   a. Epidural abscess compressing the cord
   b. Cervical spondylotic myelopathy
   c. Anterior cord syndrome
   d. Multiple sclerosis
3. Which form of multiple sclerosis has the worst prognosis?
   a. Relapsing–remitting
   b. Primary progressive
   c. Secondary progressive
4. Clinically definite ALS according to the "Escorial Criteria scale" is defined:
   a. Clinical or electrophysiologic evidence by the presence of lower motor neuron signs and upper motor neuron signs at bulbar region and two spine regions.
   b. Clinical or electrophysiologic evidence by the presence of lower motor neuron signs and upper motor neuron signs at two spine regions and upper motor neuron signs that are rostral to the lower motor neuron signs.
   c. Clinical or electrophysiologic evidence by the presence of lower motor neuron signs and upper motor neuron signs in one region or upper motor neuron signs are rostral to the lower motor neuron sign.
5. A 17-year-old female presents to your office due to a history of falls that she believes are due to lower extremity weakness. She first notices that when standing, she needs to use her hands to "walk-up" her body. Which lower motor neuron disease does she most likely have?
   a. Kugelberg-Welander disease
   b. Chronic Werdnig-Hoffmann disease
   c. Werdnig-Hoffman disease
   d. ALS
6. A 28-year-old male patient with a history of substance abuse presents to the emergency department with complaints of difficulty walking. A physical examination shows mostly intact strength in all extremities with impaired proprioception. MRI shows T2 hyperintensities posteriorly in the cord. What is the most common cause of his symptoms?
   a. Disc herniation
   b. Spinal cord infarction
   c. Nitrous oxide abuse
   d. Psychogenic

REFERENCES

1. Ross MA. Acquired motor neuron disorders. *Neurol Clin [Internet]*. 1997 Aug;15(3):481–500. https://linkinghub.elsevier.com/retrieve/pii/S0733861905703303.
2. Cifu DX.. In: Eapen BC, Johns JS, Kowalske K, Lew HL, Miller MA, Worsowicz G, eds. *Braddom's Physical Medicine & Rehabilitation*. 6th ed. : Elsevier; 2021:1049–1100.
3. Joyce N, Carter GT. Motor neuron disorders. In: Braddom RL, ed. *Physical Medicine & Rehabilitation*. 4th ed. Philadelphia: Elsevier Saunders; 2011:1041–1064.
4. Jaiswal MK. Riluzole and edaravone: a tale of two amyotrophic lateral sclerosis drugs. *Medicinal Research Reviews*. 2019;39(2):733–748.
5. Tavee J, Levin K. Myelopathy due to degenerative diseases and structural spine diseases. *CONTINUUM: American Academy Neurology*. 2015;21(1):52–66.
6. Toeldano M, Bartleson JD. Cervical spondylotic myelopathy. *Neurol Clin*. 2013;31:287–305.
7. Heary RF, Agarwal N, Ghogawala Z, Amankulor N. Spondylotic and myelopathic myelopathies. In: Kirschblum S, Lin VW, eds. *Spinal Cord Medicine*. 3rd ed. : Springer Publishing Company; 2019:635–644.
8. Lyons JL. Myelopathy associated with microorganisms. *Contin Lifelong Learn Neurol [Internet]*. 2015;21:100–120. https://journals.lww.com/00132979-201502000-00011.
9. Gorman PH, York HS, Thomas FP, Kamin SS. Nontraumatic myelopathies. In: Kirshblum S, Lin VW, eds. *Spinal Cord Medicine*. New York: Springer Publishing Company; 2018:584–605.
10. Rabinstein AA. Vascular myelopathies. *Contin Lifelong Learn Neurol [Internet]*. 2015;21:67–83. https://journals.lww.com/00132979-201502000-00009.

11. Greenberg BM, Frohman EM. Immune-mediated myelopathies. *CONTINUUM Lifelong Learning in Neurology*. 2015;21(1):121–131.
12. West TW, Hess C, Cree BAC. Acute transverse myelitis: demyelinating, inflammatory, and infectious myelopathies. *Semin Neurol.* 2012;32(2):97–113.
13. Kupershtein I, Vivies M. Spinal and spinal cord infections. In: Kirshblum S, Campagnolo DI, eds. *Spinal Cord Medicine*. 2nd ed. Philadelphia: Lipincott Williams & Wilkins; 2011:595.
14. Wu J, Ranjan S. Neoplastic myelopathies. *Contin Lifelong Learn Neurol [Internet]*. 2018;24(2):474–496. https://journals.lww.com/00132979-201804000-00008.
15. Chamberlain MC. Neoplastic myelopathies. *Contin Lifelong Learn Neurol [Internet]*. 2015;21:132–145. https://journals.lww.com/continuum/Abstract/2015/02000/Neoplastic_Myelopathies.13.aspx.
16. Hwang LS, Benzel EC. Tumors of the spinal cord and spinal canall. In: Kirshblum S, Lin VW, eds. *Spinal Cord Medicine*. 3rd ed. New York: Demos Medical Publishing; 2019:1473–1510.
17. Arnautovic K, Arnautovic A. Extramedullary intradural spinal tumors: a review of modern diagnostic and treatment options and a case of series. *Bosn J Basic Med Sci.* 2009;9(Supplement 1):S40–S45.
18. Wisoff JH. Spontaneous intraspinal hemorrhage. In: Wilkins RH, Rengachary SS, eds. *Neurosurgery*. New York: McGraw-Hill; 1996:2559–2565.
19. Ramalho J, Nunes RH, da Rocha AJ, Castillo M. Toxic and metabolic myelopathies. *Semin Ultrasound, CT MRI [Internet]*. 2016;37(5):448–465. https://doi.org/10.1053/j.sult.2016.05.010.
20. Schwendimann RN. Metabolic, nutritional, and toxic myelopathies. *Neurol Clin [Internet]*. 2013;31(1):207–218. https://doi.org/10.1016/j.ncl.2012.09.002.
21. Kumar N. Metabolic and toxic myelopathies. *Semin Neurol [Internet]*. 2012;32(02):123–136. https://www.thieme-connect.de/DOI/DOI?10.1055/s-0032-1322583.
22. Goodman BP. Metabolic and toxic causes of myelopathy. *Contin Lifelong Learn Neurol [Internet]*. 2015;21(February):84–99. https://journals.lww.com/00132979-201502000-00010.
23. Hedera P. Hereditary myelopathies. *Contin Lifelong Learn Neurol [Internet]*. 2018;24(2):523–550. https://journals.lww.com/00132979-201804000-00010.
24. Maas J. Inherited myelopathies. *Semin Neurol [Internet]*. 2012;32(02):114–122. https://www.thieme-connect.de/DOI/DOI?10.1055/s-0032-1322581.
25. Kamin S. Vascular, nutritional, and other nontraumatic conditions of the spinal cord. In: Kirshblum S, Campagnolo DI, eds. *Spinal Cord Medicine*. 2nd ed. Philadelphia: Lipincott Williams & Wilkins; 2011:608–609.
26. Tiffreau V, Rapin A, Serafi R, et al. Post-polio syndrome and rehabilitation. *Ann Phys Rehabil Med [Internet]*. 2010;53(1):42–50. https://linkinghub.elsevier.com/retrieve/pii/S1877065709002838.
27. Menant JC, Gandevia SCPoliomyelitis. *Handbook of Clinical Neurology [Internet]*. 2018;159:337–344. https://linkinghub.elsevier.com/retrieve/pii/B9780444639165000215.
28. Joyce N, Carter GT, Krivickas LS. Adult motor neuron disease. In: Kirshblum S, Campagnolo DI, eds. *Spinal Cord Medicine*. 2nd ed. Philadelphia: Lipincott Williams & Wilkins; 2011:634–635.
29. Ramaraj R. Post-poliomyelitis syndrome: clinical features and management. *Br J Hosp Med [Internet]*. 2007;68(12):648–650. https://www.magonlinelibrary.com/doi/10.12968/hmed.2007.68.12.648.
30. Beh SC, Greenberg BM, Frohman T, Frohman EM. Transverse myelitis. *Neurol Clin [Internet]*. 2013;31(1):79–138. https://linkinghub.elsevier.com/retrieve/pii/S0733861912000692.

CHAPTER

41 Myelopathy Without Specified Etiology

Mara C. Harris, Blake Fechtel, and Camilo Castillo

OUTLINE

Description/Definitions

- Myelopathies, meaning "diseases of the spinal cord" (and generally also referring to their neurologic sequelae), can be traumatic or nontraumatic.
- Myelopathies not due to trauma, spondyloarthropathy, mass, ischemia, or hemorrhage often require significant time and numerous diagnostic modalities.
- One cohort found that one-third of these patients' diagnoses changed over the 2 years following onset.[1]
- Like patients with myelopathies of a known cause, patients with "myelopathies of unspecified etiology" benefit greatly from rehabilitation services. However, they also represent a pathology where the physiatrist plays a critical part in the diagnostic team.

Epidemiology

Incidence of myelopathy: 40–80/100,000,000 per year globally[2]

- Traumatic causes make up to 90%[2]

Myelopathy of unspecified etiology

- 16%–27% of acute myelopathies.[3–6] However, some reports of unknown myelopathy have been seen in up to 60% of patients[7]

Evaluation and Diagnosis

- The diagnosis of yet unspecified myelopathy relies on four principal features (also illustrated in Table 41.1)[4]:
  - Timing of onset
  - Course of deficits
  - Imaging findings
  - Laboratory studies
- All patients presenting with myelopathy require prompt evaluation by magnetic resonance imaging (MRI); however, it is not uncommon for a patient to have myelopathic symptoms with a normal MRI[8]
  - More follow-up yields more information
  - Follow-up commonly lasts months or years as disease and imaging evolve
  - Patients often have multiple tentative diagnoses that ultimately change
  - In some cohorts, only ~50% reach a final diagnosis
  - The modalities that most contribute to a final diagnosis include repeat MRI of the brain and spine, cerebrospinal fluid, and blood testing[1,4–7,9]
  - Myelopathy of unknown etiology progresses into multiple sclerosis (MS) in a wide range of cases (up to 80%)
  - Although rare and a diagnosis of exclusion, myelopathy's nonorganic causes may be characterized by inconsistencies in history, imaging, laboratory results, and presentation inconsistencies[10]
- Fig. 41.1 highlights an algorithm that can be used as a diagnostic tool when assessing patients who have a myelopathy of unspecified etiology

History

- A detailed history investigating various risk factors, exposures, personal histories and family histories is valuable to steer subsequent investigations and reduce time to diagnosis
  - Family history of neurologic disease
  - History, risk, or symptoms of malignancy
  - History or symptoms of autoimmune diseases such as Behçet syndrome, lupus, or sarcoidosis
  - Exposure to radiation
  - Common causes of infection
  - Presence of a viral prodrome
  - Risk factors for nutrient deficiency

Table 41.1 Comparison of Principal Features of Common Myelopathies

	Average Age (years)	Major Neurological Symptoms	Clinical Outcome: Good/Fair/Poor	CSF Oligoclonal Bands: +/–[a]	Enhancement of the Cord Lesion: +/–	Multiple Cord Lesion: +/–	Brain Lesions on MRI: +/–
Multiple sclerosis	<50	Sensory deficits	Good	+	+	+/–	+
Spinal cord infarction	>50	Motor deficits and sphincter dysfunction	Poor	–	+/–	–	–
Parainfectious myelopathy	+/–50	Motor and sensory deficits	Good	–	+	–	–
Antiphospholipid syndrome	<50	Motor and sensory deficits	Fair	–	+	–	–
Myelopathy of unknown origin	<50	Sensory deficits	Good	–	+	–	–

[a]Clinical outcome according to the Lipton and Teasdall scale: +, means present: –, means absent.
Nowak DA, Mutzenbach S, Fuchs HH. Acute myelopathy. Retrospective clinical, laboratory, MRI and outcome analysis of 49 cases. *J Clin Neurosci.* 2004;11(2):145–152.
CSF, Cerebral spinal fluid.

- Keep an open mind; jumping to a premature diagnosis limits workup and delays ultimate diagnosis and disease-modifying treatment[11]

Onset and Progression

- Much like any neurologic disease, the timing of the myelopathy onset and change is often characteristic of the fundamental pathology
  - Hyperacute onset (hours to days) is generally reserved for infarction, hemorrhage, trauma, and severe neuromyelitis optica spectrum disease (NMOSD) cases
  - Acute and subacute onset (days to weeks), represents the largest group of differential diagnoses; it is the most common presentation of NMOSD. It includes acute infectious causes (abscess or postviral), MS, other autoimmune causes (such as lupus, Sjogren syndrome, or antiphospholipid syndrome), as well as functional disorders
  - Chronic and progressive onset (weeks to months) is seen more commonly among neoplastic/paraneoplastic causes, metabolic deficiencies, vascular malformations, hereditary disease, chronic infections (syphilis, HIV, human T-lymphotropic virus), and sarcoidosis[1,4–7,9]

Magnetic Resonance Imaging

- By the time physiatry is involved with the workup and care of acute myelopathies, they have generally had acute trauma, stroke, and hemorrhage imaging. As such, the **MRI with and without gadolinium** will be the most common and most valuable imaging tool in these patients.
- MRI is valuable because of the diagnostic value of the number and distribution of lesions in the CNS and identifying whether any lesions are asymptomatic (common in MS uncommon in NMOSD); diagnostic MRI imaging should always include the brain and the entire spinal cord.[9,12]
- Because many myelopathies, of unspecified etiology, are later diagnosed as MS, it is crucial to know the MRI findings atypical of MS prompting consideration of alternate pathologies (Table 41.2).[13]
- MRI findings in otherwise undiagnosed, nontraumatic myelopathies are assessed by three factors: the number (and location) of lesions, whether cord lesions are short (<3 vertebral segments in sagittal view) or long, and the axial distribution of cord lesions. The longitudinal extension of spinal impairment, the clinical correlation, and results of other complementary tests help with the diagnostic approach.[9,14]
- Testable patterns include that malignancies tend to create more eccentric lesions or lesions with irregular borders. In contrast, target lesions are more likely infectious or granulomatous (and often gadolinium-enhancing).
- The most common primary spinal cord malignancy, ependymoma, is a malignancy of the cerebral spinal fluid (CSF)-producing cells and commonly results in rostral and/or caudal cysts resulting from aberrant CSF production.
- Long, symmetric dorsal column involvement is more common in metabolic disease, particularly DNA

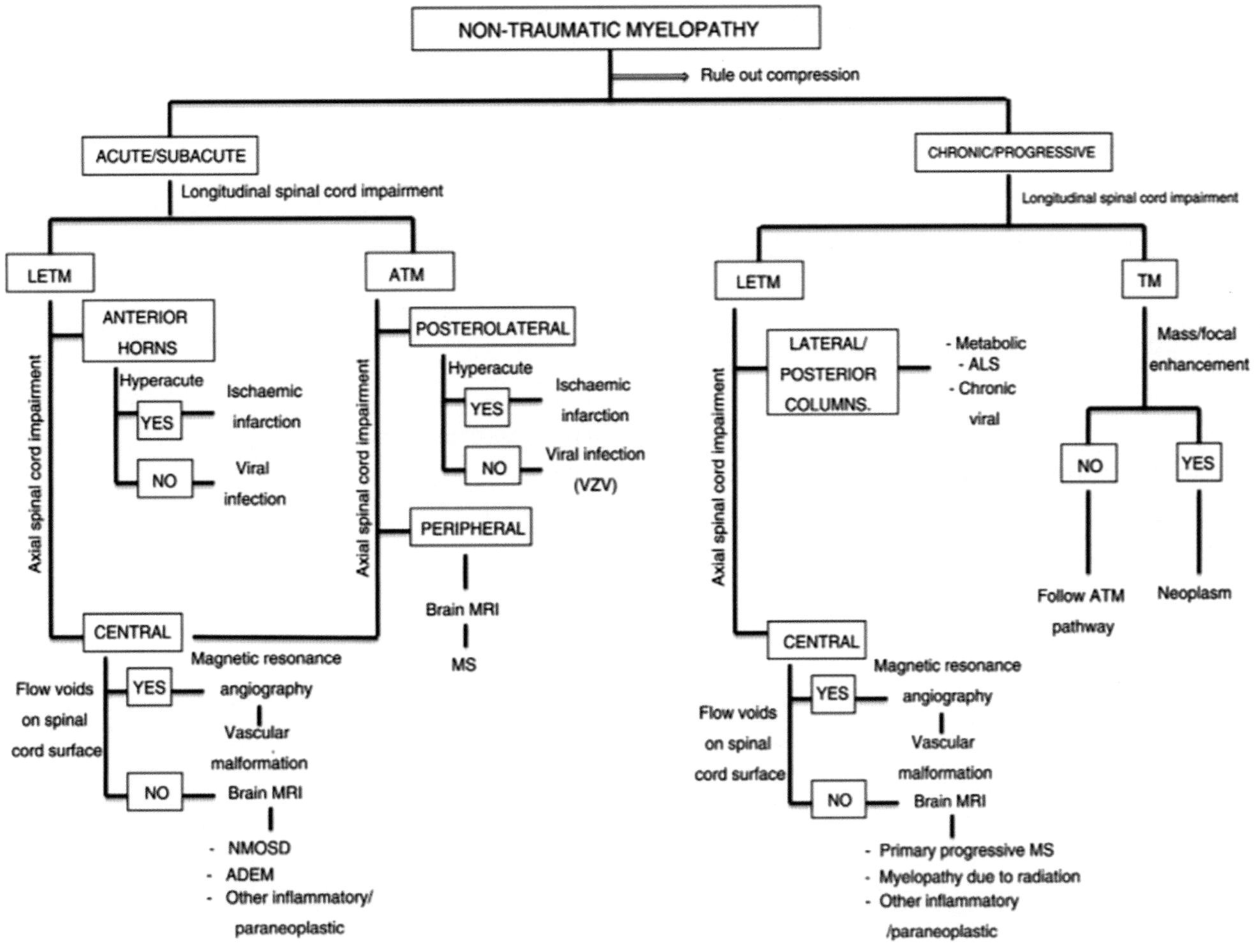

Fig. 41.1 Algorithm for Diagnostic Approach to Nontraumatic Myelopathies. *ADEM*, Acute disseminated encephalomyelitis; *ALS*, amyotrophic lateral sclerosis; *ATM*, acute transverse myelopathy; *LETM*, longitudinally extensive transverse myelitis; *MRI*, magnetic resonance imaging; *MS*, multiple sclerosis; *NMOSD*, neuromyelitis optica spectrum disorder; *TM*, transverse myelopathy. (From Herrera Herrera I, Garrido Morro I, Guzmán de Villoria Lebiedziejewski J, Ordoñez González C, Rovira À. Clinical-radiological approach to nontraumatic myelopathy. *Radiologia*. 2020;62(6):464–480. English, Spanish.)

Table 41.2 Magnetic Resonance Imaging (MRI) Findings Atypical for Multiple Sclerosis (MS)- Less Likely to Be MS in Individuals <45 Years Old

Atypical MRI Finding	Other Diagnostic Probabilities With Similar MRI Findings
Very small lesions (<3 mm)	NSWMA Vasculopathies Migraine
Absence of ovoid lesions	NSWMA Vasculopathies Migraine
Peripheric - subcortical - localization of white matter lesions rather than periventricular	NSWMA Vasculopathies Migraine
Despite the presence of a large number of subcortical lesions either no or only a few juxtacortical and/or periventricular lesions	NSWMA Vasculopathies Migraine
Absence of posterior fossa, corpus callosum and spinal cord lesions	NSWMA
Symmetrical/semi-symmetrical lesions	NSWMA inherited disorders including CADASIL
Disproportionally large corpus callosum lesions	Susac syndrome NMOSD Malignant primary brain tumors and lymphoma

Continued

Table 41.2 Magnetic Resonance Imaging (MRI) Findings Atypical for Multiple Sclerosis (MS)- Less Likely to Be MS in Individuals <45 Years Old – cont'd	
No change in successive MRIs - all MRIs are the same!	NSWMA
No gadolinium enhancement in any MRI	NSWMA Migraine Most genetic disorders
Persistent gadolinium enhancement in all MRIs	Vascular lesions, e.g., venous developmental anomalies
Continuous gadolinium enhancement in successive MRIs over many months	Neurosarcoidosis Some infectious diseases
Family members with similar "identical" MRI!	Genetic disorders
Lesions with prominent mass effect	Tumors AIIDLs Some infections Granulomatous disorders
Up/downward (edematous) extension of large brainstem lesions	NBD Tumors
Longitudinally extensive spinal cord lesions	NMOSD MOG-myelopathies Neurosarcoidosis NBD Spinal cord vascular malformations/dural fistula Tumors

AIIDLs, Atypical idiopathic inflammatory demyelinating lesions; *CADASIL*, cerebral autosomal dominant arteriopathy with subcortical infarcts and leukoencephalopathy; *CNS*, central nervous system; *MOG*, myelin oligodendrocyte glycoprotein; *NBD*, Neuro-Behçet disease; *NMOSD*, neuromyelitis optica spectrum disorder; *NSWMA*, nonspecific white matter abnormalities.
From Siva A. Common clinical and imaging conditions misdiagnosed as multiple sclerosis: a current approach to the differential diagnosis of multiple sclerosis. *Neurol Clin.* 2018;36(1):69–117.

Table 41.3 CSF Analysis

	Cell Count (cells/µl) Mean (range)	Cell Count >30 cells/µl	Protein Level (g/l) Mean (range)	Oligoclonal Bands in Cerebral Spinal Fluid
Multiple sclerosis (*n* = 31)	8.4 (0–35)	2 (6%)	0.39 (0.20–0.79)	30 (97%)
Spinal cord infarction (*n* = 4)	4.8 (0–19)	0 (0%)	0.82 (0.41–1.60)	0 (0%)
Parainfectious myelopathy (*n* = 4)	44.8 (22–57)	3 (75%)	1.22 (0.55–2.73)	0 (0%)
Antiphospholipid syndrome (*n* =1)	0	–	0.30	0(0%)
Myelopathy of unknown origin (*n* =9)	2.2 (0–8)	0 (0%)	0.44 (0.26–0.55)	1 (11%)

From Nowak DA, Mutzenbach S, Fuchs HH. Acute myelopathy. Retrospective clinical, laboratory, MRI and outcome analysis of 49 cases. *J Clin Neurosci.* 2004;11(2):145–152.

synthesis pathology, such as B12 deficiency, folate deficiency, or intrathecal methotrexate toxicity (although copper deficiency can also present in this way).

- It is worth noting that these patterns help but are generally not definitive. Some diseases (particularly sarcoidosis and NMOSD) can present in several ways, including resembling other conditions.

Laboratory Studies

- The CSF assessment for xanthochromia elevated protein, glucose, immunoglobulin's (oligoclonal bands or immunoglobulin G index), and cytology (malignant or pleocytosis) can further help steer diagnosis. This is further illustrated in Table 41.3.[4]
- If malignancy is suspect, cytology can assist with identification and diagnosis without surgery.
- Viral polymerase chain reaction (PCR) from CSF, though not particularly sensitive, may still be useful.
- Serum testing for vitamins, autoantibodies, and systemic manifestations of the myelopathy cause can help identify the cause or guide further studies.
- Of note, anti-myelin oligodendrocyte glycoprotein (anti-MOG) and anti-aquaporin four antibodies should be tested from serum rather than CSF, as serum studies are more sensitive.

Other Studies

- Some of the most challenging pathologies to identify include sarcoidosis, paraneoplastic disease, CNS manifesting systemic autoimmune, and seronegative NMOSD. This is due to the variety of ways they can present and their variation in test results throughout the course of the disease.

- Looking for the systemic manifestations may assist, such as looking for perihilar sarcoidosis, serum autoimmune antibodies, or even positron emission tomography (PET) scans for malignancy or disease lesions that are more amenable to biopsy or sampling.

Rehabilitation

Although myelopathy's etiology may remain unspecified for weeks, months, years, or indefinitely, our rehabilitation goals stay the same. Rehabilitation of spinal cord injury (SCI) patients, as a whole, focuses on three primary objectives: improving functional outcomes, promoting independence, and preventing secondary complications.[15]

- Improving functional outcomes: A patient's rehabilitation program is designed to address their specific deficits. To improve functional outcomes, patients work closely with members of the rehabilitation team to manage their functional deficits with physical skill training, including mat activities, transfers, wheelchair skills, functional electrical stimulation, standing, and ambulation.[15–18]
- Promoting independence: This can be achieved through adaptive equipment, home modifications, driving training, and vocational rehabilitation. SCI education plays a vital role in promoting independence and empowering patients to actively direct their care.[15]
- Preventing secondary complications: Secondary complications can be a significant cause of morbidity and mortality in SCI patients. A critical component of the rehabilitation process is educating patients and their caregivers on preventing and recognizing the various complications.

Prognosis

- Depending on the study, 33%–58% of myelopathy cases of unspecified etiology ultimately ended with a diagnosis while the patient was alive.[1,6,9]
- Postmortem examination allows for ultimate diagnosis in the remaining cases.[6,12]
- MS is the most common etiology, accounting for approximately 25%–50% of myelopathy cases of unspecified etiology.[6]
- Because these patients represent various diseases, the prognosis of myelopathies of unspecified etiology is also highly variable and challenging to study.
- In a study looking at long-term outcomes of patients with acute and subacute myelopathies, it was found that 74% of patients with myelopathy of unspecified etiology were able to continue the same or a similar level of vocational activity.[11]

Conclusions

- Myelopathies of unspecified origin are not uncommon
- It is important to develop a thorough and systematic approach for the evaluation of myelopathy to have the best chance of reaching a diagnosis
- In cases where the etiology remains undetermined, it is important to maintain long-term follow-up and be mindful of specific diagnostic features that may reveal themselves with time[14]

Review Questions

1. A 65-year-old single White male presents with repeated mechanical falls. On examination, motor strength is normal; however, he has marked reduced proprioception, worse in his lower extremities, and decreased sensation to vibration. He has a T2 hyperintensity lesion on MRI spanning C7 to T3 symmetrically, affecting the bilateral dorsal columns. What would you expect to see on complete blood count?
   a. Elevated white blood cells, predominately neutrophils
   b. Thrombocytopenia
   c. Microcytic anemia
   d. Macrocytic anemia
   e. Poikilocytosis
2. With the same patient, which historical detail would NOT contribute to your clinical suspicion?
   a. Poor diet and a history of numerous dental procedures using nitrous oxide
   b. Gastric bypass with chronic proton pump inhibitor and H2 blocker use
   c. Protein calorie malnutrition and chronic rheumatoid arthritis treated with methotrexate
   d. Thyroid malignancy status post radioactive iodine therapy
   e. Alcoholic with a history of foregut resection from bleeding peptic ulcer
3. A 36-year-old White female with a history of right-hand weakness and positive Hoffman sign, as well as MRI evidence of a cervical white matter lesion 3 months ago, comes to your clinic for follow-up of a new MRI. On review, their original cord lesion is unchanged or even smaller, but they have a new lesion in a white matter tract of the left parietal lobe. A thorough examination reveals her hand strength has improved mildly, and there are no new deficits. This patient's most probable diagnosis is:
   a. Amyotrophic lateral sclerosis
   b. NMOSD
   c. Paraneoplastic syndrome
   d. Multiple sclerosis
   e. Neurocysticercosis

4. A 44-year-old Black female patient presents with right lower extremity weakness and positive Babinski sign that began 2 weeks prior. On imaging, the patient has T2 hyperintensity on the dorsal subpial surface, in addition to a target-shaped lesion affecting <25% of the axial area of the cord, extending from T1–T3 with T1 gadolinium enhancement. CSF shows low glucose, elevated protein, and 10 nucleated cells. During your exam, you note a dry cough, which she attributes to seasonal allergies, even though she states it has been going on for months, despite medications. Which study would be the most reasonable next step in seeking a diagnosis?
   a. CSF viral PCR
   b. Computed tomography (CT) chest
   c. Serum anti-double-stranded DNA, anti-smith, anti-aquaporin-4, and anti-MOG studies
   d. Whole-body PET CT scan
   e. None, order intragluteal penicillin G injection and report to state public health agency
5. Twenty-five-year-old White male presents with a 3-week, progressive lower extremity numbness and weakness affecting the right more than the left. He has also had episodes of bowel and bladder incontinence. MRI shows a central gray matter lesion involving the conus medullaris extending four spinal segments. CSF studies show mildly elevated protein, four nucleated cells. What are your next diagnostic steps?
   a. CSF viral PCR studies
   b. Serum anti-MOG and anti-aquaporin-4 testing, in addition to conus angiographic studies
   c. Serum copper and ceruloplasmin concentrations
   d. CT chest
   e. Brain stem biopsy

REFERENCES

1. Gårde A, Kjellin KG. Diagnostic significance of cerebrospinal-fluid examinations in myelopathy. *Acta Neurol Scand.* 1971;47(5):555–568.
2. World Health Organization. Spinal cord injury. https://www.who.int/news-room/fact-sheets/detail/spinal-cord-injury.
3. Pinto WBV, de R, Souza PVS, de, Albuquerque MVC, de, Dutra LA, Pedroso JL, Barsottini OGP. Clinical and epidemiological profiles of non-traumatic myelopathies. *Arq Neuropsiquiatr.* 2016;74(2):161–165.
4. Nowak DA, Mutzenbach S, Fuchs HH. Acute myelopathy. Retrospective clinical, laboratory, MRI and outcome analysis of 49 cases. *J Clin Neurosci.* 2004;11(2):145–152.
5. de Seze J. Acute myelopathies: clinical, laboratory and outcome profiles in 79 cases. *Brain.* 2001;124(8):1509–1521.
6. Martí-Fábregas J, Martínez JM, Illa I, Escartín A. Myelopathy of unknown etiology. A clinical follow-up and MRI study of 57 cases. *Acta Neurol Scand.* 1989;80(5):455–460.
7. Nowak DA, Mutzenbach S, Topka H. Acute myelopathy of unknown aetiology: a follow-up investigation. *J Clin Neurosci.* 2006;13(3):339–342.
8. Wong SH, Boggild M, Enevoldson TP, Fletcher NA. Myelopathy but normal MRI: where next? *Pract Neurol.* 2008;8(2):90–102.
9. Hübbe P, Dam AM. Spastic paraplegia of unknown origin: a follow-up of 32 patients. *Acta Neurol Scand.* 2009;49(4):536–542.
10. Baker JH, Silver JR. Hysterical paraplegia. *J Neurol Neurosurg Psychiatry.* 1987;50(4):375–382.
11. Debette S, Sèze J, Pruvo J-P, et al. Long-term outcome of acute and subacute myelopathies. *J Neurol.* 2009;256(6):980–988.
12. Marshall J. Spastic paraplegia of middle age; a clinicopathological study. *Lancet.* 1955;268(6865):643–646.
13. Siva A. Common clinical and imaging conditions misdiagnosed as multiple sclerosis: a current approach to the differential diagnosis of multiple sclerosis. *Neurol Clin.* 2018;36(1):69–117.
14. Mariano R, Flanagan EP, Weinshenker BG, Palace J. A practical approach to the diagnosis of spinal cord lesions. *Pract Neurol.* 2018;18(3):187–200.
15. Cifu DX. *Braddom's Physical Medicine and Rehabilitation.* 6th ed. Elsevier; 2020.
16. Herrera Herrera I, Garrido Morro I, Guzmán de Villoria Lebiedziejewski J, Ordoñez González C, Rovira À. Clinical-radiological approach to nontraumatic myelopathy. *Radiologia.* 2020;62(6):464–480. English, Spanish.
17. Zalewski NL, Flanagan EP. Autoimmune and paraneoplastic myelopathies. *Semin Neurol.* 2018;38(3):278–289.
18. Zalewski NL, Flanagan EP, Keegan BM. Evaluation of idiopathic transverse myelitis revealing specific myelopathy diagnoses. *Neurology.* 2018;90(2):e96.

CHAPTER 42

Healthcare Maintenance for Patients With Spinal Cord Injuries/Disorders: Primary, Preventive, and Promotive Care

Mohammed B.A. Bhuiyan, Lisa A. Beck, James Milligan, Cody Unser, and Philippines Cabahug

OUTLINE

Introduction

Health maintenance of persons with spinal cord injuries/disorders (SCI/D) is commonly confined to SCI/D-related care and issues. However, they should be managed via the same continuous standard of care received by persons without SCI/D, including primary, preventive, and promotive health care. SCI medicine specialists in tertiary centers may not be abreast of current recommendations in primary care. On the other hand, health maintenance may be challenging for primary care providers who are not familiar with managing complex secondary medical complications unique to SCI/D. Studies show that although many individuals with SCI/D identify their primary care provider as their first healthcare resource, they also report unmet healthcare needs.[1] It is recommended that persons with SCI/D follow-up on their maintenance care with a physician who is knowledgeable with, but not necessarily specialized in, SCI/D. This promotes a continuum of care while attending to the unique needs of this patient population. Primary care resources available from SCI/D Systems of Care in the Veterans Health Administration (VHA), Academy of Spinal Cord Injury Professionals (ASCIP), and American Spinal Injury Association (ASIA) help deliver maintenance care for persons with SCI/D.[2,3] Evidence-based guidelines regarding health maintenance for persons with SCI do not exist. Based on current national/international guidelines, contemporary research, and published reports, a brief outline is presented below to improve health maintenance of persons with SCI/D.

Primary Care

A comprehensive evaluation, workup, and updated plan of care should be done at least annually. Ideally, individuals should have a consistent provider.[4–7] Table 42.1 provides a health maintenance checklist for annual evaluations.[2]

Adults With Spinal Cord Injuries/Disorders

Standard History and Physical Examination

Evaluate for new or ongoing medical issues, changes in function or mobility, current management, psychosocial concerns, and caregiver issues.[4,6,8]

International Standards for Neurologic Classification of Spinal Cord Injury Examination (ISNCSCI)

The ISNCSCI examination could be performed to reveal any changes in SCI/D level of injury and ASIA impairment scale classification. Common changes are due to neuropathic pain, concurrent stroke, syringomyelia, myelomalacia, new spinal issues, or complications of an existing SCI/D. Follow-up imaging studies such as magnetic resonance imaging or myelogram, as indicated, and neurosurgery consultation should be considered if warranted.[2–4,8,9]

Spinal Cord Injuries/Disorders: Focused History and Clinical Evaluation[2–4,7,9]

The following systemic evaluation relevant to SCI/D is presented here. SCI/D textbooks and concurrent chapters in this book may be referenced for further information.

Genitourinary System

Review the current neurogenic bladder management and satisfaction. Assessment for complications including urinary tract infection (UTI), stone formation, renal damage, and bladder cancer is recommended. Urology consultation and evaluation should be completed every 1–2 years.[10]

Gastrointestinal System

Gastrointestinal complications that result from SCI/D include, but are not limited to, neurogenic bowel, peptic ulcer disease, impaction, diarrhea, constipation, and incontinence. Current bowel regimen should be addressed; bowel care effectiveness may be assessed in terms of frequency, stool consistency, continence, and evacuation time. Continued education about bowel care procedure, timing, positioning, and evacuation is recommended.[11]

Cardiovascular System

Many persons with SCI/D have ongoing cardiovascular issues that warrant evaluation such as autonomic dysreflexia (AD) and orthostatic hypotension. Providers should review patient noted signs and symptoms, triggers, and current management for AD and orthostatic hypotension, and provide education as needed. Referrals to cardiology/other specialty services should be made as deemed appropriate.

Spasticity

Current management of spasticity should be reviewed, including pharmacologic and nonpharmacologic therapy. Pain and spasticity should be discussed with the patient, as they can aggravate each other.

Pulmonary System

Review current pulmonary status management, including sleep-disordered breathing. Inquire about incidence of pneumonia and other pulmonary complications, especially in persons with cervical or thoracic levels of SCI/D.

Bone Health

More than 50% of persons with SCI/D develop osteoporosis within 1 year after injury. Long-term follow-up increases the prevalence rate to >80%. Individuals must be educated and may be offered diagnostic tests in addition to medical management options.

Table 42.1 Health Maintenance Checklist for Spinal Cord Injury-Specific Health Complications[a]

GENITOURINARY
• Review bladder care/program and daily fluid intake: methods (i.e., timed-voiding; Crede maneuver, clean intermittent catheterization; indwelling urethral/suprapubic Foley catheter; s/p bladder augmentation surgery; bladder management of patients with ESRD who still make urine), effectiveness/satisfaction with management, complications (i.e., UTI, stones, incontinence), medications • Assure regular follow-up with urology (urodynamics study every 2 years; surveillance cystoscopy every 1-2 years if person with SCI has a chronic indwelling catheter, as risk of bladder cancer is higher for >10 years)
GASTROINTESTINAL
• Review bowel program: effectiveness, time, diet, oral medication, rectal interventions, complications • Assess diversion colostomy and complications; evaluate stomal function/complications; recommend periodic rectal cleaning (tap water enema every 3 months) to prevent complications, e.g., proctitis, diversion colitis, or abscess formation • Assess ostomies for tube-feeding (PEG tube/gastrostomy tube); recommend cleaning feeding tube at least once a week (flush with carbonated soda; e.g., diet soda)
AUTONOMIC DYSREFLEXIA (in individuals with injuries at T6 spinal cord segment and above)
• Assess for triggers and episodes of autonomic dysreflexia (AD), e.g., bladder, bowel, skin • Consider an AD home kit • Educate about standard AD protocol during each encounter • Consider workup for unexplained AD
SPASTICITY
• Review efficacy of pharmacological and nonpharmacological interventions for spasticity • Monitor liver function tests if on tizanidine (Zanaflex) or dantrolene (Dantrium) • Assess function and interrogate intrathecal baclofen (Lioresal) pump in those with this device; adjust dose and refill pump on time to avoid withdrawal symptoms that could be life threatening • Increased spasticity may indicate SCI complication, e.g., syringomyelia
PULMONARY
• Surveillance for signs/symptoms of sleep-disordered breathing • Review existing pulmonary assistance e.g., CPAP/BiPAP; tracheostomy tube; s/p diaphragmatic pacer; vent support (portable/regular) • Educate about maintenance of pulmonary assistive devices and complications
BONE HEALTH
• DXA at 1- to 2-year intervals • Consider physical modalities (e.g., ambulation, functional electrical stimulation) and pharmacologic management for bone health • Make aware about osteopenia/osteoporosis, which is very common in SCI

Table 42.1 Health Maintenance Checklist for Spinal Cord Injury-Specific Health Complications[a] –Cont'd

SKIN
• Full skin examination and assess risk factors for skin breakdown • Evaluation and management of any ongoing pressure injuries
MOBILITY AIDS
• Assess assistive devices (e.g., cane, walker, AFO/KFO) for patients who are ambulatory • Review precautions for fall prevention • Determine age and wear/tear of wheelchair and cushion • Include wheelchair fit in the differential for acute and chronic health concerns (e.g., pressure injury, shoulder pain) • Periodic seating evaluation (consider referral to PT/OT)
MUSCULOSKELETAL
• Screen for overuse injuries (i.e., shoulder, elbow, wrist) • Assess for complications, e.g., heterotrophic ossification; contracture
PAIN
• Assess for type (neuropathic, nociceptive), interference in life/function, management
SEXUAL AND REPRODUCTIVE HEALTH
• Assess satisfaction, barriers, and if fertility desired
SUPPORT/RESOURCES
• Assess attendant care and social support • Review home safety and equipment
ADDITIONAL CONSIDERATIONS FOR CHILDREN
• Ensure well childcare milestones are met • Begin planning transition of care for adolescence to adult care

AFO/KFO, Ankle-foot orthosis/knee-foot orthosis; *CPAP/BiPAP*, continuous positive airway pressure/bi-level positive airway pressure; *DXA*, dual-energy X-ray absorptiometry; *ESRD*, end-stage renal disease; *PT/OT*, physical therapy/occupational therapy; *SCI*, spinal cord injury; *s/p*, status post; *UTI*, urinary tract infection.

[a]Copyright permission granted by ASIA and Academy of Spinal Cord Injury Professionals.

Skin

Persons with SCI/D must be assessed for any pressure injuries, whether chronic or new in onset. Current management and progression of existing wounds, and prevention of further skin issues, should be reviewed. Consider consultation for optimizing nutrition and seating clinic for mobility equipment assessment and modifications.[12]

Mobility Aids

Most persons with SCI/D use some form of mobility assistance. Assess gait mechanics of those who are ambulatory with assistive devices (cane/walker) and consult physical therapist as needed. Manual and power mobility should be evaluated and adjusted per physical therapy and occupational therapy input to minimize musculoskeletal issues and pressure affect. Provide education on fall precautions and risks.

Musculoskeletal System

Musculoskeletal assessments of persons with SCI/D include evaluation of overuse syndrome, contracture, and abnormal posture. Up to half of persons with SCI/D develop heterotopic ossification beginning at a mean of 12 weeks after injury. Large joints below the level of injury are typically affected, most commonly the hip joint. Evaluate joint limitations/involvement, such as limited range of motion or poor seated posture. Consult to orthopedic surgery may be needed if seated posture is impaired.[13]

Pain

Chronic pain impacts about 70% of those with SCI/D. Neuropathic pain is particularly common and can significantly interfere with quality of life. Routinely review pain medications. If individuals are on narcotic pain medications, necessary protocols should be completed, including a pain contract and urine drug screening.

Sexual and Reproductive Health

Ask permission to discuss sexual health. Pharmacologic (e.g., pain meds) or psychologic factors (e.g., depression) can contribute to sexual dysfunction. Discuss concerns regarding barriers and fertility (if desired). Referrals to men's/women's health if indicated.

Support and Resources

Evaluate home safety, accessibility, and equipment. Review assistance needed and provided in the home setting. A social worker's role is vital to coordinate follow-up and services like home health aide and skilled home health services.[4,8,9,14] Provide reputable resources for SCI support groups and information.

Laboratory Workup and Imaging

In general, a standard panel of annual laboratory workup and imaging studies are recommended; this includes, but is not limited to, the list below. Additional workup may be directed per history and clinical evaluation.[3,4]

Laboratory Work-Up

Complete blood count, basic metabolic panel, cystatin-C, liver function panel, lipid panel, hemoglobin A1c, prostate specific antigen, vitamin D level, HIV/hepatitis C, urinalysis/urine culture, 24-hour urinary creatinine clearance.

Imaging Studies

Chest X-ray
Abdominal X-ray
Kidney ultrasound
Chest computed tomography (age 55–80 years; smoking history >30 pack/year and quit <15 years ago)
Abdominal ultrasound (screen for aortic aneurysm in age 65–75 years; one time if smoking history)

Psychosocial Evaluation

Depression after SCI is common yet undertreated. The Patient Health Questionnaire-9 is a reliable and valid tool to screen persons with SCI. Consider consultation for SCI/D psychology evaluation.

Spinal Cord Injuries/Disorders Education

SCI/D education should be reviewed by all providers; consider use of a designated SCI/D nurse educator to follow and provide necessary education and training.

Care Coordination

An interdisciplinary team approach is recommended to optimize continuity of care as mentioned above. A social worker's role is vital to coordinate follow-up and services like home health aide and skilled home health services.[4,8,9,14]

Comprehensive Care

Once comprehensive evaluation and workup are completed, a plan of care and follow-up are identified, and new and ongoing medical, functional, and psychosocial issues are documented. This plan is critical for maintaining good health and must be updated with the patient and their caregiver.

Children and Adolescents With Spinal Cord Injuries/Disorders[15]

Evaluation[15] and management of children and adolescents with SCI/D should follow the same standard of care as adults. Consider the presentation and complications unique to children and adolescents with SCI/D in the context of the physical, physiologic, cognitive, and psychologic changes that accompany the transition from childhood to adolescence.

Preventive care should follow recommendations set by the American Academy of Pediatrics.[16] SCI-specific considerations include:

- Anthropometrics: Scoliosis and joint contractures can lead to underestimation of height. May need to use wheelchair scale to obtain weight in those unable to stand. Monitor for scoliosis every 6 months until puberty, then yearly after that.
- Blood Pressure (BP): Check BP at each visit. Use appropriately sized cuffs. Establish baseline BP, taking into consideration normative values per age. Symptoms of AD may be vague or not communicated in young children. Elevation of systolic BP above baseline (15 mm Hg in children and 15–20 mm Hg in adolescents) may be a sign of AD. Educate the family, teachers, school nurses, and other individuals involved in the child's care about AD. Consider use of a medical alert bracelet.
- Immunizations: There is increased risk of respiratory infections in those with cervical and thoracic level lesions. Pneumococcal and annual influenza vaccination is warranted, in addition to the general immunization schedule.
- Nutrition: There is increased risk of dyslipidemia and metabolic syndrome. Monitor weight gain, lipid profile. Body mass index may underestimate obesity. Dietary counseling may be needed. Consider dual-energy X-ray absorptiometry scan to monitor adiposity. Encourage the child and family to incorporate physical activity in their daily lives (e.g., physical education classes, adaptive sports, community activities with peers).
- Increased risk for latex hypersensitivity: Ensure latex-free environment, wear medical alert identification, carry auto-injectable epinephrine. Educate child and family.
- Anticipatory guidance: Family education should include discussion of secondary health conditions, evolving equipment needs over time, pubertal changes, sexuality issues, education and return to school, and transition to adult care.

Preventive Care

A full spectrum of preventive care efforts for persons with SCI/D remains evolving and unsettled. At the very least, they should receive the same preventive care as the general population. Many of these individuals have multiple comorbidities, and it is reasonable to argue that all health preventive measures in this population are leveled as quaternary prevention. Applying the four standard levels of preventive measures will provide a framework for better understanding and delivery of optimum preventive care (Table 42.2).

Persons with SCI/D do not have an increased risk of cancer compared with the general population; however, cancer screening does not occur at the same rates. Adherence to evidence-based guidelines for cancer screening (breast, cervical, colorectal, prostate) is recommended, and considering physical and attitudinal barriers that may be encountered.[17,18]

No standard immunization guideline is available for persons with SCI/D; since SCI/D is categorized as a chronic condition, it is prudent to adopt the Centers for Disease Control (CDC) guidelines (Table 42.3).

Other vaccines to consider per CDC:

- Hepatitis B vaccination should be offered to persons with SCI/D with diabetes mellitus and age <60 years. For diabetic patients ≥60 years, vaccination may be warranted based on likelihood of acquiring hepatitis B and immune response.

Additional recommendations include varicella:

- Varicella vaccination for healthy persons >13 years of age without evidence of immunity
- Routine vaccination with the human papillomavirus vaccine for all individuals through age 26 years
- Meningococcal vaccination based on age and/or risk factor

Table 42.2 Four Levels of Prevention in SCI/D Population

Level	Primary	Secondary	Tertiary	Quaternary
SCI/D population	• Healthy, uncomplicated SCI	• Those at higher risk of complications due to having SCI/D	• Has a particular complication / disability	• Acquired a secondary disability
Goal	• Maintain health • Prevent exposure to additional risk of non-SCI-related comorbidities	• Prevent secondary illness and complications	• Prevent additional disability	• Prevent further compromise to quality of life
Measures/ Interventions	• Basic teaching about SCI/D health challenges • Access to health services • Sexual and reproductive health • Screening for cardiometabolic disease[a] • Cancer screening[a] (e.g., colorectal, prostate, breast, cervical, skin) • Immunization	• Identify AD triggers and treat • Identify and manage cardiometabolic disease risks • Annual assessment and management of neurogenic bladder • Bladder cancer screening • Periodic evaluation of bowel management • Diet and fluid management • Preventive measures for skin breakdown • Mental health evaluation	• Assessment and management of pain (neuropathic, musculoskeletal) • Recognize and manage UTI	• Identification and management of musculoskeletal issues[b] • Treatment of ongoing pressure injuries

From McColl M, Gupta S, Smith K, McColl A. Promoting long -term health among people with spinal cord injury: what's new? *Int. J. Environ. Res. Public Health.* 2017;14(12):1520; and U.S. Preventive Services Task Force (USPSTF) A and B Recommendations. https://www.uspreventiveservicestaskforce.org/uspstf/recommendation-topics/uspstf-and-b-recommendations

AD, Autonomic dysreflexia; *SCI/D*, spinal cord injuries/disorders; *UTI*, urinary tract infection.

[a]Recommendations as per United States Preventive Services Task Force.

[b]Musculoskeletal pain, muscle spasm/spasticity, osteoporosis, overuse syndrome, heterotopic ossification, contracture/ deformity.

Additional immunizations may be necessary for persons with SCI/D who are at particular risk (asplenia, adults with cancer); options for appropriate vaccinations during pregnancy are available per CDC guidelines.

Promotive Care

Like many other chronic diseases, those with SCI/D require promotive health measures to prevent and avoid unnecessary medical/functional complications. Unfortunately, there are no clear guidelines for health promotion in the SCI/D population. The following measures are an adopted version based on CDC, Whole Health Program, and contemporary SCI/D resources. It is recommended to present and discuss the following topics at least once a year, preferably during annual evaluation.[2–4,19]

- Educating individuals about avoiding unnecessary hazards/injury; these may include appropriate skin care, safe transfer technique, avoiding new maneuvers in wheelchair unless trained to do so, not to sleep in wheelchair, and not to sit close to fire or space heaters
- Helping smokers quit and promoting smoke-free environment
- Facilitating access to healthy foods and physical activity opportunities
- Promoting lifestyle change and disease self-management programs
- Promoting reproductive health
- Promoting clinical preventive services
- Promoting oral health through standard protocols
- Promoting healthy sleep

Conclusion

Better outcomes, improved quality of life, and greater life expectancy are the goals of health maintenance for persons with SCI/D. To achieve these goals, the comprehensive delivery of primary, preventive, and promotive care is highly recommended. With the advent of continued research, development, and resources, this delivery system has improved in recent years but has yet to be optimized. Recent data suggest improvement in mortality during the first year of SCI/D but not in the outcomes of long-term complications. This is likely due to inadequate maintenance of health care for this unique patient population, indicating a need for an improved care delivery model. Although this chapter reviews a very concise approach, a universal integrated standard of care is warranted for health maintenance of persons with SCI/D.

Review Questions

1. Optimal primary care for patients with SCI may include:
   a. Routine annual comprehensive health evaluation
   b. Multidisciplinary follow-up to address issues associated with long-term disability

Table 42.3 Immunizations for Adult SCI/D Patients

Vaccine	Dose	Interval	Note
Influenza	1 dose	Annually; ideally by the end of October Age 18 >years	Indicated for persons >18 years Quadrivalent; regular dose for <65 years and high dose for >65 years Contraindications: history of previous severe allergic reaction to the vaccine; history of Guillain-Barré syndrome within 6 weeks after dose of influenza vaccine (+) Egg allergy (symptoms limited to hives): can receive influenza vaccine (+) Egg allergy with symptoms other than hives (e.g., angioedema, respiratory distress): give influenza vaccine in a medical setting, supervised by a health care provider who can recognize and manage severe reactions
Pneumococcal[a]	1 or 2 doses[b]	1st dose at diagnosis	PPSV23 at onset of SCI; if PPSV23 is given <65 years old, administer 2nd dose 5 years after previous dose; if given ≥65 years old, give one dose only PCV13: 1 dose only. If immunocompetent: give PCV13 first, followed by PPSV23 1 year later. If with immunocompromising conditions: give PCV13, followed by 1 dose of PPSV23 8 weeks later
Tetanus, diphtheria, and acellular pertussis (Td/Tdap)	1 dose Tdap; Td every 10 years	Single dose of Tdap in place of Td; Td booster every 10 years for all adults >19 years	Tdap/Td vaccines do not have any serious problems; mild side effects can occur
Shingles	2 doses	1st dose at age >50 years; 2nd dose 2 to 6 months later	Recombinant zoster vaccine (RZV, Shingrix) is recommended to prevent shingles in adults >50 years; should receive even if in the past had shingles, received Zostavax, or if one is not sure if they had chickenpox There is no maximum age for getting Shingrix.
COVID-19	1 or 2 doses, depending on vaccine type	If 2 doses are required, 2nd dose at 21–28 days depending on vaccine type	Pfizer-BioNTech – 2 doses spaced apart by 21 days Moderna – 2 doses spaced apart by 28 days Johnson & Johnson – 1 single dose **Further vaccination guidelines evolving**

From Centers for Disease Control and Prevention. Immunization Schedules. https://www.cdc.gov/vaccines/schedules/index.html.
[a]Pneumococcal 23-valent polysaccharide vaccine (PPSV23); Pneumococcal 13-valent conjugate vaccine (PCV13).
[b]PPSV23: 1–2 or 3 doses depending on age and indication; PCV13: 1 dose only. Administration of PCV13 based on shared clinical decision-making.

   c. Addressing areas of unmet needs, such as psychologic concerns, sexual and reproductive health
   d. All of the above
   e. a and c only
2. Preventive care for SCI/D includes
   a. Primary and tertiary preventive measures only
   b. Quaternary preventive measures only
   c. Secondary measures only
   d. All of the above
3. Immunization protocol for persons with SCI/D is identical as patients with chronic diseases and should follow updated annual CDC recommendations.
   a. False
   b. True
4. Vaccination against pneumococcal pneumonia and influenza is recommended in persons with SCI/D, irrespective of age.
   a. False
   b. True
5. Promotive health measures for persons with SCI/D include all EXCEPT:
   a. Promoting healthy sleep
   b. Maneuvering wheelchair as per patient's choice
   c. Helping smokers quit and promoting smoke-free environment
   d. Promoting reproductive health

REFERENCES

1. Stillman M, Bertocci G, Smalley C, Williams S, Frost K. Health care utilization and associated barriers experienced by wheelchair users: a pilot study. *Disabil Health J.* 2017;10(4):502–508.
2. Primary Care Providers–SCI Healthcare Resources. https://asia-spinalinjury.org/primary-care/.
3. Clinical Practice Guidelines Spinal Cord Medicine. https://www.pva.org/research-resources/publications/.
4. Department of Veterans Affairs; Veteran Health Administration; Spinal Cord Injuries and Disorders System of Care; VHA Directive 1176; September 30, 2019.

5. Middleton JW, McCormick M, Engel S, et al. Issues and challenges for development of a sustainable service model for people with spinal cord injury living in rural regions. *Arch Phys Med Rehabil.* 2008;89(10):1941–1947.
6. McColl MA, Aiken A, McColl A, Sakakibara B, Smith K. Primary care of people with spinal cord injury: scoping review. *Can Fam Physician.* 2012;58(11):1207–1216.
7. Sezer N, Akkuş S, Uğurlu FG. Chronic complications of spinal cord injury. *World J Orthopedics.* 2015;6(1):24–33.
8. Cox RJ, Amsters DI, Pershouse KJ. The need for a multidisciplinary outreach service for people with spinal cord injury living in the community. *Clin Rehabil.* 2001;15(6):600–606.
9. DeVivo MJ. Sir Ludwig Guttmann lecture: trends in spinal cord injury rehabilitation outcomes from model systems in the United States: 1973–2006. *Spinal Cord.* 2007;45(11):713–721.
10. Al Taweel W, Seyam R. Neurogenic bladder in spinal cord injury patients. *Research and Report in Urology.* 2015;7:85–99.
11. Krassioukov A, Eng JJ, Claxton G, Sakakibara BM, Shum S. Neurogenic bowel management after spinal cord injury: a systematic review of the evidence. *Spinal Cord.* 2010;48: 718–733.
12. Kruger E, Pires M, Ngann Y, Sterling M, Rubayi S. Comprehensive management of pressure ulcers in spinal cord injury: current concepts and future trends. *J Spinal Cord Med.* 2013;36(6):572–585.
13. Goldstein B. Musculoskeletal conditions after spinal cord injury. *Phys Med Rehabil Clin N Am.* 2000;11(1):91–108. viii-ix.
14. Beatty PW, Hagglund KJ, Neri MT, Dhont KR, Clark MJ, Hilton SA. Access to health care services among people with chronic or disabling conditions: patterns and predictors. *Arch Phys Med Rehabil.* 2003;84(10):1417–1425.
15. Zebracki K, Melicosta M, Unser C, Vogel L. A primary care provider's guide to pediatric spinal cord injuries. *Top Spinal Cord Inj Rehabil.* 2020;26(2):91–99.
16. Recommendations for Preventive Pediatric Health Care Bright Futures/American Academy of Pediatrics. 2021. https://downloads.aap.org/AAP/PDF/periodicity_schedule.pdf.
17. Xu X, Mann JR, Hardin JW, Gustafson E, McDermott SW, Deroche CB. Adherence to US Preventive Services Task Force recommendations for breast and cervical cancer screening for women who have a spinal cord injury. *J Spinal Cord Med.* 2017;40(11):76–84.
18. Milligan J, Burns S, Groah S, Howcroft J. A primary care provider's guide to preventive health after spinal cord injury. *Top Spinal Cord Inj Rehabil.* 2020;26(3):209–219.
19. Centers for Disease Control and Prevention. Promoting Health for Adults. https://www.cdc.gov/chronicdisease/resources/publications/factsheets/promoting-health-for-adults.htm.

CHAPTER

Spinal Cord Injury and Aging 43

Michael Ray Ortiz

OUTLINE

Introduction

Persons with spinal cord injury (SCI) may undergo various degrees of neurological recovery acutely in the first few years after injury, followed by a seemingly prolonged period of stability. The average age at the time of injury has progressively increased from 29 years in the 1970s to approximately 43 years, based on data from 2022.[1] Individuals aging with SCI are increasingly more likely to have experienced, or will experience, age-related changes in their health and functional abilities as they grow older.[2]

Mortality and Life Expectancy

- Pneumonia and septicemia have the greatest impact on reduced life expectancy in people with SCI per 2022 data from the National Spinal Cord Injury Statistical Center database.[1]
- Death from cancer, urinary causes, digestive diseases, and suicide has remained steady or declined.
- Mortality from cardiovascular causes, metabolic causes, nervous system diseases, accidents, and mental conditions has increased.[1,3]
- More recent trends in mortality data are suggestive that more current causes of death are due to chronic conditions experienced by individuals with SCI living longer and having greater risk to natural consequences of aging.
- Advancements in both emergency and acute management, advances in rehabilitative interventions and assistive technology to enhance independence, and early identification of secondary conditions have contributed to steady improvement in life expectancy in the 20th century up to the 1980s. Life expectancy, however, has not continued to improve since then and remains below the life expectancy of the general population.[4]

Organ Systems

For a summary of differences in aging between SCI and non-SCI populations, refer to Table 43.1.

Genitourinary

- With normal human aging, there is increased urge incontinence and increased risk for urinary tract infections (UTIs) related to decline in immune function, postmenopausal changes in women, and prostatic hypertrophy in men.[5–7]
- Urologic complications continue to be common among people with SCI.[8,9]
- With SCI, the cumulative effects of detrusor–sphincter dyssynergia and elevated lower urinary tract pressure over time lead to hypertrophy of the detrusor muscle and decreased bladder compliance, which can result in development of hydronephrosis and upper tract deterioration.[10]
- There are higher rates of bladder stones, UTIs, and bladder cancer associated with the use of indwelling catheters.[11,12]
- The use of anticholinergic medications may improve health outcomes in those who manage with an indwelling catheter[13,14]; however, providers should monitor for adverse side effects of these medications, such as cognitive dysfunction, in the aging population.
- There is increased risk for developing urethral stricture and epididymoorchitis with long-term intermittent catheterization.[15]
- Risk factors for bladder cancers include recurrent UTI and use of indwelling catheters.[16,17]
- Although it is not consistently endorsed, screening cystoscopy for bladder tumors in chronically catheterized individuals with SCI may be the best option for early detection of bladder cancer.[18,19]

Table 43.1 Spinal Cord Injury and Aging

Body System	Usual Aging	Aging With Spinal Cord Injury (SCI)
Genitourinary	• ↓ Bladder capacity • ↓ Urethral compliance • ↑ Uninhibited detrusor contractions • ↑ Residual bladder volume • Gradual ↓ in kidney function • ↑ Urinary tract infections (UTIs) • ↑ Nocturia, change in diurnal urine output • Prostate enlargement • Erectile dysfunction due to comorbidities	• Intermittent catheterization • Loss of voluntary contraction • Detrusor–sphincter dyssynergia • Hypertrophy of the detrusor muscle and ↓ bladder compliance • ↑ Urinary tract pressure and resultant hydronephrosis and upper tract deterioration • Urethral stricture • Epididymitis • Indwelling catheter • ↑ UTIs • Incidence of abnormal renal function testing increases • Bladder stones • ↑ Bladder cancer (indwelling chronic catheter, smokers) • Erectile dysfunction
Gastrointestinal (GI)	• ↓ GI motility • ↓ Acid secretion • ↑ Diverticular disease • ↑ Colon cancer risk and need for colon cancer screening	• Constipation • Incontinence • GI pain • Anorectal problems (hemorrhoids, fissures, proctitis, prolapse) • Anorectal dyssynergia • ↓ Rectal expulsive force • Gallstones • ↓ Voluntary bowel control • False-positive stool testing may complicate colorectal cancer screening
Respiratory	• ↓ Chest wall and lung compliance • ↓ Alveoli • ↓ Vital capacity • Can decompensate borderline ventilators	• Impaired cough → retention of secretions, atelectasis, mucus plugs, pneumonia • Impaired ventilation (with high tetraplegia) • Sleep-disordered breathing

Cardiovascular	• ↑ Prevalence of cardiovascular disease including ischemic heart disease and peripheral arterial disease	• Early but potentially ongoing:
		  • Orthostatic hypotension
		  • Venous thromboembolism
		• Ongoing issues:
		  • Autonomic dysreflexia
		  • Diminished cardiovascular fitness
		  • Cardiovascular effects of medications in SCI
		• Influence of SCI on coronary artery disease and peripheral vascular disease
		  • ↑ Risk factors e.g., ↓ high-density lipoprotein, ↑ percent body fat and insulin resistance, ↓ physical activity
		  • Diagnostic limitations (confusing or absent signs, exercise stress test not feasible)

Metabolic/Endocrine	• Potential for polypharmacy • Impact of aging on drug pharmacokinetics (e.g., age-related decline in hepatic metabolism and renal elimination) and pharmacodynamics	• Pharmacokinetic effects of SCI/effect of SCI on drug metabolism and bioavailability (absorption, distribution, metabolism, excretion) • Effect on carbohydrate and lipid metabolism
Integumentary	• ↓ Elasticity, vascularity, and collagen content of dermis • ↓ Shear tolerance • ↑ Blisters • Skin atrophy	• ↑ Pressure injury risk (immobility, lack of sensation, spasticity) • Squamous cell carcinoma (Marjolin ulcer) risk in chronic pressure injuries
Nervous	• ↓ Vibratory sensation, muscle mass, and strength • Prolonged reaction time • ↓ Fine coordination and agility • Impaired balance/gait	• Entrapment neuropathies (median nerve at wrist, ulnar nerve at elbow) • Posttraumatic syringomyelia • Paralysis, sensory loss • May have cognitive impairment from coexisting brain injury

Table 43.1 Spinal Cord Injury and Aging –Cont'd

Body System	Usual Aging	Aging With Spinal Cord Injury (SCI)
Musculoskeletal	• Deterioration of articular cartilage • Age-related osteoporosis	• Upper extremity overuse injuries • Muscle imbalance • Chronic pain (nociceptive and/or neuropathic) • Heterotopic ossification • Disuse osteoporosis and pathologic fractures
Immune	• Age-related decline	• ↑ UTI frequency
Psychosocial	• Aging caregivers/spouse • Loss of social support • Impact on social participation	• ↑ Potential for stress, depression, isolation • Quality of life is related more with participation rather than degree of impairment

- Small studies show no added risk of prostatic cancer with SCI.[20]
- When prostatic cancer is detected, it is often at a more advanced stage/grade.[21]
- Males aging with SCI should follow age-specific prostate cancer screening.[22]
- Age-related loss of hand dexterity from arthritic changes and decreased mobility may affect self-performance of intermittent catheterization in individuals with prior adequate hand function.[23]

Gastrointestinal

- Colonic transit time is prolonged in persons with SCI, especially the left colon and rectum. Decreased gastrointestinal motility may worsen constipation.[24–26]
- Hemorrhoids and periodic rectal bleeding or trauma are common in chronic SCI.[27]
- Minor symptomatic hemorrhoidal lesions may be treated with topical therapy, whereas more severe hemorrhoids may be treated effectively with banding.[28]
- There is no evidence to suggest that persons with SCI are at increased risk for colon cancer. Frequent presence of hemorrhoids and anorectal bleeding, however, may make fecal occult testing unreliable. Persons with SCI should undergo routine screening for colorectal cancer consistent with guidelines for the general populations. The endoscopist should be familiar with the risk of autonomic dysreflexia and should be prepared to treat blood pressure elevations.[29]
- Modifications in previously established bowel programs may be required due to loss of dexterity and mobility related to aging, which may interfere with one's ability to perform digital stimulation.
- Persons with tetraplegia may be at increased risk of dental disease due to difficulty performing regular dental hygiene.

Respiratory

- Older age at time of injury is associated with higher risk of respiratory complications. There may be significant risk for respiratory tract complications (i.e., pneumonia, atelectasis) and sleep-disordered breathing.[30]
- The leading cause of rehospitalization and death in both acute and chronic SCI is respiratory disorders.[31]
- Several studies seem to show that the risk of respiratory complications is associated with increased age rather than duration of injury.[32,33]
- Clinical follow-up in persons aging with SCI should include periodic assessment of vital capacity, especially in individuals with cervical injuries who are at highest risk of respiratory complications.[34]
- Pneumococcal and annual influenza vaccinations, as well as smoking cessation, are recommended because of higher risk of pneumonia with older age.[35]
- Previously ventilator-free tetraplegics may have late-onset ventilatory failure with contributing factors including age-related decrease in chest wall and lung compliance, decreased alveoli, and decreased vital capacity. Other contributing factors may include excess weight gain, progressive thoracic kyphoscoliosis, or progressive posttraumatic syringomyelia resulting in neurologic deterioration.[23]

Cardiovascular

- Cardiovascular disease (CVD) is the leading cause of death in the general population and is one of the leading reasons of morbidity and mortality in people with long-term SCI.[3,36,37]
- The morbidity and mortality appear to be related to the level of completeness of injury and age of individual.[38,39]
- Risk factors present in SCI increasing risk of CVD include metabolic changes (c-reactive protein, lipid profile, insulin sensitivity), autonomic control (altered heart rate and blood pressure response, autonomic dysreflexia), sedentary lifestyle and lack of aerobic exercise, postinjury weight gain, and changes in body composition. General population guidelines are followed in the absence of SCI-specific CVD prevention guidelines.[35]

- Individuals with injuries T5 and above may not perceive chest pain with angina. Many present atypically with episodic dyspnea, nausea, unexplained autonomic dysreflexia, syncope, or changes in spasticity.
- Providers may encounter a challenge in differentiating heart failure from dependent edema or from lung crackles caused by atelectasis, as both are common in SCI.
- Delayed diagnosis of peripheral arterial disease in individuals with SCI is not uncommon because of lack of the cardinal symptom of intermittent claudication. Symptoms of advanced limb ischemia, such as rest pain or numbness, may be absent, and patients may first present with advanced disease.

Metabolic/Endocrine

- Changes in body composition, including reduction of lean muscle mass and increase in fat mass, along with diminished activity level, may contribute to insulin resistance and impaired glucose metabolism.[40]
- Evidence shows that persons with SCI have decreased secretion of testosterone and human growth hormones, which tends to happen prematurely, and is hypothesized to cause advanced aging.[2]
- New-onset fatigue in an aging person with SCI may be secondary to the development of hypothyroidism.
- Both SCI and aging have an effect on drug metabolism, and there are risks of drug interactions and drug-related side effects.

Integumentary

- There is loss of tissue elasticity and vascularity of the dermis and collagen, which may increase the risk of skin breakdown.[41]
- Incidence of pressure injuries increases in chronic SCI.[42,43]
- Chronic open wounds are associated with development of Marjolin ulcer and squamous carcinoma.[44]

Nervous

- There is some degree of nervous system change, including sensory loss and increase in motor deficits, with increasing age.[45]
- The incidence of entrapment neuropathies increases with duration of injury.
- There is high incidence of upper extremity entrapment neuropathies at the wrists in persons with long-term paraplegia.[46]
- The most frequent site of entrapment is the median nerve at the wrist.[47]
- Signs and symptoms of late progressive neurologic deterioration including loss of sensory and/or motor function, increasing spasticity, neuropathic pain, increasing autonomic dysfunction, and development of variable, positional Horner syndrome may be the result of posttraumatic syringomyelia.
- Decrease in balance and coordination can worsen gait issues in ambulatory persons aging with SCI.
- Age-related loss of visual acuity may reduce function in individuals previously relying on vision to compensate for sensory impairments related to SCI.

Musculoskeletal

- Degenerative arthritis in persons with SCI may worsen the ability to perform activities of daily living and mobility.
- Overuse syndromes in the upper extremities are common in persons aging with SCI. Most studies show prevalence and severity of upper extremity overuse problems are correlated with both age and duration of injury.[48]
- Shoulder and wrist pain may result from wheelchair use, including transfer activities, propulsion, and pressure relief maneuvers.[49,50]
- Ultrasonography, arthrography, and magnetic resonance imaging have better diagnostic yield of showing acromioclavicular arthrosis, impingement syndrome, rotator cuff tendinopathy, and abnormalities at the wrist than do plain radiographs in symptomatic individuals with SCI who report shoulder pain.[51–53]
- Conservative management of overuse injuries may include periodic review of daily activities and mobility mechanics. This may result in suggestions for exercise options and modified techniques for transfers and wheelchair propulsion to minimize pain.[49,50,54,55]
- When conservative management fails, surgery for impingement or rotator cuff tears may be suggested. Individuals who undergo operative treatment, however, may have a temporary impact on independence, with need for additional personal care assistance. A prolonged and possibly difficult postoperative rehabilitation period should be anticipated.[56,57]
- Osteoporosis related to paralysis and disuse is believed to be a risk factor for pathologic fracture in individuals with SCI. Age-related changes in bone metabolism may compound SCI-related osteoporosis.
- More than half of individuals with SCI will incur a fracture at some point following SCI.[58]
- Nonpharmacological interventions such as mechanical loading, functional electrical stimulation, and whole-body vibration therapy have been proposed, but long-term benefits for prevention of osteoporosis and protection from fracture require more investigation.[59]

- Pharmacologic agents such as bisphosphonates have been shown to slow bone loss in both acute and chronic SCI, but new bone formation is not evident.[58,60,61]

Immune

- The immune system is known to be influenced by factors such as depression, diminished psychosocial support, polypharmacy, neuroendocrine changes, and chronic pain, which may be coexistent in persons aging with SCI.[62]
- There is evidence of diminished immune function in people with SCI above the T10 level associated with impaired bacterial phagocytosis.[63]
- There is an increase in UTIs in persons with SCI above the age of 60 and a slight increase in frequency of infection between the 10th and 30th postinjury year.[64]

Psychosocial

- Physical changes of aging in persons with SCI may be accompanied by changes in emotional well-being, satisfaction with life, and community integration, which may be positive or negative.
- Some studies suggest depression rates decline with aging after peaking between 25 and 45 years, and in those with SCI for more than 20 years.
- Individuals with SCI have increasing needs for assistance as they age.[65]
- Aging or death of a spouse or caregiver with a decline in one's own function may lead to a loss in independence. This may lead to social isolation and reduced community participation.

Independence

- Functional decline/decreasing physical independence has been identified as an adverse outcome of long-term SCI, with research showing significant increases in the need for assistance in older individuals or those with longer duration of injury.[66,67]
- From a previous report, the average age at which additional functional assistance was first needed was 49 years for tetraplegics and 54 years for paraplegics, compared with 70 years in the general population.[65]
- Modifications in how activities are performed and/or the use of adaptive equipment and other technologies may help to preserve or maintain functional ability and independence.

Quality of Life

- Studies show depression is common among individuals with SCI, and more severe in those who are older and with longer duration of injury.[68–71]
- Life satisfaction is not necessarily negatively impacted by aging, with studies showing mixed patterns of change over time.[67,72,73]
- Aging is only one aspect of quality of life following SCI. Life satisfaction following SCI can also be related to overall general health, social support, community integration, personal factors, and level of injury and expectations of function. Identifying the various underlying factors that may contribute to declines in perceived quality of life may be difficult, and health care providers should assess the physical health, psychological status, social situation, and environment of individuals aging with SCI, as all of these have an impact on aging.[74–77]

Summary

Trends in SCI research include older age of injury, increased longevity, increased incidence of secondary health complications, and perceived decrease in independence and physical activity with aging. There remain gaps in the literature regarding many issues related to aging with SCI. Further research is needed to better understand and differentiate the effect of aging versus duration of injury. In people with SCI living longer, there is greater risk of developing chronic health conditions associated with aging. There is greater need for providers and health care teams knowledgeable about age-related changes in SCI to ensure appropriate assessment, follow-up, and management of the aging SCI population.

Review Questions

1. According to the 2022 data from the National Spinal Cord Injury Statistical Center, what has had the greatest impact on reduced life expectancy in people with SCI enrolled in the database?
   a. Pneumonia and septicemia
   b. Accidents
   c. Nervous system disease
   d. Digestive disease
2. In persons with SCI, mortality from which condition has had an increase over time?
   a. Urinary disease
   b. Cancer
   c. Cardiovascular disease
   d. Suicide
3. Risk factors for bladder cancer in persons aging with SCI include all EXCEPT:
   a. Recurrent UTIs
   b. Chronic indwelling catheters
   c. Urinary tract stones
   d. Anticholinergic medication use
4. In screening for colon cancer in patients aging with SCI, which statement is true?
   a. There is an increased risk of colon cancer compared with the general population.

b. Fecal occult blood is a reliable screening tool.
c. SCI patients should undergo earlier screening for colorectal cancer compared with guidelines for the general population.
d. Endoscopist should be familiar with the risk of autonomic dysreflexia.

5. In individuals aging with spinal cord injury, what is the most frequent upper extremity entrapment neuropathy?
   a. Median nerve at the wrist
   b. Ulnar nerve at the wrist
   c. Median nerve at the pronator teres
   d. Ulnar nerve at the elbow
6. In disuse-related osteoporosis in individuals aging with SCI, all are true EXCEPT:
   a. Bisphosphonates slow bone loss in acute and chronic SCI
   b. There is evidence of new bone formation with use of bisphosphonates
   c. Osteoporosis is thought to be an underlying factor for pathologic fracture
   d. Woman with SCI are more like likely to have long bone fractures in the lower extremities as time postinjury increases
7. With regards to quality of life in individuals aging with SCI, all are true EXCEPT:
   a. Rate of depression declines after peaking between 25 and 45 years of age
   b. Rate of depression declines among individuals greater than 20 years postinjury
   c. Risk of depression is not associated with presence of other illnesses
   d. Risk of depression is associated with significant decline in function

REFERENCES

1. Cord Spinal. *Injury Facts and Figures at a Glance. National Spinal Cord Injury Statistical Center, Facts and Figures at a Glance*. Birmingham, AL: University of Alabama at Birmingham; 2022.
2. Frontera JE, Mollett P. Aging with spinal cord injury: an update. *Physical Medicine and Rehabilitation Clinics*. 2017;28(4):821–828.
3. Savic G, DeVivo MJ, Frankel HL, Jamous MA, Soni BM, Charlifue S. Causes of death after traumatic spinal cord injury—a 70-year British study. *Spinal Cord*. 2017;55(10):891–897.
4. Charlifue S. Spinal cord injury and aging. In: Kirshblum S, Lin VW, eds. *Spinal Cord Medicine*. 3rd ed. New York: Demos Medical; 2019:987–997.
5. Ranson RN, Saffrey MJ. Neurogenic mechanisms in bladder and bowel ageing. *Biogerontology*. 2015;16(2):265–284.
6. Kline KA, Bowdish DM. Infection in an aging population. *Current Opinion in Microbiology*. 2016;29:63–67.
7. Rowe TA, Juthani-Mehta M. Diagnosis and management of urinary tract infection in older adults. *Infectious Disease Clinics of North America*. 2014;28(1):75–89.
8. McKibben MJ, Seed P, Ross SS, Borawski KM. Urinary tract infection and neurogenic bladder. *Urologic Clinics*. 2015;42(4):527–536.
9. Goldmark E, Niver B, Ginsberg DA. Neurogenic bladder: from diagnosis to management. *Current Urology Reports*. 2014;15(10):448.
10. Madersbacher G, Oberwalder M. The elderly para-and tetraplegic: special aspects of the urological care. *Spinal Cord*. 1987;25(4):318–323.
11. Drake MJ, Cortina-Borja M, Savic G, Charlifue SW, Gardner BP. Prospective evaluation of urological effects of aging in chronic spinal cord injury by method of bladder management. *Neurourology and Urodynamics*. 2005;24(2):111–116.
12. Hansen RB, Biering-Sørensen F, Kristensen JK. Bladder emptying over a period of 10–45 years after a traumatic spinal cord injury. *Spinal Cord*. 2004;42(11):631–637.
13. O'Leary M, Erickson JR, Smith CP, McDermott C, Horton J, Chancellor MB. Effect of controlled-release oxybutynin on neurogenic bladder function in spinal cord injury. *J Spinal Cord Med*. 2003;26(2):159–162.
14. Bennett N, O'Leary MA, Patel AS, Xavier M, Erickson JR, Chancellor MB. Can higher doses of oxybutynin improve efficacy in neurogenic bladder? *J Urology*. 2004;171(2):749–751.
15. Ku JH, Jung TY, Lee JK, Park WH, Shim HB. Influence of bladder management on epididymo-orchitis in patients with spinal cord injury: clean intermittent catheterization is a risk factor for epididymo-orchitis. *Spinal Cord*. 2006;44(3):165–169.
16. Gui-Zhong L, Li-Bo M. Bladder cancer in individuals with spinal cord injuries: a meta-analysis. *Spinal Cord*. 2017;55(4):341–345.
17. Ho CH, Sung KC, Lim SW, et al. Chronic indwelling urinary catheter increase the risk of bladder cancer, even in patients without spinal cord injury. *Medicine*. 2015;94(43).
18. Patil S, Prasanna KV, Chowdhury JR. To cystoscope or not to cystoscope patients with traumatic spinal cord injuries managed with indwelling urethral or suprapubic catheters? That is the question! *Spinal Cord*. 2014;52(1):49–53.
19. Sammer U, Walter M, Knüpfer SC, Mehnert U, Bode-Lesniewska B, Kessler TM. Do we need surveillance urethro-cystoscopy in patients with neurogenic lower urinary tract dysfunction? *PLoS One*. 2015;10(10):e0140970.
20. Shim HB, Jung TY, Lee JK, Ku JH. Prostate activity and prostate cancer in spinal cord injury. *Prostate Cancer and Prostatic Diseases*. 2006;9(2):115–120.
21. Scott Sr PA, Perkash I, Mode D, Wolfe VA, Terris MK. Prostate cancer diagnosed in spinal cord-injured patients is more commonly advanced stage than in able-bodied patients. *Urology*. 2004;63(3):509–512.
22. Wyndaele JJ, Iwatsubo E, Perkash I, Stöhrer M. Prostate cancer: a hazard also to be considered in the ageing male patient with spinal cord injury. *Spinal Cord*. 1998;36(5):299–302.
23. Sabharwal S. Aging with a spinal cord injury. In: Sabharwal S, ed. *Essentials of Spinal Cord Medicine*. 1st ed. New York: Demos Medical; 2014:387–393.
24. Krogh K, Mosdal C, Laurberg S. Gastrointestinal and segmental colonic transit times in patients with acute and chronic spinal cord lesions. *Spinal Cord*. 2000;38(10):615–621.
25. Leduc BE, Spacek E, Lepage Y. Colonic transit time after spinal cord injury: any clinical significance? *J Spinal Cord Medicine*. 2002;25(3):161–166.
26. Valles M, Vidal J, Clav P, Mearin F. Bowel dysfunction in patients with motor complete spinal cord injury: clinical, neurological, and pathophysiological associations. *American Journal of Gastroenterology*. 2006;101(10):2290–2299.

27. Stone JM, Nino-Murcia M, Wolfe VA, Perkash I. Chronic gastrointestinal problems in spinal cord injury patients: a prospective analysis. *American Journal of Gastroenterology*. 1990;85(9):1114–1119.
28. Cosman BC, Cajas-Monson LC, Ramamoorthy SL. Twenty years of a veterans' spinal cord injury colorectal clinic: flexible sigmoidoscopy and multiple hemorrhoid ligation. *Diseases of the Colon & Rectum*. 2017;60(4):399–404.
29. Hayman AV, Guihan M, Fisher MJ, et al. Colonoscopy is high yield in spinal cord injury. *J Spinal Cord Medicine*. 2013;36(5):436–442.
30. Hitzig SL, Tonack M, Campbell KA, et al. Secondary health complications in an aging Canadian spinal cord injury sample. *American J Physical Medicine & Rehabilitation*. 2008;87(7):545–555.
31. Burns SP. Acute respiratory infections in persons with spinal cord injury. *Physical Medicine and Rehabilitation Clinics of North America*. 2007;18(2):203–216.
32. Stolzmann KL, Gagnon DR, Brown R, Tun CG, Garshick E. Longitudinal change in FEV1 and FVC in chronic spinal cord injury. *American J Respiratory and Critical Care Medicine*. 2008;177(7):781–786.
33. Menter RR, Hudson LM. Effects of age at injury and the aging process. In: Stover SL, DeLisa JA, Whiteneck GG, eds. *Spinal Cord Injury: Clinical Outcomes From the Model Systems*. 1st ed. Gaithersburg: Aspen Publishers; 1995:272.
34. Lanig IS, Peterson WP. The respiratory system in spinal cord injury. *Physical Medicine and Rehabilitation Clinics of North America*. 2000;11(1):29–43.
35. Charlifue S, Jha A, Lammertse D. Aging with spinal cord injury. *Physical Medicine and Rehabilitation Clinics*. 2010;21(2):383–402.
36. Benjamin EJ, Blaha MJ, Chiuve SE, et al. Heart disease and stroke statistics—2017 update: a report from the American Heart Association. *Circulation*. 2017;135(10):e146–e603.
37. Osterthun R, Post MW, Van Asbeck FW, Van Leeuwen CM, Van Koppenhagen CF. Causes of death following spinal cord injury during inpatient rehabilitation and the first five years after discharge. A Dutch cohort study. *Spinal Cord*. 2014;52(6):483–488.
38. Groah SL, Weitzenkamp D, Sett P, Soni B, Savic G. The relationship between neurological level of injury and symptomatic cardiovascular disease risk in the aging spinal injured. *Spinal Cord*. 2001;39(6):310–317.
39. LaVela SL, Evans CT, Prohaska TR, Miskevics S, Ganesh SP, Weaver FM. Males aging with a spinal cord injury: prevalence of cardiovascular and metabolic conditions. *Archives of Physical Medicine and Rehabilitation*. 2012;93(1):90–95.
40. Bauman WA, Kahn NN, Grimm DR, Spungen AM. Risk factors for atherogenesis and cardiovascular autonomic function in persons with spinal cord injury. *Spinal Cord*. 1999;37(9):6 01–616.
41. Zouboulis CC, Makrantonaki E. Clinical aspects and molecular diagnostics of skin aging. *Clinics in Dermatology*. 2011;29(1):3–14.
42. McKinley WO, Jackson AB, Cardenas DD, Michael J. Long-term medical complications after traumatic spinal cord injury: a regional model systems analysis. *Archives of Physical Medicine and Rehabilitation*. 1999;80(11):1402–1410.
43. Charlifue S, Lammertse DP, Adkins RH. Aging with spinal cord injury: changes in selected health indices and life satisfaction. *Archives of Physical Medicine and Rehabilitation*. 2004;85(11):1848–1853.
44. Eltorai IM, Montroy RE, Kobayashi M, Jakowatz J, Guttierez P. Marjolin's ulcer in patients with spinal cord injury. *J Spinal Cord Medicine*. 2002;25(3):191–196.
45. Lammertse DP. The nervous system. In: Whiteneck GG, Charlifue S, Gerhart KA, eds. *Aging With Spinal Cord Injury*. 1st ed. New York: Demos Publications; 1993:129–137.
46. Davidoff G, Werner R, Waring W. Compressive mononeuropathies of the upper extremity in chronic paraplegia. *Spinal Cord*. 1991;29(1):17–24.
47. Curtin CM, Hagert CG, Hultling C, Hagert E. Nerve entrapment as a cause of shoulder pain in the spinal cord injured patient. *Spinal Cord Series and Cases*. 2017;3(1):1–3.
48. Ferrero G, Mijno E, Actis MV, Zampa A, Ratto N, Arpaia A, Massè A. Risk factors for shoulder pain in patients with spinal cord injury: a multicenter study. *Musculoskeletal Surgery*. 2015;99(1):53–56.
49. Van Straaten MG, Cloud BA, Morrow MM, Ludewig PM, Zhao KD. Effectiveness of home exercise on pain, function, and strength of manual wheelchair users with spinal cord injury: a high-dose shoulder program with telerehabilitation. *Archives of Physical Medicine and Rehabilitation*. 2014;95(10):1810–1817.
50. Tsai CY, Boninger ML, Hastings J, Cooper RA, Rice L, Koontz AM. Immediate biomechanical implications of transfer component skills training on independent wheelchair transfers. *Archives of Physical Medicine and Rehabilitation*. 2016;97(10):1785–1792.
51. Eriks-Hoogland I, Engisch R, Brinkhof MW, Van Drongelen S. Acromioclavicular joint arthrosis in persons with spinal cord injury and able-bodied persons. *Spinal Cord*. 2013;51(1):59–63.
52. Belley AF, Gagnon DH, Routhier F, Roy JS. Ultrasonographic measures of the acromiohumeral distance and supraspinatus tendon thickness in manual wheelchair users with spinal cord injury. *Archives of Physical Medicine and Rehabilitation*. 2017;98(3):517–524.
53. Akbar M, Penzkofer S, Weber MA, Bruckner T, Winterstein M, Jung M. Prevalence of carpal tunnel syndrome and wrist osteoarthritis in long-term paraplegic patients compared with controls. *Journal of Hand Surgery European Volume*. 2014;39(2):132–138.
54. Requejo PS, Mulroy SJ, Ruparel P, et al. Relationship between hand contact angle and shoulder loading during manual wheelchair propulsion by individuals with paraplegia. *Topics in Spinal Cord Injury Rehabilitation*. 2015;21(4):313–324.
55. Cratsenberg KA, Deitrick CE, Harrington TK, et al. Effectiveness of exercise programs for management of shoulder pain in manual wheelchair users with spinal cord injury. *Journal of Neurologic Physical Therapy*. 2015;39(4):197–203.
56. Robinson MD, Hussey RW, Ha CY. Surgical decompression of impingement in the weightbearing shoulder. *Archives of Physical Medicine and Rehabilitation*. 1993;74(3):324–327.
57. Goldstein B, Young J, Escobedo EM. Rotator cuff repairs in individuals with paraplegia. *American J Physical Medicine and Rehabilitation*. 1997;76(4):316–322.
58. Morse LR, Sudhakar S, Danilack V, et al. Association between sclerostin and bone density in chronic spinal cord injury. *Journal of Bone and Mineral Research*. 2012;27(2):352–359.

59. Battaglino RA, Lazzari AA, Garshick E, Morse LR. Spinal cord injury-induced osteoporosis: pathogenesis and emerging therapies. *Current Osteoporosis Reports*. 2012;10(4):278–285.
60. Gilchrist NL, Frampton CM, Acland RH, et al. Alendronate prevents bone loss in patients with acute spinal cord injury: a randomized, double-blind, placebo-controlled study. *The Journal of Clinical Endocrinology & Metabolism*. 2007;92(4):1385–1390.
61. De Brito CM, Battistella LR, Saito ET, Sakamoto H. Effect of alendronate on bone mineral density in spinal cord injury patients: a pilot study. *Spinal Cord*. 2005;43(6):341–348.
62. Nash MS, Fletcher M. The immune system. In: Whiteneck GG, Charlifue S, Gerhart KA, eds. *Aging With Spinal Cord Injury*. 1st ed. New York: Demos Publications; 1993: 159–181.
63. Campagnolo DI, Bartlett JA, Chatterton Jr R, Keller SE. Adrenal and pituitary hormone patterns after spinal cord injury. *American J Physical Medicine and Rehabilitation*. 1999;78(4):361–366.
64. Whiteneck GG, Charlifue SW, Frankel HL, et al. Mortality, morbidity, and psychosocial outcomes of persons spinal cord injured more than 20 years ago. *Spinal Cord*. 1992;30(9): 617–630.
65. Gerhart KA, Bergstrom E, Charlifue SW, Menter RR, Whiteneck GG. Long-term spinal cord injury: functional changes over time. *Archives of Physical Medicine and Rehabilitation*. 1993;74(10):1030–1034.
66. Liem NR, McColl MA, King W, Smith KM. Aging with a spinal cord injury: factors associated with the need for more help with activities of daily living. *Archives of Physical Medicine and Rehabilitation*. 2004;85(10):1567–1577.
67. Charlifue SW, Weitzenkamp DA, Whiteneck GG. Longitudinal outcomes in spinal cord injury: aging, secondary conditions, and well-being. *Archives of Physical Medicine and Rehabilitation*. 1999;80(11):1429–1434.
68. Kemp BJ, Kahan JS, Krause JS, Adkins RH, Nava GN. Treatment of major depression in individuals with spinal cord injury. *J Spinal Cord Medicine*. 2004;27(1):22–28.
69. Dryden DM, Saunders LD, Rowe BH, et al. Depression following traumatic spinal cord injury. *Neuroepidemiology*. 2005;25(2):55–61.
70. Österåker AL, Levi R. Indicators of psychological distress in postacute spinal cord injured individuals. *Spinal Cord*. 2005;43(4):223–229.
71. Krause JS, Kemp B, Coker J. Depression after spinal cord injury: relation to gender, ethnicity, aging, and socioeconomic indicators. *Archives of Physical Medicine and Rehabilitation*. 2000;81(8):1099–1109.
72. Krause JS, Broderick L. A 25-year longitudinal study of the natural course of aging after spinal cord injury. *Spinal Cord*. 2005;43(6):349–356.
73. Krause JS, Coker JL. Aging after spinal cord injury: a 30-year longitudinal study. *Journal of Spinal Cord Medicine*. 2006;29(4):371–376.
74. Lundström U, Lilja M, Gray D, Isaksson G. Experiences of participation in everyday occupations among persons aging with a tetraplegia. *Disability and Rehabilitation*. 2015;37(11):951–957.
75. McColl MA, Arnold R, Charlifue S, Glass C, Savic G, Frankel H. Aging, spinal cord injury, and quality of life: structural relationships. *Archives of Physical Medicine and Rehabilitation*. 2003;84(8):1137–1144.
76. McColl MA, Walker J, Stirling P, Wilkins R, Corey P. Expectations of life and health among spinal cord injured adults. *Spinal Cord*. 1997;35(12):818–828.
77. Weitzenkamp DA, Gerhart KA, Charlifue SW, Whiteneck GG, Glass CA, Kennedy P. Ranking the criteria for assessing quality of life after disability: Evidence for priority shifting among long-term spinal cord injury survivors. *British Journal of Health Psychology*. 2000;5(1):57–69.

CHAPTER 44

Exercise and Modalities

Ricky Hawkins

OUTLINE

Therapeutic Exercise

According to the U.S. Department of Health and Human Services, current physical activity guidelines for Americans state that "to attain the most health benefits from physical activity, adults need at least 150 to 300 minutes of moderate-intensity aerobic activity, like brisk walking or fast dancing, each week. Adults also need muscle-strengthening activity, like lifting weights or doing push-ups, at least 2 days each week."[1] In nonambulatory individuals, continued exercise is essential, because sitting has been labeled "the new smoking."

Patients with spinal cord injury (SCI) are faced with unique challenges to exercising in a rehab environment. Proper evaluation of clinical stability and functional ability will assist in determining a patient's starting point (e.g., bed mobility vs. gait). Autonomic dysregulation (including blood pressure dysregulation, a blunted heart rate response, and thermal dysregulation in those with higher levels of injury), tissue frailty/wounds, positioning needs, cognitive ability, and immediate mobility needs all require attention to allow the patient to initiate exercise with the rehab team. Another issue common in patients with early injury is quicker onset of fatigue. This reduced endurance can cause issues such as decreased time a patient is able to practice transfers or sitting balance for activities of daily living. Moreover patients with chronic SCI are especially at risk for upper extremity overuse injuries (see Chapter 23).

The benefits of exercise in SCI include improved blood pressure regulation, increased skin safety with transfers as a result of improved transfer technique, safer transfers with increased strength and endurance, and improved mood.

Range of Motion/Stretching

Maintaining good functional range of motion in a patient with SCI allows for optimized positioning, increased ease with transfers (active or passive), decreased pain, decreased risk of secondary complications such as contractures, and decreased pressure injuries. Lack of range of motion can lead to permanent loss of range of motion if tissue is allowed to progress through structural changes and become fibrotic.[5] Range-of-motion/stretching exercises are to be performed in a pain-free range, with the concept of increasing that range over time. Keep in mind that active range of motion, when available, is preferred for maximum benefit; however, in lieu of full active ability, active assisted range of motion followed by passive range of motion should be used.

Those patients with complete SCI, severe spasticity, and preexisting pressure injuries are at risk of developing of heterotopic ossification (HO). HO is suspected to occur as a result of microtrauma and stress imposed upon the musculotendinous junction, causing ossification when osteoblast-stimulating factors are released directly, or when there is local inflammatory response. HO is common in joints distal to the level of injury and seen most often in the hip. HO usually develops within the first 6 months postinjury and stabilizes within 18–24 months after injury onset. Range of motion should be performed as soon as patients are stable enough for it, as adaptive shortening followed by aggressive stretching later could contribute to HO via the above-mentioned process.[6]

Mat Activities

Mat activities are a great way to assess the patient's current ability and to monitor progress with functional mobility. Initially, depending on the patient's level of injury, a lift and sling may need to be used to transfer the patient to the mat. Bed mobility and transfer preparation tasks can be performed with increased ease due to the adjustability of the mat, as well as the increased density of the cushion on a mat table compared to a hospital bed mattress. The mat table's size allows for multiple therapists' assistance if needed and gives patients an opportunity to learn technique before also having to use strength with a technique. Patients can also work safely on pretransfer tasks, such as weight shifting in all directions, lift-offs (raising buttocks off the mat), lateral scoots, supine-to-sit-to-supine, and other tasks.

Modalities

Functional Electrical Stimulation

Following denervation of a given area, there is a marked increase in risk of pressure injuries, due to lack of blood flow, immobility, and an increase in bony prominence following muscle atrophy. Bone quality also degrades, as the forces previously placed upon bony structures are no longer applied; in turn, bone is simply reabsorbed, contributing to osteoporosis, and doubling the risk of fracture, as compared with able-bodied individuals. Following more extensive muscle atrophy, there is an increase in fatty infiltration of the muscle tissue, leading to fibrosis of muscle tissue.[2]

To mitigate the aforementioned adverse effects of SCI, functional electrical stimulation (FES) may be integrated into the rehabilitation program. FES utilizes multiple-channel electrical stimulators controlled by a microprocessor to recruit muscles in a programmed synergistic sequence that will allow the patient to accomplish a specific functional movement pattern.[3] Muscle contraction is achieved by applying a stimulus that pushes a motor unit past its excitability threshold, thus creating muscular contraction. FES demonstrates a reversal of the normal motor unit recruitment order. Motor units are typically recruited from small to large; however, due to the lower excitability threshold of larger motor units, these units are recruited first in FES.[4]

Indications for Functional Electrical Stimulation[3]

- Strengthening of muscle
- Decreasing/preventing muscular atrophy
- Decreasing/preventing edema
- Decreasing muscle spasm/guarding
- Stimulating peripheral nerve system function
- Stimulating nerve regeneration
- Increasing circulation through muscle pumping contractions
- Increasing range of motion
- Assisting with the prevention of deep vein thrombosis with inactivity

Contraindications for Functional Electrical Stimulation[3]

- Pacemakers (can be cleared by cardiology in certain cases)
- Infection
- Malignancies
- Pregnancy
- Musculoskeletal problems that would be exacerbated by muscle contraction

The benefits of utilizing FES include increased activity; endurance improvement; decreased risk of obesity, type II diabetes, cardiovascular diseases, and deep venous thromboses; and psychosocial benefits of increased activities. The likelihood of success with FES depends upon the severity of lower motor neuron injury. In cases of neurapraxia, where there is no loss of continuity of the axons, a patient is likely to have the most success. More severe cases of lower motor neuron injury, including axonotmesis and neurotmesis, where axonal continuity has been affected, are associated with reduced success with FES, due to the decrease in strength of a signal reaching the motor unit or inability (in more severe cases) of a signal to do so, moreover, patient populations will inevitably vary in response to FES. Some patients may require continued use of FES for items such as walking; on the other hand some patients may be able to progress to no longer requiring FES or only requiring an ankle foot orthosis.

Modalities Reducing Pain via the Gate Control Theory

Pain is common among the SCI population. The Gate Control Theory of pain states that nonpainful stimuli "close the gates" to the painful stimuli and keep the brain from interpreting the pain signals, since it is not reaching the brain. This theory is developed on the fact that the patient's C-fibers that transmit pain are smaller and unmyelinated, which decreases the travel rate of a painful stimulus. Aβ fibers are larger and myelinated, and thus travel at a faster rate than C-fibers, allowing a given nonpainful stimulus to "close the gates." Hot/cold packs can be used as a means of reducing pain, given this theory; another method is the use of transcutaneous electrical nerve stimulation (TENS), which induces a low-level current of electrical stimulation to reduce pain when applied appropriately.

Some contraindications to these modalities include: active infection, cancer, application in an area where inducing increased circulation would be adverse, self-use with poor sensation, pacemaker (could be cleared by cardiology in certain cases), and any other safety concern that would hinder the patient's ability to safely use the device(s).

Ultrasound

Ultrasound is another modality that can be used in the SCI population to heat tissues at a deeper level as compared to other heating modalities.[3] The thermal effects from ultrasound are similar to other heating modalities in that it can induce:

- Increased extensibility of collagen fibers in tendons and joint capsules
- Decreased joint stiffness
- Reduced muscle spasms
- Modulation of pain
- Increased localized blood flow
- Mild acute inflammatory response that could help resolve chronic inflammation

Indications for Ultrasound

- Soft tissue healing and repair
- Scar tissue
- Joint contracture
- Chronic inflammation
- Increased extensibility of collagen
- Reduction of muscle spasm
- Pain modulation
- Increased localized blood flow
- Increased protein synthesis
- Tissue regeneration
- Bone healing
- Inflammation associated with myositis ossificans
- Myofascial trigger points

Contraindications for Ultrasound

- Areas of decreased temperature sensation
- Areas of decreased circulation
- Vascular insufficiency
- Thrombophlebitis
- Eyes
- Reproductive organs
- Pelvis immediately following menses
- Pregnancy
- Pacemaker
- Malignancy
- Epiphyseal areas in young children
- Total joint replacements
- Infection

Ultrasound technology is also used in bone stimulators in a nonthermal manner to accelerate bone repair. Ultrasound has also been used in wound healing. Ultrasound has been shown to stimulate degranulation of inflammatory cells, thus facilitating the release of chemical mediators that activate other key cells in the healing process. Improved healing, however, has been more associated with early application.[3]

Nontraditional Therapies

Bodyweight-Supported Gait Training Over a Treadmill

Gait training with bodyweight support is a method utilized to allow patients with incomplete SCI to reinitiate/refine central motor programming and increase strength in a functional pattern. It will also allow earlier initiation of gait training. Typically, a gait training session will consist of two to three therapists/assistants. The patient will have one therapist on each leg to assist with transitions through gait phases, and there will usually be one person controlling speed on the treadmill for safety. Following the successful completion of a quality gait pattern at a given speed, the therapist would likely increase speed toward desired goal of community ambulation speed at 0.44–1.32 m/s. The sequential adjustments would consist of decreasing body weight support while maintaining gait quality/safety. For safety, the therapist should take into consideration the time it takes to setup and get the patient connected to the harness over the treadmill in the event that a patient experiences any kind of hypotension or other medical situation requiring return to chair/seated position.

Ambulation Using Bionic Exoskeletons

The use of exoskeletons in a therapeutic environment has been increasing as technology has improved. Such a device allows for a more consistent and natural gait pattern over time, as fatigue in the patient or therapist can alter the quality of gait pattern during bodyweight-supported treadmill training. Exoskeletons also can allow for decreased risk of overuse injuries in the assisting therapist. Programming in exoskeletons also permits a more objective monitoring of progress. Although technology has been improving and access to exoskeletons has been increasing, current research indicates that bodyweight-supported treadmill training and robotic-assisted gait training do not increase gait speed any more than standard over-ground gait training and other forms of physical therapy do.[7]

Review Questions

1. You are a physical therapist working with a patient with C8 AIS A tetraplegia. You have completed the patient's wheelchair setup and want to begin working on transfers. You have not yet assessed the patient's ability to maintain their sitting posture without back support. What would your initial activity likely consist of?
   a. Reaching from short sitting on a hospital bed
   b. Lifting their bottom just off the mat table
   c. Static sitting balance with elbows propped on stools on a mat table
   d. Short-term sitting on mat table with bilateral upper extremity support
2. A patient with chronic pain comes in for a TENS evaluation. The patient reports feeling some pain relief and states that their pain has decreased from

a 6/10 to a 3/10. What concept is responsible for the success of this intervention?
   a. Nocebo effect
   b. Gate control theory
   c. Intensive theory
   d. Specificity theory
3. A patient who has just begun using FES with physical therapy for gait assistance has to take frequent rest breaks due to fatigue of larger motor units. How could FES most contribute to this?
   a. Intensity not strong enough
   b. Reversal of motor unit recruitment
   c. Stimulation frequency is too low
   d. Incorrect location of electrodes
4. A 36-year-old patient with C6 AIS D tetraplegia has walked into your clinic for their appointment. You have been consulted for "Patient with left anterior lower extremity pain. Please evaluate for TENS." When taking the patient's history, you discover that the patient has an infected wound from a hiking accident in the area to be treated. Can you proceed with the treatment in attempts to reduce the pain?
   a. Yes
   b. No
5. Your patient has been diagnosed with heterotopic ossification and is beginning to experience some restrictiveness during progressive range of motion. What is the most appropriate treatment to start with?
   a. Heat followed with aggressive stretching
   b. Joint mobilizations (Grade 2)
   c. Gentle stretching
   d. Ice pack to the affected area

REFERENCES

1. Health.gov. 2008. [Online]. https://health.gov/sites/default/files/2019-09/paguide.pdf.
2. Gorgey A, Chandrasekaran S, Davis J, Bersch I, Goldberg G. Electrical stimulation and denervated muscles after spinal cord injury. *Neural Regeneration Research.* 2020;15(8):1397.
3. Prentice W. *Therapeutic Modalities in Rehabilitation.* 4th ed. McGraw-Hill; 2011.
4. Bickel C, Gregory C, Dean J. Motor unit recruitment during neuromuscular electrical stimulation: a critical appraisal. *European Journal of Applied Physiology.* 2011;111(10):2399–2407.
5. Kisner C, Colby L. *Therapeutic Exercise: Foundations and Techniques.* 6th ed. Philadelphia: FA Davis Company; 2012.
6. Cameron M, Monroe L. *Physical Rehabilitation.* St. Louis: Elsevier Saunders; 2007.
7. Mehrholz J, Harvey L, Thomas S, Elsner B. Is body-weight-supported treadmill training or robotic-assisted gait training superior to overground gait training and other forms of physiotherapy in people with spinal cord injury? A systematic review. *Spinal Cord.* 2017;55(8):722–729.

CHAPTER 45

Functional Mobility Following Spinal Cord Injury

Cory Wernimont and Julie Mannlein

OUTLINE

As a spinal cord injury (SCI) specialist, it is imperative to have an understanding of prognostic factors that impact potential for functional ambulation while also understanding the rehabilitation approaches to achieve these goals. Just as importantly, the physician should appreciate the various modes of wheeled mobility to promote independence. This will allow the clinician to establish short- and long-term rehabilitation goals to optimize individualized rehabilitation plans and maximize independence.

Early Mobility Goals

Bed Mobility and Upright Sitting Tolerance

Prior to initiation of higher-level mobility training, the focus of rehabilitation involves progression of bed mobility and upright sitting tolerance. The latter can be achieved with progressive vertical challenges, including dangling the legs off the side of the bed, utilization of tilt-in-space or reclining wheelchairs, and tilt tables. Blood pressure should be supported with an abdominal binder, compression stockings, and/or medications.

Pressure Relief

Once individuals begin sitting upright, they should be instructed on techniques, frequency, and duration of pressure relief, in an effort to mitigate risk of pressure injury formation. It is generally accepted to perform pressure relief for at least 1 minute for every 30 minutes of sitting,[1] with some now advocating for a 2-minute duration.[2–5] Strategies for manual pressure reliefs include:

- Wheelchair push-ups
- Anterior lean onto the thighs at an angle >45 degrees from the backrest[6,7]
- Lateral lean via hooking the arm over the back of the chair or back canes

Those without functioning triceps and/or those with a body habitus that is not conducive to manual pressure relief techniques will require alternative methods of off-loading, such as use of chairs with tilt and/or recline. Sufficient off-loading necessitates at least 45 degrees of tilt, a combination of >25 degrees of tilt with 120 degrees of recline, or >35 degrees of tilt with 100 degrees of recline.[8–10]

Transfers

Early rehabilitation should include education and training to develop safe transfer techniques, which entails training for both the patient and caregivers. Improper techniques can easily lead to traumatic and/or repetitive musculoskeletal injuries, including potentiation of skin breakdown. For those with some degree of leg strength, they may be able to progress to a stand-pivot transfer. For those without sufficient leg strength, transfer techniques will include lateral transfers, with or without a slide board. These individuals should consider alternating directions when feasible as persistent transfers in only one direction can lead to rotator cuff strain for the trailing arm.[11–13] If manual transfers are not possible, then an individual will require some form of mechanical lift, such as a manual or power sling lift, or a sit-to-stand lift.

Ambulation Following Spinal Cord Injury

Prognosis

In prognosticating for functional ambulation, which is defined as walking independently in the community with or without braces/assistive devices, the most relevant factor is the American Spinal Injury Association (ASIA) impairment scale (AIS) exam at 72 hours following the SCI.[14] Other factors influencing ambulatory potential include location of the spinal cord lesion, presence and degree of pin prick sensation, and patient age (Table 45.1).[14–18]

Clinical Prediction Tools

Identifying viable candidates for ambulation and gait training is an essential decision in mapping out rehabilitation plans. Dedicating time toward gait/locomotor training will come at the expense of spending resources toward the development of other critical skills, including refining wheelchair and transfer skills (Table 45.2).[19] Clinical prediction tools[20,21] have been developed to help clinicians anticipate who may be more likely to achieve functional ambulation. The critical variables of these tools include the following, where younger age and higher motor/sensory function are more associated with functional ambulation:

- Age greater than or less than 65
- L3 and S1 motor scores
- L3 and S1 light touch dermatomes

Approaches to Gait and Locomotor Training

As rehabilitation teams consider treatment plans, clinicians will need to determine whether to target gait training, locomotor training, or some combination of the two. **Gait training** utilizes therapist feedback in conjunction with external devices such as orthotics, exoskeleton, and/or upper extremity (UE) aides to compensate for physical deficits and promote ambulation, whereas **locomotor training** focuses on repetitive practice and strategies to induce use-dependent plasticity.[22–24] This method utilizes the afferent input created by facilitated locomotor patterns to tap into spinal cord–mediated central process generators, which in turn

Table 45.1 Predictors of Ambulation Following Spinal Cord Injury

AIS Level ~72 h After Spinal Cord Injury	Percent Functional Ambulation 1-Year Postinjury Based on Initial AIS Level	Percent Functional Ambulation 1-Year Postinjury Based on Initial AIS level and Additional Factors
AIS A	0%–5%	0%: Cervical injury 5%–8%: Thoracic/lumbar injuries
AIS B	33%	0%–33%: Only light touch preserved 66%–89%: Light touch and pin prick preserved
AIS C	75%	25%–42%: >50 years old 71%–91%: <50 years old
AIS D	80%–100%	80%–100%: >50 years old 100%: <50 years old

AIS, American Spinal Injury Association (ASIA) impairment scale.

Adapted from Scivoletto G, Tamburella F, Laurenza L, Torre M, Molinari M. Who is going to walk? A review of the factors influencing walking recovery after spinal cord injury. *Front Hum Neurosci.* 2014;8:141; Waters RL, Adkins RH, Yakura JS, Sie I. Motor and sensory recovery following incomplete tetraplegia. *Arch Phys Med Rehabil.* 1994;75(3):306–311; Ditunno P, Patrick M, Stineman M, Ditunno J. Who wants to walk? Preferences for recovery after SCI: a longitudinal and cross-sectional study. *Spinal Cord.* 2008;46(7):500–506; Burns SP, Golding DG, Rolle Jr WA, Graziani V, Ditunno Jr JF. Recovery of ambulation in motor-incomplete tetraplegia. *Arch Phys Med Rehabil.* 1997;78(11):1169–1172; Scivoletto G, Morganti B, Ditunno P, Ditunno J, Molinari M. Effects on age on spinal cord lesion patients' rehabilitation. *Spinal Cord.* 2003;41(8):457–464.

Table 45.2 Correlation Between Time Spent Completing Transfer, Wheelchair, and Gait Training During Acute Inpatient Rehabilitation Stay and Outcome Scores at One Year Postinjury

	Satisfaction With Life	Physical Independence	Mobility	Occupation	Patient Health Questionnaire (PHQ-9)	Pain
Transfer Training	Positive	Positive	Positive	Positive	Negative	No Correlation
Wheelchair Training	Positive	Positive	Positive	Positive	No Correlation	Negative
Gait Training	Negative	Negative	Negative	Negative	No Correlation	Positive

Adapted from Rigot S, Worobey L, Boninger ML. Gait training in acute spinal cord injury rehabilitation—utilization and outcomes among nonambulatory individuals: findings from the SCIRehab project. *Arch Phys Med Rehabil.* 2018;99(8):1591–1598.

induce rhythmic efferent output for reflexive gait activation, thereby stimulating neural recovery.[22–24] Locomotor training can be achieved through the use of various body weight–supported overground training, body weight–supported treadmill training, and robotic systems. The primary principles of locomotor training include[23,24]:

- Normalize stepping velocities, stance loading, and reciprocal arm swing
- Maintain upright and extended trunk/head
- Approximate hip, knee, and ankle kinematics
- Synchronize hip extension in stance and couple unloading of one limb with loading of contralateral side
- Maintain symmetrical interlimb kinematics/kinetics

For those with motor complete injuries, functional ambulation is generally only achieved in those with injuries at or below T8. These individuals generally require the support of various orthotics, with more extensive systems being required for those with thoracic injuries. Those with T8–L2 injuries will often require the use of use of a hip-knee-ankle-foot orthosis, such as a reciprocal gait orthosis, as seen in Fig. 45.1. This can enable reciprocal leg advancement with the use of a dual cable system that couples hip flexion with contralateral hip extension. This type of system requires high energy demands,[25] which can limit its use for functional daily activities. For those with volitional hip flexor control, custom fabricated knee-ankle-foot orthoses can facilitate exercise and/or home mobility. A variety of ankle-foot orthoses are available to further support those with ankle and knee weakness. These include prefabricated flexible orthoses for simple foot drop, custom-molded solid or articulated orthotics that can support the ankle and foot in multiple planes, and ground reaction force options that not only support the ankle but also provide an extension moment at the knee for those with weak quadriceps.

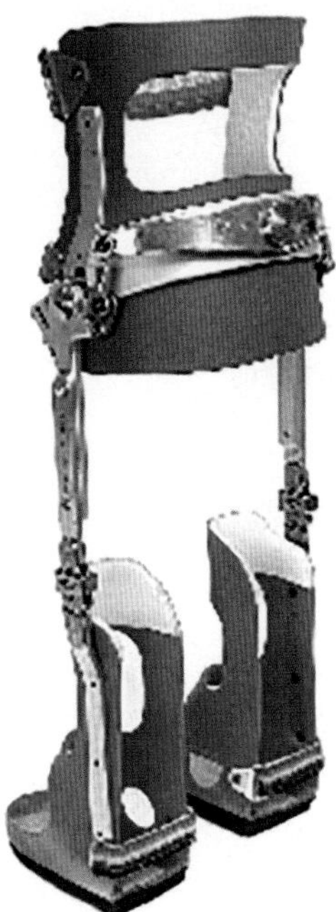

Fig. 45.1 Isocentric reciprocating gait orthosis (RGO). (Courtesy Center for Orthotic Design, Redwood City, Calif., and Fillauer Companies, Inc., Chattanooga, Tenn.)

Exoskeleton use provides an alternative solution for those with thoracic complete and lower cervical incomplete injuries. Reimbursement for these devices continues to pose a great challenge for home use, but training with them has led to independent ambulation with gait speeds sufficient for indoor use and other reported benefits, including improved spasticity and bowel management.[26,27] The five systems the U.S. Food and Drug Administration approved include the ReWalk, Ekso, Indego, Rex, and HAL (Hybrid Assistive Limb). Criteria vary slightly between devices but in general include:

- T4–T5 any AIS level or C7–T3 AIS D
- <220 lbs (100 kg); between 5 ft 0 in and 6 ft 4 in (152–193 cm)
- Sufficient UE strength and range of motion to use crutches
- Sufficient lower extremity (LE) range of motion to allow ambulation
- At least fair trunk control
- Healthy bone density
- HAL requires some degree of motor function at the hip/knee[28]

Neuromodulation and neural interfaces offer alternative strategies to support ambulation. Surface electrical stimulation units can provide ankle dorsiflexion assistance during swing phase and/or quadriceps engagement during stance. Implantable electrical stimulation systems have demonstrated ability to provide effective standing with a walker[29]; however, research continues regarding its use to promote ambulation. Implanted epidural spinal cord stimulation[30] and noninvasive epidural stimulation[31] have also demonstrated motor activation for standing and early pre-ambulation activities.

Wheelchair Mobility, Seating, and Positioning

While some individuals with SCI may achieve functional ambulation, many will require other means for independent mobility. Approximately 60% of individuals will use some form of wheelchair or scooter for more than 40 hours per week at 1-year post injury, which increases to 80% of individuals who are 30 years postinjury.[32]

When considering mobility options, the clinician must carefully consider both the type of mobility device and the seating interface. Any mobility evaluation should be performed by a team that consists of a physician with SCI expertise, a physical or occupational therapist, and an assistive technology specialist.

Specialized certifications (e.g., certified assistive technology professional, seating mobility specialist) exist in these professions.

Wheeled mobility devices come in a variety of designs and options and include manual wheelchairs (MWC), power-operated vehicles (POV)/scooters, and power wheelchairs (PWC). Justification for each will necessitate ruling out less costly and less restrictive devices for the safe, efficient, and functional use in the home.

Manual Wheelchairs

MWCs are generally configured to promote self-propulsion; however, in select situations, an individual may instead need a MWC that is pushed by a caregiver. Wheelchairs designed for independent self-propulsion include:

Standard MWC: Noncustom, heavy, limited sizes, no adjustability. Rarely used in the SCI population

Lightweight MWC: Weighs <34 lbs (15 kg), but very limited axle adjustability and positioning capability

Ultralightweight MWC: Weighs <30 lbs (13.5 kg), although frequently weighs <20 lbs (9 kg). Fully adjustable axle as well as configurable seat, back, and leg rest hanger angles. Two main styles:

- **Folding Frames:** Easily folded for transportation, but offer a less firm ride and slightly heavier
- **Rigid Frames:** Can be either a box or a cantilever style. Box style is more rigid, whereas cantilever style offers more flex, providing some degree of inherent suspension. Cantilever frames can be easier to transfer into a car due to their smaller profile

Wheelchairs designed for dependent propulsion include **manual tilt-in-space** and **reclining** wheelchairs. Although not to be used as a primary chair, **a transport chair** (equipped with four smaller wheels) offers a lightweight, narrower, and less expensive alternative for those with limited resources who require a back-up MWC.

Power Assist: A Hybrid of Manual and Power

Power assist options are considered for users who are not interested in a PWC, but who are unable to efficiently or safely propel a MWC full time due to weakness or UE injuries. Numerous studies have identified pain and injury due to UE overuse in the SCI population.[33–35] In an effort to mitigate the risk of, or account for, overuse injuries, power assist options are frequently recommended. These include pushrim-activated wheels (i.e., E-motion, Twion), rear power add-on systems (i.e., Smart Drive and Smoov), and joystick-controlled power add-on systems (i.e., E-fix).

Power Mobility

POV/Scooter: In general, a POV/scooter is not appropriate for the SCI population, given limitations in seating configurations. An exception to this can be made for high-functioning individuals with an incomplete injury who simply require powered mobility for community distances.

PWCs: For those necessitating powered mobility, PWCs are usually required. PWCs are typically classified by drive wheel configuration: rear-wheel, front-wheel, or mid-wheel drive. The placement of the drive wheel together with how the chair is programmed will change the PWC performance in various environments. Each configuration has its pros and cons, so it is important to fully assess the user's needs/goals (Table 45.3).[36]

Power Seating Functions

Power seating options use a motor to move or change a component of the seating system. These include:

Tilt-in-Space: Posteriorly tilts the seating system in space (0–55 degrees) <u>without</u> changing the angle at the hips. Benefits include increased sitting tolerance, independent management of pressure reliefs, decreased fatigue, improved postural stability, management of spasticity, pain relief, and reduced caregiver burden.

Power Recline: Allows independent adjustment of the seat-to-back angle from 80–180 degrees. Benefits include pressure reduction (especially when combined with tilt-in-space), positioning for bladder management or respiratory care, spasticity management, improved proximal stability/head control,

Table 45.3 Pros and Cons of Power Wheelchair Drive Wheel Configuration

	Pros	Cons
RWD	• Good suspension • Greater stability at higher speeds	• Larger turning radius • Front casters may limit lower extremity (LE) positioning or interfere with transfers
FWD	• Obstacle-climbing ability • Tight 90 degree turns • Improved access in front of user	• Less stability at higher speeds • Least intuitive • Instability down steep ramps
MWD	• Smallest turning radius • Most intuitive • Maneuverability • Most stable	• Drive wheel can lose traction over obstacles ("high centering") • Front casters may limit LE positioning or interfere with transfers

FWD, Front-wheel drive; MWD, mid-wheel drive; *RWD*, rear-wheel drive.

decreased fatigue, passive range of motion of hips, and improved comfort.

Power Elevating Leg Rests: Elevation of legs works most effectively in conjunction with either power tilt or power recline to allow for management of edema, spasticity, and blood pressure.

Power Seat Elevator: Allows vertical adjustment of the seat height, which can facilitate ease of transfers, improved functional reach, vocational/educational access, and social interactions.

Power Standing: Takes the user from a seated position into a partial or full stand. Standing helps to improve circulation, bowel/bladder function, digestion, and spasticity, as well as promote bone density and muscle lengthening.

Drive Controls

A crucial piece in the evaluation of power mobility is to identify access points for operation of the PWC and power seating functions. Selection of the appropriate type of drive control requires a methodical approach to identify reliable and consistently reproducible movements that can generate the output necessary to supply commands to the wheelchair. There is no required hierarchy of site selection, but usual progression begins at the hand and then moves to alternative sites such as the finger, head, foot, chin, and breath.

Drive controls are separated into two primary categories: **proportional drive** and **nonproportional drive** mechanisms. **Proportional drive**, such as joysticks, allow the user to proportionally increase their speed and/or directionality with progressively greater deflection of the joystick. The amount of deflection determines the speed (similar to a gas pedal). This requires voluntary motor control and appropriate grading of force. **Nonproportional** drive mechanisms, such as switch access, operate via a stepwise change in speed or direction. This is less fluid and reduces fine control of the wheelchair, yet provides an alternative for those without the motor control to operate a joystick (Table 45.4).

Table 45.4 Power Wheelchair Drive Controls

Proportional Drive Control	• 360 degrees directional control • Precise directional/speed control • Better control over varied terrain
Standard Joystick	• Allows for hand, chin, or foot control • Variety of joystick handle options to account for differing degrees of intrinsic hand function
Mini Joystick	• Requires less force and range of motion • Placement may be midline (finger control) or near the chin on a specialized mount or bib
RIM Control (Rehabilitation Institute of Montreal)	• Head control system with the head pad mounted to a compact joystick • User must be able to maintain constant pressure against the pad to sustain movement
Nonproportional Drive Control	• Movement controlled by directional switches • Driving is either "on" or "off" in any given direction and with stepwise speed control • Programmable options available (i.e., scanning)
Sip and Puff	• Activation via air pressure commands (sips or puffs) through a straw to dictate speed and directional control • Requires good oral motor control
Head Array	• Controlled by proximity switches in the headrest pads with activation achieved when user is within close proximity to the switch
Proximity Switch	• As above, but can be mounted in various areas of wheelchair
Fiber Optics	• Often mounted onto trays for switch activation

Adapted from Lange ML, Minkel J. Seating and wheeled mobility: a clinical resource guide. Slack Incorporated; 2018.

Seating and Positioning

Assessment Process

Assessment for any mobility device necessitates evaluation for an appropriate seating system that will optimize postural support, provide proximal stability to promote distal function, ensure comfort, protect skin integrity, and foster the greatest degree of independent functioning possible. Examination of the individual should include assessment in their current seating system, on a mat table in the seated position, and in supine to garner information about function, strength, postural control, range of motion, spasticity, skin integrity, and sizing measurements. Common sizing considerations, some of which are illustrated in Figure 45.2, include:

- Seat Width: Critical for positional support, propulsion efficiency, and optimizing access; measure the widest part of the person's hips and add 1 in (2.5 cm)
- Seat Depth: Affects weight distribution, pelvic positioning, and seating interface pressures; excessively long seat depth can pull a patient into a posterior pelvic tilt; measure along the lateral thigh from the popliteal space to the posterior buttocks and subtract 1-2 in (2.5-5 cm)
- Back Height: MWC back should be 1-2 in (2.5-5cm) below the inferior angle of the scapula for scapular clearance during self-propulsion; PWC back may need to be closer to shoulder height, especially if on a PWC with power seating; cushion will add 2-4 in (5-10 cm) to the height
- Seat-to-Foot Rest Length: Footrests that are too high will cause increased pressure on the ischia, while footrests that are too low will cause individuals to slide out of chair; measure from the medial hamstring

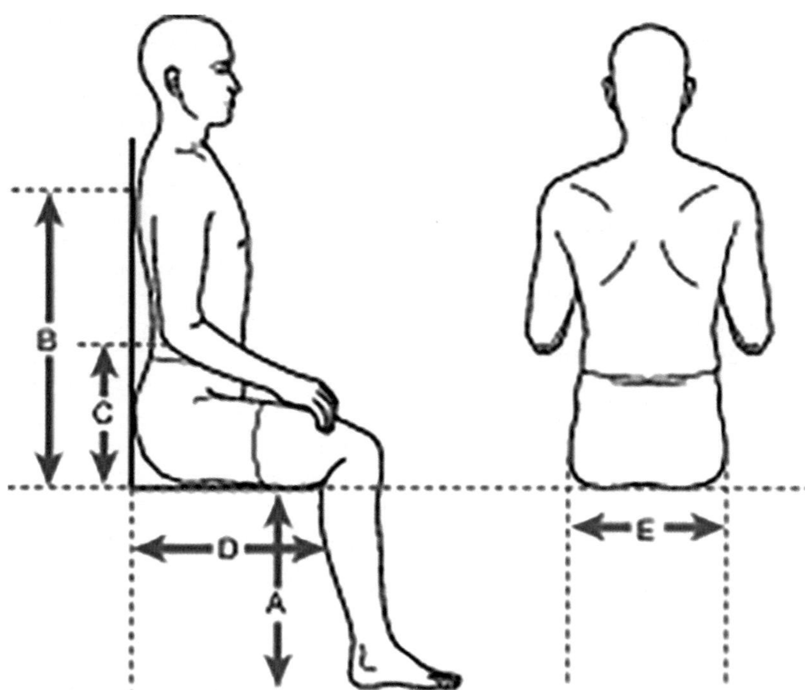

Fig. 45.2 Body measurements. A, Leg length: distance from bottom of heel to popliteal area. B, Back height: distance from buttocks to the inferior angle of the scapula. C, Armrest height: distance from buttocks to forearm with elbow at 90 degrees. D, Seat depth: distance from back of buttocks to popliteal area. E, Seat width: distance between the widest parts of the buttocks. (From: Figure 14-8, Cifu D. Braddom's Physical Medicine and Rehabilitation (Fifth Edition). Elsevier; 2016.)

tendon to the bottom of the heel and subtract the cushion height

For optimal seating in those who are full-time MWC users, further wheelchair frame configurations will need to be accounted for. The most appropriate MWC for these individuals is a properly configured, fully customizable ultralight weight wheelchair to promote safe and efficient propulsion biomechanics. Appropriate wheelchair set-up prevents UE pathology and overuse injuries.[11] Proper biomechanics include adjustment of:

- **Rear wheel axle anterior/posterior positioning** that allows vertical alignment of the shoulder to be in line with or slightly in front of the axle. With static sitting, the arm should rest to the side with the middle finger in line with the center of the axle.
- **Rear wheel axle height** configured to optimize hand placement on the rear wheel. Ideally, the elbow angle should be 100–120 degrees of elbow flexion when the hand is at the top of the handrim. Greater angles can predispose shoulder impingement, whereas angles <100 degrees result in ineffective propulsion[11,37]
- Adjustment of **backrest angle** to promote pelvic stability, account for available hip range of motion, and improve trunk balance
- Optimization of **seat slope (a.k.a. "seat dump")**, which is the difference between the front and rear seat height. This will affect balance, transfers, and wheel access
- Rear wheel **camber** will bring the top of the wheel closer to the user, which improves wheel access, lateral wheelchair stability, and maneuverability, albeit at the expense of increased overall chair width

MWC Propulsion Techniques

To preserve UE function, it is important not only to achieve ideal seating configurations but also to aim for safe propulsion techniques that reduce peak forces, decrease the rate of application of forces, and minimize the frequency of propulsive strokes. Various stroke patterns have been identified, including: (1) semicircular; (2) single-looping over propulsion; (3) double-looping over propulsion; and (4) arcing.[38,39] The single-looping over form of propulsion, which consists of having the hand above the pushrim during recovery, is the most prevalent pattern in individuals with paraplegia. However, the semicircular pattern, where the user's hand drops below the pushrim during the recovery phase, has better biomechanics. The semicircular pattern has been associated with lower stroke frequency, greater time spent in the push phase relative to the recovery phase, and less angular joint velocity and acceleration, leading to reduced repetition and more efficient propulsion.[38,39] Overall, a long, smooth wheelchair propulsive stroke should be encouraged by clinicians.[40]

Cushions

Seat cushion options are delineated by the degree of postural support and pressure relief that they offer. In justifying various cushions, a practitioner should recognize the medical needs that would give grounds for a particular category of cushion. The categories include cushions that are general use, pressure relieving, positioning, combination of pressure relieving and positioning, and custom contoured. Cushions are made of various materials to achieve varying degrees of support, pressure reduction, breathability, and adjustability. This may include materials such as foam, gel, or air with various degrees of built-in contour (Table 45.5).

Back Rests

A variety of different wheelchair backrests are also available and separated into different categories based on the degree of postural support and customization offered. These include sling/upholstery and solid backrests. The sling backrests can be made from standard upholstery or adjustable tension sling systems. Solid backrests include general use, positioning (with various degrees of contour), and custom contoured backrests. The clinical assessment will determine the correct back support based on trunk control, sitting balance, degree of postural asymmetry, transfer method, UE function, and type of wheelchair being recommended.

Table 45.5 Pros and Cons of Wheelchair Cushions

	Pros	Cons
Foam	• Inexpensive • Variety of densities • T-foam or memory foam incorporate viscoelastic properties • Pelvic stability	• Deteriorates fastest • Less pressure relieving
Visco-Elastic Fluid/Gel	• Pressure redistribution • High viscosity promotes greater stability than air cushions	• Weight • Affected by temperature (low temperatures cause transient firmness)
Air	• Pressure redistribution • Provision of micro-adjustments to optimize skin protection • Breathability • Lightweight	• Maintenance • Affected by altitude • Less pelvic stability
Honey-comb	• Lightweight • Breathability • Wicking • Pelvic stability	• Lacks adjustability • Less pressure relieving relative to viscoelastic fluid/air
Custom Contoured	• Accommodates postural asymmetries • Contouring reduces areas of high interface pressures • Pelvic stability	• Weight • Cost • Time intensive/ skilled provider • Lacks adjustability

Additional Accessories

Many accessories and positioning components are available to further optimize seating configurations. These may include variable options such as hip guides, adductor pads, abductor pads, pelvic/chest belts, thoracic lateral supports, headrests, adjustable footplates, specialized handrims, and various wheel sizes/materials. All of these can contribute greatly to maximizing patient goals and are integral to the final wheelchair prescription. Details of such items are beyond the scope of this brief review.

Review Questions

1. A 55-year-old male with C6 AIS C quadriplegia is on the inpatient rehabilitation floor and inquires, “Doctor, what are my chances to walk in a year?” As his SCI physiatrist, what are the critical dermatomes, myotomes, and age-related factors that weigh heavily in your clinical thought process when considering ambulation prognosis?
   a. T10 dermatome, L3 myotome, and age greater or less than 50 years old
   b. S4–S5 dermatome, L3 myotome, and age greater or less than 65 years old
   c. S1 dermatome, L4 myotome, and age greater or less than 50 years old
   d. S1 dermatome, L3 myotome, and age greater or less than 65 years old
2. You are in the inpatient rehabilitation gym having a discussion with the physical therapist about therapeutic options to promote neurorecovery for one of your patients with an upper thoracic motor incomplete SCI. Your goal point is to induce neuroplasticity in the hopes that the patient may continue to demonstrate ongoing neurologic recovery. In speaking with the therapist your recommendations include training that they:
   a. Utilize a body weight–supported treadmill to facilitate LE movement in any way possible, as long as the lower extremities are being engaged and moving at least small amounts voluntarily
   b. Utilize a body weight–supported overground system while tilting the patient slightly forward to leverage the stepping reflex
   c. While unloading the body with a body weight–supported system, encourage the therapist to facilitate normal stepping speeds, normal stance, and reciprocal arm swing
   d. Provide the patient with the necessary supportive orthotics to maintain an upright stance and teach compensatory gait techniques to maximize function

3. As a physiatrist working on the inpatient rehabilitation unit, which of the following would NOT be helpful to a patient with new-onset quadriplegia who is sitting up for the first time?
   a. Compression stockings
   b. Abdominal binder
   c. Close monitoring of their blood pressure
   d. Wrist/hand orthoses
4. A 34-year-old female with a C7 AIS B quadriplegia is 1 year postinjury. What form of mobility will she most likely be using for household distances?
   a. Power wheelchair with standard drive control
   b. Power scooter
   c. Optimally configured manual wheelchair
   d. Power wheelchair with alternative drive control
5. Why is it important to have the axle of an ultra-lightweight manual wheelchair as far forward as possible?
   a. Improve propulsion efficiency
   b. Reduce stress on UE joints
   c. Increase load on front casters
   d. a and b
6. What is a potential reason for someone's pelvis sitting too far forward in their wheelchair seat?
   a. Limitation in hip flexion range of motion
   b. Seat depth too short
   c. Push handles too high
   d. Increased lumbar lordosis
7. A 27-year-old female with T10 paraplegia has a history of a stage IV sacral pressure injury and significant LE spasticity. What would be the most appropriate type of wheelchair cushion for her?
   a. Custom molded
   b. 2 in (4 cm) foam cushion
   c. Pressure relieving
   d. Pressure relieving and positioning
8. A 68-year-old male with a history T8 AIS A paraplegia suffered 28 years ago following a motorcycle accident returns to your clinic and has many questions regarding techniques for adequate pressure relief. After many years of being a manual wheelchair user, he recently transitioned to a power wheelchair due to impaired shoulder function and development of a stage III right ischial pressure injury. You advise him that all the following are adequate techniques for pressure relief except:
   a. >45 degrees of recline
   b. >25 degrees of tilt with at least 120 degrees of recline
   c. >45 degrees of tilt
   d. Anterior lean with arms resting on lap and trunk leaned forward at >45 degrees
9. At which level of injury would clinicians begin considering a knee-ankle-foot orthosis as an orthosis that could realistically support functional ambulation at the home level and/or for exercise?
   a. T10 AIS B
   b. L4 AIS B
   c. L2 AIS A
   d. L3 AIS D
10. You are leading a multidisciplinary weekly team meeting for a 39-year-old male who suffered a mild traumatic brain injury, C4 AIS B quadriplegia status post C2–C7 fusion, and respiratory failure who is now weaning off of the ventilator and tolerating a Passy Muir valve. The team is weighing the various drive control options to provide him independent mobility in a power wheelchair. Which type of drive control would be a viable option for him, while allowing him to retain proportional control over the speed and directionality of his chair?
    a. Utilization of a head array with proximity switches
    b. Joystick control to be operated with his hand
    c. Sip and puff drive control
    d. Mini joystick on a swing away mount with chin access

REFERENCES

1. Nixon V. *Spinal cord injury: a guide to functional outcomes in Physical Therapy Management.* London: William Heinemann; 1985.
2. Coggrave M, Rose L. A specialist seating assessment clinic: changing pressure relief practice. *Spinal Cord.* 2003;41(12):692–695.
3. Barnett RI, Shelton FE. Measurement of support surface efficacy: pressure. *Advan Wound Care.* 1997;10(7):21–29.
4. Dicianno BE, Arva J, Lieberman JM, et al. RESNA position on the application of tilt, recline, and elevating legrests for wheelchairs. *Assistive Technology.* 2009;21(1):13–22.
5. Paralyzed Veterans of America. Guidelines CfSCMCP. Pressure ulcer prevention and treatment following injury: a clinical practice guideline for health-care providers. Paralyzed Veterans of America: Washington, DC; 2014.
6. Henderson JL, Price SH, Brandstater ME, Mandac BR. Efficacy of three measures to relieve pressure in seated persons with spinal cord injury. *Arch Phys Med Rehabil.* 1994;75(5):535–539.
7. Groah SL, Schladen M, Pineda CG, Hsieh CH. Prevention of pressure ulcers among people with spinal cord injury: a systematic review. *PM & R.* 2015;7(6):613–636.
8. Hobson DA. Comparative effects of posture on pressure and shear at the body-seat interface. *J Rehabil Res Dev.* 1992;29:21–31.
9. Jan Y-K, Crane BA, Liao F, Woods JA, Ennis WJ. Comparison of muscle and skin perfusion over the ischial tuberosities in response to wheelchair tilt-in-space and recline angles in people with spinal cord injury. *Arch Phys Med Rehabil.* 2013;94(10):1990–1996.
10. Jan Y-K, Jones MA, Rabadi MH, Foreman RD, Thiessen A. Effect of wheelchair tilt-in-space and recline angles on skin perfusion over the ischial tuberosity in people with spinal cord injury. *Arch Phys Med Rehabil.* 2010;91(11):1758–1764.
11. Paralyzed Veterans of America Consortium for Spinal Cord Medicine. Preservation of upper limb function following

spinal cord injury: a clinical practice guideline for healthcare professionals. *J Spinal Cord Medicine.* 2005; 28(5):434.

12. Perry J, Gronley JK, Newsam CJ, Reyes ML, Mulroy SJ. Electromyographic analysis of the shoulder muscles during depression transfers in subjects with low-level paraplegia. *Arch Phys Med Rehabil.* 1996;77(4):350–355.
13. Papuga MO, Memberg WD, Crago PE. Biomechanics of sliding transfer: feasibility of FES assistance. *Proceedings of the Second Joint 24th Annual Conference and the Annual Fall Meeting of the Biomedical Engineering Society.* IEEE; 2002. pp.23-26. https://doi.org/10.1109/IEMBS.2002.1053333.
14. Scivoletto G, Tamburella F, Laurenza L, Torre M, Molinari M. Who is going to walk? A review of the factors influencing walking recovery after spinal cord injury. *Front Hum Neurosci.* 2014;8:141.
15. Waters RL, Adkins RH, Yakura JS, Sie I. Motor and sensory recovery following incomplete tetraplegia. *Arch Phys Med Rehabil.* 1994;75(3):306–311.
16. Ditunno P, Patrick M, Stineman M, Ditunno J. Who wants to walk? Preferences for recovery after SCI: a longitudinal and cross-sectional study. *Spinal Cord.* 2008;46(7):500–506.
17. Burns SP, Golding DG, Rolle Jr WA, Graziani V, Ditunno Jr JF. Recovery of ambulation in motor-incomplete tetraplegia. *Arch Phys Med Rehabil.* 1997;78(11):1169–1172.
18. Scivoletto G, Morganti B, Ditunno P, Ditunno J, Molinari M. Effects on age on spinal cord lesion patients' rehabilitation. *Spinal Cord.* 2003;41(8):457–464.
19. Rigot S, Worobey L, Boninger ML. Gait training in acute spinal cord injury rehabilitation—utilization and outcomes among nonambulatory individuals: findings from the SCIRehab project. *Arch Phys Med Rehabil.* 2018;99(8):1591–1598.
20. van Middendorp JJ, Hosman AJ, Donders ART, et al. A clinical prediction rule for ambulation outcomes after traumatic spinal cord injury: a longitudinal cohort study. *Lancet.* 2011;377(9770):1004–1010.
21. Hicks KE, Zhao Y, Fallah N, et al. A simplified clinical prediction rule for prognosticating independent walking after spinal cord injury: a prospective study from a Canadian multicenter spinal cord injury registry. *Spine.* 2017; 17(10):1383–1392.
22. Hubli M, Dietz V. The physiological basis of neurorehabilitation–locomotor training after spinal cord injury. *J Neuroeng Rehabilitation.* 2013;10:5.
23. Harkema SJ. Neural plasticity after human spinal cord injury: application of locomotor training to the rehabilitation of walking. *Neuroscientist.* 2001;7(5):455–468.
24. Barbeau H, Wainberg M, Finch L. Description and application of a system for locomotor rehabilitation. *Med Biol Eng Comput.* 1987;25(3):341–344.
25. Arazpour M, Samadian M, Bahramizadeh M, et al. The efficiency of orthotic interventions on energy consumption in paraplegic patients: a literature review. *Spinal Cord.* 2015;53(3):168–175.
26. Louie DR, Eng JJ, Lam T. Gait speed using powered robotic exoskeletons after spinal cord injury: a systematic review and correlational study. *J Neuroeng Rehabilitation.* 2015;12(1):1–10.
27. Miller LE, Zimmermann AK, Herbert WG. Clinical effectiveness and safety of powered exoskeleton-assisted walking in patients with spinal cord injury: systematic review with meta-analysis. *Medical Devices (Auckland, NZ).* 2016;9:455.
28. Palermo AE, Maher JL, Baunsgaard CB, Nash MS. Clinician-focused overview of bionic exoskeleton use after spinal cord injury. *Top Spin Cord Inj Rehabil.* 2017;23(3): 234–244.
29. Triolo RJ, Bailey SN, Miller ME, et al. Longitudinal performance of a surgically implanted neuroprosthesis for lower-extremity exercise, standing, and transfers after spinal cord injury. *Arch Phys Med Rehabil.* 2012;93(5):896–904.
30. Angeli CA, Boakye M, Morton RA, et al. Recovery of overground walking after chronic motor complete spinal cord injury. *N Engl J Med.* 2018;379(13):1244–1250.
31. Sayenko DG, Rath M, Ferguson AR, et al. Self-assisted standing enabled by non-invasive spinal stimulation after spinal cord injury. *J Neurotrauma.* 2019;36(9):1435–1450.
32. National Spinal Cord Injury Statistical Center 2019 Annual Statistical Report for the Spinal Cord Injury Model Systems University of Alabama at Birmingham: Birmingham, Alabama2019 [updated December 2019]. https://www.nscisc.uab.edu.
33. Yang J, Boninger ML, Leath JD, Fitzgerald SG, Dyson-Hudson TA, Chang MW. Carpal tunnel syndrome in manual wheelchair users with spinal cord injury: a cross-sectional multicenter study. *Am J Phys Med Rehabil.* 2009;88(12): 1007–1016.
34. Dyson-Hudson TA, Kirshblum SC. Shoulder pain in chronic spinal cord injury, part 1: epidemiology, etiology, and pathomechanics. *J Spinal Cord Med.* 2004;27(1):4–17.
35. Alm M, Saraste H, Norrbrink C. Shoulder pain in persons with thoracic spinal cord injury: prevalence and characteristics. *J Rehabil Med.* 2008;40(4):277–283.
36. Lange ML, Minkel J. Seating and wheeled mobility: a clinical resource guide. Slack Incorporated; 2018.
37. DiGiovine C, Rosen L, Berner T, Betz K, Roesler T, Schmeler M. RESNA Position on the Application of Ultralight Manual Wheelchairs Arlington, VA: Rehabilitation Engineering & Assistive Technology Society of North America; 2012. https://www.resna.org/Portals/0/Documents/Position%20Papers/UltraLightweightManualWheelchairs.pdf.
38. Shimada SD, Robertson RN, Bonninger ML, Cooper RA. Kinematic characterization of wheelchair propulsion. *J Rehabil Res Dev.* 1998;35(2):210–218.
39. Boninger ML, Souza AL, Cooper RA, Fitzgerald SG, Koontz AM, Fay BT. Propulsion patterns and pushrim biomechanics in manual wheelchair propulsion. *Arch Phys Med Rehabil.* 2002;83(5):718–723.
40. Boninger ML, Impink BG, Cooper RA, Koontz AM. Relation between median and ulnar nerve function and wrist kinematics during wheelchair propulsion. *Arch Phys Med Rehabil.* 2004;85(7):1141–1145.

CHAPTER 46

Activities of Daily Living

Kathryn Beckner, Karen DeMarco, and Heather Kloepping

OUTLINE

Activities of Daily Living

Activities of daily living require basic performance skills and include activities to take care of one's own self-care and body. Daily living activities are divided into two categories: basic activities of daily living (ADLs) and instrumental activities of daily living (IADLs). Basic ADLs consist of self-care tasks, such as eating, grooming, bathing, dressing, and toileting. IADLs consist of advanced performance skills, including taking care of children and pets, household cleaning, grocery shopping, meal preparation, laundry, financial management, community mobility, and driving.[1]

Functional Independence Measure

The functional independence measure (FIM) is an evaluation instrument assessing the level of independent functioning on a variety of physical and cognitive tasks.[2] The FIM is commonly used in inpatient or subacute rehabilitation facilities to assess progress toward functional goals and/or to communicate to families or other treatment staff the level of care and assistance an individual may require. ADLs are evaluated with use of FIM scores on a rating scale of 1–7 (Table 46.1).

Projected Functional Outcomes and Adaptive Equipment/Functional Orthoses

Functional outcomes and goals can be projected based on neurological level of injury (NLI) of a person with spinal cord injury (SCI). Moreover, level of injury can inform adaptive equipment, durable medical equipment, assistive devices, and orthotics that are anticipated to be of utility. The level of injury categories depict anticipated ADL FIM scores and equipment requirements (Table 46.2).[1] Of note, these projected functional outcomes and equipment needs assume that a person has a motor complete SCI.

Architectural Adaptations

ADA Guidelines

The Americans With Disabilities Act of 1990 (ADA) provides requirements for public accommodations of commercial facilities.

Table 46.1 Functional Independence Measure Scoring Tool

FIM Score	Description
Score 7: Independent	Patient performs all tasks of an activity within a reasonable amount of time and without modification, assistive devices, or aids
Score 6: Modified Independent	Patient performs activity with more than a reasonable amount of time and/or requires modification, assistive device, or aid; or involves safety considerations for which the patient accepts responsibility
Score 5: Supervision/ Set Up	Patient receives standby assistance, cueing, or coaxing from helper; helper sets up needed items or applies orthosis or assistive/ adaptive devices
Score 4: Minimal Assistance	Patient expends 75% or more of the effort and requires no more help than touching (contact guard assistance)
Score 3: Moderate Assistance	Patient expends 50% to 74% of the effort and requires more help than touching
Score 2: Maximum Assistance	Patient expends 25% to 49% of the effort
Score 1: Total Assistance	Patient expends less than 25% of the effort, requires assistance from two helpers, or does not perform the activity

Table 46.2 Projected Functional Outcomes and Required Adaptive Equipment/Functional Orthoses Based on the NLI of a Person with SCI

NLI	Projected Functional Outcomes	Adaptive Equipment/Functional Orthoses
C1–C4	• Total assistance for all self-care ADLs • Independently instruct caregivers on ADLs • May be independent with power wheelchair mobility via alternative drive controls such as head array, sip and puff, or chin control • Power tilt pressure relief • Total assistance with manual wheelchair mobility, including pressure reliefs • Use of mobile arm supports	• Pressure-relieving cushion • Tilt-in-space manual wheelchair • Tilt-in-space shower/commode chair • Ceiling lift or portable lift • Mouth sticks • Voice-activated technologies such as smart phones, computers, and electronic aids to daily living (EADL) units • Switch access to control assistive technology devices such as computers, tablets, e-readers, and cell phones • Splinting: elbow extension splints (static or dynamic), wrist drop orthoses with or without universal cuff, resting hand splints • Typing aides, page turners • Hospital bed with specialty air mattress
C5	• Total assistance for self-care ADLs, might be able to use equipment with set up for eating and grooming • May be independent with power wheelchair mobility and pressure reliefs utilizing upper extremity/hand control • Total assistance with tilt-in-space manual wheelchair unless independent with manual pressure reliefs; can then utilize ultralightweight manual wheelchair	• Addition of ability to use long opponens splint • Pressure-relieving cushion • Splinting: elbow extension splints (dynamic or static), wrist drop orthoses with universal cuff attachment, resting hand splints • Standard vs. tilt-in-space shower/commode chair • Ceiling lift or portable lift • Universal cuffs/universal holders • Universal cuff adapted utensils for feeding and grooming • Bioness H200 neuroprosthesis • Hospital bed with specialty mattress
C6	• Addition of tenodesis, ability to use wrist extension for passive hand grasp and wrist flexion for hand release • Set up level for eating, grooming, and upper body bathing and dressing; assistance for lower body dressing, lower body bathing, and toileting • Independent with power wheelchair mobility and pressure reliefs utilizing upper extremity/hand control • Independent with ultralightweight manual wheelchair mobility indoors, some to total assistance required outdoors	• Tenodesis splint • Power assist add-on for manual wheelchair • Pressure-relieving cushion • Drop arm bedside commode, rolling rehabilitation shower/commode chair • Resting hand splints, wrist cock-up splint • Short opponens splint • Ceiling lift, portable lift, or transfer board • Button hook/zipper pull • Adapted universal cuff catheter inserter • EADLs • Hospital bed with specialty mattress
C7–C8	• Independent or modified independent (use of equipment) for eating, grooming, upper body dressing and upper body bathing; assistance for lower body dressing, lower body bathing, and toileting • Independent with power wheelchair mobility and pressure reliefs • Independent with ultralightweight manual wheelchair mobility indoors and level outdoor terrain, some assistance with uneven outdoor terrain	• Specialty backrest with postural supports in manual wheelchair • Pressure-relieving cushion • Transfer board • Built-up handles on utensils • Resting hand splints • Button hook/zipper pull • Long-handled equipment such as dressing stick, sock aide, reacher, long-handled sponge • Rolling shower/commode chair, drop arm bedside commode • Long-handled equipment for bowel care: digital stimulator, suppository inserter • Hospital bed with specialty mattress
T1–S5	• Independent or modified independent (use of equipment) with ADLs • Independent with ultralightweight manual wheelchair mobility and pressure reliefs	• Specialty backrest with postural supports in manual wheelchair • Pressure-relieving cushion • Transfer board • Long-handled dressing equipment: reacher, dressing stick, sock aide, long-handled sponge, leg lifter • Long-handled equipment for bowel care: digital stimulator, suppository inserter • Drop arm bedside commode, rolling shower/commode chair, raised toilet seat with grab bars, tub transfer bench • Hospital bed and/or bedrails for standard bed • Sexual aides: e.g., Intimate Rider; liberator shapes, body bouncer, plush wedges

ADLs, Activities of daily living.

An ADA-compliant ramp must follow a 1:12 ratio for rise and run: for each 1 in (2.5 cm) of rise, there must be 12 in (30 cm) of run. A 1:12 ratio is required, but a 1:16 or 1:20 is preferred.[1] An ADA ramp must be at least 36 in (9 ratio 1 cm) wide. Extended ramp runs require intermittent landings. ADA requires level landings at the top and bottom of a ramp.

ADA provides the following guidance for wheelchair turning space: "the space required for a wheelchair to make a 180-degree turn is a clear space of 60 in (152.4 cm) diameter or a T-shaped space," as illustrated in Fig. 46.1A and B.[3]

The exact turning radius of a wheelchair depends on the wheeled mobility device and the end user's technique to turn (Fig. 46.1A vs. Fig. 46.1B).[3] The space needed to maneuver a manual wheelchair versus a power wheelchair is impacted by the overall length and width of the chair.[4]

Architectural Recommendations In the Home

In making architectural recommendations for the wheelchair user in the home environment, it is important to consider the needs of end user, the needs of the caregiver (if necessary), environmental factors, and cost considerations. If the home is not owned by the end user, there are often limited structural adaptations available.

The entrance of a home must be accessible for a wheelchair user's ingress/egress. The initial considerations in accessing an ingress/egress are the exterior terrain of the home, the exterior approach to the home, the presence of handrails, and the number of steps to enter.[1]

For safety and emergency preparedness, it is recommended that the user have two accessible forms of ingress/egress at different locations in the home. One ingress/egress should be located off the end user's sleeping area (bedroom or room adapted for bedroom).[4]

The recommended width of the entrance doorway is 36 in (91 cm). The recommended door width for doors throughout the home is 32 in (81 cm).[4] If 36- and 32-in door widths are not available, the door width should accommodate the end user's wheelchair, which varies depending on the width of the wheeled mobility device. The end user's hand function should be considered in determining the type of doorknobs most appropriate at the entrance and throughout the home. Lever-style doorknobs are most appropriate for the end user with limited hand function.

The accessibility of light switches, thermostats, and other wall-mounted controls should be considered in the home evaluation. These controls should be within reach from a seated position. Power wheelchair users may have a power seat function to adjust and increase their seated height, but a manual wheelchair user does not have height adjustability built into their mobility device.

The kitchen should be set up for access from a seated position with the following general considerations: sink accessibility, counter height, cabinet height, oven/stove height, placement of oven/stove knobs, and access to appliances. A roll-under sink provides the greatest level of ease and accessibility for a wheelchair user. It is recommended to consider covering the pipes for safety considerations.[1]

A first-floor bedroom is recommended for full-time wheelchair users. There are multiple considerations for

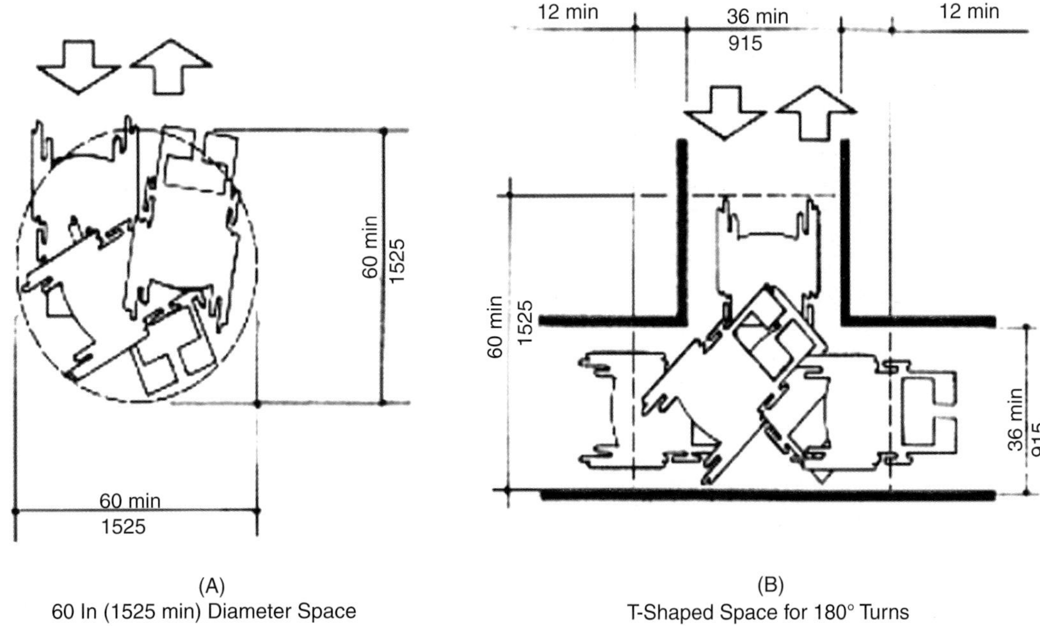

Fig. 46.1 Guidance for Wheelchair Turning Space Provided by the Americans With Disabilities Act.(A) Circular turn. (B) T-shaped turn.

a second-floor bedroom for a wheelchair user: a means by which to access the second floor, the need for a wheelchair on the second floor, and emergency evacuation considerations.

The bathroom recommendations vary depending on the level of injury, associated level of independence, needs of the end user, and needs of the caregiver (if applicable). Durable medical equipment may be needed to supplement the architectural adaptations of the home to provide a safe setup of the bathroom and promote the highest level of independence. The following are basic setup considerations[1]:

- Sink setup and height
  - Access to faucet from seated position
- Toilet setup and surrounding space to set up a transfer
  - Toilet height
- Tub/shower setup and surrounding space to set up a transfer
  - Shower stall
  - Tub only
  - Tub/shower combination
  - Roll-in shower
- Access to outlets from seated position

Wheelchair users may need to complete toileting and bathing tasks outside the bathroom if they do not have bathroom access or cannot safely or independently access this space.

Smooth, hard floor surfaces provide the greatest ease of propulsion in a manual wheelchair and limited interference with a power wheelchair. It is recommended that plush carpet be removed, as it creates a resistive surface that may significantly impact the ease of propulsion. It is recommended that throw rugs be removed, as they may create a trip hazard and get caught in the wheels of a manual or power wheelchair.

An occupational therapy evaluation is recommended for a full home evaluation and assessment of end user's function, functional needs, and home environment.

Environmental Control Technology

The goal of assistive technology in the SCI population is to support or restore function, quality of life, and independence post injury. Electronic aids to daily living (EADLs) are devices that can be used to control one's surrounding environment. EADLs include control of electronic devices within the end user's environment.[1]

The EADL needs of the end user vary depending on the level of injury and ability to independently interact with their surrounding environment. EADLs provide a range of increased access to and control of devices and the surrounding environment to include but not limited to:

- Call bell access
- Hospital bed function operation
- Cell phone access
- Landline phone access
- Smart phone access and control of applications
- Computer access and control of programs
- Lights on/off
- Thermostat control
- Television operation and control
- Stereo operation and control
- Security camera access and operation
- Automatic door opener operation
- Household appliance operation

EADLs for the SCI population range from consumer products to advanced medical-grade technology. The needs of the end user, the desired outcome, and the products available determine which type of technology is most appropriate.

EADLs are operated in a variety of ways. The means of control is based on the end user's functional ability and task-specific needs. EADLs may be switch controlled, remote controlled, voice activated, or touch activated.[1]

An occupational therapy evaluation is recommended for a full EADL evaluation to explore functional tasks and access methods for the end user based on their goals, needs, and functional ability.

Tendon Transfers

Definition: The detachment of a functioning muscle-tendon unit from its insertion and reattachment to another tendon or bone to substitute for the function of a paralyzed muscle or injured tendon, in order to restore active elbow extension, key grip, and finger grasping.[5]

Goals of Upper Extremity Reconstruction

- Promote improved upper extremity (UE) function to facilitate increased independence with functional tasks and ADLs without the need for adaptive equipment or orthoses.
- Decrease burden of care on caregivers.
- Improve patient perceived satisfaction and quality of life.
- The patient's goals and direct involvement in the decision-making process for surgery are key to a successful outcome after surgery.
- Having a specific functional goal in mind prior to surgery facilitates a more successful outcome.
- Realistic goals and expectations should be discussed upfront with each patient.[6–9]

Surgeon's Classification of the Tetraplegic Upper Extremity

- International classification for surgery of the hand in tetraplegia (ICSHT) was developed to identify

candidates for UE restoration surgery. It provides more specifics regarding available active muscle function. The number and type of procedures that can be performed are based on international standards for neurologic classification of SCI (ISNCSCI): the more muscles available for transfer, the more options for reconstructing specific functions.
- Therapists should also implement assessment of an individual's function over the three domains of the international classification of functioning, disability and health using validated outcome measures for individuals with SCI (e.g., FIM, the spinal cord independence measure, manual muscle testing).[6]

Candidates for Surgery

- Generally must be motor C5 or greater
- Neurological stability—typically, transfer not complete until at least 1-year postinjury, but evaluation can occur before to establish baseline and to provide education
- Plateau of functional gains with traditional therapies
- Good motivation with appropriate and realistic goals for improved function
- Good caregiver support to help with stretching, splinting, and exercises
- Good compliance with recommendations with use of stretching, splinting, and exercises
- Supple joints free of contractures
- Well-controlled spasticity
- Good general health[7]

Muscle Strengths Required for Tendon Transfer

- A donor muscle must have a muscle grade strength of at least 4, because after transfer, there is a loss of some strength, often one muscle grade.[6]

Priority Hierarchy for Restoration

1. Elbow extension
2. Wrist extension
3. Lateral pinch and release (key pinch)
4. Palmar grasp and release[7]

Common Surgical Reconstruction Options

- **Elbow extension:** Two options: (1) Posterior deltoid to triceps (2) Biceps to triceps. Typically, biceps to triceps tendon transfer is an easier surgery and easier to rehabilitate.
  - Goals of surgery:
    1. Increase active range of motion for elbow extension with gravity eliminated and against gravity, to allow for increase in available space that the upper extremity is able to reach for functional tasks.
    2. Patient identified goals of surgery include propelling a wheelchair, improving functional transfers, balancing in wheelchair, dressing, driving a vehicle, and positioning arms when lying down.
  - Functional outcomes—improvements with:
    1. Bed mobility
    2. Transfers
    3. Safety with driving
    4. Balance in sitting
    5. Weight shifting
    6. Overhead reach
    7. Manual wheelchair use
    8. Acts as an antagonist to the brachioradialis to prevent elbow contracture
- **Wrist extension:** Brachioradialis (BR) to extensor carpi radialis brevis
  - Goal of Surgery: Achieve stronger wrist extension to facilitate improved tenodesis grasp. Typically performed in conjunction with key pinch surgery, such as flexor pollicis longus (FPL) tenodesis or split distal FPL tenodesis (see below)
  - Functional outcomes:
    1. Typically can achieve 2 kg of increased passive pinch strength through tenodesis
    2. Increased independence with ADLs such as feeding and grooming without need for orthoses or adaptive equipment
    3. Picking up objects
    4. Handwriting
    5. Opening and closing zippers
    6. Pressing buttons on remotes
    7. Sustained grasp of objects
- **Lateral pinch:** BR to FPL or FPL tenodesis or split distal FPL tenodesis
  - Goal of surgery: Improve tenodesis pinch or active key pinch for ADL tasks
  - Functional outcomes:
    1. Typically can achieve 2 kg of increased pinch strength
    2. ADLs such as feeding and grooming without need for orthoses or adaptive equipment
    3. Picking up objects
    4. Handwriting
    5. Opening and closing zippers
    6. Pressing buttons on remotes
    7. Sustained grasp of objects
- **Palmar grasp:** Extensor carpi radialis longus to flexor digitorum profundus (FDP) or pronator teres to FDP
  - Goal of surgery: To restore some active grasp for someone with preserved function of both radial wrist extensors

- Functional outcomes:
  1. Improved power grasp
  2. Improved hook grasp
  3. Gross grasp of objects
  4. Brushing hair
  5. Using telephone
  6. Driving
  7. Self-catheterization[6]

Postoperative Rehabilitation Course

Recommend initial inpatient rehabilitation stay at a specialty center, as it is difficult to find specialized therapy treatments in outpatient clinics.

- Typically immobilized in cast for 3–4 weeks to allow tendon healing.
- Adapting patient's environment around short-term limitations of casted/splinted UE (e.g., moving power wheelchair joystick position, relearning ADLs with opposite UE, or training caregivers to assist with ADLs).
- Regain active and passive range of motion based on criteria guidelines; typically, will wear removable splint to immobilize and protect the tendon transfer when outside of therapy.
- Muscle reeducation of transferred muscle for new muscle action.
- Use of functional electrical stimulation or biofeedback as required.
- Instruction to use transferred muscle as much as possible.
- Learning/practice of functional tasks and ADLs.
- Improvements in function after tendon surgery shown to continue for up to 12 months post-surgery.[6]

Review Questions

1. A 30-year-old male with a spinal cord injury utilizes a power wheelchair independently and utilizes tenodesis grasp with his right hand to drink from a cup with setup. What is his anticipated level of injury?
   a. C5
   b. C6
   c. C7
   d. C8
2. The minimum required ratio for an ADA-compliant ramp is:
   a. 1:10
   b. 1:12
   c. 1:16
   d. 1:20
3. All wheelchairs (manual and power) have the same length and width that impact home accessibility.
   a. True
   b. False
4. An EADL is used to ______________________.
   a. Provide toileting hygiene
   b. Passively stretch an upper extremity
   c. Control one's surrounding environment and electronic devices within the environment
   d. Apply electric stimulation to a muscle
5. In the hierarchy of recommended tendon transfers, ________________ is recommended first.
   a. Elbow extension
   b. Wrist extension
   c. Lateral pinch
   d. Palmer grasp
6. What is the biggest predictor for successful outcome after tendon transfer?
   a. Direct patient involvement in decision-making for surgical intervention
   b. Length of time since injury
   c. Functional goal focused
   d. a and c

REFERENCES

1. Pedretti LW, Pendleton HM, Schultz-Krohn W, eds. *Pedretti's Occupational Therapy: Practice Skills for Physical Dysfunction.* 7th ed. St. Louis: Elsevier; 2013.
2. *Uniform Data System for Medical Rehabilitation. The FIM System Clinical Guide, Version 5.2.1.* Buffalo: UDSMR; 2018.
3. Department of Justice ADA Title III Regulation 28 cfr part 36(1991) [Internet]. https://www.ada.gov/reg3a.html#anchor33.
4. Veterans Benefits Administration. Handbook for Design: A Guide for Specially Adapted Housing and Special Housing Adaptation Projects [Internet]. [Updated 2019 June]. https://www.benefits.va.gov/HOMELOANS/documents/docs/sah_handbook_for_design.pdf.
5. Liew SK, Shim BJ, Gong HS. Upper limb reconstruction in tetraplegic patients: a primer for spinal cord injury specialists. *Korean J Neurotrauma.* 2020;16(2):126–137.
6. Dunn JA, Sinnot KA, Rothwel AG, Mohammed KD, Simcock JW. Tendon transfer surgery for people with tetraplegia: an overview. *Arch Phys Med Rehabil.* 2016 Jun;97(6):S75–S80.
7. Sharma J. Most desired function of persons with tetraplegia and the role of upper extremity reconstruction. Lecture presented at: VISN-6 SCID 2019: Trends and Advancements in Care; Virginia; 2019
8. U. S. Access Board. Ramps and curb ramps [Internet]. https://www.access-board.gov/ada/guides/chapter-4-ramps-and-curb-ramps.
9. Johanson ME. Rehabilitation after surgical reconstruction to restore function to the upper limb in tetraplegia: a changing landscape. *Arch Phys Med Rehabil.* 2016 Jun;97(6):S71–S74.

CHAPTER 47

Communication and Spinal Cord Injury

Katelyn Barley and Stacy Gross

OUTLINE

The ability to communicate is critical to spinal cord injury (SCI) rehabilitation. Speech-language pathologists (SLP) should lead the evaluation and treatment of speech production, motor speech, voice, communication, and cognitive–communication deficits that may result from SCI and secondary injury or insult (e.g., traumatic brain injury [TBI]) or as a result of the initial injury (e.g., need for a tracheostomy). The need for treatment by a SLP is common in this population, and early intervention is vital. Establishing and enabling communication can improve psychological well-being, increase compliance, and provide the patient the opportunity to direct care.

Speech Production in Patients With Tracheostomy

A significant portion of patients with cervical and thoracic SCI initially require a tracheostomy for prolonged mechanical ventilation and airway management secondary to impaired respiratory function. Although speech is normally produced by a steady exhalation of air passing through the vocal folds and allowing one to phonate, with a tracheostomy, the majority of air passes through the tracheostomy tube below the vocal folds. Some air may leak to the vocal folds, but it is typically not forceful enough to generate phonation. An SLP, with the support of a respiratory therapist, can evaluate the patient with a tracheostomy to determine the most appropriate way to generate voicing.

Speech With Tracheostomy on Mechanical Ventilation[1]

- Partial or full cuff deflation for "leak" speech
- Talking tracheostomy tube
- Speaking valve in-line with ventilator circuit (cuffless tracheostomy or deflated cuff)

Speech With Tracheostomy Without Mechanical Ventilation[1]

- Partial or full cuff deflation for "leak" speech
- Finger occlusion of tracheostomy (cuffless tracheostomy or deflated cuff)
- Speaking valve on hub of tracheostomy tube (cuffless tracheostomy or deflated cuff)

When placed on the hub of a tracheostomy tube or in-line with the ventilator circuit, a speaking valve redirects airflow through the vocal folds rather than through the tracheostomy in order to enable voice. A Passy Muir valve is a frequently used one-way speaking valve (Fig. 47.1).[2] In addition to allowing voice, speaking valves provide benefits to the swallow function and secretion management. Contraindications for speaking valve use include airway obstruction, unstable medical or pulmonary status, and inability to tolerate full cuff deflation. It is imperative to have the cuff fully deflated on a cuffed tracheostomy before initiation of a speaking valve or digital occlusion of the tracheostomy. Once a patient is deemed appropriate, the medical team may consider capping the tracheostomy to progress toward eventual decannulation of the tracheostomy tube.

Protocols for decannulation may vary by setting. However, these criteria are generally accepted[3]:

- Acceptable arterial blood gases
- Free of respiratory distress following ventilator liberation
- Stable vital signs and absence of fever, sepsis, or untreated infections

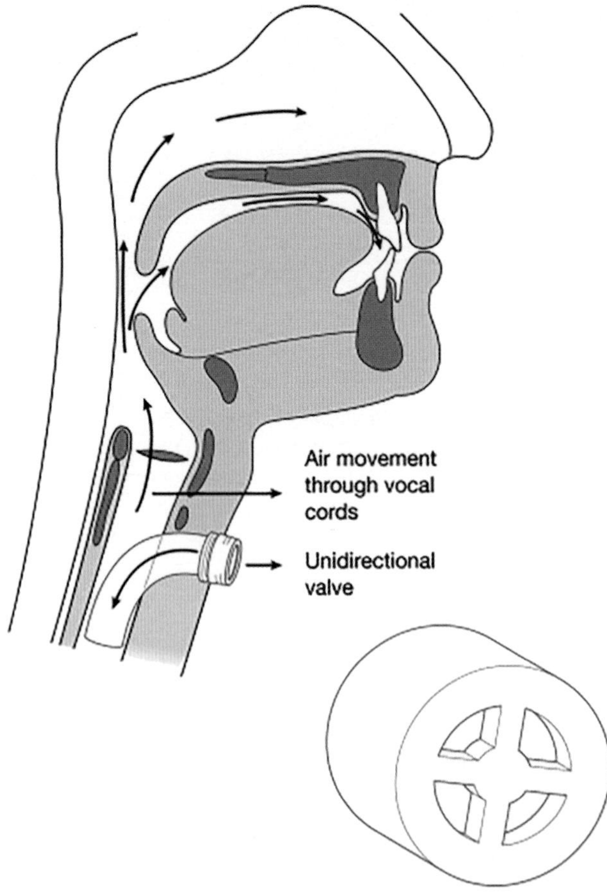

Fig. 47.1 Functioning of a Passy-Muir tracheostomy speaking valve. Figure Coutsey: Redrawn from Manzano JL, Lubillo S, Henriquez D, et al: Verbal communication of ventilator dependent patients, *Crit Care Med* 21:512–517, 1993.

- Oxygen saturation of ≥90% with cap in place with or without supplemental oxygen
- Absence of known upper airway obstruction or airway disorder
- Ability to clear secretions with manually assisted (Quad) cough
- No need for deep suctioning for ≥48 hours

Speech and Voice Disorders

Following an SCI, patients may experience impairments in speech and voice as a result of impaired respiratory support. These changes are particularly seen in those with cervical SCI as a result of respiratory dysfunction. Muscular strategies for producing inspiratory and expiratory forces change following injury to the cervical spinal cord.[4] Weakness or paralysis of respiratory muscles because of the injury can lead to deficits in respiratory, phonatory, and prosodic aspects of speech production. Additionally, deficits may occur at the laryngeal level because of intubation trauma and/or recurrent laryngeal nerve palsy.

Patients report the following as common experiences post-SCI[5,6]:

- Running out of air and voice when talking
- Reduced utterance length
- Straining to produce voice
- Changes in vocal quality throughout the day
- Breathy, rough, harsh, and/or hoarse vocal quality
- Difficulties being heard over long distances
- Difficulties being heard in noisy environments
- Fatigue in conversation

Research has established the ability to communicate effectively as a key facilitator to adjustment and community integration following SCI.[7] Although vocal impairments are generally reported to be mild-to-moderate following SCI, these deficits may have a significant impact to daily life. A patient's voice outcomes and the magnitude of their limitations may be dependent on physical aspects of injury, coping strategies, and vocal demands.[8]

Patients should be monitored to identify those who would benefit from an SLP's service. Identifying patients early on can minimize maladaptive voice behaviors, such as vocal strain, which can lead to further impairments and limitations in participation. SLPs evaluate respiration, phonation, articulation, resonance, and prosody of the patient's speech to determine a treatment plan. Assessment relies on patient report and maximum performance speech tasks.

Once impairments are identified, SLPs can develop interventions for rehabilitation or compensation. Impaired respiratory–phonatory control can be directly targeted using abdominal binders or respiratory strength training devices such as expiratory muscle strength training.[4,9] Patients can receive immediate benefit through compensatory strategies, such as communication strategies or the use of a personal voice amplifier. Speech strategies address overall intelligibility through slowing rate of speech, over articulating, and improving breath support.

Dysarthria

Dysarthria is a motor speech disorder caused by muscle weakness. The muscles that are used to produce speech (tongue, larynx, surrounding muscles) are either damaged, paralyzed, or weakened. Many neuromuscular conditions, including multiple sclerosis (MS) or amyotrophic lateral sclerosis (ALS), can result in dysarthria. Dysarthria can be present in greater than 80% of patients with ALS at any point during disease progression.[10] Mixed flaccid-spastic dysarthria is the most common type of dysarthria for this population, due to both lower and upper motor neuron involvement. The most severe characteristics include imprecise consonants, hypernasality, harshness, and slow rate of speech.[11] It is imperative that SLP involvement begin at initial diagnosis and continue as speech and intelligibility decreases with worsening dysarthria. In patients with ALS, the ultimate goal is to optimize communication for as long as possible, starting with speech strategies and progressing to more complex speech-generating devices.

Approximately 40%–50% of patients with MS can present with dysarthria throughout their disease process.[11] The severity of dysarthria is generally related to the severity of neurologic deficits. The presentation of dysarthria in this population is variable, but most frequently identified as spastic, ataxic, or mixed spastic-ataxic.[11] Some common characteristics include impaired loudness control, harshness, and articulatory breakdown. Because the presentation of MS is so variable, a thorough assessment by an SLP is warranted in order to develop individualized treatment programs.

Augmentative and Alternative Communication[12]

Many patients with SCI, especially those with severe SCI and debilitating, progressive diseases such as ALS and MS, can benefit from augmentative and alternative communication (AAC). Aided AAC systems can range from basic to high-tech. Patients with more mild speech issues use basic AAC to supplement their verbal speech. AAC used in this way is considered *augmentative*. Systems may include pen and paper, whiteboard, letter board, or picture board. Those with more severe impairments, such as ALS, can benefit from a speech-generating device as an *alternative* to verbal speech. These advanced systems can even include integrated environmental control units. It is not uncommon to use multiple types of AAC depending on the communication partner, setting, and need.

An SLP will assess the patient's communication ability, communication needs, and cognitive ability to determine the most suitable form of AAC. Of note, patients with ALS and MS can present with accompanying cognitive deficits that may impact their ability to utilize more complex communications systems effectively. In this population, the SLP will also consider mobility and positioning limitations to determine the best means of selection for the AAC.

Direct Selection

Patient points directly with a body part or tool
- Touch, typically by finger
- Use of a stylus, mouth stick, or computer mouse
- Laser pointer
- Head tracking
- Eye gaze

Indirect Selection

Patient selects a target from a set of choices
- Visual scanning with a switch
- Auditory scanning with a switch
- Partner-assisted scanning

Electronic Aids to Daily Living

Electronic aids to daily living (EADLs) provide control of one's environment through alternative access while increasing their level of function, typically within their home. A patient with limited functional mobility and/or dexterity can benefit from the use of an EADL device to improve the interaction with their environment. EADLs have different transmission methods including infrared (i.e., television or universal report), radio frequency (i.e., garage door opener), and home automation system (i.e., table lamp). Most any electronic devices (lights, fans, air conditioning, televisions, and telephones) and many mechanical devices can be controlled (hospital beds, window blinds, and doors). Like AAC devices, alternative access methods to a smart device may be required due to a patient's upper extremity limitation; however, not all smart devices have accessibility features.

Cognitive–Communication Deficits

Rehabilitation for a patient with SCI can be complicated by a dual diagnosis of TBI. The SLP plays a critical role in addressing the resulting cognitive–communication impairments that may affect learning of SCI-specific information. Additionally, patients without a documented or suspected TBI may also require cognitive–communication support due to a diagnosis affecting new learning, such as language or learning disabilities, dementia, or attention deficit disorders.[13]

Potential Cognitive Impairments

- Orientation
- Memory
- Attention
- Organization and sequencing
- Speech processing
- Problem solving and reasoning
- Pragmatics
- Executive functioning
- Safety, insight, and judgment

With support, these patients can plan and execute rehabilitation strategies to perform or direct their care. Following an assessment of a patient's cognitive–communication abilities, an SLP can provide treatment and share rehabilitation strategies with the team.

Supports for Cognition

- External aids, such as signs, calendars, or environmental cues
- Applications, such as alarms, timers, reminders, to-do lists, calendars, or voice memos
- Timers for pressure relief or medication management
- Written instructions for care, such as transfers
- Schedules or planners
- Memory book
- Smart pen
- Providing rest breaks during therapy

Review Questions

1. The following are important factors to consider when determining whether a patient is an appropriate candidate for use of a speaking valve EXCEPT
   a. Tolerating several hours of tracheostomy collar
   b. Able to tolerate cuff deflation
   c. Ability to manage secretions
   d. Whether the patient requires supplemental oxygen
2. Which of the following is NOT a common problem that may impact phonation following SCI?
   a. Fatigue
   b. Decreased breath support
   c. Limited jaw range of motion secondary to cervical collar
   d. Intubation trauma
3. In neurodegenerative conditions such as ALS, regular SLP follow-up services are critical to monitoring speech function for all the following reasons EXCEPT
   a. It allows time to learn how to use an AAC device before it is needed
   b. Determine if/when AAC may be required
   c. Adjust access methods as disease progresses to accommodate new limitations
   d. Medicare requires consistent follow-up
4. Which of the following options restores speech by allowing air through the stoma and then redirecting airflow through the vocal folds?
   a. Passy Muir speaking valve
   b. Digital occlusion
   c. Capped tracheostomy tube
   d. All of the above
5. A patient with an SCI presents with harsh, breathy voice 1 month following anterior cervical discectomy and fusion. Which of the following is the most likely cause of dysphonia?
   a. Postoperative edema
   b. Recurrent laryngeal nerve palsy
   c. Vocal fold nodules
   d. Poor vocal hygiene
6. An SLP is consulted to enable communication for a patient with C4 complete quadriplegia with a cuffless tracheostomy. Which of the following would be the most appropriate method for enabling communication?
   a. Verbal speech via digital occlusion of the tracheostomy
   b. Verbal speech following speaking valve placement
   c. Speech-generating device with direct selection via eye gaze
   d. Alphabet board with indirect selection via partner-assisted scanning

REFERENCES

1. Hess DR. Facilitating speech in the patient with a tracheostomy. *Respir Care.* 2005;50(4):519–525.
2. PassyMuir. PassyMuir Tracheostomy & Ventilator Swallowing and Speaking Valves patient education handbook. Irvine, CA: PassyMuir, n.d.
3. Pelton JL. *Adult Tracheostomy Decannulation for Non-Ventilated Patients.* Lincoln, NE: Madonna Rehabilitation Specialty Hospital–Lincoln, Respiratory Therapy; 2018. https://www.passy-muir.com/wp-content/uploads/2019/09/AH_Adult-Trach-Decann.pdf.
4. Hoit JD, Banzett RB, Brown R, Loring SH. Speech breathing in individuals with cervical spinal cord injury. *J Speech Hear Res.* 1990;33(4):798–807.
5. Ward EC, Jarman L, Cornwell PL, Amsters DI. Impact of voice and communication deficits for individuals with spinal cord injury living in the community. *Int J Lang Commun Disord.* 2016;51(5):568–580.
6. Wall LR, Nund RL, Ward EC, Cornwell PL, Amsters DI. Experiences of communication changes following spinal cord injury: a qualitative analysis. *Disabl Rehabil.* 2020;42(16):2271–2278.
7. Boschen KA, Tonack M, Gargaro J. Long-term adjustment and community reintegration following spinal cord injury. *Int J Rehabil Res.* 2003;26(3):157–164.
8. Johansson K, Seiger A, Forsen M, Nilsson JH, Hartelius L, Schalling E. Assessment of voice, speech and communication changes associated with cervical spinal cord injury. *Int J Lang Commun Disord.* 2018;53(4):761–775.
9. Sapienza CM, Wheeler KW. Respiratory muscle strength training: functional outcomes versus plasticity. *Semin Speech Lang.* 2006;27(4):236–244.
10. Tomik B, Guiloff RJ. Dysarthria in amyotrophic lateral sclerosis. *Amyotroph Lateral Scler.* 2010;11(4):4–15.
11. Duffy JR. *Motor Speech Disorders: Substrates, Differential Diagnosis, and Management.* 3rd ed. St. Louis, MO: Elsevier; 2013.
12. Beukelman D, Mirenda P. *Augmentative and Alternative Communication: Supporting Children and Adults with Complex Communication Needs.* 4th ed. Baltimore, MD: Paul H. Brookes Publishing Co; 2013.
13. Gordan W, Spivak-David D, Adornato V, et al. SCIRehab Project series: the speech language pathology taxonomy. *J Spinal Cord Med.* 2009;32(3):307–318.

CHAPTER 48

Participation/Living With Spinal Cord Injury

Katharine Tam

OUTLINE

Rehabilitation empowers individuals with a spinal cord injury (SCI) to return to their communities as active participants. Community reintegration is defined as the full inclusion and participation within the physical and psychosocial environment.[1] This concept can be further understood through discussion on community access and return to recreation and sports activities, work, and social relationships.

Recreation and Sports Activities

Involvement in recreation and sports activities has many physical and psychosocial benefits. Rehabilitation professionals help increase patient awareness of opportunities and strategies for safe participation at the community and national level.

Benefits

Participation in sports by persons with SCI is associated with increased community integration.[2] Engagement in physical exercise is associated with higher quality of life, decreased secondary health conditions including pressure injuries, and lower healthcare costs including fewer physician visits per year, rehospitalizations, and medical complications over time.[1,3,4] Exercise is associated with improved cardiac health as demonstrated in a small study of persons with chronic paraplegia and improved lipid profiles after 3 months of upper extremity circuit training.[5] Other small studies of 6-week exercise programs demonstrated decreased fasting insulin[6] and decreased pain symptoms.[7]

Access

Engagement in physical exercise is low among persons with SCI.[8] Accessibility to physical activity facilities remains limited.[9–11] Sports and recreation programming for the SCI community is an important facilitator for physical activity and should be year-round with opportunities for persons with varied levels of athleticism and physical abilities.

Equipment Considerations

Adaptive sport equipment should be individualized for the participants to support varied levels of impairments across different neurologic levels and severity of SCI. Common equipment considerations that facilitate safe participation in sports activities include:

- Seating and positioning
  - Enhanced trunk stability[12,13]
    - Increased posterior slope ("dump"): rear floor-to-seat height lower than front floor-to-seat height
    - Center of mass is transferred posteriorly
    - Increased pressure at the back support
  - Pressure injury prevention[14]
    - Increased posterior slope increases risk for pressure injury
    - Risk can be reduced with proper weight-bearing distribution at the posterior thighs
- Camber: angle of the wheels in relation to the vertical where distance between the top of the wheels is less than the bottom.[15,16]
  - Increased turning responsiveness and stability
  - Contact protection with close positioning of the hands to athlete's body

Medical Precautions

Persons with SCI who participate in sports and recreation are at slightly higher risk for injuries than able-bodied athletes, and most injuries involve the upper limbs.[17–19] Table 48.1 lists common medical complications that clinicians should consider in athletic participants with SCI.[20,21]

Table 48.1 Medical Considerations for Athletic Participants With Spinal Cord Injury

SCI Concern	Medical Considerations	Precautions
Thermo-regulation	Hyperthermia and hypothermia Impaired sweating and shivering response below level of injury	Cooling with cold water immersion, air circulation with fans, iced towels, partially frozen hydration[a] Maintaining warmth with layers, warm packs, warmers, waterproof clothing, regular breaks from winter elements
Sensation	Sunburn	Utilize sunscreen, shade, UV-protective clothing
	Pressure injury	Awareness of high pressures, friction, shear, and moisture that commonly increase risk for pressure injury Utilize prevention strategies from nonsporting seating: high pressure avoidance and increased contact for pressure distribution
Bone health	Fractures Decreased bone density increases risk of fracture from minor injuries	Monitor for signs of fracture: irregular body positioning, erythema, edema, ecchymosis, dysreflexia Stabilize until evaluation with imaging
Autonomic dysfunction (SCI at/above T6)	Severe hypotension Impaired cardiovascular response Deceased maximum heart rate Impaired sympathetic innervation of heart	Utilize perceived exertion scales (e.g., Borg) rather than maximum heart rate as training parameter
	Athletic doping with dysreflexia Decreased perceived exertion and increased performance due to sympathetic reflexes	Maintain awareness of the International Paralympic Committee banned practice of "boosting": the intentional use of noxious stimuli to cause dysreflexia. Risks include severe hypertension, seizure, stroke, cerebral hemorrhage, death[b]

[a]Forsyth P, Pumpa K, Knight E, Miller J. Physiological and perceptual effects of precooling in wheelchair basketball athletes. *J Spinal Cord Med.* 2016;39(6):671–678.
[b]Mazzeo F, Santamaria S, Iavarone A. "Boosting" in paralympic athletes with spinal cord injury: doping without drugs. *Funct Neurol.* 2015;30(2):91–98.

Community Access

The ability to participate in activities at the community level is influenced by access to transportation and accessibility of the built environment. Participation in community activities is correlated with subjective quality of life,[22] and further impacted by individual factors including family support, self-esteem, informational support, and coping style.[23,24]

Transportation

Access to transportation facilitates participation. Options for individuals with SCI include public transportation, wheelchair-taxi, taxi, or an adapted vehicle. Ownership of an adapted vehicle was associated with increased independence in driving.[25] The benefits of driving after an SCI include increased mental well-being, quality of life, life-satisfaction, employment, and community reintegration.[26–30] Higher activities of daily living (ADL) independence at hospital discharge, paraplegia, and longer duration of injury were among the significant predictors of driving an adapted vehicle after SCI.[29] The highest level of neurologic impairment at which driving remained feasible was C6 AIS A[30] or C5 with highly specialized equipment.[31,32] Waiting several months to a year may allow for maximum neurologic return and optimize cost-effective modifications.[21] Vehicle modifications may include hand-operated controls, lift systems, ramps, and adaptive seating.[29,33,34] Table 48.2 illustrates expected independence level with driving and likely adaptations needed by neurologic level of injury.[32,35] This table is abstracted from an extensive table of expected outcomes published by the Consortium for Spinal Cord Medicine that further denotes expected levels of independence with other essential ADLs that would impact independence with driving. Referral to a drivers rehabilitation specialist can facilitate predriving assessment, vehicle evaluation and prescription, appropriate wheelchair selection if there is an intention to use the wheelchair as a seat in the vehicle, and ensure safe return to driving.[21] Predriving assessment includes a review of an individual's medical history, functional capacity, vision, reaction time, and necessary mobility equipment.[31]

Universal Design

Wheelchair mobility skills and accessible built environments work in tandem to allow for community access after SCI. The Americans with Disabilities Act of 1990 prohibited discrimination against persons with

Table 48.2 Expected Functional Outcomes for Driving and Adaptive Equipment Needs by Neurologic Level of Injury

Level of Injury	Independence With Driving	Adaptive Equipment
C1–C4	Total assist	Attendant-operated van with lift, tie-downs, etc. Accessible public transportation
C5	Independent with highly specialized equipment Some assist with accessible public transportation Total assist with attendant-operated vehicle	Highly specialized modified van with lift
C6–C7	Independent driving from wheelchair	Modified van with lift, sensitized hand controls, and tie-downs for wheelchair
C8	Independent with car if independent with transfer and wheelchair loading Independent driving modified van from captain's seat	Car with hand controls Modified van with lift and hand controls
T1–T12	Independent in car including loading and unloading wheelchair Independent driving modified van from captain's seat	Car with hand controls Modified van with lift and hand controls
L1–S5	Independent in car including loading and unloading wheelchair	Car with hand controls depending on degree of lower extremity function

disabilities and increased community access by requiring reasonable accommodations to enable access to public and nonresidential spaces.[36,37] The Americans with Disabilities Act Accessibility Guidelines provide basic standards for building requirements.[38,39] Accessibility laws did not include private homes, and individuals with SCI will often require home modifications prior to returning home. More inclusive design philosophies have emerged. Universal design is a "paradigm where people of all abilities are included in the intended population of users of a product or environment" and may be known as inclusive design, design for all, life span design, or barrier-free design.[40] Considerations for access to the community include barrier-free entrances, appropriate doorway and hallway widths, accessible bathrooms, elevators, curb-cuts, parking spaces with access aisles, and accessible public transportation. Access to a broader community beyond an individual's local environment was addressed by the 1986 Air Carrier Access Act, which prohibits discrimination against people with physical or mental impairments, and requires boarding assistance and aircraft accessibility features in newly built aircrafts.[41] Seat cushions for pressure relief should be brought onto the aircraft, along with all necessary medication and equipment.[31]

Vocational Rehabilitation

Employment after SCI is an important component of community reintegration. The average rate of return to work after SCI is approximately 35%.[42] Longer duration of injury is associated with higher employment rate, and peaks at 10 years postinjury.[43–45] Vocational rehabilitation professionals can help individuals return to education or work after an SCI. Vocational rehabilitation is "a multi-professional approach that is provided to individuals of working age with health-related impairments, limitations, or restrictions with work functioning and whose primary aim is to optimize work participation."[46]

Benefits

Persons with SCI perceive employment as necessary for social integration and an important contributor to an individual's social identity.[47,48] Qualitative literature demonstrated employment was associated with financial health, social security, development of valued social roles, moral duty, social participation, and distraction.[47,50] Quality of employment mattered, and social welfare jobs that were understimulating were considered meaningless and less preferable than unemployment.[50] Quantitative studies, which were mostly correlational, suggest employed individuals with SCI may benefit from reduced depression and handicap, enhanced quality of life, community integration, independence, subjective well-being, satisfaction with life, and survival.[51–56]

Return-to-Work Interventions

Returning to employment after SCI may be a challenging and daunting goal, which rehabilitation specialists should address early in the rehabilitation process by providing reassurance that employment is possible. A rehabilitation team can maximize an individual's return-to-work by optimizing health conditions, minimizing secondary SCI complications, maximizing functional independence, and providing education on vocational interventions. State vocational rehabilitation agencies are available in every state and territory in the

United States, and support persons with disabilities seeking employment with a wide range of services that include preemployment transition, training, job search assistance, job placement assistance, benefits counseling, transportation, and rehabilitation technology.[21] The Department of Veterans Affairs provides vocational, education, and training programs to eligible Veterans. Other SCI literature-supported vocational interventions (Table 48.3) include the Individual Placement and Support,[57–59] Resource Facilitation,[60] and Early Intervention models.[61–64] These models incorporate the foundational principles of competitive employment as a primary outcome, integration of vocational and healthcare services, patient-centered job choice, and follow-up support.[21]

Social Issues

Psychosocial and adjustment issues have an important impact on community participation. Relationship outcome, peer group acceptance, and family resources may have a greater influence on functional outcome than neurologic level of injury.[31,65] Marriages after SCI have similar emotional quality compared to those in the general population and better marital adjustment as compared to preinjury marriages. Rate of divorce after SCI is higher among preinjury marriages and often occur within 3 years of injury.[66] Relationships may be affected by caregiver burdens, as spouses who are caregivers report higher levels of stress, burnout, fatigue, resentment, and depression as compared with spouses who are not caregivers.[67]

Table 48.3 Spinal Cord Injury Employment Interventions

Intervention	Strategy
Individual placement and support	Employment specialist is integrated in spinal cord injury interdisciplinary team. Primary objective: competitive employment Services: (1) rapid engagement in job search, (2) benefits counseling, (3) ongoing support to maintain employment
Resource facilitation	Vocational resource facilitator initiates early intervention services during inpatient phase of spinal cord injury rehabilitation and maintains supportive contact after transition to outpatient phase. Services: Inpatient phase: (1) assess vocational interests and skills, (2) integrate employment goals with therapy goals Outpatient phase: (3) make referrals to address identified psychosocial and health barriers, (4) address accessible work environment and accommodations, (5) educate stakeholders about SCI
Early intervention	Initiating vocational goals during acute rehabilitation to foster hope for return-to-work Strategy: (1) establish vocational rehabilitation relationship during inpatient setting, (2) establish vocational identity, (3) explore vocational options, (4) establish vocational goals, (5) job support, (6) service development

Review Questions

1. How do persons with SCI perceive return to employment?
   a. Employment is necessary for social integration
   b. Unemployment is preferable to unchallenging social welfare jobs
   c. Employment is an important contributor to one's social identity
   d. All of the above
2. What is the average rate of return to work after SCI of 10 years?
   a. 10%
   b. 25%
   c. 35%
   d. 45%
3. Which of the following occurs with increased posterior slope of an SCI athlete's wheelchair seating?
   a. Increased pressure at the back support
   b. Increased coccyx and sacral pressure
   c. Decreased risk for pressure injury
   d. Decreased trunk stability
4. Which of the following are significant predictors for return to driving?
   a. Paraplegia
   b. Longer duration of injury
   c. Higher motor score on International Standards for Neurological Classification of SCI
   d. a and b
   e. All of the above
5. Which of the following is a false statement about SCI athletic doping by "boosting"?
   a. It can lead to severe hypertension, seizure, cerebral hemorrhage, and death
   b. The International Paralympic Committee has no official statement on athletic doping
   c. Performance is enhanced by activation of sympathetic reflexes
   d. It can be triggered by kinking an indwelling catheter

REFERENCES

1. Stiens SA, Kirshblum SC, Groah SL, McKinley WO, Gittler MS. Spinal cord injury medicine. 4. Optimal participation in life after spinal cord injury: physical, psychosocial, and economic reintegration into the environment. *Arch Phys Med Rehabil.* 2002;83(3 Suppl 1):S72–S81, S90-S98.

2. Hanson CS, Nabavi D, Yuen HK. The effect of sports on level of community integration as reported by persons with spinal cord injury. *Am J Occup Ther.* 2001;55(3):332–338.
3. Anneken V, Hanssen-Doose A, Hirschfeld S, Scheuer T, Thietje R. Influence of physical exercise on quality of life in individuals with spinal cord injury. *Spinal Cord.* 2010;48(5):393–399.
4. Curtis KA, McClanahan S, Hall KM, Dillon D, Brown KF. Health, vocational, and functional status in spinal cord injured athletes and nonathletes. *Arch Phys Med Rehabil.* 1986;67(12). 862-5.
5. Nash MS, Jacobs PL, Mendez AJ, Goldberg RB. Circuit resistance training improves the atherogenic lipid profiles of persons with chronic paraplegia. *J Spinal Cord Med.* 2001;24(1):2–9.
6. Kim DI, Taylor JA, Tan CO, et al. A pilot randomized controlled trial of 6-week combined exercise program on fasting insulin and fitness levels in individuals with spinal cord injury. *Eur Spine J.* 2019;28(5):1082–1091.
7. Wilbanks SR, Rogers R, Pool S, Bickel CS. Effects of functional electrical stimulation assisted rowing on aerobic fitness and shoulder pain in manual wheelchair users with spinal cord injury. *J Spinal Cord Med.* 2016;39(6):645–654.
8. Dearwater SR, LaPorte RE, Robertson RJ, Brenes G, Adams LL, Becker D. Activity in the spinal cord-injured patient: an epidemiologic analysis of metabolic parameters. *Med Sci Sports Exerc.* 1986;18(5):541–544.
9. Rimmer JH, Padalabalanarayanan S, Malone LA, Mehta T. Fitness facilities still lack accessibility for people with disabilities. *Disabil Health J.* 2017;10(2):214–221.
10. Johnson MJ, Stoelzle HY, Finco KL, Foss SE, Carstens K. ADA compliance and accessibility of fitness facilities in western Wisconsin. *Top Spinal Cord Inj Rehabil.* 2012;18(4):340–353.
11. Cardinal BJ, Spaziani MD. ADA compliance and the accessibility of physical activity facilities in western Oregon. *Am J Health Promot.* 2003;17(3):197–201.
12. Maurer CL, Sprigle S. Effect of seat inclination on seated pressures of individuals with spinal cord injury. *Phys Ther.* 2004;84(3):255–261.
13. Cooper RA, De Luigi AJ. Adaptive sports technology and biomechanics: wheelchairs. *PM R.* 2014;6(8 Suppl): S31–S39.
14. Darrah SD, Dicianno BE, Berthold J, McCoy A, Haas M, Cooper RA. Measuring static seated pressure distributions and risk for skin pressure ulceration in ice sledge hockey players. *Disabil Rehabil Assist Technol.* 2016;11(3):241–246.
15. Mason BS, van der Woude LH, Goosey-Tolfrey VL. The ergonomics of wheelchair configuration for optimal performance in the wheelchair court sports. *Sports Med.* 2013;43(1): 23–38.
16. Laferrier JZ, Rice I, Pearlman J, et al. Technology to improve sports performance in wheelchair sports. *Sports Technology.* 2012;5(1-2):4–19.
17. Derman W, Schwellnus M, Jordaan E, et al. Illness and injury in athletes during the competition period at the London 2012 Paralympic Games: development and implementation of a web-based surveillance system (WEB-IISS) for team medical staff. *Br J Sports Med.* 2013;47(7):420–425.
18. Willick SE, Webborn N, Emery C, et al. The epidemiology of injuries at the London 2012 Paralympic Games. *Br J Sports Med.* 2013;47(7):426–432.
19. Webborn N, Willick S, Reeser JC. Injuries among disabled athletes during the 2002 Winter Paralympic Games. *Med Sci Sports Exerc.* 2006;38(5):811–815.
20. Webborn N, Van de Vliet P. Paralympic medicine. *Lancet.* 2012;380(9836):65–71.
21. Kirshblum S, Lin VW. *Spinal Cord Medicine.* Demos Medical Publishing; 2018.
22. Dijkers MP. Correlates of life satisfaction among persons with spinal cord injury. *Arch Phys Med Rehabil.* 1999;80(8):867–876.
23. Whiteneck G, Meade MA, Dijkers M, Tate DG, Bushnik T, Forchheimer MB. Environmental factors and their role in participation and life satisfaction after spinal cord injury. *Arch Phys Med Rehabil.* 2004;85(11):1793–1803.
24. Song HY. Modeling social reintegration in persons with spinal cord injury. *Disabil Rehabil.* 2005;27(3):131–141.
25. Post MW, van Asbeck FW, van Dijk AJ, Schrijvers AJ. Services for spinal cord injured: availability and satisfaction. *Spinal Cord.* 1997;35(2):109–115.
26. Conroy L, McKenna K. Vocational outcome following spinal cord injury. *Spinal Cord.* 1999;37(9):624–633.
27. Siösteen A, Lundqvist C, Blomstrand C, Sullivan L, Sullivan M. The quality of life of three functional spinal cord injury subgroups in a Swedish community. *Paraplegia.* 1990;28(8):476–488.
28. Tsai IH, Graves DE, Lai CH. The association of assistive mobility devices and social participation in people with spinal cord injuries. *Spinal Cord.* 2014;52(3):209–215.
29. Norweg A, Jette AM, Houlihan B, Ni P, Boninger ML. Patterns, predictors, and associated benefits of driving a modified vehicle after spinal cord injury: findings from the National Spinal Cord Injury Model Systems. *Arch Phys Med Rehabil.* 2011;92(3):477–483.
30. Kiyono Y, Hashizume C, Matsui N, Ohtsuka K, Takaoka K. Car-driving abilities of people with tetraplegia. *Arch Phys Med Rehabil.* 2001;82(10):1389–1392.
31. Scelza WM, Kirshblum SC, Wuermser LA, Ho CH, Priebe MM, Chiodo AE. Spinal cord injury medicine. 4. Community reintegration after spinal cord injury. *Archives of Physical Medicine and Rehabilitation.* 2007;88(3):S71–S75.
32. Cifu DX. *Braddom's Physical Medicine and Rehabilitation.* 6th ed. Philadelphia: Elsevier; 2021.
33. Biering-Sørensen F, Hansen RB, Biering-Sørensen J. Mobility aids and transport possibilities 10–45 years after spinal cord injury. *Spinal Cord.* 2004;42(12):699–706.
34. Henriksson P, Peters B. Safety and mobility of people with disabilities driving adapted cars. *Scandinavian J Occupational Therapy.* 2004;11(2):54–61.
35. Consortium for Spinal Cord Medicine Outcomes following traumatic spinal cord injury: clinical practice guidelines for health-care professionals. *J Spinal Cord Med.* 2000;23(4): 289–316.
36. Civil Rights Division USDoJ. Information and technical assistance on the Americans with Disabilities Act. https://www.ada.gov/ta-pubs-pg2.htm.
37. Department of Justice Nondiscrimination on the basis of disability by public accommodations and in commercial facilities. Final rule. *Fed Regist.* 1991;56(144). 35544-35691.
38. Architectural and Transportation Barriers Compliance Board Americans with Disabilities Act (ADA) accessibility guide-

lines for buildings and facilities. Final guidelines. *Fed Regist.* 1991;56(144). 35408-3542.
39. Architectural and Transportation Barriers Compliance Board Americans with Disabilities Act (ADA) accessibility guidelines for buildings and facilities; play areas. Final rule. *Fed Regist.* 2000;65(202). 62498-6529.
40. Joines S. Enhancing quality of life through Universal Design. *NeuroRehabilitation.* 2009;25(4):313–326.
41. Transportation UDo. About the Air Carrier Access Act Tuesday, January 27, 2015. https://www.transportation.gov/airconsumer/passengers-disabilities.
42. Young AE, Murphy GC. Employment status after spinal cord injury (1992–2005): a review with implications for interpretation, evaluation, further research, and clinical practice. *Int J Rehabil Res.* 2009;32(1):1–11.
43. Krause JS, Kewman D, DeVivo MJ, et al. Employment after spinal cord injury: an analysis of cases from the model spinal cord injury systems. *Archives of Physical Medicine and Rehabilitation.* 1999;80(11):1492–1500.
44. Krause JS, Saunders L, Staten D. Race-ethnicity, education, and employment after spinal cord injury. *Rehabilitation Counseling Bulletin.* 2009;53(2):78–86.
45. Ottomanelli L, Sippel JL, Cipher DJ, Goetz LL. Factors associated with employment among veterans with spinal cord injury. *J Vocational Rehabilitation.* 2011;34:141–150.
46. Escorpizo R, Reneman MF, Ekholm J, et al. A conceptual definition of vocational rehabilitation based on the ICF: building a shared global model. *J Occup Rehabil.* 2011;21(2):126–133.
47. Meade MA, Reed KS, Saunders LL, Krause JS. It's all of the above: benefits of working for individuals with spinal cord injury. *Top Spinal Cord Inj Rehabil.* 2015;21(1):1–9.
48. Schedin Leiulfsrud A, Ruoranen K, Ostermann A, Reinhardt JD. The meaning of employment from the perspective of persons with spinal cord injuries in six European countries. *Work.* 2016;55(1):133–144.
49. Schedin Leiulfsrud A, Reinhardt JD, Ostermann A, Ruoranen K, Post MWM. The value of employment for people living with spinal cord injury in Norway. *Disability & Society.* 2014;29(8):1177–1191.
50. Hay-Smith EJ, Dickson B, Nunnerley J, Anne Sinnott K. "The final piece of the puzzle to fit in": an interpretative phenomenological analysis of the return to employment in New Zealand after spinal cord injury. *Disabil Rehabil.* 2013;35(17):1436–1446.
51. Chapin MH, Holbert D. Employment at closure is associated with enhanced quality of life and subjective well-being for persons with spinal cord injuries. *Rehabilitation Counseling Bulletin.* 2010;54(1):6–14.
52. Gorzkowski JA, Kelly EH, Klaas SJ, Vogel LC. Girls with spinal cord injury: social and job-related participation and psychosocial outcomes. *Rehabil Psychol.* 2010;55(1):58–67.
53. Leduc BE, Lepage Y. Health-related quality of life after spinal cord injury. *Disabil Rehabil.* 2002;24(4):196–202.
54. McColl MA, Stirling P, Walker J, Corey P, Wilkins R. Expectations of independence and life satisfaction among ageing spinal cord injured adults. *Disabil Rehabil.* 1999;21(5-6):231–240.
55. Hess D, Meade M, Forchheimer M, Tate D. Psychological well-being and intensity of employment in individuals with a spinal cord injury. *Topics in Spinal Cord Injury Rehabilitation.* 2004;9(4):1–10.
56. Ottomanelli L, Barnett SD, Goetz LL. A prospective examination of the impact of a supported employment program and employment on health-related quality of life, handicap, and disability among veterans with SCI. *Qual Life Res.* 2013;22(8):2133–2141.
57. Ottomanelli L, Lind L. Review of critical factors related to employment after spinal cord injury: implications for research and vocational services. *J Spinal Cord Med.* 2009;32(5):503–531.
58. Trenaman LM, Miller WC, Escorpizo R, Team SR. Interventions for improving employment outcomes among individuals with spinal cord injury: a systematic review. *Spinal Cord.* 2014;52(11):788–794.
59. Ottomanelli L, Goetz LL, Suris A, et al. Effectiveness of supported employment for veterans with spinal cord injuries: results from a randomized multisite study. *Arch Phys Med Rehabil.* 2012;93(5):740–747.
60. Trexler LE, Trexler LC, Malec JF, Klyce D, Parrott D. Prospective randomized controlled trial of resource facilitation on community participation and vocational outcome following brain injury. *J Head Trauma Rehabil.* 2010;25(6):440–446.
61. Krause JS. Years to employment after spinal cord injury. *Arch Phys Med Rehabil.* 2003;84(9):1282–1289.
62. Fadyl JK, McPherson KM. Understanding decisions about work after spinal cord injury. *J Occup Rehabil.* 2010;20(1):69–80.
63. Ottomanelli L, Barnett SD, Goetz LL. Effectiveness of supported employment for veterans with spinal cord injury: 2-year results. *Arch Phys Med Rehabil.* 2014;95(4):784–790.
64. Middleton JW, Johnston D, Murphy G, et al. Early access to vocational rehabilitation for spinal cord injury inpatients. *J Rehabil Med.* 2015;47(7):626–631.
65. Holicky R, Charlifue S. Ageing with spinal cord injury: the impact of spousal support. *Disabil Rehabil.* 1999;21(5-6):250–257.
66. Kreuter M. Spinal cord injury and partner relationships. *Spinal Cord.* 2000;38(1):2–6.
67. Post MW, Bloemen J, de Witte LP. Burden of support for partners of persons with spinal cord injuries. *Spinal Cord.* 2005;43(5):311–319.

CHAPTER

49 Rehabilitation Team

Ellia Ciammaichella

OUTLINE

The core of spinal cord injury/disorders (SCI/D) medicine is the rehabilitation team. It is person-centered and involves a dynamic and interprofessional collaborative practice of clinicians throughout the continuum of care. The person-centered approach places the individual with SCI/D at the center of the team, and they are actively engaged in goal setting and decision-making. In cases of pediatric-onset SCI/D, the person-centered approach may also be family centered.[1] Conceptually, the person-centered approach is associated with better outcomes, improved quality of life, higher satisfaction, and lower costs; however, implementation is limited due to lack of consensus and minimal guidelines.[2]

The rehabilitation team is dynamic because it accommodates the entire continuum of care from initial injury or diagnosis through hospitalization, home, and outpatient services. With each transition of service, needs evolve and thus the members of the team evolve as well. The rehabilitation team is an interprofessional collaborative practice, such that each team member works within and out of their comfort zone to engage and collaborate with all members when developing and implementing treatment strategies to target rehabilitation goals. In contrast, a multidisciplinary approach involves many members caring for the same patient but working in parallel and predefined silos. Some disciplines that participate in the rehabilitation team include the physiatrist, rehabilitation nursing, physical therapy, occupational therapy, speech language pathology, recreational therapy, music therapy, neuropsychologist, respiratory therapy, nutritionist, orthotist, case manager, social worker, SCI/D educator, peer support specialist, vocational rehabilitation counselor, schoolteacher, chaplain, and other physician specialties.

Patient Safety

As persons with SCI/D advance through the continuum of care, there are certain safety risks that can be anticipated. Most noticeable are common secondary complications that can be prevented or minimized through education and surveillance. SCI/D education is the cornerstone of acute inpatient rehabilitation, so persons with SCI/D are highly encouraged to participate in such a program. Furthermore, studies show a statistically significant reduction in length of stay and decreased overall mortality when care is provided by specialized SCI centers.[3]

Transitions of service are a common area of communication failure and disjoints the continuity of care. Additionally, the fragmented electronic medical records and pure plethora of data within it may exacerbate the situation. Therefore, to bridge the transition, a structured document that is succinct and provides necessary information to transfer care is recommended. A physician-to-physician sign-out is also recommended.

Lack of local SCI/D subspecialists is common, so the community physician may be the person's primary medical professional to provide their medical needs. There has been a joint effort by the Academy of Spinal Cord Injury Professionals (ASCIP) and American Spinal Injury Association (ASIA) to provide "Primary Care Providers SCI Healthcare Resources" that are specifically created for community physicians.[4] The primary barrier has been information dissemination.

Other patient safety concerns are the common access barriers to healthcare. Accessibility requires both physical access as well as psychosocial access. For example, common screening tests such as weight evaluation, mammograms, pap smears, and colonoscopies may be overlooked by the physician or may be inaccessible to the person with SCI/D. An approach called "Universal Design"[5] is the design of an environment that minimizes barriers regardless of a person's size, age, or ability, and may be a good approach to minimizing access barriers.[6]

Unfortunately, the available social support systems are often fragmented and difficult to find. Social support is defined as "an exchange of resources between individuals intended to enhance the well-being of the recipient."[7] It can be instrumental (tangible), emotional (exchange with a close friend), companionship (sense of belonging), or informational (advice from a peer).[8] Research suggests that social support systems are positively related to life satisfaction, subjective well-being, and quality of life.[7]

Another safety risk is the poor emphasis on reintegration into society. Early rehabilitation programs emphasize rehabilitation of physical impairments but place less emphasis on reintegration into society, such as returning to employment. Employment assists in economic self-sufficiency and is associated with "financial satisfaction and better health."[9,10] Unfortunately, the average unemployment rate of persons with SCI/D is 68%, which is over 10 times higher than the national unemployment rate.[11,12] Psychosocial challenges to reintegration include lack of or fragmented psychosocial services,[11] financial disincentives, implicit bias, workplace discrimination, and inaccessibility. Conversely, positive modifiable factors that influence employment after SCI/D include postinjury education, fewer secondary health complications, driving independence, strong wheelchair skills, and having a strong work value. Some studies suggest that vocational training, on-site vocational rehabilitation counseling during inpatient rehabilitation, use of service dogs, job placement services, and supported employment programs for veterans positively influence being employed after SCI/D.[10]

Another barrier is unconscious or implicit bias, which is defined as an underlying automatic and involuntary association that a person makes between a specific social group (persons with SCI/D) and an attribute (ability to work or care for themselves). Since it is implicit, the bias is unspoken and sometimes contrary to a person's explicit beliefs. Implicit bias is often difficult to identify, but can be implied in action. For example, when a bystander instinctively begins pushing a person in a wheelchair, this implicitly suggests that the person in the wheelchair needed help to mobilize. Unfortunately, implicit bias is a significant barrier for persons with SCI/D in obtaining appropriate medical care, and diminishes their quality of life and ability to integrate into society. Although there is a social movement to identify and eliminate implicit bias by encouraging diversity and inclusion, there is currently no evidence-based universal approach.[13]

Medicolegal Issues

Medicolegal issues as they relate to SCI/D may include appropriate treatment, capacity, end of life, and medical negligence. Providing appropriate treatment is highly dependent on each injured person's circumstance, such as availability of local resources, religious beliefs and values, and medical decision-making capacity. Depending on the geographic location and age of the injured person, the injured person is transported to the nearest hospital with resources to treat the anticipated injuries. According to the bioethical principle of autonomy, the injured person having medical decision-making capacity above the age of majority is provided with the necessary information to make an informed decision. A physician diagnoses that an injured person has capacity when they can understand the benefits, risks, and alternatives to a proposed medical course of action, including lack of treatment.[14] Capacity is distinguished from competency, which is a legal determination by a judge. If the injured person lacks capacity, then a surrogate is identified and provided necessary information to make an informed decision on the injured person's behalf. A surrogate is generally the health power of attorney, also known as advance directive, advance health care directive, durable power of attorney for health care, or medical power of attorney directive. If a health power of attorney does not exist, a surrogate is determined by law (usually the most immediate family member). On the other hand, if exigent circumstances require immediate medical care before a surrogate can reasonably be contacted, the emergency exception to informed consent applies, and medical care is provided on the premise that a reasonable person would not refuse necessary medical care.[15]

Due to the severity of trauma, there are situations where physicians are placed in an ethical dilemma when bioethical principles of autonomy (right to make an informed decision), benevolence (do good), nonmaleficence (do no harm), and justice (equal treatment) collide.[16] There are situations where lack of or withdrawal of treatment is appropriate. Prior to making this decision, the medical team must provide balanced and impartial information on the benefits, risks, and alternatives, including lack of treatment, to the decision maker. It is essential that physiatrists and SCI/D subspecialists are consulted early on, as they can provide expertise in long-term outcomes and make a substantial impact on determining medical futility. Given this information, if treatment is considered futile, the physician is not obligated to perform it. Medical futility as defined by scholar Griffin Trotter and adopted by the American Medical Association occurs when "there is a goal, there is an action and activity aimed at achieving this goal, and there is virtual certainty the action will fail in achieving this goal."[17] If "virtual certainty" does not exist, the treatment is not considered futile. However, if a treatment is considered medically futile, the physician must engage in dialogue and discuss alternatives that respectfully guide future discussions.

Medical negligence may occur during care of persons with SCI/D. The law of medical negligence is generally governed by state tort statutes. Usually, medical negligence requires that the medical professional have a duty of care, breached the duty, the breach of which caused the injury, and the injury having identifiable damages. The duty is generally created with a physician–patient relationship. However, there are situations where duty of care is assumed by law or creation of peril. For example, physicians assume a duty to continue care until emergency medical services arrive if they voluntarily assist someone. The breach of duty may be an action or inaction, and occurs when the physician does not provide a standard of specialist care. The breach must be the actual or "but for" cause of the injury. In other words, no other action was the cause of the injury. Occasionally, however, it may be enough that the breach is a "substantial factor" in the injury. The breach must also be reasonably foreseeable or proximate cause of the injury. Finally, damages must be identifiable and have occurred due to the breach.[18]

Social Resources

Since the most common cause of SCI/D is trauma from a motor vehicle collision, automobile insurance, uninsured motorist coverage, and health insurance will likely be important resources for medical expenses. Depending on the geographical location of injury, fault may or may not be important. Automobile insurance is generally the primary payer. Once automobile insurance limits are exhausted and claims paid out, then health insurance will generally cover the remaining medical expenses. Often, complications arise because automobile insurance pays through reimbursement, and may require the injured person initially pay the medical expenses. Additionally, health insurance may delay payments until the automobile insurance claim is paid out. Moreover, lack of automobile insurance may preclude health insurance coverage.

If the injury occurred on the job, Workers' Compensation may provide wage replacement benefits, medical treatment expenses, vocational rehabilitation, and disability and death benefits. However, in exchange, the injured employee waives all related negligence claims, although they can generally sue for any intentional injury. Every state in the United States mandates Workers' Compensation except for Texas. Minimum requirements vary with each state.

If the injured person is a Veteran eligible for benefits through the U.S. Department of Veterans Affairs (VA), they can enroll into the VA SCI/D system of care. This provides lifelong, coordinated, team-based, comprehensive care. Approximately 42,000 veterans with SCI/D are eligible for care at VA health care facilities.[19] The injury need not be service-connected; however, if the SCI/D is a service-connected disability, the Veteran may also be eligible for Veterans Benefits Administration disability compensation benefits, which can include compensation for loss of income as well as grants to maximize independence, such as adaptive automobile or housing grants.

The Social Security Act of 1935 and amendments also provide benefits. They provide Social Security Disability Insurance, a benefit for those who have paid Social Security taxes with sufficient work credits, and Supplemental Security Income, which is based on financial need. The Social Security Amendments of 1965 created Title XVIII as Medicare for persons 65 years and older and Title XIX as Medicaid for low-income persons.

While Medicare was initially created for the elderly, it was expanded in 1973 to include eligibility based on disability. Once disability benefits from Social Security or the Railroad Board are collected for 24 months, a person is automatically eligible for Medicare Part A (hospital insurance) and Part B (outpatient medical coverage). These benefits are referred to as Traditional or Original Medicare, and a monthly premium and coinsurance may be required. With Traditional Medicare, Part D (outpatient medication coverage) is optional. Traditional Medicare can also be substituted for Medicare Part C, commonly referred to as managed Medicare or Medicare Advantage Plan. In this option, the plan can apply network and coverage restrictions and out-of-pocket costs, but may provide additional benefits such as routine vision or dental care and outpatient medication coverage. With Medicare Part C, the policyholder must pay any monthly premium for Part A and Part B and any additional premium for Part C.[20]

Low-income persons may be eligible for state-based health programs such as Medicaid, Children's Health Insurance Program (CHIP), and Basic Health Program (BHP). Medicaid provides health coverage to low-income people and benefits. CHIP assists families with income too high to qualify for Medicaid. BHP assists people who have fluctuating income above and below Medicaid and CHIP eligibility criteria. While there are certain mandatory benefits, programs vary by state.

Advocacy

Since the SCI/D population has unique needs and is substantially affected by implicit bias, it is imperative that SCI/D medicine subspecialists devote time and resources to advocacy. Topics of interest include: promoting accessibility through "universal design"; calling out implicit bias and promoting health equity; improving opportunities for education, sports, employment, and other avenues of social integration; improving common causes of healthcare failures such as transitions of care; promoting alternative means of transportation; exploring alternative modes of healthcare (such as telehealth); and supporting preventive education to reduce the occurrence of SCI/D. Advocacy can be done at the local level such as within family gatherings, employment, neighborhood associations, and little league. It can also be done at the county, state, and national levels through medical and nonmedical organizations and legislation.

The most common barrier to success in advocacy is failure to engage in advocacy. To overcome this, it is recommended to break down an advocacy opportunity into steps. First, choose a topic that drives the individual and identify opportunities for improvement. Second, explore possible solutions. Networking through meetings and social media can hone both the definition of the problem and assist in exploring possible solutions. This dynamic process may necessitate reevaluating the topic and requires the most research. Third, select a possible solution. Fourth, apply the solution and reevaluate the problem. This often requires knocking on doors and networking. Remember, focus on facts. Like the Plan-Do-Study-Act cycle of quality improvement, this process requires multiple iterations. Advocacy takes time and patience.

Practice Management

Practice management includes continuing education, medical licensing and board certification, financial management, and the practice of medicine. Continuing education in SCI/D medicine is supported through the sharing of information in organizations such as ASIA, ASCIP, VA, United Spinal Association, Christopher & Dana Reeve Foundation, Canadian/American Spinal Research Organizations, and Facing Disability.

While medical licensing is state-dependent and does not limit practice scope, board certification is often required to practice in a specific specialty. Subspecialty certification in SCI Medicine is currently only offered through the American Board of Physical Medicine and Rehabilitation. A physician becomes board eligible in SCI Medicine by (1) holding a current board certification by a member board of the American Board of Medical Specialties, (2) having an unrestricted, current, and valid license to practice medicine in at least one jurisdiction in the United States, its territories, or Canada, and (3) completing a 12-month Accreditation Council for Graduate Medical Education–accredited fellowship in SCI Medicine. Board eligibility in SCI Medicine lasts for 7 years from completion of fellowship. Most board-certified SCI Medicine subspecialists are physiatrists.[21]

In the field of SCI/D, financial management is often dictated by insurance and grants. The most common insurance includes Medicare, Medicaid, VA benefits, Workers' Compensation, and private insurance. As many persons with SCI/D require specialized types of durable medical equipment (DME) called complex rehabilitation technology (CRT), SCI/D subspecialists must be proficient in obtaining CRT for their patients. For example, Traditional Medicare often requires (1) a face-to-face examination by a physician, (2) a standard written order (which includes the beneficiary's name, order date, general description of the item, dispensed quantity, treating physician's name or NPI and treating physician's signature), (3) a certification of medical necessity, (4) a home assessment, and (5) delivery documentation. In addition, Traditional Medicare limits coverage of DME to that needed within the home, and can only be provided once the policyholder is no longer institutionalized.

Finally, the mode of practicing medicine is ever-changing and depends on the needs of the person. The SCI/D subspecialist may work in the inpatient setting as either a consult physician or primary physician within the acute medical, acute inpatient rehabilitation, long-term acute care hospital, or skilled nursing facility. The SCI/D subspecialist may also work in the outpatient setting at a clinic with face-to-face visits or virtually with the use of specialized technology. The SCI/D subspecialist may also visit patients at home. In the future, there may be other modes of medicine including the use of artificial intelligence.

Review Questions

1. True or false: The term *interprofessional* and *multidisciplinary* are interchangeable when describing the rehabilitation team.
2. The following are risks for patient safety EXCEPT:
   a. Transitions of service
   b. Fragmented social support systems
   c. Implicit bias
   d. Healthcare safety nets
3. True or false: Medical decision-making capacity is a legal decision determined by a judge.
4. True or false: Implicit bias cannot be contrary to a person's explicit beliefs.
5. True or false: In the context of SCI/D, medical futility is easy to determine.
6. True or false: Advocacy can be big or small.

REFERENCES

1. Hostler SL. Pediatric family-centered rehabilitation. *Journal of Head Trauma Rehabilitation*. 1999;14(4):384–393.
2. Yun DW, Choi JS. Person-centered rehabilitation care and outcomes: a systematic literature review. *International Journal of Nursing Studies*. 2019;93:74–83.
3. Parent S, Barchi S, LeBreton M, Casha S, Fehlings MG. The impact of specialized centers of care for spinal cord injury on length of stay, complications, and mortality: a systematic review of the literature. *J Neurotrauma*. 2011;28(8):1363–1370.
4. Academy of Spinal Cord Injury Professionals, Inc. Primary Care Providers - SCI Healthcare Resources [Internet]. American Spinal Injury Association. 2020. https://asia-spinalinjury.org/primary-care/.
5. UN General Assembly, Convention on the Rights of Persons with Disabilities: resolution/adopted by the General Assembly, 24 January 2007, A/RES/61/106. https://www.refworld.org/docid/45f973632.html.
6. The Centre for Excellence in Universal Design [Internet]. Centre for Excellence in Universal Design. 2020. https://universaldesign.ie/.
7. Müller R, Peter C, Cieza A, Geyh S. The role of social support and social skills in people with spinal cord injury—a systematic review of the literature. *Spinal Cord*. 2011;50(2):94–106.

8. Semmer NK, Elfering A, Jacobshagen N, Perrot T, Beehr TA, Boos N. The emotional meaning of instrumental social support. *International Journal of Stress Management*. 2008;15(3):235–251.
9. Escorpizo R, Smith EM, Finger ME, Miller WC. Work and employment following spinal cord injury. In: Eng JJ, Teasell RW, Miller WC, et al., eds. *Spinal Cord Injury Rehabilitation Evidence*. Version 6.0. Vancouver; 2018:1-35. https://scire-project.com/wp-content/uploads/S6-Work-Employment-Chapter-_RE_AC_MF_RE-MQ-Apr-11-2019.pdf.
10. Vogel LC, Klaas SJ, Lubicky JP, Anderson CJ. Long-term outcomes and life satisfaction of adults who had pediatric spinal cord injuries. *Archives of Physical Medicine and Rehabilitation*. 1998;79(12):1496–1503.
11. National Spinal Cord Injury Statistical Center. *Facts and Figures at a Glance*. Birmingham: University of Alabama at Birmingham; 2020.
12. The Employment Situation. News Release, Bureau of Labor Statistics. US Dept of Labor; 2022. https://www.bls.gov/news.release/pdf/empsit.pdf.
13. Hausmann LR, Myaskovsky L, Niyonkuru C, et al. Examining implicit bias of physicians who care for individuals with spinal cord injury: a pilot study and future directions. *The Journal of Spinal Cord Medicine*. 2014;38(1):102–110.
14. Barstow C, Shahan B, Roberts M. Evaluating medical decision-making capacity in practice. *Am Fam Physician*. 2018;98(1):40–46.
15. Berg JW. *Informed Consent: Legal Theory and Clinical Practice*. Oxford: Oxford University Press; 2007.
16. Beauchamp TL, Childress JF. *Principles of Biomedical Ethics*. New York: Oxford University Press; 2019.
17. Kasman DL. When is medical treatment futile? *Journal of General Internal Medicine*. 2004;19(10):1053–1056.
18. Wecht CH, Wecht CH. *Preparing and Winning Medical Negligence Cases*. Huntington: Juris Pub; 2009.
19. Fyffe DC, Williams J, Tobin P, Gibson-Gill C. Spinal cord injury veterans' disability benefits, outcomes, and health care utilization patterns: protocol for a qualitative study. *JMIR Research Protocols*. 2019;8(10). e14039.
20. Oh JW. *Maximize Your Medicare: Qualify for Benefits, Protect Your Health, and Minimize Your Costs*. New York: Thorndike Press; 2020.
21. American Board of Physical Medicine and Rehabilitation [Internet]. ABPMR. https://www.abpmr.org/Subspecialties/SCIM.

Answers to Review Questions

Chapter 1 Neurophysiology of the Spinal Cord

1. **A:** Pacinian corpuscles lie deep in the subcutaneous tissue and are responsible for responding to high-frequency vibrations (>40 Hz) on the skin. These receptors quickly adapt, so intermittent vibratory stimuli tend to be more effective at drawing attention than sustained vibration (and also improve battery life). Merkel receptors respond to low-frequency pressure details such as texture. Ruffini corpuscles detect skin stretch and joint rotation. Meissner corpuscles detect fine point discrimination and tapping as well as low-frequency vibration, so they may play a minor role in transmitting the vibration sensation.
2. **B:** The anterior horn is generally organized so that motor neurons for axial muscles are medial, those for distal muscles are lateral, those for extensors are anterior, and those for flexors are posterior. Astrocytomas are rare intradural, intramedullary tumors that tend to arise eccentrically in the gray matter, whereas ependymomas develop from ependymal cells along the central canal, and hemangioblastomas tend to develop posteriorly or posterolaterally.
3. **D:** The anterior spinal artery is at risk of infarction during aortic repair surgeries, resulting in anterior cord syndrome. Signs include flaccid paraplegia (due to damage of anterior horn cells that stimulate muscles) and impairment in the sensory modalities–pain (including somatic and visceral types) and temperature, and crude touch–transmitted via the anterior and lateral spinothalamic pathways. Vibration and proprioception information is carried afferently via the posterior columns and classically is unaffected.
4. **C:** The majority of corticospinal fibers decussate in the medulla and travel inferiorly to the target alpha motor neurons in the contralateral anterior horn of the spinal cord. Therefore, the ipsilateral leg (right) will be affected. At the time of trauma, the patient is experiencing spinal shock with a flaccid limb. However, corticospinal fibers are axons of upper motor neurons, and damage to them would eventually result in spasticity. The intact lumbosacral cord suggests the lower motor neuron cell bodies and axons are intact, so a superimposed lower motor syndrome featuring persistent flaccidity would not be expected.
5. **A:** The patient is experiencing autonomic dysreflexia likely due to excess bladder pressure. Autonomic dysreflexia is characterized by unbalanced net parasympathetic effect above the level of the lesion (in this case C8) and net sympathetic activity below the level neurological level of injury (NLOI). The parasympathetic nervous system postganglionic neurons are mostly cholinergic and would be responsible for flushing, or dilation of the vessels above the NLOI. The abdominal vascular bed, also referred to as splanchnic vessels, undergoes vasoconstriction from net sympathetic stimulation if affected during a dysreflexia event. It is unlikely that a hypersensitivity reaction to a catheter would present as described. The adrenoreceptors ($\alpha1$, $\alpha2$, $\beta1$, $\beta2$) respond to postganglionic sympathetic neurons. While sympathetic stimulation to the heart may increase during autonomic dysreflexia in a patient with C8 NLOI, the effect on heart rate is overshadowed by vagal activation from the parasympathetic surge above the NLOI. The overall effect tends to yield normal or below-normal heart rate.

Chapter 2 Neuroanatomy

1. C: The atlantoaxial joint provides approximately 50% of cervical rotation.
2. 1 A: In the thoracolumbar spine, the intermediolateral column contains the cell bodies of preganglionic sympathetic neurons. Motor neuron cell bodies are in the ventral horn of the gray matter. Preganglionic parasympathetic neurons are found in the brainstem and the sacral intermediolateral column. Lastly, second-order neurons for the spinothalamic tract are found primarily in the substantia gelatinosa of the dorsal horn of the gray matter.
3. C: The C8 nerve root would be damaged in a C7–T1 fracture/dislocation. Due to there being an extra cervical nerve root compared with cervical vertebrae, C8 must come out below the C7 vertebra.
4. B: The artery of Adamkiewicz most commonly branches off on the left side between T8–L2 to provide primary blood supply to the anterior spinal artery. Occlusion of this artery would lead to flaccid paraplegia and impaired pain/temperature sensation.
5. A: The pia mater forms the filum terminale.

Chapter 3 Epidemiology, Risk Factors, and Genetics

1. **C:** Smoking is not a known risk factor for SCI. However, age is a risk factor for SCI, as SCI varies by age. Incidence is lowest for the pediatric group, highest for individuals in their late teens and twenties, and increasing for individuals older than 65 years of age. Alcohol is also a risk factor for SCI with

between 22% and 50% of patients presenting with new SCI reporting alcohol use at the time of injury. Race is also a risk factor for SCI with the White to non-White prevalence and incidence ratios being approximately 1.5.

2. **B:** A, C, and D are incorrect. The annual incidence of SCI in the United States is approximately 54 cases per million or 17,810 new SCI cases per year.
3. **C:** Motor vehicle accidents are the leading cause of injury, followed by falls. Acts of violence (primarily gunshot wounds) are the third most common cause of SCI. Sports/recreation activities are the fourth most common cause of injury.
4. **B:** Incomplete tetraplegia is the most common type of injury, followed by incomplete paraplegia and complete paraplegia. Complete tetraplegia is the least common type of injury.
5. **B:** The leading cause of death following SCI is respiratory disease. Infectious diseases are the second most common cause of death. In the past 45 years, rates of cancer and heart disease have been declining.

Chapter 4 Prevention of Spinal Cord Injury

1. **A:** Rugs in a walkway can become a tripping hazard. Therefore, it is recommended to remove these if an elderly person lives in the home. Supervised exercise programs, tapering of psychotropic medications, and environmental modifications including addition of grab bars in the bathroom are all supported strategies to reduce falls in the elderly.
2. 2. **C:** Folic acid 4000 μg daily is the recommended dose for those who are planning or could become pregnant. The dose is increased to 4000 μg or 4 mg daily if, as in this case, the mother has had a child with a neural tube defect.
3. **C:** Treatment of neuropathic pain. The goal of tertiary prevention is to prevent the transition from disability into handicap. Both answers B and D are examples of primary prevention, which is prevention of an accident that could cause traumatic SCI. Answer A is an example of secondary prevention or limiting/reversing initial damage.

Chapter 5 Clinical and Basic Research

1. **B:** Research in the laboratory and in animal models that may lead to advances in SCI treatment.
2. **D:** It inhibits glial cell containment of the injured area and preservation of the brain–spinal cord barrier.
3. **C:** Chondroitin sulfate proteoglycans.
4. **A:** Oligodendrocytes.

Chapter 6 Prehospital Evaluation and Management

1. **C:** 72 hours.
2. **A:** This is the classic pattern for neurogenic shock. Hypotension, decreased cardiac output, decreased heart rate, decreased systemic vascular resistance.
3. **C:** A MAP of >85–90 for 7 days.
4. **B:** A high-speed motor vehicle accident is an example of a high-risk factor for the Canadian C-Spine Rule.
5. **A:** The five elements of the primary survey include airway management, breathing and ventilation, circulatory management, disability assessment, and exposure. Establishment of an airway with intubation is indicated in a patient with GCS less than or equal to 8. The use of manual in-line stabilization is recommended if intubation is necessary in the trauma patient with suspected spinal cord injury.
6. **D:** There is no definitive evidence to support the routine use of any neuroprotective agents, such as steroids, in acute traumatic spinal cord injury.

Chapter 7 Neurological Assessment and Classification

1. **A:** In this case, there is no preservation of sensory function, as there is no sensation noted in the S4–S5 dermatome including light touch, pinprick, and deep anal pressure. Additionally, there is no preservation of motor function as seen by the absence of voluntary anal contraction. Therefore, this patient meets the criteria for AIS A.
2. **D:** The neurologic level of injury is determined as the lowest level from both the left and right sides that has both normal sensation and motor function. Therefore, C6 is the neurologic level of injury. Since voluntary anal contraction is present, the patient is at least an AIS C. To determine between AIS C and AIS D, the number of key muscles below the neurologic level of injury are counted. Since greater than half the key muscles below the neurologic level of injury have a grade of ≥3, the patient is an AIS D.
3. **B:** The testing of nonkey muscles can be helpful in distinguishing between an AIS grade of B or C.
4. **C:** The motor level is determined by the lowest key muscle that has a grade of 3 on the manual muscle test. However, all muscles above this level need to have a grade of 5. In this scenario, the right motor level is C8, as all muscles above this level have a grade of 5. On the left, the level is C7. Although the left C8 has a grade of 3, not all levels above C8 have a grade of 5. The overall motor level for this case is C7.
5. **B:** In this case, there is sensory function preservation at S4–S5. Therefore, the patient is not a complete injury (AIS A). However, there is no motor preservation as seen by the absent voluntary anal

contraction. Additionally, there is no motor function more than three levels below the motor level. Therefore, this falls under the classification of AIS B.

6. **D:** The ASIA examination is best performed within 72 hours to 1 week after initial injury.

Chapter 8 Neuroimaging

1. **B:** Plain films miss a large percentage of clinically significant spine fractures, and thus CT scans, which can be performed rapidly and in unstable patients, have replaced X-rays to screen for suspected vertebral fractures. MRIs demonstrate spinal cord injury and other pathology quite well, but are inferior for fracture detection to CT scans, take much longer to perform, and cannot be obtained in patients who are unstable and require equipment (such as ventilators) during the scan, or in patients who have certain implanted devices (among other contraindications for MRI).
2. **D:** Diffusion weighted imaging (DWI) can detect early ischemia in the brain and spinal cord, which appears normal on T2 and STIR sequences until spinal cord edema is present.
3. **A:** Subacute early intramedullary hemorrhage (3–7 days after hemorrhage) is hyperintense on T1-weighted (T1W) imaging and hypointense on T2-weighted (T2W) imaging. Spinal cord edema and demyelination are hyperintense on T2W images but not on T1W. Although syringomyelia can be seen on T1W images, the fluid-filled cavity is not hyperintense.
4. **C:** With the presence of edema after anterior spinal cord infarcts, involvement of the anterior horn cells, which are particularly vulnerable to ischemia, can be seen on T2-weighted sequences. On axial views, the hyperintense anterior horns give the "owl eye sign."
5. **D:** Although the initial physical exam is the single best predictor of neurological outcome, T2 sagittal imaging findings of parenchymal hemorrhage, transection, and longer length of injury within the spinal cord correlate with a poorer neurologic recovery, whereas no spinal cord abnormality on MRI is associated with favorable outcomes.

Chapter 9 Electrodiagnostics in Spinal Cord Injury

1. **D:** All of the above: median, ulnar, radial.
2. **C:** C8–T1 cervical root avulsion.
3. **B:** Distal spinal muscular atrophy.
4. **B:** Electrodiagnostic studies are important for patient selection and stratification for clinical trials.
5. **D:** C5–T1 and L3–S1 (because these innervate limb muscles).
6. **C:** A single anterior horn cell innervates a single muscle fiber. (One anterior horn cell may innervate 200 to over 1600 muscle fibers.)

Chapter 10 Functional Assessments

1. **B:** The functional independence measure (FIM) quantifies a patient's function based on two primary categories; motor and cognitive–communicative. Each item is measured on a 7-point scale in which a higher score indicates a greater independence. The FIM is used during inpatient rehabilitation to track progress from admission to discharge.
2. **A:** The WISCI is a functional capacity assessment that measures improvements in walking in patients with acute and chronic SCI. It is a standardized assessment that takes into account the level of assistance needed in walking, as well as use of assistive devices and braces, in ambulation of a standard 10 m distance. Scores on this assessment range from 0–20, with 0 being unable to stand or participate in assistive walking and 20 being ambulation without any assistance or assistive devices.
3. **C:** ISNCSCI is the gold standard for diagnosis and prognosis of spinal cord injury. The assessment uses key sensory and motor exam components to determine a patient's neurologic level of injury as well as the severity of injury as described by the American Spinal Injury Association (ASIA) Impairment Scale (AIS), which is then used to set functional goals.
4. **D:** The SCIM is a comprehensive functional rating scale that both assesses abilities in areas of self-care, respiration and sphincter management, and mobility and defines quantitative goals for functional restoration of primary daily activities. SCIM items are scored by observing the patient performing a task and choosing the score most compatible with the patient's performance from those listed in the SCIM evaluation sheet next to the scoring criterion definition.
5. **B:** The PARA-SCI measures the type, frequency, duration, and intensity of physical activity performed by persons with SCI who use a wheelchair as their primary mode of mobility. It can be used among people with paraplegia or tetraplegia and aims to facilitate collection of epidemiologic data to develop health-promoting physical activity guidelines and interventions for patients with SCI.

Chapter 12 Cardiovascular Issues in Spinal Cord Injury: Neurogenic Shock, Spinal Shock, and Orthostatic Hypotension

1. **C:** The patient's parasympathetic nervous system is being unopposed by the sympathetic nervous system; B does not explain the bradycardia, A is cardiogenic shock, D is septic shock.
2. **A, D, F, H:** Hallmarks of neurogenic shock include bradycardia and hypotension, which result in

decreased cardiac output and decreased peripheral perfusion, causing cool and clammy extremities and a lowered body temperature.

3. **A, C, E, F:** are all correct. There is loss of vasomotor tone, increased venous pooling due to vascular failure to vasoconstrict, which results in decreased cardiac preload which is nurse anonymous to decrease venous blood return to the heart.
4. **C:** Atropine is an anticholinergic agent that will help prevent bradycardia, which can result in hypoperfusion and progress to asystole. Adenosine is used for arrhythmias. Warfarin is used to anticoagulate. Norepinephrine is used as a pressor to vasoconstrict.
5. **A:** Fluid resuscitation is the correct answer. Fluid resuscitation is initial intervention for neurogenic shock followed by use of pressors.
6. **B:** Neurogenic shock will have hypotension, bradycardia, and hypothermia.
7. **B:** is the correct answer. This person clinically has orthostatic hypotension, which is common in higher-level injuries. Make the patient lie down and check blood pressure; start intravenous fluids if necessary. Could also consider addition of compressive wear, or pharmacological therapy, but given the number of symptoms, the person needs to return to a supine position. Making a person sit upright is for autonomic dysreflexia. ECG is for ruling out arrhythmia, where symptoms may be unrelated to sit vs. supine. Oral hypotensives are not always indicated, as they have greater side effects and slower onset than the correct answer.
8. **B:** The most appropriate management is: CT of the abdomen/pelvis and chest should be done. Patient is tachycardic, not bradycardic, and thus appears to be in hypovolemic shock. Hypovolemic shock is associated with tachycardia and hypotension (neurogenic shock is associated with bradycardia). It is important to rule out other ongoing causes, such as blood loss, that can result in the same clinical picture. The diagnosis of neurogenic shock should only be made when other causes of shock have been excluded. Intravenous fluids are likely important and would be the initial treatment for neurogenic shock.
9. **B:** Temporary loss or depression of all or most **spinal** reflex activity below the level of the injury; A is neurogenic shock, D is septic shock. C is incorrect, as hypertension should not be seen in spinal shock.
10. **C:** 85–90 mm Hg is currently the recommended standard. Theoretically, this will aid in maintaining cord perfusion.

Chapter 13 Autonomic Dysreflexia

1. **C:** Parasympathetic hyperactivity. AD occurs due to sympathetic hyperactivity, which leads to vasoconstriction that is more profound in SCI above the T6 neurological level and cannot be modulated by descending inhibition from above.
2. **B:** Tachycardia. Clinical presentation of AD includes hypertension, sweating (typically below the level of injury), headache, and anxiety. Reflex bradycardia is sometimes exhibited due to parasympathetic (via vagal nerve) activity.
3. **E:** Orthostatic hypotension. Hypertension, not hypotension, is the hallmark presentation of AD, and may lead to cerebral or retinal hemorrhage. Seizures and atrial fibrillation have been reported as complications of AD.
4. **A:** Placing patient in the supine position. Placing the patient in a sitting (rather than supine) position is recommended during treatment of AD as this can lower the cerebral blood pressure.

Chapter 14 Pulmonary Issues After Spinal Cord Injury

1. **True:** The incidence of respiratory complications is the main cause of morbidity and mortality in the patients with acute spinal cord injury. This can range from 36% to 83%. Approximately two-thirds of patients with acute SCI will experience complications such as atelectasis, pneumonia, and respiratory failure, which will lead to mechanical ventilation.
2. **D:** Above C5 AIS A: The degree of respiratory dysfunction will depend on the extent and level of the neurological injury, in such a way that high cervical and thoracic injuries are at the highest risk. Various studies have suggested an increasing trend in cervical injuries, in particular C1–C4 injuries, with an increased rate of SCI resulting in mechanical ventilation dependency. Complete lesions above C5 usually require intubation in virtually 100% of cases.
3. **E:** Acute spinal cord injury above T12 neurologic level of injury will cause some form of respiratory impairment. In cervical and high paraplegia, expiratory muscles are more impaired due to the impairment of absence of abdominal muscles. The loss of expiratory musculature causes an impairment in the ability to produce effective coughing, leading to the subsequent accumulation of secretions. This results in carbon dioxide retention and loss of cough mechanism that can lead to respiratory failure if not addressed.

   Acute SCI causes loss of sympathetic tone that leads to parasympathetic predominance manifested by increased vascular congestion, decreased mucociliary activity, increased production of secretions, and bronchospasm that facilitates the onset of atelectasis.
4. **D:** The preservation of diaphragmatic function should be a primary objective in all patients undergoing

mechanical ventilation. Diaphragmatic dysfunction is a common cause of weaning failure. In high cervical and thoracic injuries, ventilation will depend almost exclusively on the functioning of the diaphragm, which will be responsible for providing 90% of the tidal volume.

Chapter 15 Sleep Disorders in Individuals With Spinal Cord Injury

1. **B:** Obstructive sleep apnea is defined by greater than 90% loss of airflow with continued or increased thoracic and abdominal effort for at least 10 seconds. Central sleep apnea is defined as greater than 90% loss of airflow with absent thoracic and abdominal effort for at least 10 seconds. Cheyne-Stokes breathing is a form of central sleep apnea and represents exaggerated response to hypoventilation or rise in partial pressure of carbon dioxide (pCO_2) that leads to a rapid increase in ventilation and subsequent rapid decline in pCO_2. The rapid decrement in pCO_2 results in a loss of respiratory drive and consequent apneic period. During the apnea, oxygenation decreases while pCO_2 gradually rises above the apneic threshold, resulting in eventual resumption of breathing. Ventilation oscillates between apnea and hyperpnea in a crescendo–decrescendo pattern usually lasting between 30 seconds to several minutes. Tetraplegics are more likely to have sleep apnea compared to paraplegics. Prevalence among adults with paraplegia is not significantly different from what is seen in the general population.
2. **B:** Melatonin is used to treat circadian rhythm sleep–wake disorders. Sleep disordered breathing can be treated with fixed continuous pressure (CPAP), auto-PAP (APAP), bilevel pressure (BiPAP) for high pressure requirements, adaptive servo-ventilation (ASV) for CSA, oral appliances for mild or moderate OSA, upper airway surgery, and retrognathia and hypoglossal nerve stimulation.
3. **A:** PLM is defined as periodic episodes of repetitive and highly stereotyped limb movements involving great toe and ankle dorsiflexion, often accompanied by knee and hip flexion; B is periodic leg movement syndrome (PLMS), C is periodic limb movement disorder (PLMD), and D is restless leg syndrome (RLS).
4. **C:** Individuals with SCI do not have nocturnal decrease in blood pressure (BP) or significant BP variability over 24 hours compared with controls. They also do not have significant variability in circadian rhythm of leg resistance and flow, whereas lower resistance and higher flow values during sleep have been observed in the general population. People with SCI have lower 24-hour heart rate (HR) values compared to able-bodied individuals, but their circadian HR profile is similar to that in the general population. People with SCI have lower energy expenditure and sleeping metabolic rate compared to control individuals, despite decreased fat-free mass.
5. **B:** Initial treatment should start with proper sleep hygiene, and comorbid conditions should also be addressed. Pharmacological therapy, such as hypnotic medications, should be used only after cognitive-behavioral therapy for insomnia (CBT-I) has been attempted given concerns for fall risk and impaired cognition. Dopamine agonists such as ropinirole or pramipexole can be used to treat PLM if symptoms persist despite physical exercise and iron supplementation.

Chapter 16 Thromboembolism/Deep Vein Thrombosis

1. **C:** Risk factors found to increase the chance of VTE in patients with SCI include complete injuries, prior VTE, age, concomitant lower extremity fractures, and paraplegia. SCI patients with paraplegia have been found to be at higher risk for VTE than those with tetraplegia. A retrospective study consisting of 16,000 SCI patients found an odds ratio of 1.8 for developing VTE when comparing those with complete paraplegia versus complete tetraplegia. Another retrospective analysis separated over 18,000 SCI patients into five SCI groups, with high thoracic injuries (T1–T6) found to be at highest risk and high cervical injuries (C1–C4) to be one of the lowest groups at risk for VTE.
2. **B:** Most recent guidelines suggest that at least 8 weeks of thromboprophylaxis should be administered to minimize risk of VTE. A notable decrease in episodes of VTE was seen in studies, indicating this time frame may be most appropriate for those without additional factors requiring prolonged thromboprophylaxis, such as prior VTE or malignancy.
3. **D:** Utilization of duplex ultrasound as a screening tool for DVT in asymptomatic patients has not been found to be sensitive. Additionally, it is difficult to determine how to treat asymptomatic patients with abnormal findings seen on duplex ultrasound, as these findings are of uncertain clinical significance. Given the patient's new injury and 2-week course of LMWH, he should continue on with prophylactic anticoagulation while in rehabilitation, with a goal of 8 weeks of therapy.
4. **A:** Though there has not been specific research surrounding prophylactic anticoagulation for patients with chronic SCI, these patients are believed to be at equivalent, or increased, risk for VTE as compared with patients without SCI who may be admitted for similar reasons. For this reason, Ms. Smith should be anticoagulated with the same prophylactic dosing

that would be given to a patient without SCI who was admitted with sepsis.

5. **C:** The three main components thought to predispose patients with new SCI to VTE include venostasis, hypercoagulability, and endothelial injury. These are the major contributing factors known to make up the Virchow triad.
6. **D:** A retrospective study conducted by Maung et al. found that the risk of VTE does differ with the level of SCI. Patients with high thoracic injuries (T1–T6) were found to be at highest risk of VTE and those with high cervical injuries (C1–C4) were found to be at lowest risk.
7. **C:** Per 2016 Consortium Clinical Practice Guidelines, vitamin K antagonists, LMWH, or DOACs are appropriate in the postacute rehabilitation stage. DOACs and vitamin K antagonists are not appropriate to be given in the acute period after new SCI. Goal of INR for vitamin K antagonist should be 2.0–3.0.

Chapter 17 Neurogenic Bowel

1. **E:** All of the above are causes of diarrhea in persons with SCI.
2. **C:** Areflexic NBD bowel care typically involves manual removal of stool one or more times each day. Repeated digital stimulations and suppositories are less effective than in reflexic NBD. Enemas are generally discouraged.
3. **B:** Her examination is consistent with spinal shock, which can last days to weeks. Areflexic bowel care is indicated. With a complete (AIS A) injury, her prognosis for recovery of anal sensation is low after 72 hours or 1 week. Enemas are a last resort.
4. **C:** Despite absent sensation, symptoms of AD are present, which indicate a focus of irritation. Index of suspicion for acute abdomen should be high. In chronic SCI, causes include obstruction due to intraabdominal adhesions, sigmoid or cecal volvulus, pancreatitis, cholelithiasis, and others. Urgent imaging is warranted, possibly followed by hospital admission, nasogastric suction, NPO status, and surgical consultation.
5. **B:** Time spent on bowel care and caregiver burden are less following stoma. AD can still occur but is less after stoma. A trial of transanal irrigation could be performed. Ostomy reversal is generally possible but frequently chosen by people with SCI.

Chapter 18 Dysphagia and Common GI Issues After SCI

1. **D:** Patients with dysphagia can potentially involve many members of a medical team, such as the ones above. The listed complaints are more consistent with an esophageal dysphagia than oropharyngeal and thus better managed by a gastroenterologist.
2. **D:** It is a common misbelief that a fully inflated cuff prevents aspiration. Because the cuff of a tracheostomy tube sits below the level of the vocal folds, any material that collects on the cuff is considered to be aspiration. In addition, a fully inflated cuff may still allow some material to slip below the cuff.
3. **B:** In a systematic review by Iruthayarajah et al., age, cervical spine surgery, and presence of a tracheostomy tube were found to be the most significant factors in determining risk of dysphagia in patients with spinal cord injury. Xerostomia caused by medications can be a cause of dysphagia in the oral stage but is less significant.
4. **C:** The patient has undergone surgical intervention with body plaster cast placement, likely causing him to lie supine for prolonged periods of time. In addition, he has lost 25 lbs since the injury and has now developed nausea and vomiting worse after meals. The most likely diagnosis is Superior Mesenteric Artery Syndrome. The best first initial treatment is conservative management with small, frequent meals in the upright body position.
5. **D:** HIDA scan is indicated if the diagnosis of acute cholecystitis remains unclear following ultrasound. MRCP and ERCP is indicated when there is concern for concurrent choledocolithiasis from a stone in the common bile duct (elevated AST, ALT, total bilirubin). CT has low specificity for diagnosing acute cholecystitis.

Chapter 19 Neurogenic Bladder

1. **B:** Although all the topics mentioned are a part of a detailed urologic history, determining a patient's baseline urine production is critical, as some dialysis patients are oliguric but may appear to be anuric when an acute neurogenic bladder is present. This may result in inappropriate elimination management strategies and lead to complications associated with urinary retention.
2. **C:** The risk of spreading malignant cells from the closed system of the bladder into the retroperitoneum contraindicates suprapubic tube use.
3. **A:** Tamsulosin and other alpha 1a selective antagonists may have higher rates of retrograde ejaculation.
4. **B:** Answer C describes voiding symptoms; answer D describes post-micturition symptoms. Answer A is not considered to be a key feature of LUTS.
5. **D:** Patients with traumatic brain injury may suffer suprapontine lesions, and autonomic dysreflexia can be seen in patients with suprasacral lesions.

Chapter 20 Urological Conditions in Persons With Spinal Cord Injury

1. **B:** The finding of detrusor–sphincter dyssynergia is most likely to be observed in a patient with a suprasacral spinal cord injury. During voiding there is discoordination of the normal physiology of voiding. The external sphincter, along with the pelvic floor musculature, should relax during the micturition process. In this scenario, the patient's external sphincter is closed or partially closed and forces the bladder to contract against a closed sphincter.
2. **D:** All persons that experience a spinal cord injury should be scheduled for urodynamics after spinal shock has abated and a new baseline is reached. Although this procedure does have limitations, it is the best way for providers to understand the physiology of bladder filling, storage, and emptying.
3. **A:** This patient's current bladder management is satisfactory from a urologic standpoint. However, he is having secondary issues due to pooling of urine in his diaper. Application of a condom catheter would be the best option with least morbidity. To achieve this, the patient should undergo a malleable penile prosthesis, which would allow for proper application. Additionally, the penile prothesis would make sexual activity easier for this patient. An augmentation cystoplasty and botulinum neurotoxin injection are unwarranted, as the patient has adequate bladder capacity and low bladder pressures. Appendicovesicostomy and an artificial urinary sphincter are not good options due to poor hand dexterity.
4. **E:** Counsel the patient on asymptomatic bacteriuria. This patient most likely has asymptomatic bacteriuria. Persons with indwelling catheters and those that perform intermittent catheterization are likely to have chronic bacterial colonization of their bladder. Urine cultures should only be drawn in the setting of symptoms or if the patient is planning to undergo an invasive urologic procedure. If treatment must be initiated, a longer course of antibiotics (10–14 days) should be prescribed. Suprapubic catheter and cystoscopy are not indicated. Prophylactic antibiotics are rarely warranted in persons with SCIs due to increased resistance and rapid recolonization of the bladder when discontinued.
5. **D:** Ureteroscopy and laser lithotripsy. Stones larger than 10 mm are unlikely to pass with medical expulsive therapy. Extracorporeal shock wave lithotripsy and percutaneous nephrolithotomy are contraindicated due to chronic anticoagulation. Urodynamics is not an appropriate method to treat kidney stones. Ureteroscopy can be safely performed without cessation of anticoagulation.

Chapter 21 Sexuality and Reproduction After Spinal Cord Injury

1. **B:** Reflexogenic orgasms require an intact sacral reflex arc (S2–S4).
2. **C:** This is thought to be due to the fact that the spinothalamic outflow (which is part of the psychogenic efferent pathway) that transmits pinprick sensation for T11–L2 lies very close to the sympathetic cell bodies.
3. **B:** There have been some suggestions that there are alternate afferent pathways via the vagus nerve that can bypass the spinal cord and help generate orgasm.
4. **D:** A significant number of individuals are unable to ejaculate and often require methods to assist.
5. **D:** Phosphodiesterase type 5, with assistance of nitrous oxide (NO), reduces inactivation of cGMP, thus promoting smooth muscle relaxation. This, in turn, can lead to hypotension, headaches, and flushing.

Chapter 22 Women's Health After Spinal Cord Injury

1. **C:** Autonomic dysreflexia is a hypersensitivity response to noxious stimuli below level of injury. It can be triggered anytime during pregnancy and delivery. AD will persist until noxious stimuli have been removed.
2. **D:** Higher risk for UTIs; up to 59% due to hydronephrosis, areflexic or overactive bladder, and frequent cauterizations. Try to avoid indwelling catheters due to increased risk of infection, but may be needed in the first and third trimesters to help with AD. Chronic UTIs during pregnancy can lead to early births.
3. **D:** Spasticity is a symptom of upper motor neuron disorder, resulting from intact spinal reflexes persisting below the level of the injury. Some women will see an increase in spasticity during pregnancy. Oral baclofen is used in the medical management of spasticity during pregnancy. Clonidine and tizanidine are contraindicated. Oral baclofen has been associated with neonatal withdrawal symptoms such as irritability, poor feeding, and seizures.
4. **A:** Typically, injuries T10 and below are able to perceive labor and feel contractions. Uterine contractions travel into the spinal cord at T10 (via Frankenhauser plexus). Women with injuries below this, such as at T11–T12, will also feel pain with labor contractions. Even still, labor pain in individuals with SCI above this level can be perceived as referred pain to the upper extremities, increased spasticity, autonomic dysreflexia, and nonspecific pain.
5. **C:** Injuries above T4 can lead to delayed ability to breastfed in complete injuries due to the fact that the afferent pathway of milk ejection reflex is initiated by infant suckling and is carried from receptors in the breast via dorsal roots from T4–T6.

Chapter 23 Musculoskeletal Disorders

1. **B:** Urgent MRI should be considered to evaluate for acute rotator cuff tear in this patient who is dependent on his upper extremities for mobility and ADLs.
2. **B:** The rear axle should be as far forward as possible without compromising stability to decrease stroke frequency, rate of rise, and the push angle.
3. **C:** Initial treatment with tendon sheath corticosteroid injections have the best outcome.
4. **D:** NSAIDs have not been shown to have efficacy in the treatment of carpal tunnel syndrome.
5. **D:** For manual wheelchair propulsion the seat height should be adjusted so that the elbow angle is between 100–110 degrees.
6. **C:** Supracondylar femur.
7. **D:** Fractures in chronic SCI are typically extra-articular.
8. **A:** There is no compelling evidence that vitamin D, calcium, bisphosphonates, routine DEXA scans, and/or standing activities help prevent lower extremity fractures in SCI.
9. **E:** Autonomic dysreflexia does not show a positive correlation with shoulder contractures in chronic SCI.
10. **D:** Knee flexion deformities need a very thorough MSK examination, as hip flexion deformities and/or ankle equinus deformities can cause knee flexion deformities. Performing only a hamstring tenotomy may not be beneficial for treatment in this scenario.

Chapter 24 Heterotopic Ossification

1. **B:** After SCI, HO most commonly develops around the hip, followed by the knee, elbow, shoulder, and rarely also in smaller joints of the hands and feet.
2. **C:** HO usually occurs 3–12 weeks after injury with peak incidence around 8 weeks.
3. **A:** In early HO, triple-phase bone scan is more sensitive than X-ray. Bone scan evaluates for the increased uptake of osteotropic radionucleotides and may reveal HO as early as 2.5 weeks after injury.
4. **B:** Serum ALP is the most commonly ordered lab when HO is suspected but is not specific. It can be elevated in HO, but sometimes may not be elevated. It can also be elevated with nonspecific trauma, surgery, or abdominal conditions.
5. **A:** Surgical excision of HO usually occurs when ectopic bone appears completely matured on bone scan, which can take up to 12–18 months to occur.

Chapter 25 Spine Fractures, Dislocations, and Instability

1. **C:** At the thoracolumbar junction. This includes all populations including pediatric and adult. Pediatric spine injuries account for 2%–5% of all spine injuries, and are more common in the cervical spine. Adult thoracolumbar injuries include high-energy injuries as well as ground-level falls as in the geriatric population. Biomechanically, the transition from a relatively stable thoracic spine to a mobile lumbar spine contributes to a higher percentage of injuries in this region.
2. **D:** All of the above. Any condition that results in spinal instability could be included in the category.
3. **C:** White and Panjabi's description of spinal instability was and still is utilized in clinical practice but did not necessarily help with treatment decision-making. SINs is specifically designed for neoplastic disease only. Levine Edward classification is used to describe C2 pars interarticularis (hangman's) fractures. TLICS uses fracture morphology, soft tissue integrity, and neurological status to suggest treatment options.
4. **C:** When Denis performed a retrospective analysis of over 200 sacral fractures, he noted that zone I injuries resulted in about 6% incidence of neurologic injury, zone II about 30%, and zone III about 55%.
5. **A:** Relatively poorly developed spinal ligaments and muscles compared with adults, more horizontally sloped facet joints in the subaxial spine, and a relatively larger sized head-to-body ratio than adults increase the risk of cervical spine injury in children compared with adults.
6. **B:** In the pediatric population, the most common cause of spinal *cord* injury is penetrating injury, followed by sports injuries. The most common cause of spinal *column* injury is motor vehicle accidents followed by falls and then pedestrian injuries.

Chapter 26 Spine Complications

1. **C:** PTS is most commonly asymptomatic. When symptoms are present, pain is often the first symptom. Weakness may occur but is often a late finding.
2. **D:** Charcot spine is believed to be caused by loss of sensation and protective reflexes in a joint with preserved motion.
3. **D:** As neurologic exam is unchanged and there is minimal angulation of the spine, there is no indication for surgical referral, advanced imaging, or bracing. Repeating imaging at regular intervals would be warranted to monitor for curve progression.
4. **C:** MRI is the gold standard for diagnosis of posttraumatic syringomyelias.
5. **A:** Pseudarthrosis is the result of abnormal spinal motion at a site of previous spinal fusion.

Chapter 27 Spinal Orthoses

1. **D:** Additional potential complications include anxiety, pulmonary function compromise, psychological dependence, muscle weakness, dysphagia, and osteoporosis. There are some additional potential complications associated with the Halo device, which include pin loosening, pin site infection/abscess, and vertebral "snaking" due to lack of total contact.
2. **B:** At a minimum, three points of contact are required for immobilization with a goal of offloading the area of pathology, transferring forces to unaffected areas, and limiting motion in the desired plane(s). Orthoses, such as a custom-molded TLSO, can also be designed for "total contact."
3. **A:** Flexion/extension restriction is typically between 40%–90% with less control of movement in other planes.
4. **E:** The mass of body segments, force moments generated by physical activity, and muscle tension all contribute to axial load. The greatest forces are typically produced by muscle tension.
5. **B:** These fractures commonly result from fragility, such as osteoporosis, or trauma. Some single-level compression fractures may be treated with extension-based exercise and ambulation alone. Extension orthoses (such as Jewitt or CASH) are typically used for bracing.

Chapter 28 Posttraumatic Syringomyelia

1. **C:** Plain films of the spine to evaluate for scoliosis causing asymmetric sitting pressures. Scoliosis and other progressive spinal deformities can cause unequal distribution of sitting pressures, thus potentially causing too much pressure over a bony prominence. Consider scoliosis in all SCI patients with PTS, and vice versa.
2. **D:** Rapid cognitive decline is not associated with posttraumatic syringomyelia.
3. **C:** Sensory dissociation. Selective loss of pain and temperature due to central syrinx obstructing spinothalamic tracts.
4. **D:** Contrast-enhanced MRI. MRI is the gold standard for diagnosis of PTS. T1- and T2-weighting is able to differentiate between normal spinal cord tissue, edema, CSF, and myelomalacia.
5. **D:** Pain is the most common presenting symptom. Atrophy and weakness may be a late finding.

Chapter 29 Spasticity

1. **A:** Increasing inhibitory feedback to spinal reflexes. Baclofen is a GABA-B agonist at mono- and polysynaptic spinal reflexes, i.e., presynaptic inhibition.
2. **D:** Tonic, phasic. Clonus is a rhythmic pattern of muscle contraction provoked by sudden stretch activating muscle spindles reflexes. Tension produced activates Golgi tendon organs, in turn relaxing the muscle; the contraction of the affected muscle stretches the antagonist, creating a cycle of alternating contraction in the agonist/antagonist pair.
3. **C:** Start trimethoprim/sulfamethoxazole and monitor for subsequent improvement in her spasticity. Prior to making changes to pharmacotherapy plan or starting new medications for spasticity, correctable causes should be treated.
4. **D:** Stretching three times per day and physical therapy. Acute spinal cord injury patient with expected UMN pattern; initial management should focus on nonpharmacologic interventions.
5. **B:** Baclofen 5 mg TID. Baclofen is a good initial choice in patients with normal renal function and lack of improvement despite nonpharmacologic interventions. It is recommended to initiate with a low dose and titrate as needed.
6. **A:** Tell the patient to go to the nearest ED and to take a dose of oral baclofen if available in case of pump failure, as this is a potentially life-threatening condition. Baclofen withdrawal due to pump or catheter malfunction is an emergency with risk of serious adverse events and death. Initial management should include the use of oral baclofen to reduce the risk of withdrawal seizures while evaluation of the pump/catheter is pursued.
7. **A:** Chemodenervation with Botox to the FCU. FCR patient with focal spasticity creating functional impairment despite nonpharmacologic and pharmacologic interventions is a good candidate for chemodenervation.

Chapter 30 Thermoregulation and Sweating

1. **C:** The hypothalamus provides central control of thermoregulation.
2. **D:** Afferent skin temperature sensation. Afferent signals are regulated by environmental (temperature) changes on peripheral thermoreceptors.
3. **D:** T8. Injuries above T8 can be associated with temperature dysregulation due to impaired sympathetic control below the level of injury.
4. **B:** 1–2 °F. With a complete SCI, the efferent relay system from the hypothalamus to cause vasoconstriction to preserve heat is impaired.
5. **A:** Ice bath/whole-body water immersion. Can be dangerous and there is a risk of drowning.

Chapter 31 Traumatic Brain Injury and Spinal Cord Injury

1. **A:** Cervicogenic headaches can be very common after a TBI. A thorough neck and cervical spine exam

should be performed. Oftentimes with cervicogenic headache, pain is felt on the posterior of the skull radiating from the neck. Occipital nerve block procedure should be considered.

2. **B:** Valproic acid is an appropriate choice. Patient's symptoms prior to injury are representative of undiagnosed bipolar disorder. Valproic acid is often used to treat bipolar disorder; in addition, it is often used to treat agitation in the setting of TBI and also seizure treatment.
3. **D:** Further history. It is of utmost importance when dealing with cognitive dysfunction to obtain a clear baseline prior to the injury, as many patients may have had similar difficulties premorbidly. In this case, the patient may have a premorbid diagnosis or history consistent with ADHD. This should be ruled out prior to further workup. Additionally, given the short time course since injury and initial negative findings on CT head, neuroimaging would be unlikely to show any abnormalities at this time.
4. **C:** Vision impairment is very common after sustaining a TBI. This patient likely sustained a mTBI, which is presented through the vision disorder. The patient likely is experiencing double vision that is then causing headaches. The request for dimmed lights will likely require tinted lenses, as the patient is experiencing photosensitivity.
5. **C:** Cranial nerve injuries are commonly sustained as a result of the TBI. Cranial nerve I is the olfactory nerve and is the most commonly injured cranial nerve when a person sustains a TBI. This nerve helps to facilitate smell. Impaired smell affects proper taste. This often leads to insufficient food and calorie intake. Oftentimes, by adding more spices and salt to food, a patient will increase their food intake.

Chapter 32 Neuromodulatory and Disease-Modifying Agents

1. **A:** Functional electrical stimulation (FES) applies electrical currents to neural tissue in a synchronized fashion to restore impaired function. Patients with spinal cord injury and lower motor neuron sparing are candidates for FES. Electrodes can be placed anywhere along the LMN anterior horn cell → spinal root → peripheral nerve → neuromuscular junction.
2. **C:** Large nerve fibers are stimulated first as opposed to small diameter fibers because large fibers typically innervate large motor units and are activated with less current. Sensory nerve fibers may be activated as well, causing pain; this can be seen with use of transcutaneous electrodes.
3. **B:** A closed system uses sensors to provide feedback to the command control unit. Sensory feedback signals from limbs can be obtained from externally placed goniometers (measure joint position) and potentiometers (measure joint motion) placed at various joints. This allows the command control unit to calculate the velocity and acceleration of movement and adjust output commands in real time.
4. **C:** Implanted electrodes are ideal for long-term use because they allow for stimulation of specific muscles, providing good muscle recruitment with low current requirements. Implanted electrodes are surgically placed adjacent to a nerve (epineural), around a nerve via cuff, at the motor point on the muscle surface (epimysial), or within the muscle itself (intramuscular).
5. **B:** The standard of care for multiple sclerosis is prompt treatment after diagnosis is made and involves shared decision-making and education, as there are many considerations when selecting a disease modifying therapy.

Chapter 33 Pressure Ulcers/Injuries: Prevention, Treatment, and Management

1. **A:** All pressure injuries are considered chronic wounds. An acute wound heals in an orderly, timely, and durable manner and does not require long-term follow-up. Acute wounds have an identifiable mechanism of injury such as trauma or surgery. Some sources suggest the trajectory for acute wound healing is complete within 4 weeks. Chronic wounds do not progress through healing in an orderly manner; they commonly plateau or stall at some point due to various pathologic conditions, and, consequently, predictable tissue repair does not occur.
2. **D:** Pressure injury risk assessment tools provide a tangible way to quantify potential risk so that interventions may be reserved for those at highest risk and avoid unnecessary interventions and higher financial expenditures on those who may not need them.
3. **A:** A pressure injury is defined as an area of localized injury to the skin and/or underlying soft tissue that usually occurs over a bony prominence or is related to the use of a medical or other device, and it is the result of pressure or pressure in combination with shear.
4. **B:** One of the treatment priorities once a pressure injury is diagnosed is to eliminate the pressure to the wound. The SCI population spends extended times sitting; this often means bedrest to unload ischial or sacrum/coccyx pressure injuries.
5. **B:** A pressure injury is defined as an area of localized injury to the skin and/or underlying soft tissue that usually occurs over a bony prominence or is related to the use of a medical or other device, and it is the result of pressure or pressure in combination with shear.

Chapter 34 Nutritional and Body Composition Assessments After Spinal Cord Injury

1. **D:** Dramatic loss of muscle mass and bone mass with a significant increase in total body fat, visceral fat, and intramuscular fat in the paralyzed legs. Due to the critical illness response after a spinal cord injury, proteins are catabolized, there is a resistance to anabolic signals, various stress-triggered mechanisms accelerate the skeletal muscle mass loss below the level of injury, and there is a relative preservation of fat tissue.
2. **A:** Basal metabolic rate, dietary-induced thermogenesis, activity energy expenditure. Energy expenditure can be broken down into three components: basal metabolic rate (BMR), dietary-induced thermogenesis, and activity energy expenditure in which the BMR is the energy required to maintain homeostasis and metabolic activities of cells at rest and is the largest component of daily energy expenditure.
3. **C:** 1.5–2 g/kg. Attempting to achieve a positive nitrogen balance with aggressive nutrition support is generally unsuccessful and can result in overfeeding, so usually up to 2 g protein/kg ideal body weight is adequate to prevent substrate overload. Protein intake recommendations for those with stage 1–2 pressure injuries are 1.2–1.5 g/kg and stage 3–4 pressure injuries are 1.5–2 g/kg.
4. **C:** Low carbohydrate, high protein, low fat and saturated fat. Studies have shown that individuals with SCI tend to consume excess energy for their estimated needs despite a lower overall caloric intake. Excess protein intake, excess carbohydrate intake, and excess dietary fat and saturated fat intake may lead to slowness of the metabolism, increase the circulating cortisol, and induce a state of hypercatabolism. General nutrition guidelines are to consume a heart-healthy diet with fruits, vegetables, whole grains, low-fat dairy, poultry, fish, beans/legumes, and nuts while limiting sweets and red meats. Research has shown improvement in overall nutritional status when macronutrients are adjusted with a lower carbohydrate intake consisting of whole grains, fruits, and low-fat dairy products; a higher protein intake of low-fat meats and fish, eggs, legumes, and nuts while limiting red meat and fat intake to <30% total calories with <6% from saturated fats.

Chapter 35 Endocrine/Metabolic

1. **C:** TNF-α, IL-6, CRP are biomarkers that are indicative of systemic inflammation, whereas answer A contains anabolic hormones or their derivatives. Answer B contains markers of lipid metabolism (LDL-C and HDL-C) as well as the protein that is the receptor for IGF-1 (IGFBP-3).
2. **B:** Although spasms are involuntary muscle contractions, they are nonetheless muscle contractions that mitigate disuse atrophy. This can stave off increases in intramuscular fat. Spasms are not, however, indicative of voluntary motor return, and there is nothing unique about spastic vs. voluntary motor contractions that would cause spasms to release proteins affecting lipid metabolism.
3. **C and D:** Both answers C and D contain components that can be entered into the formulas described earlier in the chapter, whereas answers A and B contain components that have not (in combination) been found to be significantly predictive of BMR.
4. **A:** Skeletal muscle is the main organ that metabolizes glucose, whereas items in answers B–D do not directly affect metabolism of glucose specifically.
5. **B:** While interventions like aerobic training and dietary changes may improve one's metabolic profile, only neuromuscular or functional electrical stimulation has been shown to improve metabolic profile by inducing hypertrophy of the paralyzed muscles below the injury level.

Chapter 36 Infections With Spinal Cord Injury

1. **B:** Pneumonia is the most common cause of death in SCI at a rate of 30%–50%. UTI is the most common cause of infection overall in SCI.
2. **C:** Bone biopsy is the gold standard for diagnosing osteomyelitis through histopathologic analysis. Nuclear scintigraphy is highly sensitive for excluding osteomyelitis, but its specificity for osteomyelitis is much lower.
3. **A:** SCI patients with indwelling vascular lines have been found to have an elevated risk for gram-negative colonization in comparison with the general population.
4. **D:** Despite the patient having an unremarkable workup for positive blood cultures, the next best step is to evaluate for occult abscess due to the risk of inadequate source control with only antibiotic treatment.
5. **C:** If *Proteus* is cultured, it should be treated due to the presence of urease, which splits urea to form ammonia and carbon dioxide and causes increased urine pH and precipitation of ions and urolithiasis formation. The presence of VRE in the urine is often representative of asymptomatic bacteriuria not requiring antibiotics.

Chapter 37 Evaluation and Management of Pain After Spinal Cord Injury

1. **C:** Dysesthetic pain syndrome is caused by incomplete SCI with preservation of the dorsal column

and absence of the STT and is described in 5% of patients with SCI pain.
2. **A:** Musculoskeletal pain, a nociceptive pain syndrome, can also include above-the-level pain and visceral pain, whereas below the level pain is typically neuropathic pain.
3. **E:** Both have been described as the most severe in published reports. Below-the-level pain is significantly more common (40%–60% of patients with SCI pain), whereas visceral pain is seen in 10%–20%.
4. **C:** Tricyclic antidepressants and gabapentinoids.
5. **D:** All of the above.
6. **C:** Targeted transforaminal epidural steroid injections can directly address neuropathic pain from nerve root involvement at the level of injury.
7. **A:** Corticospinal tracts. Dorsal columns carry information related to proprioception and discriminative touch.
8. **D:** The onset time is often 1.5–2 years and must be differentiated from surgical causes such as syrinx and postlaminectomy pain syndrome.
9. **F:** The delayed onset of SCI below the level pain can coincide with the two conditions. An MRI with contrast can often differentiate this.
10. **C:** B explains dysesthetic pain syndrome, A explains pain upregulation usually due to wide dynamic range neurons, D explains phantom pain classically and many other neuropathic pain states more generally but not spasticity.

Chapter 38 Psychological Aspects of Spinal Cord Injury

1. **B:** Sertraline; SSRIs, of which sertraline is one, and SNRIs are considered first-line agents for psychopharmacologic treatment of generalized anxiety disorder. Benzodiazepines have fallen out of favor due to potential for tolerance and dependence. Beta-blockers can be used to treat anxiety, though they are not considered first-line agents.
2. **D:** Hospitalization can help reduce risk of suicide by helping patient maintain safety. The other three options are all factors that increase someone's suicide risk.
3. **A:** Trauma-focused psychotherapy; there is insufficient evidence that indicates medication is effective in treating symptoms of acute stress disorder.
4. **B:** Psychotherapy and pharmacotherapy; research supports the combination of psychotherapy and pharmacotherapy as more effective than either alone.
5. **B and C:** Clinical Practice Guidelines recommend screening of all SCI rehabilitation patients prior to discharge. Brief counseling from treatment providers has been shown to improve outcomes for alcohol and tobacco users.
6. **B:** Patients disabled due to conversion have similar problems as patients with primarily organic conditions when it comes to biopsychosocial functioning and can benefit from interdisciplinary rehabilitative services.

Chapter 39 Traumatic Myelopathy

1. **C:** C5 is the most common level of spinal cord injury.
2. **D:** Bilateral facet injury is a flexion type of injury and is always unstable as vertebral body >50% displaced on X-ray, causing significant spinal canal narrowing. The posterior longitudinal ligament is also disrupted in this type of injury.
3. **D:** Halo-vest immobilizer is the most restrictive and not removable compared with cervical collars. Halo-vest is used for patients with unstable cervical fractures for 8–12 weeks. Most common complications from halo are pin loosening and local infection.
4. **C:** An injury to spinal levels T12-L2 (rarely T11) will impact the spinal cord at the level of the conus, resulting in CMS.
5. **B:** If a patient is suspected to be in spinal shock, the first sign of emerging from it is a delayed Babinski reflex. The upgoing toe occurs about 1 second AFTER the stroke on the sole.
6. **D:** The NLI is C6, given that it is the most caudal segment with bilaterally normal sensory and motor function. Even though there is no sacral sparing in this case, it would be incorrect to state that the patient is complete or has an AIS A type of injury as this would not be an accurate description of the individual's injury. In light of the substantial preservation of both motor and sensory function below C6, it is very unlikely that the cervical SCI has led to a total absence of function in the lowest sacral area that would lead to it being classified as a complete injury. For this reason, in this case, the AIS is ND. The International Standards Committee recommends describing the exam results in the comment box, including the fact that this individual likely has a C6 incomplete injury and an L2 complete injury. If a classification variable cannot be determined, an ND should be documented, as is the case on this occasion as it relates to the AIS and ZPPs.

Chapter 40 Nontraumatic Myelopathies

1. **D:** Hypotension may decrease perfusion to the spinal cord via the anterior spinal artery causing an "anterior spinal cord injury syndrome." Those syndromes are characterized by weakness and decreased pain and temperature with preserved proprioception below the injury level.
2. **B:** Cervical spondylotic myelopathy is the most common cause of spasticity and gait disbalance in patients >55 years of age.

3. **B:** Primary progressive is the type of multiple sclerosis with the worst prognosis.
4. **A:** This is the correct definition.
5. **A:** Kugelberg-Welander disease.
6. **C:** Patient presents with posterior column deficits that raise concern for nitrous oxide abuse causing subacute combined degeneration in the setting of substance abuse.

Chapter 41 Myelopathy Without Specified Etiology

1. **D:** Symmetric dorsal columns lesion on MRI suggests metabolic or toxic cause, particularly subacute combined degeneration due to B12 deficiency, folate deficiency, or methotrexate toxicity. These deficiencies often (though not always) result in macrocytic anemia due to impaired DNA synthesis.
2. **D:** Common causes of subacute combined degeneration include inadequate B12 absorption, which relies on stomach acid to attach B12 to protein R for absorption in the proximal small intestine. Nitrous oxide inactivates B12, and in nutritionally borderline patients can inactivate B12 and push patients into functional deficiency. Thyroid function does not have a significant correlation with dorsal column degeneration.
3. **D:** Asymptomatic white matter lesions are a hallmark of multiple sclerosis. Furthermore, the most common pattern of disease is relapsing–remitting. Previously unidentified lesions are much less likely to be truly asymptomatic in NMOSD. ALS does not typically affect the parietal lobe and does not generally present with a remitting pattern. Neurocysticercosis, or brain tapeworm, typically involves ring-enhancing (target) lesions not specific to white matter tracts.
4. **B:** CT for sarcoidosis lesion that would be more easily biopsied. A short, ring-enhancing lesion that does not involve the gray matter and involves the subpial surface limits the most likely differential to parasitic, sarcoid, or tuberculosis. With the chronic cough, evaluation for neoplasm would also be reasonable. CT of the chest would highlight possible masses or perihilar granulomas that could serve as better targets for tissue diagnosis than the CNS's direct biopsy. Autoimmune myelopathies are less likely to be ring-enhancing, tend to be longer than three segments, and involve more than one-fifth of the cord's axial area, including the gray matter. Syphilis also does not tend to be ring-enhancing. Usually, it involves more than one-half of the axial area of the cord.
5. **B:** Isolated conus lesions longer than three segments typically are either vascular, necessitating angiographic analysis, or NMOSD. In this example, the gray matter involvement and CSF studies are more suggestive of NMOSD.

Chapter 42 Healthcare Maintenance for Patients With Spinal Cord Injuries/Disorders: Primary, Preventive, and Promotive Care

1. **D:** All of the above.
2. **D:** All of the above.
3. **B:** True.
4. **B:** True.
5. **B:** Maneuvering wheelchair as per patient's choice.

Chapter 43 Spinal Cord Injury and Aging

1. **A:** Pneumonia and septicemia have been shown to have the greatest impact on reduced life expectancy in people with SCI.
2. **C:** There is increasing mortality for cardiovascular, metabolic, and nervous system diseases, as well as accidents and mental conditions. Death from cancer, urinary, and digestive diseases, and suicide are remaining steady or declining.
3. **D:** The risk factors for development of bladder cancer in patients with SCI include recurrent UTI, use of indwelling catheters, urinary tract stones, and cigarette smoking. For individuals managed with indwelling catheters, anticholinergic medication use may improve health outcomes.
4. **D:** There is no evidence to suggest that there is added risk of colon cancer in persons with SCI. Fecal occult blood is not a reliable screening tool due to the frequent presence of hemorrhoids, rectal prolapse, and other distal rectal pathology. SCI patients should undergo routine screening consistent with guidelines for the general population. Endoscopists should be familiar with risk of autonomic dysreflexia and how to treat it.
5. **A:** The most frequent site of upper extremity nerve entrapment is the median nerve at the wrist. Entrapment of the ulnar nerve at the wrist and elbow is also common.
6. **B:** There is no evidence of new bone formation with use of bisphosphonates in the treatment of osteoporosis in chronic SCI.
7. **C:** Risk of depression in the older population is associated with presence of other illnesses.

Chapter 44 Exercise and Modalities

1. **D:** Short-term sitting on mat table with bilateral upper extremity support. The mat table will give you the most stable platform compared with a hospital bed. You also want to give the patient a nondynamic activity without assistive tools if the goal is to assess their ability to maintain sitting posture without back support.

2. **B:** Gate control theory. Nonpainful stimuli "close the gates" to the painful stimuli and keep the brain from interpreting the pain signals, since it is not reaching the brain.
3. **B:** Reversal of motor unit recruitment. FES causes motor unit recruitment to be reversed starting with larger, stronger, but highly fatigable motor units.
4. **B:** No. TENS promotes blood flow to the applied area. Active infections are contraindicated due to the risk of spreading infection.
5. **C:** Gentle stretching. Slow, gentle stretching is best applied due to the decreased risk of microtrauma and possible increased ossification compared with aggressive stretching. Range of motion should be preserved as much as possible to prevent further complications.

Chapter 45 Functional Mobility Following Spinal Cord Injury

1. **D:** Several clinical prediction tools have been developed utilizing both five sets of data points and three sets of data points. The critical findings on the ASIA exam include the L3 and S1 myotomes, as well as the L3 and S1 dermatomes. Although it has been shown that an age of 50 may be an important marker for ambulation potential, the prediction formulas utilize an age cutoff of 65.
2. **C:** To promote neuroplasticity, the clinical team will want to utilize locomotor training to promote neural recovery. Locomotor training uses techniques as shown in answer C, while additionally encouraging an upright head/trunk, approximating hip/knee/ankle kinematics, synchronizing hip extension in stance with contralateral limb unloading, as well as maintaining symmetrical interlimb kinematics/kinetics. Gait training utilizes support devices and compensatory techniques to achieve maximal function, with less focus being on neuroplasticity.
3. **D:** Progressive sitting tolerance for new quadriplegics is often supported with use of an abdominal binder and compression stockings to reduce postural hypotension and excessive pooling of blood in the abdominal viscera and lower extremities. This is done with close monitoring of blood pressure by the clinicians. Wrist/hand orthoses may actually hinder the patient's ability to participate with sitting balance activities.
4. **C:** Having functioning triceps would allow this patient to easily self-propel an optimally configured ultralightweight manual wheelchair. A power scooter would not be appropriate due to the lack of seating system support needed, and a power wheelchair would not be necessary, thus allowing them the convenience and transportability of a manual wheelchair vs. power.
5. **D:** Rear axle position of a manual wheelchair has been studied extensively and has been found to be one of the most important factors in preservation of UE function. The goal is to adjust the rear axles as far forward as possible without compromising the stability of the user. Furthermore, reducing the amount of weight on the front casters typically makes the chair roll more easily.
6. **A:** Limitations in hip flexion range of motion (ROM) will prevent the pelvis from achieving a neutral position, causing the pelvis to rotate rearward, the trunk to become kyphotic, and the hips to slide forward. During the hip ROM assessment, the examiner should identify the point at which hip ROM is exceeded and pelvis rotates rearward.
7. **D:** Being that this patient has an existing wound on her seating surface as well as significant LE spasticity, she will require BOTH a pressure-relieving and positioning cushion. This will offer her LE positioning components to optimize her seated stability as well as properly distribute her seating interface pressures to facilitate wound healing.
8. **A:** Answers B, C, and D are all adequate and effective methods for pressure relief. Additionally, tilting back >35 degrees in combination with 100 degrees of recline is also an alternative option. Reclining in isolation can actually induce further shear, placing the patient at risk for skin breakdown.
9. **C:** Patients who demonstrate control of hip flexors to advance their lower extremities may be able progress to ambulating short distances, albeit with high energy demands, with knee-ankle-foot orthoses, to support weakness in their knees and ankles. An individual with a T10 motor complete injury will require a more supportive device such as a reciprocating gait orthosis. Individuals with lower injuries (answer B) and/or much more incomplete (answer D) will require much less bracing (in these cases, most likely some form of ankle-foot orthosis).
10. **D:** Options A and C are both viable options for the patient but would provide nonproportional switch access with stepwise speed and directional control. Most joysticks provide proportional drive control; however, a patient with C4 ASIA B quadriplegia would not be able to access the joystick with their hand unless they had sparing of motor function into at least the C5 myotomes.

Chapter 46 Activities of Daily Living

1. **B:** A patient with a C6 level of injury may utilize tenodesis, or the ability to use wrist extension for passive hand grasp.
2. **B:** An ADA-compliant ramp must follow a 1:12 ratio for rise and run: for each 1 inch of rise, there must be 12 inches of run. A 1:12 ratio is required, but a 1:16 or 1:20 is preferred.

3. **B:** Home door widths should accommodate the end user's wheelchair, which varies depending on the width of the wheeled mobility device.
4. **C:** Electronic aids to daily living (EADLs) are devices that can be used to control one's surrounding environment.
5. **A:** The hierarchy of recommended tendon transfers is as follows: 1. Elbow extension 2. Wrist extension 3. Lateral pinch and release (key pinch) 4. Palmar grasp and release.
6. **D:** The patient's goals and direct involvement in the decision-making process for surgery are key to a successful outcome after surgery. Having a specific functional goal in mind prior to surgery facilitates a more successful outcome.

Chapter 47 Communication and Spinal Cord Injury

1. **D:** Patients can still utilize and tolerate a Passy Muir valve (PMV) even if they require supplemental oxygen. This is not a main factor in considering patients for speaking valve use. Patients must be able to tolerate cuff deflation and be able to manage their own secretions to consider PMV use.
2. **C:** While limited jaw range of motion can impact articulation, it should not affect the patient's ability to phonate.
3. **D:** Although Medicare does require SLP evaluation and recommendations for specific AAC equipment, there are not specific guidelines regarding frequency of assessment/follow-up.
4. **A:** Both digital occlusion and capping of the tracheostomy tube block airflow through the stoma in order to restore a closed system. Air will flow through the nose and mouth and down to the lungs prior to returning through the vocal folds and allowing phonation. In comparison, a Passy Muir speaking valve allows air to flow through the stoma on inhalation. Upon exhalation, air is redirected through the vocal folds enabling voice.
5. **A:** While recurrent laryngeal nerve palsy can account for long-term dysphonia following anterior cervical surgery, the prevalence is considered to be rare. More likely, the patient has continued postoperative edema causing a harsh, breathy voice. Vocal fold nodules and/or poor vocal hygiene may also account for dysphonia but are less likely in a patient who had no vocal issues prior to surgery.
6. **B:** Although a communication partner can digitally occlude the patient's tracheostomy, the patient is unable to do it themself as a result of their SCI. The patient can achieve greater independence in communication with the use of a speaking valve, assuming good tolerance. While the use of eye gaze accounts for the patient's limited mobility, a complex speech-generating device is more appropriate for long-term use. Partner-assisted scanning would also be appropriate for the patient's ability but take a considerable amount of time and limit independence.

Chapter 48 Participation/Living With Spinal Cord Injury

1. **D:** All of the above.
2. **C:** 35%.
3. **A:** Increased pressure at the back support.
4. **D:** A and B.
5. **B:** The International Paralympic Committee has no official statement on athletic doping.

Chapter 49 Rehabilitation Team

1. **False:** While an interprofessional team is a collaborative practice, a multidisciplinary team involves the same patient, but members work separately.
2. **D:** Healthcare safety nets are not a risk factor. Common safety risks include lack of prevention of secondary complications, transitions of services, fragmented social support systems, limited emphasis on reintegration into society, and implicit bias.
3. **False:** Capacity is a medical diagnosis by a physician. A patient has decision-making capacity when they can understand the benefits, risks, and alternatives to a proposed medical course of action, including lack of treatment. Competency, on the other hand, is a legal determination by a judge.
4. **False:** Implicit bias is automatic and involuntary, so it is not easily understood or controlled. In comparison, explicit bias is voluntary and known by the person. Because of this, implicit bias can be contrary to a person's explicit belief.
5. **False:** Medical futility requires that there is "virtual certainty" that the action will fail to treat the condition. Note that this is different than being "virtually certain" that the SCI/D will not be cured or that the injured person will have limited independence despite the treatment provided. Thus, it is essential that the SCI/D subspecialist provides their expertise in outcomes to guide the medical team.
6. **True:** Advocacy can happen locally through church or little league. Advocacy can happen nationally through organizations and political affiliations. All advocacy makes a huge impact.
7. **False:** Traditional Medicare has specific requirements, including the five-element order. However, other insurance programs may not require the five-element order. This emphasizes the complexity in ordering CRT and the variations that insurance places in obtaining key equipment for persons with SCI/D.

Index

Note: Page numbers followed by f indicate figures and t indicate tables.